ADULT NEUROGENESIS

Adult Neurogenesis

Stem Cells and
Neuronal Development
in the Adult Brain

Gerd Kempermann

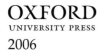
OXFORD
UNIVERSITY PRESS
2006

OXFORD
UNIVERSITY PRESS

Oxford University Press, Inc., publishes works that further
Oxford University's objective of excellence
in research, scholarship, and education.

Oxford   New York
Auckland   Bangkok   Bogotá   Buenos Aires   Cape Town   Chennai
Dar es Salaam   Delhi   Hong Kong   Istanbul   Karachi   Kolkata
Kuala Lumpur   Madrid   Melbourne   Mexico City   Mumbai   Nairobi
São Paulo   Shanghai   Singapore   Taipei   Tokyo   Toronto

Published by Oxford University Press, Inc.
198 Madison Avenue, New York, New York, 10016

www.oup.com

Oxford is a registered trademark of Oxford University Press

Library of Congress Cataloging-in-Publication Data
Kempermann, Gerd.
Adult neurogenesis : stem cells and neuronal development in the adult brain /
Gerd Kempermann.
p. cm.
Includes bibliographical references and index.
ISBN-13: 978-0-19-517971-2
ISBN: 0-19-517971-4
1. Developmental neurobiology.   2. Neural stem cells.   I. Title.
QP363.5.K466 2005
612.6'4018—dc22   2005040868

9 8 7 6 5 4 3 2 1

Printed in the United States of America
on acid-free paper

For Uta, Georg, and Rusty

Preface

Adult neurogenesis, that is, the generation of new neurons in the adult brain, has progressed through various stages of study in the short period of 30 years between 1965 and the mid-1990s. First it was regarded as an impossibility, then as a curiosity, later as an exception to otherwise steadfast rules, and finally as an accepted phenomenon of mammalian neurobiology. This book is meant to provide an introduction to this burgeoning field.

Of course, what the reader will find on these pages is not all that could or perhaps should be said about adult neurogenesis. The ideal was to draw a coherent picture, but as anybody knows who has embarked on such an endeavor, this effort occasionally leads to a biased view. This was not intended and in fact, every attempt was made to avoid the unfair treatment of other people's results. The arguments laid down in this book have been tested in discussions with many colleagues, some of whom are mentioned in the Acknowledgements. If I have stepped on anyone's toes, please accept my apologies. The goal was certainly not to hurt toes, but to provide a critical and scientifically sound argument. It is, of course, the proverbial shoulders of giants that I have stood on. By now, the giants should, with all due respect, be rather used to this treatment. But I am well aware that I have also used the less trained shoulders of many students and postdoctoral researchers, whose work has contributed to what we now know about adult neurogenesis. They might rightfully feel more injustice if I have misrepresented their work. By no means do I intend to suggest that I have delivered the definitive interpretation. But what I do hope to convey is my enthusiasm for this field of research. So what the reader will find here is one scientist's take on the world of adult neurogenesis. I hope this view comes equipped with good enough arguments to withstand the critique that no doubt will follow. Everything presented here is meant to be an invitation for discussion. Should the book be well received, future editions will incorporate ensuing discussion, so that the community's views, rather than a personal opinion, will take shape and be taught to the next generation of neuroscientists.

Acknowledgments

My first thank you goes to the two people who brought me into the field of adult neurogenesis. I would like to thank Fred H. Gage for his continued support and the many challenging discussions over the past 10 years, and H. Georg Kuhn, with whom I did my first experiments on adult neurogenesis. H. Georg Kuhn also commented on versions of the manuscript for this book. So did Theo D. Palmer, my desk neighbor at the Salk Institute, whose contributions during many discussions have been extremely valuable in shaping the ideas presented here. I would also like to thank former Gage lab colleague, Daniel Peterson, whose advice on many methodological issues is unsurpassed. I am very grateful that two pioneers of the field of adult neurogenesis, Joseph Altman and Pasko Rakic, took the time to comment on parts of the manuscript. I thank the following colleagues who contributed images to this book and allowed their reproduction: Harish Babu, Christiana Cooper-Kuhn, Peter Eriksson, Fred H. Gage, Alexander Garthe, Rainer Glass, Sebastian Jessberger, Helmut Kettenmann, Zaal Kokaia, David Kornack, Monika Kott, Golo Kronenberg, H. Georg Kuhn, Olle Lindvall, Gudrun Lutsch, Jeffrey D. Macklis, Pasko Rakic, Constanze Scharff, Sophie Scotto-Lomassese, Barbara Steiner, Li Ping Wang, and Andreas Wodarz. In addition, I received very useful comments on particular questions from Harish Babu, Alexander Garthe, Sophie Scotto-Lomassese, and Tracey Shors.

I would also like to thank colleagues in my lab in Berlin, who patiently accepted that time and again work on this book took priority over their immediate problems. Needless to say, without such a wonderful team the endeavor would not have been possible. My work in Berlin has been primarily funded by the Max Delbrück Center for Molecular Medicine (MDC) Berlin Buch as member institute of the Helmholtz Association of National Research Centers and by VolkswagenStiftung. Together with the Department of Neurology at Charité, University Medicine Berlin, these institutions provided the excellent environment, in which not only research on adult neurogenesis but also a book project could develop. For this I would particularly like to thank Ulrich Dirnagl, Karl Max Einhäupl, Detlev Ganten, and Helmut Kettenmann.

I thank Astrid Poppenhusen for her good advice as literary agent. I am also grateful to Fiona Stevens and Nancy Wolitzer at Oxford University Press, who led this project through the various stages of realization.

Figure 1-3 (which is also found as the cover image) was drawn by Jared Travnicek. His work and the inclusion of many other illustrations would not have been possible without the generous financial support of Helmut Lingen, Cologne.

Finally, I would like to thank my wife Uta for her love, patience, and support.

Contents

ADULT NEUROGENESIS

1

Introduction

New neurons! A thought of great suggestive power.

To renew continuously—this is what bone marrow, skin, and intestines do all the time. As Pasko Rakic of Yale University likes to say in his lectures, "with respect to my skin, I am a new man every year." Intestinal epithelia do not live to experience very many warm meals before they are replaced. Blood donation is a safe experience because we can rely on our bone marrow to replace our donation within a short period of time. Blood, skin, and intestines are the classic regenerative tissues. Intuitively we are not always particularly appreciative about their lifesaving cellular turnover. But when it became clear in the 1990s that something very similar is possible in the brain, even if it occurs on a minute scale, the finding was hailed as a fundamental breakthrough. Peter Eriksson's 1998 study (Eriksson et al., 1998), in which he reported that new neurons are generated in the hippocampus of adult humans, moved the field of adult neurogenesis from heresy to where it is now: not quite into orthodoxy but at least firmly established. The *New York Times* hailed the discovery of ongoing neurogenesis in the adult brain as the most important research result from the "Decade of the Brain," which spanned the years 1990 to 1999 (Blakeslee, 2000). In fact, adult neurogenesis was discovered much earlier. Nevertheless, the decade of the brain saw an impressive surge in scientific and public awareness of the phenomenon of neurogenesis in the adult mammalian brain, and the wealth of studies published certainly constituted a major scientific advancement.

The journalistic blessing by the *New York Times* and other newspapers and magazines also contributed, however, to some widely held misconceptions about the recent history of this exciting field of science. Research on adult neurogenesis was firmly rooted in general progress throughout the twentieth century in developmental neurobiology, stem cell biology, and research on brain plasticity. Nonetheless, few scientific developments have caught the imagination of the scientific community and the public as much as the so-called stem cell revolution. Adult neurogenesis—that is, the generation and development of new neurons in the adult brain—is a highly visible and intriguing part of this revolution. It is the stem cells of the adult brain that drive adult neurogenesis.

The fundamental change that modern stem cell biology has introduced to science is similar to the paradigm shift caused by the sequencing of the genome: our view changed from a deductive perspective, which we have

3

become accustomed to in science, to an essentially open situation. Genes and stem cells are to a large degree characterized by their potential. This causes a reversed perspective that is much more difficult to deal with than the classical method, working backwards along a chain of causes. Within the realm of stem cell research, adult neurogenesis appears to be something like an island of classical perspective within a sea of contexts that fall apart. Understanding of this circumscribed process will allow insights into a strange new world. But we should not deceive ourselves—even the old view was not straightforward. High-dimensional regulatory networks with seemingly fuzzy or chaotic properties within a cell and on a systems level have always made it impossible to speak in a strict and simple sense of "causes." Therefore, what on the surface we perceive as a paradigm shift is actually a shift in perception itself and in awareness. And while it is true that adult neurogenesis is a scientific question very much at the heart of this type of new scientific problem, it is also obvious that what seemed to be a short footnote to neurobiology has become one of the most intriguing questions in science today.

WHAT IS ADULT NEUROGENESIS?

Adult neurogenesis is the production of new neurons in the adult brain (Fig. 1–1). The term comprises a complex process, beginning with the division of a precursor cell (or potentially even before) and ending with the existence of a new functioning neuron (Fig. 1–2). Neurogenesis is much more than just the division of a precursor cell. It is a process, not an event. It involves decisions at the precursor cell level, such as whether symmetric divisions (with identical daughter cells) or asymmetric divisions (with two different daughter cells) occur. After asymmetric division, various factors

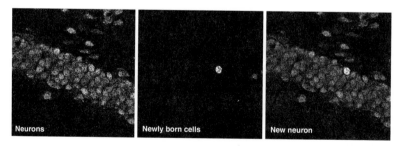

Figure 1–1. New neurons in the adult brain. Both neurons and newly generated cells can be visualized with immunohistochemistry. The third image shows the co-localization of both markers in one granule cell of the adult dentate gyrus. The method of "birth-dating" cells and thereby mark them as new is based on the incorporation of a tagged false base (bromodeoxyuridine, BrdU) into the DNA of dividing stem or progenitor cells (see Chapter 7 for further explanation).

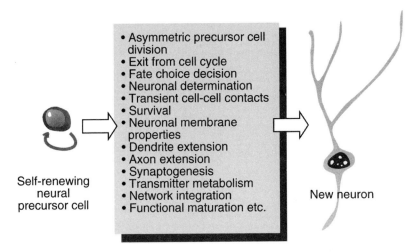

Figure 1–2. Neurogenesis is a process, not an event. In the context of neuronal development in the adult brain, the term *neurogenesis* has undergone an important shift in meaning. Whereas the old usage of the word, influence by the conditions in the developing nervous system, tended to equate proliferation of neural precursor cells with neurogenesis, this limited use of the word is not helpful in the context of adult neurogenesis. Adult neurogenesis is regulated at many different stages of cell development, most of the newly generated cells die, and gliogenesis appears to originate from the same proliferating precursor cells. Here the term *neurogenesis* thus comprises all necessary steps, starting with division of a precursor cell and resulting in the existence of a functionally fully integrated new neuron.

determine when the progeny is to become a neuron. Neurogenesis includes securing the survival of the new cell because only part of the daughter cells survives. Neurogenesis involves migration of the differentiating progeny and the differentiation process itself—that is, the turning on and off of genes according to a neuronal profile. It entails sending out the cellular processes: dendrites and axon that make connections and form synapses. It involves the fulfillment of electrophysiological criteria of neuronal function: the presence of sodium currents and the ability to generate action potentials. And there are even more steps and criteria we could rightfully subsume to "neurogenesis," in everyday research and in most contexts, all of these criteria can and need not be demonstrated. It is nonetheless important to realize that in our discussion of neurogenesis, all of these steps and criteria are meant.

For the purpose of this book, adult neurogenesis is essentially considered a process in vivo. This is in accordance with how the term is widely used, but of course the development of new neurons can be studied in cell culture, and this has been done very successfully. Hynek Wichterle, Tom Jessell, and coworkers (2002), for example, have been able to recapitulate all of the many regulatory steps that guide embryonic stem cells toward becoming motor neurons. This is perhaps the most straightforward way to demonstrate neurogenesis. It is conceivable that in the future we might see something similar in the context of adult neurogenesis. The approach taken by Tom Jessell's group is a prime example of what is possible in controllable and reductionistic experimental systems. However, it is also an unusually complete example in which the applicability to the in vivo context will be immediately clear. This is not the case with all in vitro studies.

A brain region that can generate neurons is called a "neurogenic" region. *Neurogenic* implies two things: first, the presence of immature precursor cells from which new neurons can develop, and second, a microenvironment that is permissive for neurogenesis to occur. In the adult mammalian brain there are two known neurogenic regions, the hippocampus and the olfactory system. In these two regions a sizable amount of adult neurogenesis can be found (Fig. 1–3, Color Plate 1). In the hippocampal dentate gyrus new granule cells are produced, and in the olfactory bulb new interneurons are produced in the granule cell layer and the periglomerular region (Fig. 1–4). We refer to the rest of the brain as "non-neurogenic," although this categorization might ultimately turn out to be premature. Currently the key factor considered for neurogenic permissiveness, which is whether the local microenviron-

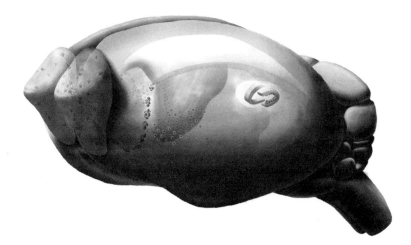

Figure 1–3 (Color Plate 1). The two neurogenic regions in the adult brain. Only two regions of the adult mammalian brain appear to be neurogenic under physiological conditions. Precursor cells residing in the lateral walls of the lateral ventricle give rise to new interneurons in the olfactory bulb. Neurogenesis in the adult hippocampus generates new excitatory granule cells throughout life. Both forms of adult neurogenesis originate from different precursor cell populations, are independently regulated, and serve entirely different functions. See Chapter 8 for details on the distinction between neurogenic and non-neurogenic regions, the key criteria for this distinction, and also their limitations. Illustration by Jared Travnicek.

Comparison of adult-born neurons

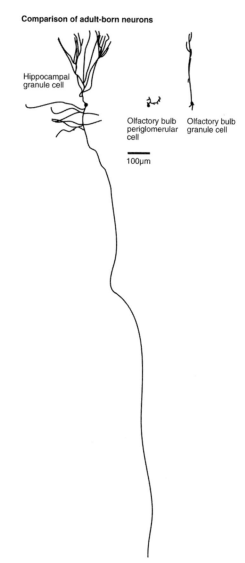

Hippocampal
granule cell

Olfactory bulb
periglomerular
cell

Olfactory bulb
granule cell

100μm

Figure 1–4. The three types of neurons generated in adult neurogenesis. In adult neurogenesis, excitatory hippocampal granule cells and inhibitory interneurons are produced in the olfactory bulb, here drawn to scale. New interneurons in the olfactory bulb are found in the granule cell layer of the bulb and in the periglomerular regions. The periglomerular interneurons of the olfactory bulb come in two neurotransmitter phenotypes. Whereas all interneurons are GABAergic, 5% of these cells also use dopamine as neurotransmitter.

ment allows an implanted neural precursor cell to develop into a neuron. So far, transplantation into the adult brain has yielded neurons only in the olfactory system and the hippocampus, although the same precursor cells could give rise to neurons under appropriate in vitro conditions (Gage et al., 1995; Suhonen et al., 1996; Herrera et al., 1999; Shihabuddin et al., 2000; Lie et al., 2002).

There are numerous single reports of adult neurogenesis occurring outside the hippocampus and the olfactory system, but none of these reports has passed the stage of being anecdotal. One study that stirred excitement during the decade of the brain, reporting neurogenesis in the neocortex of adult primates (Gould et al., 1999, 2001), was not confirmed by other laboratories (Kornack and Rakic, 2001a; Rakic, 2002; Koketsu et al., 2003). The adult brain has been good for so many surprises with respect to adult neurogenesis, however, that one should not dismiss these observations prematurely. Technical concerns or extremely low numbers of observations are nonetheless serious issues. We will discuss the question of neurogenesis in non-neurogenic regions in greater detail in Chapter 8. One thing is important to consider, however: it seems that under pathological conditions, much more is possible than under normal ones. There is reasonable evidence of induced adult neurogenesis in neurogenic and non-neurogenic regions as a response to brain damage, most notably ischemia (Arvidsson et al., 2002). But this reactive neurogenesis, which will be our topic in Chapters 8 and 12, seems to occur on a minute scale. The term *non-neurogenic* should thus be taken with a grain of salt: non-neurogenic regions are brain areas that under normal conditions do not show overt signs of neurogenesis, as in the hippocampus and olfactory system, but might do so under special conditions. The litmus test remains the implantation experiment.

Thus, to refine the definition for this book, adult neurogenesis is the generation of new neurons in the central nervous system of adult mammals. We will touch only briefly on neurogenesis in invertebrates and lower vertebrates, including birds, although adult neurogenesis in songbirds is a particularly interesting topic. This will be covered according to its relevance to the mammalian situation, not with the intent to provide extensive coverage. For many decades, preceding the first reports of adult neurogenesis in mammals, adult neurogenesis in nonmammalian species including birds has been hardly controversial. It is not the phenomenon of new neurons in the adult brain that has stirred controversy but the question as to the extent that the same could occur in mammals.

Adult here means at the earliest stage that mammals become sexually mature. This definition is important because a large part of brain development occurs postnatally. Although *adult* is of course after birth, the term *postnatal* in this context implies after birth but before sexual maturity. The neurons of the cerebellum, for example, are generated almost entirely after birth—in humans as late as 12 years of age. The hippocampus, too, is to a large degree formed postnatally. But this postnatal neurogenesis can be clearly set apart from adult neurogenesis. Postnatal neurogenesis is a direct continuation of embryonic and fetal neurogenesis. Adult neurogenesis is a very restricted process that occurs in a cellular environment that otherwise has terminated its development. Postnatal neurogenesis is the rule for many brain parts; adult neurogenesis is the exception even within brain regions.

This book deals with adult neurogenesis in the central nervous system (CNS) only, with one notable exception: the olfactory epithelium, which will be covered in the first part of Chapter 5. The olfactory epithelium lies outside the CNS, although the axons of the receptor neurons, which routinely are generated anew throughout life, project to the olfactory bulb inside the CNS. The reason for making this exception is that adult neurogenesis of the olfactory epithelium might very well constitute a functional unit with adult neurogenesis in the olfactory bulb. Also, adult neurogenesis of the olfactory epithelium shares many similarities with cerebral adult neurogenesis and it generates massive numbers of new neurons, many more than in any other neurogenic region. This feature alone makes it interesting as a model system for adult neurogenesis in general.

Adult neurogenesis has also been reported for the peripheral nervous system (Ciaroni et al., 2000; Geuna et al., 2000; Namaka et al., 2001). The literature, however, is still rather scant and is not covered in this book.

ADULT NEUROGENESIS IN THE HIPPOCAMPUS AND OLFACTORY SYSTEM

In the adult hippocampus, a population of precursor cells resides in the subgranular zone (SGZ) (Fig. 1–5). For earlier anatomists the area that today is referred to as SGZ was simply the border between the granule cell layer of the dentate gyrus and the hilus (or plexiforme layer or CA4). The term *subgranular zone* was coined by Joseph Altman in a study on neurogenesis in the cat in 1975 (Altman, 1975). The progeny of these continuously dividing cells migrate varying distances into the granule cell layer. They then extend their dendrites, as do all other granule cells, into the molecular layer and send an axon along the mossy fiber tract to area CA3, the projection area of the granule cells. Within a couple of weeks and by all known standards, the new granule cells become virtually indistinguishable from their older siblings. The entire process of development is regulated in an activity-dependent fashion, and numerous individual factors have been identified that can influence adult neurogenesis.

In the adult olfactory system, the population of precursor cells is found in the subventricular zone (SVZ) in the temporal walls of the lateral ventricles (Fig. 1–6). Here progeny migrate over a long distance along the rostral migratory stream to the olfactory bulb, where they differentiate into interneurons—one population in the granule cell layer of the bulb and two populations with different neurotransmitter phenotypes in the periglomerular layer. Manipulation of the olfactory system influences neurogenesis in the olfactory bulb, and first theoretical considerations have tried to place neurogenesis in this system into a functional context. The olfactory system also comprises the olfactory epithelium, which is part of the peripheral nervous system and in which massive adult neurogenesis occurs.

Even at this superficial level of description, numerous differences between neurogenesis in the hippocampus and that in the SVZ become obvious. Most dramatic is the quantitative difference. In rodents, neurogenesis

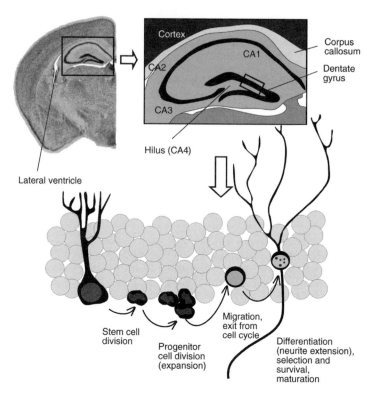

Figure 1–5. Adult hippocampal neurogenesis. Neural precursor cells reside in the border zone between the granule cell layer and the hilus, the subgranular zone (SGZ). The SGZ is a neurogenic niche that, in addition to containing neural precursor cells, also provides the microenvironment in which neuronal development can occur. Neurogenesis progresses from division of a radial glia-like stem cell over rapid divisions of intermediate progenitor cells to production of postmitotic immature and mature granule cells. All cues for all stages of development must be present and accessible for the developing neurons. The mature new granule cells extend their dendrites into the molecular layer, where they, like all other granule cells, receive input from the entorhinal cortex and send their axon along the mossy fiber pathway to hippocampal region CA3.

has been estimated to be many-fold higher in the olfactory bulb than in the dentate gyrus. In humans it might be the other way around (Sanai et al., 2004). But qualitative differences might be more interesting; functionally, very distinct types of neurons are produced. It seems, however, that the precursor cells from one region, after implantation into the other region, behave in a location-specific manner and generate the other phenotype. In this scenario the local microenvironment is important in defining the specific developmental path that neurogenesis takes. At the same time, other studies have suggested that despite all this, the progenitor cell populations

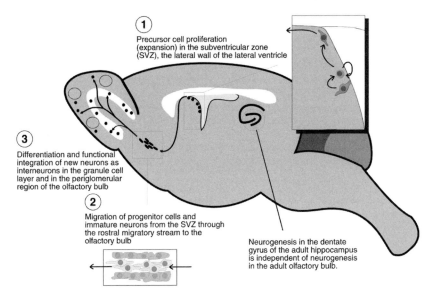

Figure 1–6. Adult neurogenesis in the olfactory bulb. Neural precursor cells reside in the subventricular zone (SVZ), the lateral wall of the lateral ventricles. Stem cells generate transiently amplifying progenitor cells, which generate migratory neural progenitor cells, which travel along the rostral migratory stream to the olfactory bulb, where they terminally differentiate and integrate functionally into the local network. Neurogenesis in the adult olfactory bulb and that in the hippocampus are completely independent processes.

in both regions are not identical. This makes matters even more complex: how much of adult neurogenesis lies in the precursor cells and how much is dictated by the cellular microenvironment?

OPEN QUESTIONS IN ADULT NEUROGENESIS

Adult neurogenesis is scientifically interesting for two reasons that to some degree are independent. In the context of brain function in health and disease, the ability of the brain to make new neurons is important. At the same time, adult neurogenesis can be used as a model system for investigating central questions in applied stem cell biology. The focus, then, is to study factors controlling the development of new neurons under conditions prevailing in the adult brain and discern what has to be achieved if stem cells or immature neurons are implanted in the brain. For most of the young history of neurobiology, the adult brain was essentially considered to be non-neurogenic, if not antineurogenic. But the adult brain routinely does exactly what tissue engineers intend to do in (stem) cell-based therapy for the brain: make new neurons.

But how does the brain do it? And why does it go to all the trouble of maintaining this complex machinery? Or is adult neurogenesis an atavism, an empty-running leftover from evolution? What is adult neurogenesis good for? Is there anything special about the new neurons besides their later birth? How are they integrated into the existing networks? How could they possibly contribute to brain function? How is adult neurogenesis regulated? How does the brain "know" that more neurons are needed, and how is this demand translated into signals a precursor cell can "understand"? Which genes govern this process? Which cascades of receptor and messenger molecules control neurogenesis? What is the relationship between adult neurogenesis and embryonic neurogenesis? What is the nature of the stem and progenitor cells underlying adult neurogenesis? And which role does their local microenvironment play? Why is adult neurogenesis restricted to only few brain regions? What defines a neurogenic region as neurogenic? Do the neurogenic regions differ from each other? And why would the neurogenic regions of the brain rely on a mechanism to produce new neurons, whereas the rest of the brain seems to do perfectly fine without it? Unless, of course, there is damage, and the inability of the adult brain to repair itself on the cellular level becomes obvious. Has adult neurogenesis anything to do with regeneration? Or is it at least a futile attempt at this? And vice versa: what happens if adult neurogenesis fails? Could the failure of adult neurogenesis have anything to do with degeneration? Are there neuroplastic diseases and stem cell disorders of the brain? Can adult neurogenesis be stimulated and employed to improve regeneration?

WHY A BOOK?

Obviously, a great number of questions remain open. And it is no wonder that so many people have become interested in adult neurogenesis. That the mammalian brain can make new neurons, but under normal conditions does so only in a few privileged regions and otherwise apparently neglects this potential for regeneration, is a stunning phenomenon. This is clearly still a blank spot on the map of neuroscience—*"hic sunt leones"* ("here are the lions"), as the medieval cartographers wrote when they did not know how to fill in the map. Today it is often, "here are the stem cells," when we do not know either. But at least we have become much better at asking the questions. The fact that we do not know much does not imply that we will not know anything. The field is literally exploding and researchers are beginning to appreciate the vast range of this topic. Progress in research on adult neurogenesis will require interdisciplinary approaches. It was only recently that everybody stood in awe, realizing that there are indeed new neurons in the adult brain. But the days of sheer phenomenology are over. To address the full range of questions outlined above will require contributions from numerous disciplines. The publication of a book on this topic seems the perfect way to prepare the grounds for such endeavors.

Also, acting as a reviewer for scientific journals I have become painfully aware that some researchers, obviously unaware of the literature, are trying to reinvent the wheel again and again. I have seen articles in which questions were asked that were largely answered many years before. Even the highest-ranking journals have published confirmatory studies, which is nice for the impact-seeking authors but distorting the perception of priorities in intellectual contributions. A cohesive book on the topic might help to avoid such mistakes by bringing together the key discoveries and concepts of the field. It cannot replace a thorough reading of the original articles, but it can draw the bigger picture and chart the field in general so that useless replications are avoided.

Some readers might argue that this book will already be outdated the day it appears. But it is not meant primarily to be an up-to-date review of the literature. Indeed, any such attempt would be futile. The emphasis of this book is more on concepts and on the links between the various fields that are relevant to adult neurogenesis. Nevertheless, every effort has been made to adequately mirror the state of relevant knowledge in late 2004. Adult neurogenesis is difficult to grasp, because it draws from many areas of neuroscience. This interdisciplinary nature of the field makes research on adult neurogenesis fascinating because it enables researchers to take a fresh look at many long-known phenomena of neurobiology. How, for example, does the existence of adult hippocampal neurogenesis influence concepts on how the hippocampus functions? None of the older theories on learning and memory (and other hippocampal functions) had to consider the fact that the underlying network could be altered by adult neurogenesis.

A REVOLUTION IN OUR HEADS?

The impending integration of new neurons into many older and well-established concepts does not mean that everything in the field will fundamentally change. After all, the adult brain does regenerate poorly and does not seem to make use of the regenerative potential resting in its more or less abundant stem cells. Does it have a good reason for this poor performance or is this just the path evolution coincidentally took? There is a risk in any new and burgeoning field that it overestimate its relevance. But here I am only asking for a careful and realistic consideration. The overview given in this book should help with this consideration, to learn what adult neurogenesis is about and, perhaps even more importantly, what it is not about. I believe though that research on adult neurogenesis could make some critical and relevant contributions to a number of fields of neurobiology because it touches on a line of thought that previously was absent: the possibility of plasticity on the level of neuronal numbers. This type of phenomenon simply was not supposed to occur in a good mammalian brain. In a way, this argument is similar to a line from a poem by Christian Morgenstern: *"daß nicht sein kann, was nicht sein darf"* ("that what must not be, cannot be").

With today's knowledge it is easy to wonder about some previous views prevalent in neurobiology that disregarded the mere possibility of plasticity on the level of neurons. Joseph Altman first described adult neurogenesis in the rodent hippocampus in 1965 (Altman and Das, 1965). His landmark study was preceded by two other articles, 2 and 3 years earlier, in which he suggested the possibility of adult neurogenesis with somewhat weaker evidence (Altman, 1962, 1963). Michael Kaplan first reported neurogenesis in the adult olfactory bulb in 1977 (Kaplan and Hinds, 1977). Even Fernando Nottebohm's exciting work in the 1980s on adult neurogenesis in songbirds (Goldman and Nottebohm, 1983) did not fundamentally change the general perception of adult neurogenesis as some sort of oddity or perhaps evolutionary atavism. Nottebohm stated in a 2001 interview in *The New Yorker*: "The view that neurons in the adult brain come and go was considered the view of a lunatic" (Specter, 2001). This seems to be only partially true, however, because Nottebohm's work on adult neurogenesis in songbirds received widespread attention and appraisal. Still, with respect to the situation in mammals, the phrase might capture something of the spirit of that time. For adult mammalian neurogenesis it took more than 30 years after the initial description until, along with the discovery of neural stem cells in the adult brain by Brent Reynolds and Sam Weiss (Reynolds and Weiss, 1992) and by Perry Bartlett and colleagues (Richards et al., 1992), research on adult neurogenesis in mammals found its plausible basis, became widely accepted, and was steered into the mainstream.

Today, however, the principal and somewhat stubborn skepticism of the earlier days has given way to the unspoken belief that essentially everything is possible. Out of this rising enthusiasm many things are dangerously taken at face value. Not all supposedly new neurons, detected immunohistochemically after ischemia or some other type of lesion, make this a finding of reactive neurogenesis. Such images alone are also not the proof of an exploitable potential for self-repair and regeneration only waiting to be stimulated by some clever drug, leading to restoration of function. Before we can really make such a claim, a number of important questions will have to be answered. And these questions are the same ones that come to mind with respect to physiological adult neurogenesis.

THE MYTH OF THE "NO NEW NEURONS" DOGMA

The reluctance of the scientific world to embrace the idea of new neurons in the adult brain is often referred to as obedience to the so-called no-new-neurons dogma. Literally, a dogma is teaching *ex cathedra*, the final word on a fundamental issue in which, when all arguments have been heard, no logical decision can be made. The body of dogmata is the catalog of fundamental sentences in theology, upon which everything else is built, but which by definition can neither be proven nor falsified.

While dogma is from the domain of theology, natural sciences know axioms. Unlike dogma, axioms do not involve a decision and a binding statement made by an authority. Since the Renaissance natural science has been built on empery, not on a body of thought from the authorities.

In the history of science, many discoveries have taken a long time to become accepted. In hindsight it is tempting to mock the ignorant contemporaries who did not recognize the obvious truth. But this is a dangerous attitude that blocks a clear view of how science works, and it is unfair to criticize those who quarreled and remained skeptical; science is based on skepticism. This does not exclude, unfortunately, the possibility that otherwise justified skepticism could be misused.

In some sense, Altman's discovery of adult neurogenesis was a discovery made before its time. Some of the reasons for its lukewarm welcome in the world of science are obvious. The evidence then for new neurons was based on autoradiographically detected grains from tritiated thymidine over cells that had to be morphologically identified as neurons. These were not pyramidal neurons in the cortex or Purkinje cells in the cerebellum, clearly identifiable neurons even by plain morphological standards, but "microneurons" and "granule cells." Modern glial biology has shown how complex and neuron-like astrocytes might be. In maintaining the standard that extraordinary claims require extraordinary evidence, it was quite in order that even Altman's meticulous studies were greeted with skepticism. Nevertheless, the editors of *Science, Nature,* and *The Journal of Comparative Neurology* did publish his work. The influence remained limited, partially because the finding could not be reconciled with the otherwise available concepts of neurobiology of the time. The great anatomists, from His, to Cajal, and to Spielmeyer, along with many others asked themselves whether neurons could divide, but they never found evidence of this. And they were right— even today we remain convinced that neurons do not divide. But at the time of Altman's pioneering work, the concept of stem cells in the adult brain did not yet exist. Without stem cells the idea of adult neurogenesis conflicted with the central principles of neuroscience known in the 1960s as much as they do with those known today. Altman was well aware of this discrepancy and reasoned that precursor cells might exist in the brain. There was no authority that proclaimed the dogma of no new neurons. Rather, the finding was at odds with the knowledge of the time, and even those who found it interesting had no means to technically take the issue further.

There is, however, a disturbing aspect to this story. Even though nobody was in a position to issue a *"No new neurons"* dogma, it seems that people took a dogmatic position and made political use of the fact that neurogenesis could not be proven. In 2001, Michael Kaplan, who in the late 1970s had published a series of studies on adult neurogenesis in which he used electron microscopy to prove the neuronal nature of the newly generated cells, wrote a commentary on his personal history in the field of adult neurogenesis: "But in any revolution, whether political or scientific, there are crusades and battles: not all are winners. In the midst of a revolution one must chose allegiance, and during the 1960s and 1970s, those who chose to support the notion of neurogenesis in the adult brain were ignored or silenced" (Kaplan, 2001). These are strong accusations, but a scholarly historical investigation of this phase of neurogenesis research has yet to be done. The historical account that follows in Chapter 2 of this book is meant to track the development of evidence for adult neurogenesis, not the many other aspects of history.

Pasko Rakic's influential 1985 article, "Limits of Neurogenesis in Adult Primates," also published by *Science*, is often taken as one of the *ex cathedra* writings that, as one comment phrased it, "single-handedly held the field of neurogenesis back by at least a decade" (Specter, 2001). But this is neither true nor fair, and a phrase from a journalistic article should not be taken as a scientific statement. The arguments discussed in Rakic's paper had to be raised against far-reaching conclusions from Altman's, Kaplan's, and even Nottebohm's data. If such valid skepticism was used against the people, not their data, then this is certainly not in order. The stem cell field of today, however, with its disturbing, quick pushes into clinical applications, aptly shows how easy it is to get carried away by suggestive ideas derived from premature extrapolation of single scientific observations. When new tools became available, Rakic was ready to embrace the idea that adult neurogenesis occurs in the neurogenic zones of the adult brain (Kornack and Rakic, 1999; Kornack and Rakic, 2001b). But most of his arguments raised in 1985 remain valid and important. In 2005 there is still no convincing evidence of physiological neurogenesis in most parts of the brain, and the dilemma between stability and plasticity applied by Rakic in his comment on neuronal development and plasticity remains one of the fundamental issues in neuronal network theory.

Finally, science is not about being 100% right every time. To the contrary, it is a responsibility of the community to raise arguments against the impressions elicited by a new observation, even if one might turn out to be wrong in this skepticism. Opportunism in science is as bad as everywhere else. Enthusiasm about a scientific topic should never lead to a watering down of the standards. It is no coincidence that research on adult neurogenesis took off only when the link to neural stem cells could be made and when immuno-histochemistry, confocal microscopy, and stereological quantification tools enabled a clearer picture of what was going on in the neurogenic zones.

When it was reported that adult stem cells might be able to cross organ and germ layer borders so that "blood" could make "brain" and "brain" could make "blood," these findings were received with skepticism by some (Anderson et al., 2001) but not most investigators. Overall, these findings were hardly questioned and immediately found their way into visions of medicine of the future: with stem cells everything would be possible. However, new data strongly supported the critics, and although it cannot be categorically ruled out that transdifferentiation is principally possible, it is not what it first seemed to be. The rather blind surrender to a suggestive idea on the basis of limited evidence turned out to be the wrong choice.

The scientific community's opinion on adult neurogenesis took the slow path that many new ideas in science must take. There is nothing inherently wrong with this. One can argue about style here and there, and there might have been misuse of scientific arguments to influence research politics, but the general course along which science progressed in this case is not refutable. Some ideas, such as the double helix, find their terrain well prepared. When they are first brought up, their explanatory power is so extensive that many open questions are immediately resolved; other important discoveries are made ahead of the questions to which they are the answers.

We should thus bury the *no-new-neurons* dogma because it is misleading: nobody spoke *ex cathedra* that there are no new neurons, and the apparent lack of neurogenesis in the adult brain has never been an axiomatic rule. It simply reflected the state of knowledge at the time. The rest of the story was human nature—moving too slowly in some places, too quickly in others.

WHAT TO EXPECT IN THIS BOOK

Chapter 2 gives a historic account and summarizes the development of the concept of plasticity, the fundamental capacity of the brain to alter its structure in response to function. This discussion might at first glance seem to be a typical historic digression but this is hardly the case. Adult neurogenesis is a plastic event that takes place in the context of other signs of plasticity. Like other instances of plasticity, neurogenesis is intricately linked to function, thus it does not make sense to view adult neurogenesis in isolation. The concepts of plasticity set the stage for the description of how adult neurogenesis was discovered and how it was discussed.

In Chapter 3 we describe the *conditio sine qua non* of adult neurogenesis: stem or progenitor cells with the potential to generate new neurons. The term *stem cell* has suffered inflationary use in recent years. A clear picture of what is actually meant by "stemness" is important to understand some fundamental principles underlying adult neurogenesis. This endeavor is not at all trivial, as the discussion of numerous conflicting concepts of stem cells in the adult brain will show. Although many important things can be said about them, stem cells of the brain still remain rather elusive creatures.

Chapter 4 reviews general aspects of brain development. Neural stem cell biology is essentially developmental biology, but developmental neurobiology is also to a large degree stem cell biology. Adult neurogenesis is neuronal development under the conditions of the adult brain. To understand to what degree adult neurogenesis is a recapitulation of embryonic and fetal neurogenesis and is an independent process with its own rules and mechanisms, a review of some principles of neural stem cell biology in brain development is necessary. We will place adult neurogenesis in the context of neuronal development in the embryonic and early postnatal brain. What is similar and what is different between these two forms of neuronal development? Whereas embryonic development occurs in a microenvironment that is itself developing, adult neurogenesis has to proceed in a cellular milieu that is in general hostile to neuronal development. Adult neurogenesis has to implement and maintain its own permissive microenvironment. Also, embryonic neuronal development is massively parallel, allowing us to determine with relative precision which brain parts are generated at which gestational time point. In the adult, however, all stages of neuronal development can be found next to each other. How can regulatory cues address the correct target cells only?

Chapters 5 and 6 will give a detailed description of what is known about neurogenesis in the adult mammalian olfactory system and hippocampus. The emphasis here is on analysis of the "naked" process itself, not its regulation or function. Still, thoughts about plasticity (from Chapter 2) and stem cells (from Chapter 3) allow determination of where regulation might set in.

Chapter 7 deals with the experimental techniques used to investigate adult neurogenesis in vivo. There are several principal issues and technical pitfalls that have to be considered when designing experiments on adult neurogenesis and analyzing the data. The selection of marker proteins to identify different populations of cells is crucial, as is the proper use of confocal microscopy to examine the expression of these marker antigens in vivo. Other important questions are how adult neurogenesis can be quantified and how it can be compared between different experimental conditions. Many of the problems in interpreting seemingly contradictory findings on adult neurogenesis arise at least in part from methodological problems.

With that in mind, Chapter 8 will turn to a discussion of adult neurogenesis outside the neurogenic regions. For this we will revisit the concept of the stem cell niche as the microenvironment that enables precursor cell activity and neurogenesis. How do neurogenic regions differ from non-neurogenic ones? Does adult neurogenesis physiologically occur in the cortex and elsewhere outside the hippocampus and the olfactory system? This issue has been discussed controversially and is to some degree a debate on methods. But there is more to the discussion than methodological issues. The previous chapters feed into hypotheses on what might be happening in the adult cortex.

Chapter 9 discusses the regulation of adult neurogenesis. Factors that have been shown to affect adult neurogenesis are discussed here. It will become obvious that from the present range of data, no unambiguous picture of how adult neurogenesis is regulated can be drawn. This situation does not, however, preclude the deduction of some very fundamental principles and the development of a number of testable hypotheses.

Chapter 10 addresses the potential function of adult neurogenesis. This can be done on different conceptual levels. *Function* here can mean the function of the individual new cell or the cell within the context of its neuronal network, as well as the relevance of the entire process of neurogenesis for brain function and cognition.

Chapter 11, on comparative biology, is the shortest of all the chapters, reflecting how little is known about adult neurogenesis in this context. Nevertheless, a comparative approach can be extremely powerful. How much can we learn about adult neurogenesis by studying the fruitfly and zebrafish? Adult neurogenesis is well preserved throughout evolution, but there are some fundamental changes between adult neurogenesis in rodents and that in other vertebrates. Why can lizards regenerate entire brain parts, but "higher animals" cannot? Is adult neurogenesis advantageous or disadvantageous? Is it just an alternative mechanism, the use of some principle originally developed for something else, or something that has been shaped under direct evolutionary pressure? We will discuss adult neurogenesis in songbirds in some detail and consider how much we know about adult neurogenesis in humans.

The last chapter deals with medical aspects of adult neurogenesis. What happens if adult neurogenesis fails? What role does adult neurogenesis play in the pathogenesis of neurological disorders? We will also discuss the therapeutic consequences that might arise from such a role and the lessons that can be learned from adult neurogenesis for neurotransplantation approaches.

A HYPOTHESIS

The general hypothesis underlying this book is that adult neurogenesis is a particularly prominent manifestation of a far more general principle of neurobiology: the idea that brain development never ends and that plasticity can be taken as continued development. As we will see, quantitatively, adult neurogenesis is minute over the largest periods of adulthood. Most of what we call adult neurogenesis actually occurs fairly early in life. But the point is that it never seems to end and that it remains regulated by activity and many other factors. Because neurons are involved, adult neurogenesis receives and deserves particular interest. But adult neurogenesis also needs to be seen in the context of other aspects of cell genesis throughout life and in connection with the many other aspects of plasticity, for example, on the level of neurites and synapses or in glial cells.

REFERENCES

Altman J (1962) Are new neurons formed in the brains of adult mammals? Science 135:1128–1129.

Altman J (1963) Autoradiographic investigation of cell proliferation in the brains of rats and cats. Anat Rec 145:573–591.

Altman J (1975) Postnatal development of the hippocampal dentate gyrus under normal and experimental conditions. In: The Hippocampus (Isaacson RL, Pribram KH, eds), pp 95–122. New York: Plenum Press.

Altman J, Das GD (1965) Autoradiographic and histologic evidence of postnatal neurogenesis in rats. J Comp Neurol 124:319–335.

Anderson DJ, Gage FH, Weissman IL (2001) Can stem cells cross lineage boundaries? Nat Med 7:393–395.

Arvidsson A, Collin T, Kirik D, Kokaia Z, Lindvall O (2002) Neuronal replacement from endogenous precursors in the adult brain after stroke. Nat Med 8:963–970.

Blakeslee S (2000) A decade of discovery yields a shock about the brain. New York Times, January 4 p 1.

Ciaroni S, Cecchini T, Cuppini R, Ferri P, Ambrogini P, Bruno C, Del Grande P (2000) Are there proliferating neuronal precursors in adult rat dorsal root ganglia? Neurosci Lett 281:69–71.

Eriksson PS, Perfilieva E, Björk-Eriksson T, Alborn AM, Nordborg C, Peterson DA, Gage FH (1998) Neurogenesis in the adult human hippocampus. Nat Med 4:1313–1317.

Gage FH, Coates PW, Palmer TD, Kuhn HG, Fisher LJ, Suhonen JO, Peterson DA, Suhr ST, Ray J (1995) Survival and differentiation of adult neuronal progenitor cells transplanted to the adult brain. Proc Natl Acad Sci USA 92:11879–11883.

Geuna S, Borrione P, Fornaro M, Giacobini-Robecchi MG (2000) Neurogenesis and stem cells in adult mammalian dorsal root ganglia. Anat Rec 261:139–140.

Goldman SA, Nottebohm F (1983) Neuronal production, migration and differentiation in a vocal control nucleus of the adult female canary brain. Proc Natl Acad Sci USA 80:2390–2394.

Gould E, Reeves AJ, Graziano MS, Gross CG (1999) Neurogenesis in the neocortex of adult primates. Science 286:548–552.

Gould E, Vail N, Wagers M, Gross CG (2001) Adult-generated hippocampal and neocortical neurons in macaques have a transient existence. Proc Natl Acad Sci USA 98:10910–10917.

Herrera DG, Garcia-Verdugo JM, Alvarez-Buylla A (1999) Adult-derived neural precursors transplanted into multiple regions in the adult brain. Ann Neurol 46:867–877.

Kaplan MS (2001) Environment complexity stimulates visual cortex neurogenesis: death of a dogma and a research career. Trends Neurosci 24:617–620.

Kaplan MS, Hinds JW (1977) Neurogenesis in the adult rat: electron microscopic analysis of light radioautographs. Science 197:1092–1094.

Koketsu D, Mikami A, Miyamoto Y, Hisatsune T (2003) Nonrenewal of neurons in the cerebral neocortex of adult macaque monkeys. J Neurosci 23:937–942.

Kornack DR, Rakic P (1999) Continuation of neurogenesis in the hippocampus of the macaque monkey. Proc Natl Acad Sci USA 96:5768–5773.

Kornack DR, Rakic P (2001a) Cell proliferation without neurogenesis in adult primate neocortex. Science 294:2127–2130.

Kornack DR, Rakic P (2001b) The generation, migration, and differentiation of olfactory neurons in the adult primate brain. Proc Natl Acad Sci USA 98:4752–4757.

Lie DC, Dziewczapolski G, Willhoite AR, Kaspar BK, Shults CW, Gage FH (2002) The adult substantia nigra contains progenitor cells with neurogenic potential. J Neurosci 22:6639–6649.

Namaka MP, Sawchuk M, MacDonald SC, Jordan LM, Hochman S (2001) Neurogenesis in postnatal mouse dorsal root ganglia. Exp Neurol 172:60–69.

Rakic P (2002) Neurogenesis in adult primate neocortex: an evaluation of the evidence. Nat Rev Neurosci 3:65–71.

Reynolds BA, Weiss S (1992) Generation of neurons and astrocytes from isolated cells of the adult mammalian central nervous system. Science 255:1707–1710.

Richards LJ, Kilpatrick TJ, Bartlett PF (1992) De novo generation of neuronal cells from the adult mouse brain. Proc Natl Acad Sci USA 89:8591–8595.

Sanai N, Tramontin AD, Quinones-Hinojosa A, Barbaro NM, Gupta N, Kunwar S, Lawton MT, McDermott MW, Parsa AT, Manuel-Garcia Verdugo J, Berger MS, Alvarez-Buylla A (2004) Unique astrocyte ribbon in adult human brain contains neural stem cells but lacks chain migration. Nature 427:740–744.

Shihabuddin LS, Horner PJ, Ray J, Gage FH (2000) Adult spinal cord stem cells generate neurons after transplantation in the adult dentate gyrus. J Neurosci 20:8727–8735.

Specter M (2001) Rethinking the brain. The New Yorker, July 23, pp 42–53.

Suhonen JO, Peterson DA, Ray J, Gage FH (1996) Differentiation of adult hippocampus-derived progenitors into olfactory neurons in vivo. Nature 383:624–627.

Wichterle H, Lieberam I, Porter JA, Jessell TM (2002) Directed differentiation of embryonic stem cells into motor neurons. Cell 110:385–397.

2

History

Adult neurogenesis was discovered relatively late in the twentieth century. The first reports on neurogenesis in the hippocampus came from Joseph Altman in 1962, 1963, and 1965 (Altman, 1962a, 1963; Altman and Das, 1965a, 1965b). The first report on neurogenesis in the adult olfactory bulb was from Michael Kaplan in 1977 (Kaplan and Hinds, 1977), although Joseph Altman had published two studies on postnatal neurogenesis in the olfactory bulb in 1965 and 1969 (Altman and Das, 1965b; Altman, 1969). Only in the early 1990s, beginning with the first studies identifying stem cells in the adult brain (Reynolds and Weiss, 1992; Kilpatrick and Bartlett, 1993; Palmer et al., 1995), did research on adult neurogenesis gain momentum.

To appreciate the phenomenon of adult mammalian neurogenesis, one must know the essentials of neurobiology. Without a working knowledge of cells and their ability to divide or nerve cells and their inability to divide, one can never grasp the excitement that arose about adult neurogenesis. When cells and cell divisions were discovered in the nineteenth century, naturally related questions arose. Can all cells divide? Is division a characteristic feature of cells? Consequently, can neurons divide as well? Because it was soon found out that they cannot, adult neurogenesis was simply put out of the question. When adult neurogenesis was first reported it just appeared to be mysterious, to put it mildly. Given the general state of biological knowledge at the time, adult neurogenesis, if the reports on it were to be taken seriously at all, must have seemed an oddity, a strange exception to a plausible rule.

Today, when stem cells are the talk of the town and adult neurogenesis has gone mainstream, it is important not to forget that these phenomena have their roots in something that was long considered an oddity. Carl Sagan has aphoristically defined science as "the marriage of skepticism and wonder" (Sagan, 1995). In the case of any scientific topic and adult neurogenesis in particular it is important not to lose the ability to marvel at what we see and the distance to question what we believe we have seen. A historical perspective makes this dual responsibility easier.

CELLS AS THE STRUCTURAL PRINCIPLE OF ALL LIVING THINGS

Today it is difficult to think of biology other than as a science of cells. In some sense, cells are the unit of biology. But cells are something that can only be seen under the microscope and thus were completely unknown until optical

22

lenses and microscopes were invented. Ancient biology was a biology of material, forces, and spirits. For Aristotle, the most important authority on ancient biology, there was uninterrupted continuity between living and non-living matter. Earth and sea could "spontaneously" generate organisms (Mazzarello, 1999). This idea was not refuted until the eighteenth century, when Lazzaro Spallanzani and others showed that only organisms could produce other organisms. Where the antique philosopher–biologists had been convinced that "nature does not jump" (*natura non saltat*), these empiricists claimed that there is in fact a gap between living and nonliving things. With the invention of the microscope a whole new universe was made accessible to human curiosity. Researchers began to look for the smallest units of life. In 1676 Antoni van Leeuwenhoek, the inventor of the microscope, reported to the Royal Society that moving and thus presumably living particles ("animalcules") could be seen in pond water (Dobell, 1960).

Robert Hooke was the English Leonardo da Vinci. A true Renaissance man, born in 1635, he made contributions to almost all fields of science, from physics (Hooke's law, an equation describing the elasticity of a spring) and chemistry, to astronomy, architecture, and engineering. His greatest biological achievement was the first description of the "cell" as the constituent of plants. He used his own improvement of Antony van Leeuwenhoek's microscope. Studying a piece of cork he could "exceedingly plainly perceive it to be all perforated and porous, much like a honey-comb . . . these pores or cells . . . were indeed the first microscopical pores I ever saw, and perhaps, that were ever seen, for I had not met with any writer or person that had made any mention of them before this" (Micrographia, Observation XVIII, 1665). The "pores" reminded him of the cells of monks in their monastery, and the analogy stuck. Preceding this discovery was the first description of red blood "corpuscles" by Jan Swammerdam (Winsor, 1980).

After Hooke it took almost 200 years until the recognition was made that all living things are entirely composed of cells and, even more importantly, that development depends on cells, because cells give rise to cells. It is amazing that none of the first describers of cells developed a theory around this discovery. The significance of the observation was not appreciated until much later (see Wolpert, 1995). The first speculative steps toward a cell theory were made in 1805 by Lorenz Oken, who proposed that plants and animals are conglomerates of tiny living "infusoria," which, however, he did not equate with cells but rather with the animalcules of Leeuwenhoek. In 1832, Christian Gottfried Ehrenberg recognized that fungi and "infusoria" propagated by division (Ehrenberg, 1832), Again, the link to multicellular organisms was not made. An important next milestone was the discovery of the cell nucleus by Robert Brown in 1833 (see references in Watermann, 1982).

Around 1838–1839, the botanist Matthias Jacob and the physician Theodor Schwann met in the laboratory of famous physiologist Johannes Müller in Berlin, where they discussed their view that organisms are made up of cells. They did not publish their work together, but are jointly recognized today as the fathers of cell biology. Schwann stated that "the elementary parts of all tissues are formed of cells." Even more importantly, he suggested that the "universal principle of development . . . is the formation of cells." Neither Schleiden nor Schwann, however, came to terms with the origin of cells. They adhered to the view, influentially propagated in Schwann's major written works, that cells could generate *de novo* and arise within or even outside other cells (Watermann, 1982).

In 1858 the German pathologist Rudolf Virchow coined the term "cellular pathology." Key to his work was his statement, "Every animal appears as a sum of vital units, each of which bears in itself the complete characteristics of life." His famous dictum, *omnis cellula e cellula* ("every cell is from a cell"), and its implications for medicine made his theory one of the most influential ideas in biology. Virchow implied that "cells make cells," in health and disease, and that therefore the brain (or any other organ) could not be taken as static, but as a product of development (Virchow, 1859).

In 1766 Abraham Trembley was the first to report the direct observation that "animalcules" could reproduce. There is not one single name to attach to the discovery that cell divisions underlie growth and development. This concept became increasingly accepted toward the end of the nineteenth century. Another scientist from Berlin, Robert Remak, is credited with the first proposal of a theory of cell propagation by cell divisions: "The cells . . . multiply by continuous division, which starts at the nucleus" (Remak, 1852, 1855). Rudolf Albrecht von Kölliker reported cell divisions in the early vertebrate embryo that yielded cells that went on to differentiate into the many different types of cells found in the mature organism. In some sense, this is the birth of the idea of stem cells. In the 1860s von Kölliker and others began to interpret embryology in light of the new cell theory.

The discovery of mitosis as the mechanism of cell division was extremely protracted (Gourret, 1995). It is said to have begun with the work of Hermann Fol, Otto Bütschli, and Eduard Strasburger, who around 1873 first described intranuclear figures that correspond to the mitotic apparatus, as it is called today.

CELLS OF THE NERVOUS SYSTEM

Neurons and Glia

It turned out to be tremendously difficult to study cells in the brain. The major breakthrough came in 1873, when Camillo Golgi announced his now-famous staining method, a silver impregnation that miraculously (the reason is still not completely known) stained only selected neurons, thus raising them above the overwhelmingly dense background. The structure of the nervous tissue became accessible.

As far as we know, Rudolf Virchow was the first to distinguish between neurons and glia. He coined the term *glia*, a Greek term for *Nervenkitt*, or nerve glue (Virchow, 1846). Camillo Golgi's silver impregnation methods allowed the visualization of individual glial cells and the description of astrocytes. Golgi was also the first to describe radial fibers that extended between the ventricular and pial surface of the neural tube (Golgi, 1886). However, another new staining method, introduced by Weigert in 1895, led to the dismissal of the idea of glial cells as individual entities. Rather, this became the period of the "glial syncytium," some sort of continuous cytoplasm with interspersed nuclei, engulfing all nerve cells (Hardesty, 1904). The idea gained much influence but was never fully accepted. In 1913 Ramon y Cajal used his gold–chloride–sublimate staining to prove that glial cells were indeed individual cells. He distinguished neurons (the "first element") from astrocytes (the "second element"). A group with small rounded nuclei did not fall into either category and became the so-called third element of Cajal. P. Del Rio-Hortega discovered that this third group of cells consisted of oligodendrocytes and another class of cells, for which he coined the term "microglia" (Rio-Hortega, 1919). He made the case that microglia alone be considered the third element and oligodendrocytes be grouped with astrocytes. Thus, by 1921 the major cell classes of the central nervous system had been described, and the general pattern of lineage relationships as we know it today was in place.

Dividing Cells in the Central Nervous System

To understand growth of the embryo and the development of organs, mapping of mitotic figures became an important tool. In 1881, Altmann described mitotic figures in the walls of the neural tubes (Altmann, 1881) and in 1896, Ludwig Merk from Graz wrote "Mitosen im Centralnervensysteme—ein Beitrag zur Lehre vom Wachstum desselben." This large, comparative study of many species contained the observation that the numbers of cell divisions change over time, and secondary centers of cell division might take the place of the proliferative plane near the ventricle. He also described the characteristic pattern of cerebellar development: after an initial phase of cell division near the ventricle, the granule cell layer is formed in an outside–inside fashion (Merk, 1896).

The first description of germinal cells (*Keimzellen*) in the developing nervous system goes back to Wilhelm His (1889), who, along with the Spaniard Santiago Ramon y Cajal and the Italian Camillo Golgi, was the greatest neuroanatomist of the time. These three laid the foundation of modern neurobiology. Wilhelm His placed particular emphasis on developmental aspects (much of them studied in salmon). These early investigations were based on the light-microscopic identification of mitoses and meticulous anatomical analyses.

His described how neuroepithelial cells of the neural tube (the "medullary canal" in his nomenclature) produced "germinal cells" and differentiated cells, including the "spongioblasts." The idea was that germinal cells produced neuroblasts, which generated nerve cells. The "spongioblasts," in contrast, were equivalent to what today is called radial glia and were thought to produce glia only. In 1897 Alfred Schaper reported that not only the epithelial cells of the tube but also the germinal cells could give rise to spongioblasts. Schaper also introduced the "indifferent cell," or "medullo-blast," a sort of parenchymal germinal cell, separated from the ventricular epithelium. He proposed that these cells retained the capabilities of the spongioblasts after migration into the tissue (Schaper, 1897).

Wilder Penfields seminal work in 1932 neuroglia contains a schematic drawing that summarizes the knowledge about lineage relationships at that time (Penfield, 1932) (Fig. 2–1). Today it seems that *cum grano salis* both spongioblastic and medulloblastic lineages, which were thought to be mutually exclusive at Penfield's time, can be found in the adult brain. A plausible hypothesis is that spongioblasts would relate to the precursor cells of the dorsal brain, generating principal neurons and astrocytes, the "medulloblasts" to the precursor cells of the ventral brain, giving rise to interneurons and oligodendrocytes. This analogy is somewhat deceptive and remains problematic, because the term *medulloblast* has additional controversial connotations. In 1938 John Kershman argued that medullo-blasts would only exist in the cerebellum, where they could give rise to medulloblastomas. Today we know the tumor entity of medulloblastomas as primitive neuroectodermal tumors of roof of the fourth ventricle, but the medulloblast as a cell entity has disappeared altogether. However, the proposal of an "indifferent" apolar parenchymal cell as a "bipotential un-differentiated element" (Kershman, 1938) as suggested by Schaper has regained appeal with the discovery of NG2-expressing parenchymal precursor cells. Some NG2-cells have been found to be multipotent ex vivo, and in vivo can express markers of multiple lineages (Belachew et al., 2003). Remarkably, Schaper suggested that some of the indifferent cells remained in a bipotent state until late in life and might perhaps provide the material for "regeneration processes" in the brain (Kershman, 1938).

Much later than in the context of the rare medulloblastoma and despite an early theory about the origin of "subependymomas" (Globus and Kuhlen-beck, 1944), it was recognized that proliferative cells in the ventricular walls of adult primates might be the origin of gliomas (Lewis, 1968).

CAN NEURONS DIVIDE?

Independent of the evolving understanding of the course of brain development and the lineage relationship between the major classes of cells in the brain, it was generally accepted that cell genesis almost completely ceased after embryogenesis and was absent in the adult. Wilhelm Spielmeyer, in his *Histopathologie des Nervensystems* (1922), wrote, "in general, the ganglion cells of the postembryonic period do not have a capability for cell division." But he did mention the possible exception of retinal ganglion cells, in which

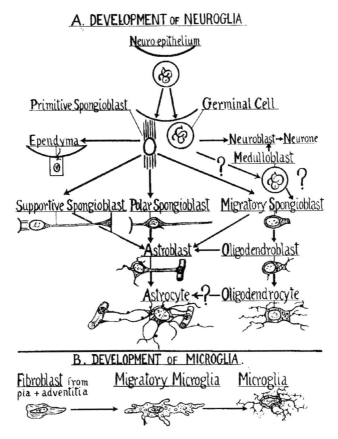

Figure 2–1. Penfield's scheme of cellular origin in the central nervous system. In 1932 Wilder Penfield published this drawing in his work on neuroglia (Penfield, 1932). Several types of cells in this scheme, for example, the "medulloblast" and the "spongioblast," did not appear in most later systematics. Modern precursor cell biology, however, leads to a new appreciation of the lineage relationships proposed during Penfield's time. The "spongioblast," for example, first described by Schaper in 1897, shows intriguing similarities to the proposed precursor cells of the brain tissue outside the neurogenic regions, many of them expressing the proteoglycan NG2 and nestin. Such historical links remain speculation at present but they indicate that adult precursor cell biology has its roots in the work of classical early twentieth-century neuroanatomy.

Schreiber and Wengler induced mitoses by injections of "Scharlachöl." Nevertheless, Schreiber and Wengler (1908, 1910) remained skeptical of whether they had observed complete mitoses and they carefully weighed the evidence.

Regeneration in the central nervous system of amphibians had long been known and described by Müller, Masius and van Lair, and others. Reports about similar observations in mammals by Brown-Séguard and Dentans were already disputed at the time. Some authors claimed that among the proliferative response found after needle stick injuries to the adult mammalian cortex dividing ganglion cells could be detected. Others argued against these conclusions. Vitzous' bold claims of complete regeneration of the monkey visual system after ablation of large areas of the visual cortex were greeted with great skepticism (see references in Schreiber and Wengler, 1910). Thus at the end of the nineteenth century, the topic of neuronal regeneration had already been heavily discussed. Intriguingly, many of the arguments have since remained the same: how can we prove the neuronal nature of a cell that has undergone division? How can we prove lineage relationships?

An alternate theory, the idea of amitotic nuclear divisions in nerve cells, was discussed with fervor but refuted early on. Cell division became generally accepted as the only path of growth in animals. It was also recognized that with demonstration of a true mitosis of ganglion cells, proof of possible neuronal regeneration would be made, the implications of which did not go unnoticed (Schreiber and Wengler, 1910). Regarding this possibility, Ramon y Cajal made the following rather pessimistic statement: "Once development was ended, the fonts of growth and regeneration of the axons and dendrites dried up irrevocably. In the adult centers, the nerve paths are something fixed, and immutable: everything may die, nothing may be regenerated" (Ramon y Cajal, 1928).

This statement, found in the introduction to reviews on adult neurogenesis, is considered the origin of the no-new-neurons dogma. The problematic implications of the term *dogma* in this context have been discussed in Chapter 1. In addition, even this short historical outline underscores that Cajal's statement was not a lonely decision *"ex cathedra"* but one that reflected his conclusions from ongoing scientific discussions of that time. He found that there was not enough evidence to support the idea that neurons could divide.

THE ORIGINS OF STEM CELL BIOLOGY

The term *stem cell* first arose in the scientific literature of the nineteenth century, but its use was not defined, and conflicting terms for what we would consider a stem cell today were common. Although a history of stem cell biology remains to be written, one aspect of it is important for our context.

The modern, multifaceted idea of stem cells arose largely in the context of the first work on human in vitro fertilization in the early 1960s (Edwards, 2001). R.G. Edwards, who became the father of in vitro fertilization, began to study cells isolated from mammalian embryos and blastocysts and their development in vitro. Explants of inner cell masses from blastocysts showed outgrowth into many cellular lineages in culture (Cole et al., 1966). Implantation of such embryonic stem cells derived from mice into blastocysts originating from mice of a different strain produced the first mouse chimeras, which were highly obvious because of their mixes of coat color patterns (Gardner, 1968). The same general principle underlies today's transgenic animals. Peter Hollands (1987) used embryonic stem cells to repopulate the bone marrow of irradiated mice. This report bridged the work on embryonic stem cells with E.D. Thomas's pioneering work in hematology. For certain types of leukemia and other disorders, bone marrow transplantation or the transplantation of bone marrow stem cells has become clinical routine (Thomas, 1999). The rise of embryonic stem cells, with their unlimited capacity for self-renewal and differentiation into various cell types, has sparked the hope that embryonic stem cells might be used for cell replacement beyond the hematopoetic system.

In the nervous system, cell transplantation had been tried with varying but mostly limited success. Parallel to a severe setback to such treatment, the widespread but pointless use of adrenal transplants to treat Parkinson disease (Madrazo et al., 1987), Olle Lindvall, Anders Björklund first succeeded in treating Parkinson's patients with striatal implants of fetal mesencephalic tissue (Lindvall et al., 1987). Despite ongoing controversies about this treatment strategy (Freed et al., 2001, 2003; Hagell et al., 2002), the reports can be taken as proof of principle that neuronal replacement therapy is possible in humans. Because one of the major obstacles in realizing neural cell replacement therapy is the availability of graftable cells, stem cells, with their theoretically unlimited expandability, would provide an ideal source for cells used in neural transplantation.

The greatest hopes in neural transplantation coincided with the reemerging interest in adult neurogenesis and the discovery of neural precursor cells in the adult brain. Consequently, stem cells in the adult brain have never been considered solely an interesting biological fact. As predicted by Schreiber and Wengler in 1910, the evidence of successful mitoses in the brain was immediately regarded as evidence of regeneration and has had important medical implications. The discovery of actively proliferative neural stem cells in the early 1990s is inseparable from the general rise in stem cell–based medicine. In many reports on adult neurogenesis, the two views on stem cells intermingle—the perspective of developmental biology on the one hand and the perspective of regenerative medicine on the other. There is nothing wrong with either of these perspectives, but the two different conceptual frameworks in stem cell biology can cause profound misunderstandings (see also Anderson, 2001). Research on adult neurogenesis might benefit from the booming interest in stem cells, but despite the many important and interesting medical implications of adult neurogenesis, it remains mostly an area of developmental biology.

THE IDEA OF PLASTICITY

The impact of the study of adult neurogenesis on the neurosciences can only be truly appreciated in the light of the concept of plasticity. The term *plasticity* represents the observation that the brain alters its structure, depending on its activity. Plasticity is how form follows function in the brain. The earlier neuroanatomists, in particular Ramon y Cajal, did not consider the brain to be static, even if they saw how poorly it regenerated. They did not have the tools to see the reciprocal link between function and structure that is characteristic for the brain. Today we know that a static brain would be dead. Brain function depends on plasticity. Ironically, then, it was not the anatomists but the psychologists who first favored a rigid, hardwired brain structure. The behavorists who dominated psychology in the first decades of the twentieth century exemplify how ideology allows one to ignore obvious facts, silence opposing arguments through shear influence and power, and thereby prevent progress. The behaviorists declared that all learning was based on a simple relationship between input and output. A reflex, such as the patellar tendon reflex, is the prototype of this relationship. All behavior could be reduced to such units of reflex-like responses. Learning was essentially pavlovian and based only on conditioning, that is, stimuli of different kinds were linked to motoric outputs. This reduction of learning to motoric behavior should have made investigators skeptical, even during the heyday of the theory, and is only one of the many bizarre features of behaviorism. Behaviorism began to be questioned when psychiatrist Hans Berger from Jena demonstrated the electroencephalogram (EEG) in 1924. The complexity and restlessness of this continuous and widespread brain activity were impossible to explain in terms of behaviorism. In the behavioristic mindset, brain activity between input and output did not exist, nor did activity independent of input or motoric output. The behavioristic brain could be thought of as hardwired, and of course failed to explain signs of recovery after damage and functional plasticity.

The great thinker in the neurosciences whose work marks the transition from this narrow perspective to modern cognitive neurobiology is Donald Hebb, known mostly for his famous "Neurophysiological postulate." The key sentence in his book "The organization of behavior: A Neurophysiological theory" 1949, is : "When an axon of cell A is near enough to excite cell B and repeatedly or persistently takes part in firing it, some growth process or metabolic change takes place in one or both cells such that A's efficiency, as one of the cells firing B, is increased." In essence, what Hebb implied was a basis for learning on the level of synapses. If activity in two cells were closely enough related in time, this activity would strengthen their connection. Contiguity between pre- and postsynaptic activity leads to permanent structural changes, which is plasticity. Hebb postulated that plasticity was fundamental to learning and long-term memory and thereby essentially the basis for cognition and brain function in general.

It was later found that for this principle to work, it had to account for both strengthening and weakening of connections with equal specificity. In 1973, Tim Bliss and Terje Lomo discovered long-term potentiation (LTP), which became generally accepted as the electrophysiological correlate to learning. The induction of LTP is indeed hebbian (Kelso et al., 1986). But so is its counterpart, long-term depression (LTD), the long-lasting weakening of a neuronal connection. Whether LTP or LTD occurred could depend solely on the temporal spacing of the stimuli. If cell A fired shortly before B, LTP was found; if cell A fired shortly after B, LTD resulted (Markram et al., 1997). This is called the "temporally asymmetric" form of Hebb's rule and helps explain the constant formation and dismantling of connections in the brain that underly cognitive processes. Hebb postulated plasticity as the fundamental principle of how the brain works.

While "Hebb's synapse" became the most influential part of his work, Hebb did not stop at the level of single cell–cell interactions. He postulated further that information was not stored in single synapses but that the synapses formed the basis of autonomously "reverberating activity" in what Hebb called "cell assemblies." This not only introduced the idea of neuronal networks but also proposed that self-sustained activity in such networks, independent of concurrent input, underlay cognition. Intrinsic activity as much as extrinsic input could feed into the network activity. An implicit consequence of this idea is that continuous brain activity, as seen on the EEG, is paralleled by an equally continuous structural plasticity.

The often-quoted thesis of Hebb's postulate is immediately preceded by an equally interesting sentence: "Let us assume that the persistence or repetition of reverberatory activity (or trace) tends to induce lasting cellular changes that add to its stability." Literally, there is no reason to believe that these changes should be restricted to synaptic changes. Consequently, adult neurogenesis relates to this aspect of Hebb's idea on how the brain and mind work. New cells obviously add new synapses, but they also provide new knots in the network and they might change not only the size (quantity) but also the quality of neuronal cell assemblies. Adult neurogenesis might thereby become a matter more of qualitative change than of adding greater quantities of cells, in the sense of increasing processing power in our computer by putting in extra memory.

Hebb was interested in more than the basic rules of learning and their underlying neurophysiological principles. He also stimulated the field of developmental psychology by studying experimentally how early experience influenced cognitive abilities later in life. In his most influential activity in this field, he compared rats kept in laboratory cages with rats he had reared at home (supposedly as pets for his children) and found long-lasting positive effects on learning and memory (Hebb, 1947). He concluded that experience shapes neuronal development and, consequently, cognition. The finding was reported in a 43-line abstract in *American Psychologist* and is indeed not much more than an anecdote: group sizes were small and no proper controls had been included; no exact data can be found in the text. However, in 1952, Bernard Hymovitch, a Ph.D. student working with Hebb, published a replication and confirmation of Hebb's observation with larger groups and better controls and thus proved the initial claim to be correct.

With this work, Hebb became the father of research on the effects of "enriched environments," an experimental setup that in the late 1950s to the mid-1970s became a central paradigm in developmental psychology. It allowed investigators to address experimentally the fundamental question of how we become what we are. How much of us is inherited and how much is acquired by education? Or in terms of biology, how much of an individual is determined by his or her genes and how much by interaction with the environment? Especially in pedagogic debates during this period exact numbers were stated with confidence in terms of the percentage of a person that was inherited and how much came from education. Depending on the individual position in this debate, the percentage could range between 0% and 100%. Today we know that development is a continued interaction between genes and environment and that at every single moment, any living organism is 100% genes and 100% environment, with environment beginning essentially on the cellular level and constituting everything outside the genome itself. This insight originated partly from the studies of enriched environments, because in the laboratory situation one could keep the genetic influence constant by using inbred strains of rodents. Twin studies in humans complemented this line of research and allowed investigators to address issues that were more specifically human. With the rise of molecular biology, the molecular basis of the constant interaction between genes and environment was discovered, providing another crucial aspect of what constitutes plasticity.

Mark Rosenzweig, a psychologist at the University of California, Berkeley, built an amazing and influential scientific empire on the initial observation of effects of environmental enrichment on behavior as Hebb had reported it. Together with E.L. Bennett and colleagues, he published a large series of studies in the 1960s in which he showed manifold and dynamic changes, after environmental enrichment, in numerous measures describing the brain (Bennett, 1976; Rosenzweig and Bennett, 1996; Rosenzweig, 2003). Most notably, they made the conceptual link between "activity," or experience, and gross alterations in brain structure. They showed that environmental enrichment profoundly influences the anatomy and physiology of the brain.

Even the question was asked whether environmental enrichment could influence the amount of brain cell, neurons, and glia. One of the early studies by Joseph Altman, who later was the first to describe adult neurogenesis, addressed the question of whether environmental enrichment could stimulate the production of new neurons in the adult brain (Altman and Das, 1964). He and later others (Diamond et al., 1966) reported more glia in some brain regions, but no increased neuronal numbers. The question was timely and important, but the methods of that time did not allow reliable quantification as the basis of discovering a significant increase in cell numbers. Adult neurogenesis itself had not even been described.

An enriched environment is "the complex combination of social and inanimate stimulation" (Rosenzweig and Bennett, 1996) and usually consists of a large group of animals living in a large cage with toys and exchangeable tunnels, bridges, and other equipment. These mice are compared with animals living under the usual, rather spartan conditions of laboratory housing. This simple manipulation has far-reaching effects on the brain and its function. Because of the special laboratory situation, however, it has often been claimed that enriched environments do not really reflect "enrichment" but actually bring "impoverished" animals back to normal (Cummins et al., 1977). Although there is some truth to this critique, for research rodents, laboratory caging has become the "natural" habitat for hundreds of generations. They do not survive when left out in the wild, and there is good evidence that they experience enrichment as rather stressful and the regulatory cages as normal. Besides this qualification, in addressing the many questions about learning, the differences that can be seen between enriched and control animals are much more important than determining how the finding relates to feral conditions. The most important general conclusion to be drawn from this wealth of studies is that activity can regulate many aspects of neuronal development and function in the adult brain. The magnitude of the effect and its detailed relationship to specific stimuli or stressors are important but secondary to the result that such regulation is occurring at all. Related to the experimental paradigm of environmental enrichment are studies on voluntary physical activity, another paradigm with numerous and impressive effects on the brain. Here the findings from active rodents compared to those from animals in standard cages might intuitively seem more directly applicable to the situation of modern humans with their sedentary lifestyle.

The effects of environmental enrichment and physical activity on brain morphology and function have shown that the brain is not static and its development is never finished. There is a large body of literature (not reviewed here) on the structural reorganization after brain lesions. Many clinical observations confirm this idea (Wilson et al., 2002; Colcombe et al., 2004). The studies of animals in enriched environments delivered the systems and behavioral framework for research on synaptic and cellular plasticity. Adult neurogenesis and its activity- and experience-dependent regulation is therefore not an island of plasticity in a sea of static connections. Rather, adult neurogenesis fits seamlessly into a larger vision of the brain as an ever-changing structure that is constantly developing and refining its structure in response to functional demands.

THE HISTORY OF RESEARCH ON ADULT NEUROGENESIS

Prehistory

A study reported in 1912 by Ezra Allen from McGill University is considered to be the first account of cell divisions in the adult rodent brain. Allen showed mitotic figures in the wall of the lateral ventricles of albino rats up to 120 days of age and depicted the germinal and mantle layers (roughly corresponding to ventricular and subventricular zones) of the ventricular wall at up to 2 years of age (Fig. 2–2) (Allen, 1912).

An extensive characterization of the ventricular wall during late human embryonic development came from Swedish pathologist Erik Rydberg in 1932. He adhered to the prevailing concept of the time and described spongioblasts and germinal cells as well as "migratory spongioblasts," which were thought to produce oligodendrocytes or even to be bipotent and generate oligodendrocytes and astrocytes. His book is a neuropathological account of birth defects. From today's perspective it is amazing to see how elaborate the descriptive approach to brain anatomy and pathology and thus to neurobiology of the time had become. The 1930s were a turning point in that the classical neuroanatomic studies of, for example, Korbinian Brodman, Oskar Vogt, and their contemporaries had reached their limits. On the level of what was accessible by the mid 1930s, the brain had essentially been charted. There were nevertheless still many gaps in descriptions of the germinative zones of the adult brain.

In John Kershman's (1938) work on Schaper's "medulloblast and the medulloblastoma," Kershman introduced the term *subependymal layer* for the cell layers immediately below the *ependymal zone*. Work by Globus and Kuhlenbeck (1944) indicated that the human subependyma persisted into adult life and might be the occasional origin of tumors (the entity of subependymomas is indeed recognized by the modern World Health Organization classification of brain tumors). The hippocampus as a germinative zone of the adult brain, however, had gone completely unnoticed and did not enter the picture until work by Joseph Altman in 1963.

Revision of Nomenclature by the Boulder Committee

In 1970 a committee of 11 distinguished neuroscientists, called the "Boulder Committee" after their meeting place in Boulder, Colorado, published a consensus declaration for a revised nomenclature of the ventricular wall

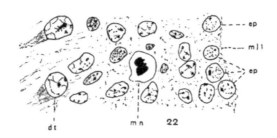

Figure 2–2. Dividing cell in the adult rodent subependymal layer. The first known depiction of cell divisions in the wall of the lateral ventricles is found in the work of Ezra Allen (1912) and shows mitotic figures in the subependymal layer of a 120-day-old rat.

in the embryonic central nervous system (Boulder Committee, 1970). This nomenclature replaced the original nomenclature of His (1889, 1904) and its many modifications over the past 80 years. The description by the Boulder Committee contains an interesting paragraph summarizing the state of knowledge at the beginning of the 1970s:

> No basis exists today for assigning more specific names to cells of the innermost two zones than is indicated by the terms *ventricular cell* and *subventricular cell*. All ventricular cells are identical in structure and behavior by every available criterion, though it is quite possible that different clones will be shown to exist among them. Subventricular cells fall into two classes based on cell size and nuclear morphology; cells of both classes proliferate and the possible relationships remain to be worked out.

The Boulder Committee thus canonized the term *subventricular zone* (SVZ) as we know it today and recognized different populations of dividing (precursor) cells in the SVZ. They did not explicitly apply this knowledge to the situation in the adult, although they referred to the older studies mentioned above that had suggested the persistence of a germinative matrix into adulthood.

From Descriptive Anatomy to Biological Experiments

The first study in which dividing cells were not only identified by the presence of mitotic figures but actively labeled came from Messier, Leblond, and Smart, also at McGill. They used tritiated thymidine that was incorporated into the DNA of dividing cells and detected by autoradiography. They reported that "in the cerebrum, reactions were most frequent in clusters of cells underlying the ependyma of the lateral ventricle." Labeled cells were also found in other brain regions, for example, as satellite cells of neurons, and the question was raised of whether occasional neurons that showed the label were in fact dividing (Messier et al., 1958).

In 1959 William Bryans used colchicine injections to arrest mitoses and thereby increase the likelihood of finding them in the adult brain. He was able to confirm earlier reports and concluded that "it is conceivable that division of cells within the sub-ependymal region may represent a continuous source of glia in the adult rat" (Bryans, 1959).

In a number of studies Smart continued the work with tritiated thymidine and in 1961 published the first extensive survey on DNA synthesis in the adult mouse brain, concluding that glial cells might divide throughout the parenchyma (Smart and Leblond, 1961). Smart also studied the subependymal layer of 35-day-old mice in greater detail and saw DNA synthesis and mitotic figures. He estimated the number of newly generated cells and wondered whether cell death might balance this production of cells. He reported that "the number of pycnotic nuclei correspond with the number of metaphases" and concluded that "in any case, the evidence was that subependymal cells do not add a significant number of new cells to the cell population of the adult brain" (Smart, 1961).

Leblond and Smart clearly had the methods to find adult neurogenesis. But no new neurons arise in the subependymal layer of the ventricular wall and consequently they could not find them there. They underestimated cell migration away from the site of cell division and did not study the olfactory bulb. Similarly, their reports do not mention DNA synthesis and mitoses as signs of cell proliferation in the hippocampus.

Joseph Altman

Despite the fact that essentially all previous evidence hinting at the possibility of adult neurogenesis was obtained in the SVZ, adult neurogenesis was first discovered in the hippocampus by Joseph Altman. Altman deserves credit for a remarkably complete and insightful initial description.

In 1962, Joseph Altman was a scientist in the Psychophysiological Laboratory at Massachusetts Institute of Technology. He applied the tritiated thymidine method to study cell divisions (DNA synthesis) in the adult brain. The initial results were interesting but far from clear. In 1962, Altman injected tritiated thymidine directly into the brain and found H3-thymidine incorporation into glial cells primarily around the lesion site. These cells survived up to 2 months after the injury (Altman, 1962b).

Altman had no bias for the SVZ. Like Messier and Leblond, he found occasional labeling in parenchymal cells along with the morphology of neurons. Could these indeed be neurons? In 1962 he published an article in *Science*, asking, "Are new neurons formed in the brains of adult mammals?" Remarkably, for an article published in *Science*, his answer was only, perhaps. Altman wrote that the absence of mitoses in the adult neurons "does not definitely rule out neogenesis of neurons in the adult, for new neurons might arise from non-differentiated precursors such as ependymal cells" (Altman, 1962a). He went on to describe the following: "In addition to the numerous labeled glia cells, which presumably underwent proliferation in response to the lesions, a few labeled glia cells, some labeled neuroblasts, and also labeled nuclei of some neurons were observed in brain regions not necessarily associated with the lesion area." An example of a labeled neuron shown in the article might look suspiciously like a satellite cell (see Chapter 7), and the term *neuroblast* in this context is rather elusive. But the study introduced the appropriate methods, asked the right questions, and proposed a clear idea that precursor cells might generate new neurons. Despite the provocative title, the 1962 *Science* article did not contain proof of adult neurogenesis and today appears as a remarkable indication of the things to come.

The next big step was a study published in 1963 in *Anatomical Record* (Altman, 1963). Here, tritiated thymidine was given systemically to rats and cats. Again, labeled glia was found and also some possible neurons in the cortex. Most strikingly, however, "a proliferative region of granule cells was identified in the dentate gyrus of the hippocampus." Figure 2–3 is taken from this article and shows the first depiction of adult neurogenesis in history. The study also contains proliferating cells in the SVZ and their migration below the corpus callosum.

As discussed in later chapters, adult cortical neurogenesis under physiological conditions has not yet been convincingly replicated. Satellite glia and methodical factors might account for these false-positive results. However, Altman recognized the problem of satellite cells and reported labeled cortical cells that he thought were unambiguously neurons with no satellite cells identifiable. It is probably understandable that this claim was not

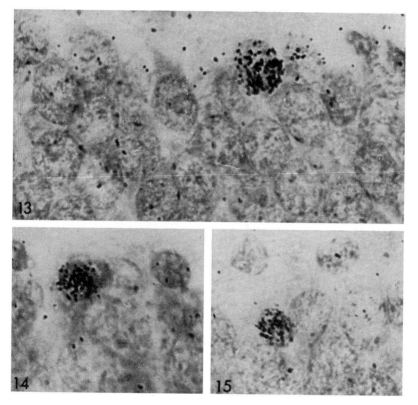

Figure 2–3. Altman's first image of an adult-generated neuron. Joseph Altman used tritiated thymidine to label proliferating cells and visualized the incorporation by autoradiography. In 1963 he published a study (from which this image is taken) providing the first known depiction of adult neurogenesis (Altman, 1963). The picture shows grains from the blackened photoemulsion over hippocampal granule cells in an adult rat. Similar images and a wealth of related data are found in second study done 2 years later, which is generally taken as the first report on adult neurogenesis (Altman and Das, 1965a). Reprinted with kind permission of Joseph Altman and the publisher.

unanimously accepted. The convincing power of a few autoradiographic grains was not great enough. That neurogenesis appeared to be a rather widespread phenomenon in the adult brain directly contradicted the preceding work by Smart, Leblond and Messier, and this discrepancy certainly did not help acceptance of the work.

Although the 1963 study contained the first images of a newly generated granule cells, Altman's 1965 study published in the *Journal of Comparative Neurology*, "Autoradiographic and Histological Evidence of Postnatal Neurogenesis in Rats," is widely considered to be the inaugural article of the field of adult neurogenesis (Altman and Das, 1965a). The co-author of this fundamental paper was Gopal D. Das. It is a remarkably complete study that did not stop with the mere demonstration of tritiated thymidine in granule cells. The pictorial evidence of adult hippocampal neurogenesis is similar to that in the 1963 study. Altman and Das showed that neurogenesis was restricted to the granule cell layer and that no new neurons were found in the hilus and the CA fields. They also reported that new cells survived at least 2 months after labeling, that neurogenesis showed a steep age-dependent decline with very high levels early postnatally, and that adult hippocampal neurogenesis could be detected at least up to an age of 8 months in the rat. In addition to the labeled granule cells they also found smaller labeled cells with dark nuclei and hypothesized that these cells might be the local precursor cell population. One strength of this study was that it sought evidence of neuronal development and did not deliver a mere snapshot in time. Another strength was that adult neurogenesis was demonstrated with a second method that was independent of the use of tritiated thymidine. The second half of the article gave a careful analysis of changes in the anatomy of the dentate gyrus over time and the changes in its cellular composition. Here, Altman and Das showed that postnatal and adult hippocampal neurogenesis caused a sixfold increase in the number of granule cells between 6 days after birth and the age of 3 months. They found that the decrease in the number of undifferentiated cells in the granule cell layer gradually gave way to increasing numbers of neurons. This independent confirmation based on absolute cell counts set the study apart from the earlier and most of the later studies. It also made the evidence for neurogenesis in the adult hippocampus considerably stronger than that in the case of supposed signs of adult cortical neurogenesis.

In addition to the data on hippocampal neurogenesis, the 1965 article also contained more information on cell proliferation in the subependymal zone. Here a strong decrease in labeled cells was observed over time after the injection of tritiated thymidine. The authors concluded "these facts would suggest a high rate of cell proliferation in adult rats in this region and the migration of labeled cells to as yet undetermined in regions." In a second 1965 study, the authors published first evidence that cells postnatally generated in the subependymal zone would migrate to the olfactory bulb and mature into neurons there (Altman and Das, 1965b). In 1969, Altman was the first to describe in detail the "rostral migratory stream," the route of migration between the SVZ and olfactory bulb (Altman, 1969).

In summary, the first report on adult hippocampal neurogenesis was an unusual piece of scientific work. Its true value could only be recognized much later, but even for its time the evidence for adult neurogenesis seemed to be strong. With today's knowledge it is amazing to see how many important questions were asked and answered in this first study. One would think that these arguments in favor of adult neurogenesis would be hard to argue against, even at the time they were published. But despite all this evidence, adult neurogenesis was not accepted for almost another 30 years (Gross, 2000).

Although not all of Altman's initial observations on adult neurogenesis have been replicated by others, the core set of data has been confirmed. Some possible reasons for the striking lack of acceptance of Altman's discovery were mentioned in Chapter 1. For Altman the response from the scientific community, characterized by Fernando Nottebohm (2002) as "stiff resistance," turned into an unfortunate mix of justifiable skepticism and valid critique on the one hand and ignorance and sometimes even outright hostility on the other. This part of the history of research on adult neurogenesis remains to be investigated. Although Altman made many more important contributions to research on brain development, he stopped publishing on adult neurogenesis in the 1970s. His wife, Shirley Bayer, however, published a number of reports that built on the initial observations and, for example, described the net growth of the rodent dentate gyrus (Bayer et al., 1982; Bayer, 1985).

Michael Kaplan

It took another 15 years until another researcher took up studies on adult neurogenesis with the same dedication as Altman's. Michael Kaplan published an extensive series of studies on adult neurogenesis in the hippocampus, the olfactory bulb, and the cortex, most notably the visual cortex. Kaplan's great contribution was the use of electron microscopy to prove the neuronal nature of cells labeled with tritiated thymidine. His most important study, published together with James Hinds in 1977, showed adult neurogenesis in the hippocampus and the olfactory bulb of 3-month-old rats. In his electron-microscropic investigations, Kaplan described microtubules in long processes, synapses, and the characteristic karyoplasm of the labeled granule cells. In 1984 Kaplan identified the proliferative "neuroblast" in the subgranular zone and found that, a few hours after labeling with radioactive thymidine, these cells had somatic synapses and small neurites (Kaplan and Bell, 1984). Despite the terminology *neuroblast*, however, what Kaplan seemed to suggest were dividing neurons. In the absence of stem cells in the adult brain and consequently a clear concept of neuroblasts in adulthood, his assumption was not greeted with much enthusiasm and support. Kaplan also published a careful and extensive characterization of neurogenesis in the olfactory bulb, demonstrating the long-term survival off newly generated neurons (Kaplan et al., 1985).

In 1983 Kaplan used tritiated thymidine to label dividing cells in the subependymal layer of an almost 5-year-old rhesus monkey, but had to conclude that the cells incorporated only minute amounts of radioactivity (Kaplan, 1983).

Kaplan's greatest interest, however, was in neurogenesis in the visual cortex. As an undergraduate he investigated the effects of environmental enrichment on cell generation in the adult rat and found layer IV neurons labeled. Although the study was never published, Kaplan later gave an account of it in a 2001 article on the current paradigm shift in neurogenesis research. Kaplan also did a study giving electron-microscopic evidence of neurogenesis in the visual cortex of adult rats (Kaplan, 1981). The evidence was perhaps not as strong as in the case of hippocampus and olfactory bulb, because the cells have a less distinctive morphology, but this alone could not explain the discrepancy with the extensive studies published by Pasko Rakic on cell genesis in the adult monkey cortex. Rakic found no evidence of neurogenesis in the adult monkey brain, as reflected in the title of his 1985 article, "Limits of Neurogenesis in the Adult Primate." Many later studies by other groups also could not confirm the existence of adult cortical neurogenesis (Kornack and Rakic, 2001a; Ehninger and Kempermann, 2003; Koketsu et al., 2003).

In hindsight, Kaplan might have detected the dividing parenchymal precursor cells in the non-neurogenic regions of the adult brain, many of which express the proteoglycan NG2 (see Chapter 8) and show both glial and some immature neuronal features. They often have a stellate or bipolar appearance. Synapses have not yet been reported on them, but the characterization of this peculiar cell population is still in flux. In the electron-microscopic image, Kaplan might thus have detected neuronal features on a cell that light microscopically does not appear truly neuronal and according to current knowledge does not qualify as a functioning neuron. He would have been both right and wrong at the same time. The existence of a tissue precursor cell showing both glial and neuronal characteristics was clearly beyond the reach of that time.

Kaplan left the field of neurogenesis disappointed. Justified skepticism toward his data from cortex seems to have spoiled the recognition of his achievements in research on adult neurogenesis in the hippocampus and olfactory bulb. Kaplan felt marginalized and excluded. Thus he became "both excited and jealous" (Kaplan, 2001) when, in 1998, Peter Erickssson published his report on neurogenesis in the adult human brain (Eriksson et al., 1998). Kaplan claims to have suggested a similar project to the ethics community of his university in 1982 but he could not carry it out (Kaplan, 2001). Because he had intended to use radioactively labeled thymidine in brain cancer patients and did not have the immunohistochemical and microscopic tools of the Ericksson study, success would have been questionable and the data would likely have remained controversial. His idea counts nonetheless, and reflects the many innovative lines along which Kaplan thought to increase knowledge about adult neurogenesis.

Fernando Nottebohm

The next major step in research on adult neurogenesis was taken in 1983 with Fernando Nottebohm's work on neuronal replacement in the brains of songbirds. In canaries the males have elaborated and complex song repertoires, whereas the females sing much less. Treatment with testosterone, however, increases the females' singing (Nottebohm, 1980). In the 1970s it was found that gender difference in song behavior paralleled sexually dimorphic anatomy. Some of the nuclei of the canary song system are much larger in males than in females. When females receive testosterone, their altered singing behavior is associated with a growth of certain nuclei in the song system, including the archistriatum and the high vocal center (HVC) (Nottebohm, 1980). In males, these same nuclei grow and shrink during the course of the year, with their volume correlating with the seasons in which the birds depend on their singing (Nottebohm, 1981). In the spring, with the beginning of the breeding season and when the birds learn their songs, the volume of the HVC is largest. Nottebohm first assumed that these changes were due to fluctuations in the neuropil and primarily reflected synaptic growth and pruning. But was this sufficient to explain the large volume changes? Nottebohm applied the method of birthmarking dividing cells with tritiated thymidine and discovered a large number of labeled cells of neuronal appearance in the HVC (Goldman and Nottebohm, 1983). Somewhat against the initial hypothesis, however, was the finding that the ratio of labeled cells among the neurons of the HVC was the same for males and females. Nottebohm and his colleague Steven Goldman reasoned that these marked neurons might reflect a neuronal turnover.

Like Altman and Kaplan, Nottebohm first used microscopic techniques to identify labeled neurons. With electon microscopy, synapses were detected on labeled neurons (Burd and Nottebohm, 1985). The breakthrough experiment, however, was a truly revolutionary functional study and probably marked the turning point in the acceptance of adult neurogenesis by a wider audience. In canaries treated with tritiated thymidine 4 weeks earlier, random electrophysiologic recordings were made in the HVC. The chance of hitting a labeled cell was about 1 in 10. After recording, the cells were filled with horseradish peroxidase, which could be detected histochemically after autoradiography for the radioactive thymidine. Indeed, about 10% of the filled cells were marked with silver grains and thus identified as new (Paton and Nottebohm, 1984). Nottebohm later wrote, "I believe this experiment, combining autoradiography, fine anatomical description, and neurophysiological recordings established the credibility of past and

future claims that new neurons continued to be added to the adult vertebrate brain" (Nottebohm, 2002).

In adult birds neurogenesis occurs throughout the telencephalon and is
not restricted to a few neurogenic zones as in mammals. Like in mammals,
however, cell proliferation in the adult avian brain is largely concentrated
on the walls of the ventricles. Here, a great number of radial glia-like cells
were found whose long processes projected into the gray matter and provided
a guidance structure along which the new neurons could migrate (Alvarez-
Buylla et al., 1987; Alvarez-Buylla and Nottebohm, 1988). Arturo Alvarez-
Buylla, who later applied these insights from the avian brain to mammalian
neurogenic regions, found that the radial glial cells even divided asymmetrically, with their long process remaining in place (Alvarez-Buylla et al., 1990).
Strikingly, the HVC is not penetrated by radial fibers, leaving open the possibility that another population of precursor cells causes the production of
the projection neurons in this region.

Thus, by 1990 the work on songbirds had not only shown activity-
dependent regulation of adult neurogenesis and functional integration of
new neurons but also prepared the groundwork for studies on the identity
(and possible heterogeneity) of precursor cells in the adult brain.

Neurogenesis in the Adult Hippocampus

The third rediscovery of adult hippocampal neurogenesis (after Altman's
and Kaplan's) was made by Heather Cameron and Elizabeth Gould, working with Bruce McEwen at Rockefeller University in New York (Gould et al.,
1992; Cameron et al., 1993). These researchers were interested in the effects
of stress and the accompanying hormonal changes on the brain (Gould
et al., 1991). They wondered why the dentate gyrus did not seem to be sensitive to stress-induced cell death as found in other hippocampal regions.
In line with Altman's observations and the findings of Nottebohm and coworkers, they hypothesized that adult hippocampal neurogenesis might
result in regeneration of the dentate gyrus, balancing the amount of cell
death. They combined the classical thymidine method with immunohistochemistry for neuronal marker neuron-specific enolase (NSE), thereby
applying a straightforward double-labeling method (Cameron et al., 1993).
Adult hippocampal neurogenesis was confirmed by the new method. In the
following years, the group published a series of studies on the negative
regulation of adult hippocampal neurogenesis by stress and increased corticosterone levels. In contrast to the initial idea, stress, with its detrimental
consequences for some hippocampal neuronal populations, also decreased
adult neurogenesis and did not induce regenerative neurogenesis. Adrenalectomy and thus the removal of all stress hormones caused adult neurogenesis to increase (Cameron and Gould, 1994). The advance was thus not
only methodical, it also included the demonstration that adult hippocampal

neurogenesis in mammals could be regulated, albeit in these cases mainly down-regulated. These studies coincided with the discovery of neural precursor cells in adult mammals (Reynolds and Weiss, 1992), providing a broader conceptual basis for the acceptance of adult neurogenesis.

Two more methodical milestones brought the field to where it is today. Modifying a method developed by Gratzner in 1982 and first applied to adult olfactory neurogenesis by Frank Corotto and colleagues in 1993 (see below), Georg Kuhn, working with Fred H. Gage at the University of California and later the Salk Institute in La Jolla in 1996, replaced tritiated thymidine with the immunohistochemically detectable thymidine analog bromodeoxyuridine (BrdU) to label proliferating cells in the adult hippocampus and used confocal microscopy and double- and triple-labeling paradigms to investigate the newly born cells. The facilitated identification of new neurons also made quantification more reliable and feasible and prepared the ground for many later studies on the regulation of adult neurogenesis (Kuhn et al., 1996). In 2001, Henriette van Praag and coworkers, also at Fred H. Gage's laboratory, used a retrovirus labeled with the green fluorescent protein (GFP) to visualize newly generated cells in living tissue slices and were thus able to confirm that newborn neurons in the adult rodent hippocampus become functional granule cells (van Praag et al., 2002).

In addition, the late 1990s saw a series of publications in which adult neurogenesis climbed up the evolutionary ladder and was first described in primates (Gould et al., 1997, 1999; Kornack and Rakic, 1999). The work in nonhuman primates was followed in 1998 by Peter Eriksson's and Fred H. Gage's study showing evidence of adult hippocampal neurogenesis in humans (Eriksson et al., 1998) (Fig. 2–4, Color Plate 2).

Neurogenesis in the Adult Olfactory Bulb

Parallel to Cameron and Gould's work on adult hippocampal neurogenesis were two independent rediscoveries of neurogenesis in the adult olfactory bulb (Corotto et al., 1993; Luskin, 1993). At the University of Missouri at Columbia Frank Corotto and Joel Maruniak, were the first to use the BrdU method, albeit without confocal microscopy, to show that proliferating cells from the SVZ migrated into the olfactory bulb, where they expressed NSE and Calretinin (Corotto et al., 1993). Marla Luskin, from Emory University, used a retrovirus carrying the β-galactosidase gene to mark the progeny of proliferative precursor cells in the SVZ and reported how the cells use a narrow migratory pathway to reach the olfactory bulb, where they differentiate into two types of interneurons (Luskin, 1993). Using a similar method, Steven Levison and James Goldman at Columbia University showed that SVZ precursor cells postnatally also give rise to astrocytes and oligodendrocytes in striatum and cortex (Levison and Goldman, 1993). Also in

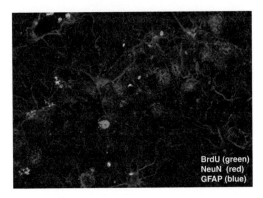

BrdU (green)
NeuN (red)
GFAP (blue)

Figure 2–4 (Color Plate 2). Neurogenesis in the adult human hippocampus. Peter Eriksson, neurologist in Gothenbury, Sweden, identified terminally ill patients who had received injections of bromodeoxyuridine (BrdU) for tumor staging purposes. He received their informed consent and after their death was able to examine their brains. He applied the same histologic methods that are routinely used to visualize adult neurogenesis in rodents. The confocal micro-scopic image shows the human dentate gyrus; BrdU is green, NeuN is red, as-trocytic marker GFAP is blue. One granule cell is double-labeled for BrdU and NeuN and thereby identified as a new neuron (compare with Fig. 1–1). Re-printed from Eriksson et al. (1998), with permission of the authors and *Nature Medicine*.

1993, Carlos Lois and Arturo Alvarez-Buylla of Rockefelleer University reported the neurogenic potential of SVZ precursor cells in explant cultures, directly linking adult neurogenesis with stem cell biology (Lois and Alvarez-Buylla, 1993). The same authors published their account of olfactory bulb neurogenesis in vivo in 1994 and in the following years went on to charac-terize the migration of the precursor cells. They identified the particular mechanism of *chain migration* by which the newborn cells move along each other in the rostral migratory stream to reach the olfactory bulb (Lois et al., 1996). Since then, Alaverez-Buylla and Fiona Doetsch have characterized the microanatomical structure of the SVZ and identified the different pre-cursor cell types in this region (Doetsch et al., 1997, 1999, 2002).

Neurogenesis in the adult primate olfactory bulb was first demonstrated by David Kornack and Pasko Rakic of Yale University (Kornack and Rakic, 2001b). A direct demonstration for the human brain is still lacking, although some indirect evidence has been reported (Bedard and Parent, 2004). In specimens from adult human brain, however, a structure of the SVZ was found that clearly differed from that of other mammals and no signs of chain migration into the olfactory bulb were seen (Sanai et al., 2004). Neurogenesis in the adult olfactory bulb might thus be either completely absent in hu-mans (or at least be very rare) or originate from precursor cells residing in the olfactory bulb.

REFERENCES

Allen E (1912) The cessation of mitosis in the central nervous system of the albino rat. J Comp Neurol 22:547–568.

Altman J (1962a) Are new neurons formed in the brains of adult mammals? Science 135:1128–1129.

Altman J (1962b) Autoradiographic study of degenerative and regenerative proliferation of neuroglia cells with tritiated thymidine. Exp Neurol 5:302–318.

Altman J (1963) Autoradiographic investigation of cell proliferation in the brains of rats and cats. Anat Rec 145:573–591.

Altman J (1969) Autoradiographic and histological studies of postnatal neurogenesis. IV. Cell proliferation and migration in the anterior forebrain, with special reference to persisting neurogenesis in the olfactory bulb. J Comp Neurol 137:433–457.

Altman J, Das GD (1964) Autoradiographic examination of the effects of enriched environment on the rate of glial muliplication in the adult rat brain. Nature 204:1161–1163.

Altman J, Das GD (1965a) Autoradiographic and histologic evidence of postnatal neurogenesis in rats. J Comp Neurol 124:319–335.

Altman J, Das GD (1965b) Post-natal origin of microneurons in the rat brain. Nature 207:953–956.

Altmann (1881) Über Embryonales Wachstum. Leipzig.

Alvarez-Buylla A, Buskirk DR, Nottebohm F (1987) Monoclonal antibody reveals radial glia in adult avian brain. J Comp Neurol 264:159–170.

Alvarez-Buylla A, Nottebohm F (1988) Migration of young neurons in adult avian brain. Nature 335:353–354.

Alvarez-Buylla A, Theelen M, Nottebohm F (1990) Proliferation "hot spots" in adult avian ventricular zone reveal radial cell division. Neuron 5:101–109.

Anderson DJ (2001) Stem cells and pattern formation in the nervous system: the possible versus the actual. Neuron 30:19–35.

Bayer SA (1985) Neuron production in the hippocampus and olfactory bulb of the adult rat brain: addition or replacement? Ann NY Acad Sci 457:163–172.

Bayer SA, Yackel JW, Puri PS (1982) Neurons in the rat dentate gyrus granular layer substantially increase during juvenile and adult life. Science 216:890–892.

Bedard A, Parent A (2004) Evidence of newly generated neurons in the human olfactory bulb. Brain Res Dev Brain Res 151:159–168.

Belachew S, Chittajallu R, Aguirre AA, Yuan X, Kirby M, Anderson S, Gallo V (2003) Postnatal NG2 proteoglycan-expressing progenitor cells are intrinsically multipotent and generate functional neurons. J Cell Biol 161:169–186.

Bennett EL (1976) Cerebral effects of differential experience and training. In: Neural Mechanisms of Learning and Memory (Rosenzweig MR, Bennett EL, eds), pp 279–287. Cambridge, MA: MIT Press.

Bliss TV, Lomo T (1973) Long-lasting potentiation of synaptic transmission in the dentate area of the anaesthetized rabbit following stimulation of the perforant path. J Physiol 232:331–356.

Boulder Committee (1970) Embryonic vertebrate central nervous system: revised terminology. The Boulder Committee. Anat Rec 166:257–261.

Bryans WA (1959) Mitotic activity in the brain of the adult rat. Anat Rec 133:65–71.

Burd GD, Nottebohm F (1985) Ultrastructural characterization of synaptic terminals formed on newly generated neurons in a song control nucleus of the adult canary forebrain. J Comp Neurol 240:143–152.

Cameron HA, Gould E (1994) Adult neurogenesis is regulated by adrenal steroids in the dentate gyrus. Neuroscience 61:203–209.

Cameron HA, Woolley CS, McEwen BS, Gould E (1993) Differentiation of newly born neurons and glia in the dentate gyrus of the adult rat. Neuroscience 56:337–344.

Colcombe SJ, Kramer AF, Erickson KI, Scalf P, McAuley E, Cohen NJ, Webb A, Jerome GJ, Marquez DX, Elavsky S (2004) Cardiovascular fitness, cortical plasticity, and aging. Proc Natl Acad Sci USA 101:3316–3321.

Cole RJ, Edwards RG, Paul J (1966) Cytodifferentiation and embryogenesis in cell colonies and tissue cultures derived from ova and blastocysts of the rabbit. Dev Biol 13:385–407.

Corotto FS, Henegar JA, Maruniak JA (1993) Neurogenesis persists in the subependymal layer of the adult mouse brain. Neurosci Lett 149:111–114.

Cummins RA, Livesey PJ, Evans JG (1977) A developmental theory of environmental enrichment. Science 197:692–694.

Diamond MC, Law F, Rhodes H, Lindner B, Rosenzweig MR, Krech D, Bennett EL (1966) Increases in cortical depth and glia numbers in rats subjected to enriched environment. J Comp Neurol 128:117–126.

Dobell C (1960) Antony van Leeuwenhoek and His "Little Animals." New York: Dover.

Doetsch F, Caille I, Lim DA, Garcia-Verdugo JM, Alvarez-Buylla A (1999) Subventricular zone astrocytes are neural stem cells in the adult mammalian brain. Cell 97:703–716.

Doetsch F, Garcia-Verdugo JM, Alvarez-Buylla A (1997) Cellular composition and three-dimensional organization of the subventricular germinal zone in the adult mammalian brain. J Neurosci 17:5046–5061.

Doetsch F, Verdugo JM, Caille I, Alvarez-Buylla A, Chao MV, Casaccia-Bonnefil P (2002) Lack of the cell-cycle inhibitor p27Kip1 results in selective increase of transit-amplifying cells for adult neurogenesis. J Neurosci 22:2255–2264.

Edwards RG (2001) IVF and the history of stem cells. Nature 413:349–351.

Ehninger D, Kempermann G (2003) Regional effects of wheel running and environmental enrichment on cell genesis and microglia proliferation in the adult murine neocortex. Cereb Cortex 13:845–851.

Ehrenberg CG (1832) Über das Entstehen des Organischen aus einfacher Materie, und über die organischen Molecüle und Atome, insbesondere als Erfahrungsgegenstände. Poggendorff's Annalen der Physik und Chemie 24:1–48.

Eriksson PS, Perfilieva E, Björk-Eriksson T, Alborn AM, Nordborg C, Peterson DA, Gage FH (1998) Neurogenesis in the adult human hippocampus. Nat Med 4:1313–1317.

Freed CR, Greene PE, Breeze RE, Tsai WY, DuMouchel W, Kao R, Dillon S, Winfield H, Culver S, Trojanowski JQ, Eidelberg D, Fahn S (2001) Transplantation of embryonic dopamine neurons for severe Parkinson's disease. N Engl J Med 344:710–719.

Freed CR, Leehey MA, Zawada M, Bjugstad K, Thompson L, Breeze RE (2003) Do patients with Parkinson's disease benefit from embryonic dopamine cell transplantation? J Neurol 250 (Suppl 3):III44–46.

Gardner RL (1968) Mouse chimeras obtained by the injection of cells into the blastocyst. Nature 220:596–597.

Globus JH, Kuhlenbeck H (1944) The subependymal cell plate (matrix) and its relationship to brain tumors of the ependymal type. J Neuropathol Exp Neurol 3:1–35.

Goldman SA, Nottebohm F (1983) Neuronal production, migration and differentiation in a vocal control nucleus of the adult female canary brain. Proc Natl Acad Sci USA 80:2390–2394.

Golgi C (1886) Sulla fina anatomia degli organi centrali des sisterna nervoso. Milan: Hoepli.

Gould E, Cameron HA, Daniels DC, Woolley CS, McEwen BS (1992) Adrenal hormones suppress cell division in the adult rat dentate gyrus. J Neurosci 12:3642–3650.

Gould E, McEwen BS, Tanapat P, Galea LAM, Fuchs E (1997) Neurogenesis in the dentate gyrus of the adult tree shrew is regulated by psychosocial stress and NMDA receptor activation. J Neurosci 17:2492–2498.

Gould E, Reeves AJ, Fallah M, Tanapat P, Gross CG, Fuchs E (1999) Hippocampal neurogenesis in adult old world primates. Proc Natl Acad Sci USA 96:5263–5267.

Gould E, Woolley CS, McEwen BS (1991) Naturally occurring cell death in the developing dentate gyrus of the rat. Comp Neurol 304:408–418.

Gourret JP (1995) Modelling the mitotic apparatus. From the discovery of the bipolar spindle to modern concepts. Acta Biotheor 43:127–142.

Gratzner HG (1982) Monoclonal antibody to 5-bromo- and 5-iododeoxyuridine: a new reagent for detection of DNA replication. Science 218:474–475.

Gross CG (2000) Neurogenesis in the adult brain: death of a dogma. Nat Rev Neurosci 1:67–73.

Hagell P, Piccini P, Bjorklund A, Brundin P, Rehncrona S, Widner H, Crabb L, Pavese N, Oertel WH, Quinn N, Brooks DJ, Lindvall O (2002) Dyskinesias following neural transplantation in Parkinson's disease. Nat Neurosci 5:627–628.

Hardesty I (1904) On the development and nature of the neuroglia. Am J Anat 3:229–268.

Hebb DO (1947) The effects of early experience on problem-solving at maturity. Am Psychol 2:306–307.

Hebb DO (1949) The Organization of Behavior: A Neurophysiological Theory. New York: John Wiley & Sons.

His W (1889) Die Neuroblasten und deren Entstehung im embryonalen Mark. Arch Anat Physiol Anat Abt :249–300.

His W (1904) Die Entwicklung des menschlichen Gehirns während der ersten Monate. p 176. Leipzig: S. Hirzel.

Hollands P (1987) Differentiation and grafting of haemopoietic stem cells from early postimplantation mouse embryos. Development 99:69–76.

Hymovitch B (1952) The effects of experimental variation on problem solving in the rat. Comp Physiol Psychol 45:313–321.

Kaplan MS (1981) Neurogenesis in the 3-month-old rat visual cortex. J Comp Neurol 195:323–338.

Kaplan MS (1983) Proliferation of subependymal cells in the adult primate CNS: differential uptake of DNA labelled precursors. J Hirnforsch 24:23–33.

Kaplan MS (2001) Environment complexity stimulates visual cortex neurogenesis: death of a dogma and a research career. Trends Neurosci 24:617–620.

Kaplan MS, Bell DH (1984) Mitotic neuroblasts in the 9-day-old and 11-month-old rodent hippocampus. J Neurosci 4:1429–1441.

Kaplan MS, Hinds JW (1977) Neurogenesis in the adult rat: electron microscopic analysis of light radioautographs. Science 197:1092–1094.

Kaplan MS, McNelly NA, Hinds JW (1985) Population dynamics of adult-formed granule neurons of the rat olfactory bulb. J Comp Neurol 239:117–125.

Kelso SR, Ganong AH, Brown TH (1986) Hebbian synapses in hippocampus. Proc Natl Acad Sci USA 83:5326–5330.

Kershman J (1938) The medulloblast and the medulloblastoma. Arch Neurol Psychiatry 40:937–967.

Kilpatrick TJ, Bartlett PF (1993) Cloning and growth of multipotential neural precursors: requirements for proliferation and differentiation. Neuron 10:255–265.

Koketsu D, Mikami A, Miyamoto Y, Hisatsune T (2003) Nonrenewal of neurons in the cerebral neocortex of adult macaque monkeys. J Neurosci 23:937–942.

Kornack DR, Rakic P (1999) Continuation of neurogenesis in the hippocampus of the macaque monkey. Proc Natl Acad Sci USA 96:5768–5773.

Kornack DR, Rakic P (2001a) Cell proliferation without neurogenesis in adult primate neocortex. Science 294:2127–2130.

Kornack DR, Rakic P (2001b) The generation, migration, and differentiation of olfactory neurons in the adult primate brain. Proc Natl Acad Sci USA 98:4752–4757.

Kuhn HG, Dickinson-Anson H, Gage FH (1996) Neurogenesis in the dentate gyrus of the adult rat: age-related decrease of neuronal progenitor proliferation. J Neurosci 16:2027–2033.

Levison SW, Goldman JE (1993) Both oligodendrocytes and astrocytes develop from progenitors in the subventricular zone of postnatal rat forebrain. Neuron 10:201–212.

Lewis PD (1968) Mitotic activity in the primate subependymal layer and the genesis of gliomas. Nature 217:974–975.

Lindvall O, Backlund EO, Farde L, Sedvall G, Freedman R, Hoffer B, Nobin A, Seiger A, Olson L (1987) Transplantation in Parkinson's disease: two cases of adrenal medullary grafts to the putamen. Ann Neurol 22:457–468.

Lois C, Alvarez-Buylla A (1993) Proliferating subventricular zone cells in the adult mammalian forebrain can differentiate into neurons and glia. Proc Natl Acad Sci USA 90:2074–2077.

Lois C, Alvarez-Buylla A (1994) Long-distance neuronal migration in the adult mammalian brain. Science 264:1145–1148.

Lois C, Garcia-Verdugo J-M, Alvarez-Buylla A (1996) Chain migration of neuronal precursors. Science 271:978–981.

Luskin MB (1993) Restricted proliferation and migration of postnatally generated neurons derived from the forebrain subventricular zone. Neuron 11:173–189.

Madrazo I, Drucker-Colin R, Diaz V, Martinez-Mata J, Torres C, Becerril JJ (1987) Open microsurgical autograft of adrenal medulla to the right caudate nucleus in two patients with intractable Parkinson's disease. N Engl J Med 316:831–834.

Markram H, Lubke J, Frotscher M, Sakmann B (1997) Regulation of synaptic efficacy by coincidence of postsynaptic APs and EPSPs. Science 275:213–215.

Mazzarello P (1999) A unifying concept: the history of cell theory. Nat Cell Biol 1:E13–15.

Merk L (1896) Die Mitosen im Centralnervensysteme. Denkschriften der königlichen Akademie der Wissenschaften, math-naturwissenschaftliche Classe 53:79–118.

Messier B, Leblond CP, Smart I (1958) Presence of DNA synthesis and mitosis in the brain of young adult mice. Exp Cell Res 14:224–226.

Nottebohm F (1980) Testosterone triggers growth of brain vocal control nuclei in adult female canaries. Brain Res 189:429–436.

Nottebohm F (1981) A brain for all seasons: cyclical anatomical changes in song control nuclei of the canary brain. Science 214:1368–1370.

Nottebohm F (2002) Neuronal replacement in adult brain. Brain Res Bull 57:737–749.

Palmer TD, Ray J, Gage FH (1995) FGF-2-responsive neuronal progenitors reside in proliferative and quiescent regions of the adult rodent brain. Mol Cell Neurosci 6:474–486.

Paton JA, Nottebohm FN (1984) Neurons generated in the adult brain are recruited into functional circuits. Science 225:1046–1048.

Penfield W (1932) Neuroglia: normal and pathological. In: Cytology and Cellular Pathology of the Nervous System (Penfield W, ed), pp 423–479. New York: Hoeber.

Rakic P (1985) Limits of neurogenesis in primates. Science 227:1054–1056.

Ramon y Cajal S (1928) Degeneration and Regeneration of the Nervous System. New York: Hafner.

Remak R (1852) Über extracelluläre Entstehung thierischer Zellen und über die Vermehrung derselben durch Theilung. Archiv für Anatomie, Physiologie und wissenschaftliche Medicin :137–176.

Remak R (1855) Untersuchungen über die Entwicklung der Wirbelthiere. Berlin: G. Reimer.

Reynolds BA, Weiss S (1992) Generation of neurons and astrocytes from isolated cells of the adult mammalian central nervous system. Science 255:1707–1710.

Rio-Hortega P (1919) El tercer elemento de los centros nerviosos. Bol Soc Esp de Biol 9:69.

Rosenzweig MR (2003) Effects of differential experience on the brain and behavior. Dev Neuropsychol 24:523–540.

Rosenzweig MR, Bennett EL (1996) Psychobiology of plasticity: effects of training and experience on brain and behavior. Behav Brain Res 78:57–65.

Rydberg E (1932) Cerebral injury in newborn children consequent to birth trauma. Acta Pathol Microbiol Scand Suppl 10:1–247.

Sagan C (1995) The Demon-Haunted World. New York: Random House.

Sanai N, Tramontin AD, Quinones-Hinojosa A, Barbaro NM, Gupta N, Kunwar S, Lawton MT, McDermott MW, Parsa AT, Manuel-Garcia Verdugo J, Berger MS, Alvarez-Buylla A (2004) Unique astrocyte ribbon in adult human brain contains neural stem cells but lacks chain migration. Nature 427:740–744.

Schaper A (1897) Die frühesten Differenzierungsvorgänge im Zentralnervensystem. Archiv für Entwicklungsmechanismen 5:81.

Schreiber L, Wengler F (1908) Über die Wirkungen des Scharlachöls auf die Netzhaut. Mitosenbildung in Ganglienzellen. Centralblatt für allgemeine Pathologie 19:529.

Schreiber L, Wengler F (1910) Über die Wirkungen des Scharlachöls auf die Netzhaut. Mitosenbildung in Ganglienzellen. Graefes Archiv für Ophthalmologie: 74.

Smart I (1961) The subependymal layer of the mouse brain and its cell production as shown by radiography after thymidine-H3 injection. Comp Neurol 116:325–347.

Smart I, Leblond CP (1961) Evidence for division and transformation of neuroglia cells in the mouse brain as derived from radioautography after injection of thymidine-H3. J Comp Neurol 116:349–367.

Spielmeyer W (1922) Histopathologie des Nervensystems. Berlin: Julius Springer.

Thomas ED (1999) Bone marrow transplantation: a review. Semin Hematol 36:95–103.

van Praag H, Schinder AF, Christie BR, Toni N, Palmer TD, Gage FH (2002) Functional neurogenesis in the adult hippocampus. Nature 415:1030–1034.

Virchow R (1846) Über das granulierte Aussehen der Wandungen der Gehirnventrikel. Allgemeine Zeitschrift für Psychiatrie 3:242–250.

Virchow R (1859) Die Cellularpathologie in ihrer Begründung auf physiologische und pathologische Gewebelehre. Berlin: Verlag von August Hirschfeld.

Watermann R (1982) Schwann's microscopic research and his cell theory. Contribution on his 100th anniversary [in Germany]. Z Mikrosk Anat Forsch 96:1032–1043.

Wilson RS, Mendes De Leon CF, Barnes LL, Schneider JA, Bienias JL, Evans DA, Bennett DA (2002) Participation in cognitively stimulating activities and risk of incident Alzheimer disease. JAMA 287:742–748.

Winsor MP (1980) Swammerdam, Jan. In: Dictionary of Scientific Biography, Vol. 13 (Gillespie C, ed), pp 168–175. New York: Scribner.

Wolpert L (1995) Evolution of cell theory. Phil Trans R Soc Lond B 349:227–233.

3

Neural Stem Cells

Adult neurogenesis originates from precursor cells in the adult brain. In this sense, neural stem cell biology is the basis of neuronal development in the adult brain. The idea that stem cells are an indispensable prerequisite of adult neurogenesis might today seem self-evident. But stem cells have only recently become household names. For decades, concepts of brain plasticity fared well without accommodating stem cells. Although early reports on adult neurogenesis pondered the thought of precursor cells giving rise to the neurons, this idea remained more or less speculation (Altman and Das, 1965; Kaplan, 1983). Adult neurogenesis largely appeared to be an exception to the rule that neurons are strictly postmitotic and should not divide. It is thus no coincidence that research on adult neurogenesis and its acceptance in the scientific community gained ground only when neural stem cells were discovered in the early 1990s (Reynolds and Weiss, 1992; Richards et al., 1992; Kilpatrick and Bartlett, 1993, 1995; Palmer et al., 1995; Ray et al., 1995). The existence of stem cells made adult neurogenesis more plausible than dividing neurons, which were hard to accept.

Historically, stem cell biology was restricted to embryology and to the biology of organs with inherent regenerative ability. The hematopoetic system is the quintessential regenerative organ, the skin and the intestines being other examples. Only with the demonstration of precursor cells in organs considered to be non-regenerating, such as the lung, the liver, and finally the heart and the brain, were stem cells viewed increasingly as a ubiquitous phenomenon in the body. Visions of exploiting the regenerative potential of these cells for new therapeutic approaches for incurable disorders made the issue of the identity and nature of stem cells pressing.

What are the different types of stem cells in the adult organism? How can they be distinguished? How do they relate to stem cells in embryogenesis? How much of what is found in one type of stem cell applies to another? Are there common rules that apply to all forms of stem cells? Is there one grand, unifying theory of stem cell biology and, if so, what consequences does this have for the different functional contexts and potential applications in which stem cells are found? How do neural stem cells fit into the greater context of stem cell biology?

Whereas in the hematopoetic system all different mature cell types originate from one single stem cell, it is not known whether the entire brain originates from one single type of neural stem cell (Fig. 3–1). Consequently, it is not known whether such a neural precursor cell of the highest potential

50

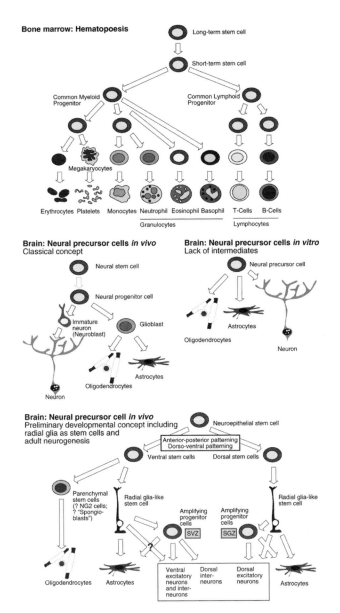

Figure 3–1. Stem cell hierarchies. In hematology, there is a detailed hierarchy of the various mature cell types and the progenitor cells from which the former are derived. Although many questions remain open, the individual cell types can be comparatively well defined by sets of key surface markers. A widely used schema of precursor cell hierarchy in the adult brain (middle left) appears to be comparatively crude. In contrast to the situation in hematology, it is not known whether the stem cell that ranks highest in the hierarchy persists in adulthood. Most in vitro systems (middle right) do not reflect the proposed situation in vivo. As discussed in this chapter, the exact lineage relationships within the precursor cell progeny of the adult brain are still undetermined. The bottom panel depicts a possible lineage relationship based on developmental criteria and involves the remaining neurogenic precursor cell populations in the adult subventricular zone (SVZ) and subgranular zone (SGZ). Compare the schema presented in this figure with the partially conflicting concepts in Figures 2–1, 3–4, 3–8, and 3–11.

persists in the adult brain (as it does in the bone marrow for the hematopoetic system).

THE CARDINAL FEATURES OF ALL STEM CELLS: SELF-RENEWAL AND MULTIPOTENCY

Neural stem cells are undifferentiated cell that divide and from which development of the nervous system (or parts of it) originates. Adult neurogenesis is thus a concrete manifestation of stem cell biology.

Stem cells are characterized by two key properties: their ability to undergo unlimited self-renewal by division and the potency to generate at least two different cell types (McKay, 1997; van der Kooy and Weiss, 2000; Weissman et al., 2001). The ability to generate a diversity of differentiated cells is called "multipotency." The term *multipotency* has a second, more restricted meaning in stem cell biology, referring to the concrete range of developmental potential of somatic, or "adult," stem cells (see below). Many researchers in the field consider the multipotency criterion unneccessary and base their definition and assessment of "stemness" solely on self-renewal. In this concept, *unipotent* stem cells can exist, giving rise to only one type of differentiated cell.

This definition is a minimal definition, but in many instances it remains unclear whether even the most basic criteria are met. Often, *stem cell* is a bona fide label whose concrete meaning and implications depend on the context. Particularly in the popular media, the term *stem cell* often represents some medical silver bullet and has thus accrued so many everyday connotations, that talking about stem cells scientifically sometimes becomes difficult. Fortunately, in most contexts the damage due to the superficial usage of *stem cells* is limited, as long as it is understood that no specific statements about these cells are made. *Stem cells* in this sense is a generic term for one cell that can "make" a complex piece of bodily tissue. This meaning is not wrong, but it is insufficient.

Self-renewal is the most important criterion of stemness and means that cell division generates at least one identical copy of the mother cell. If the division yields two identical copies, the division is called "symmetric." *Asymmetric* divisions produce one new stem cell that is identical to the mother cell and one cell that is more determined for a certain lineage of cellular differentiation than the stem cell. These daughter cells have reduced stem cell properties and are referred to as "progenitor cells."

Strictly speaking, symmetric division does not have to generate two cells identical to the mother cell. A division would still be symmetric if just the two daughter cells were identical but different from the mother cell. However, when stem cells are defined, it is implied that daughter and mother cells are identical. If a stem cell were to divide in such a way that none of the daughter cells were an identical copy of the mother cell, another mandatory criterion of stem cells would be violated: the unlimited nature of its self-renewal.

In theory, unlimited self-renewal makes stem cells eternal; in reality, however, it is difficult to prove unlimited self-renewal even for the life span of the organism. The unlimited self-renewal of stem cells is conceptually set against a limited self-renewal of the progenitor cells (Weissman et al., 2001; Seaberg and van der Kooy, 2003). Irrespective of their limited self-renewal, progenitor cells are usually more proliferative than stem cells and can vastly expand the number of new cells. They are thus referred to as "transit-amplifying" or "transiently amplifying" progenitor cells. Because self-renewal of progenitor cells is by definition not unlimited, symmetric division of progenitor cells can generate two daughter cells that are identical to each other but different from the mother cell. During brain development, precursor cells can go through a terminal symmetrical division that leads to the existence of two differentiating cells (Takahashi et al., 1996; Cai et al., 2002).

The neuroepithelial cells, the stem cells in the wall of the neural tube in embryonic development, divide symmetrically during the initial expansion phase (Fig. 3–2). They divide asymmetrically to produce neuronally determined progenitor cells in asymmetric neurogenic divisions. Such progenitor cells, detached from the surface of the ventricle, can divide symmetrically

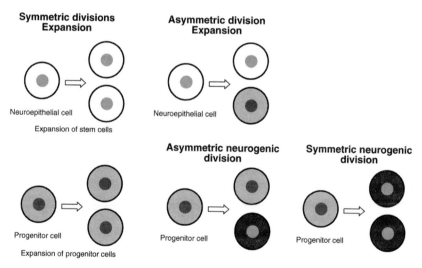

Figure 3–2. Asymmetric divisions. Asymmetric division is one hallmark of stem cells. The key criterion for stem cells is self-renewal. Every stem cell thus has to generate one new stem cell during its division. To produce differentiating progeny at the same time, asymmetric divisions have to occur. Progenitor cells are the progency of stem cells and have limited stem cell properties, most notably limited self-renewal. Symmetric division of progenitor cells can produce two daughter cells that are different from the mother cell. The schema presented here is based primarily on the work of Wieland Huttner and colleagues (Wodarz and Huttner, 2003; Kosodo et al., 2004).

into two cells that are both differentiating into neurons. This constitutes a symmetric neurogenic division (Kosodo et al., 2004). Consequently, these progenitor cells are not self-renewing and thus are not considered stem cells.

Conceptually, the distinction between stem and progenitor cells is important (Seaberg and van der Kooy, 2003), because many conclusions in stem cell biology and research on adult neurogenesis are based on the inferred properties and the assumed potential of the precursor cells. The immediate progeny of stem cells are progenitor cells, not differentiated cells. Progenitor cells in turn generate differentiated cells. Cells with different degrees of stemness (self-renewal and multipotency) can be identified in the brain (and elsewhere), but in a concrete situation it is usually not possible to categorize a cell as either a stem cell or a progenitor cell. Often the term *progenitor cell* is used as the more parsimonious label, implying that it remains undetermined whether the given cell is in fact capable of unlimited self-renewal and the potential to generate multiple cell lineages. However, to avoid confusion, the term *precursor cell* should be favored as umbrella term encompassing both stem and progenitor cells.

The second defining criterion of stem cells besides self-renewal is multipotency. The potential for differentiation into different cell types can be subdivided into a number of categories of potency, or potential (Fig. 3–3).

The fertilized egg, the zygote, is considered totipotent because it can produce an entire organism, including the trophoblast, the placenta. The zygote is thus often considered the ultimate stem cell. However, the zygote violates the stem cell definition of unlimited self-renewal because it loses its totipotency after two or three divisions. There are no totipotent cells beyond these earliest stages of development.

Further divisions lead to the morula and the blastocyst stage, which begins at approximately the 64-cell stage. A cavity forms and the wall of the little cyst thickens at one side. This local accumulation of cells is called the inner cell mass.

EMBRYONIC STEM CELLS

Embryonic stem (ES) cells are pluripotent and are found in the inner cell mass of the blastocyst. The trophoblast, from which the placenta originates, is not part of the inner cell mass but surrounds it. *Pluripotency* is consequently defined as the ability to generate cells of all body tissues, but not the trophoblast. If an ES cell is implanted into the uterus it cannot give rise to a complete new organism because it cannot generate the placenta.

The potential therapeutic use of ES cells has stirred stem cell debates in many countries. Because ES cells are pluripotent and can be propagated in vitro with relative ease, they hold great promise for regenerative medicine. They could provide a source for implantable cells in cell replacement therapies, possibly a strategy to treat incurable diseases. Another goal is to generate cell lines from human ES cells that carry specific mutations to develop

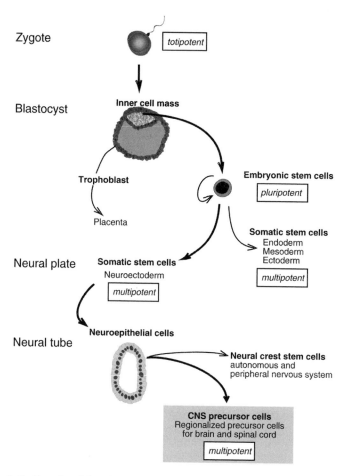

Figure 3–3. Levels of developmental potential. In the course of development, the potential of stem cells to generate different types of cells becomes increasingly restricted. Adult neurogenesis orginates from multipotent tissue-specific (or somatic) precursor cells. A few studies indicate, however, that rare more-than-multipotent cells might persist in the adult brain and bone marrow (Rietze et al., 2001; Jiang et al., 2002). These cells would be able to differentiate into cells of more than one germ layer. It is not known whether such cells play a physiological role.

better cell models of human disease. Such cell lines would be ideally suited to test new drugs and learn about disease-specific signaling mechanisms (see Chapter 12). Embryonic stem cells are not controversial because of their pluripotency, and the use of ES cells is not controversial per se; what is controversial is the use of *human* ES cells or of pluripotent cells, as long as these have to be derived from human embryos. The stem cell debate is largely not a debate over stem cells but over the ethical status of the human embryo.

In many contexts, *embryonic stem cells* and *pluripotent cells* have become synonyms, which is problematic. Whereas ES cells are pluripotent, it is not clear whether pluripotent cells are indeed only found in the embryonic inner cell mass. Some examples of more-than-multipotent cells have been reported and are discussed below (Rietze et al., 2001; Toma et al., 2001; Jiang et al., 2002).

In cell culture, neural precursor cells have been successfully generated from ES cells (Thomson et al., 1998; Brustle et al., 1999; Mujtaba et al., 1999; Lee et al., 2000; Reubinoff et al., 2000; Westmoreland et al., 2001; Zhang et al., 2001; Aubert et al., 2002). Sequential protocols have been devised that allow the development of neural cells in vitro (Castelo-Branco et al., 2003; Perrier and Studer, 2003). Upon implantation into the developing or adult brain, these precursors behave like those neural precursor cells that can be derived from later developmental stages. The implanted ES cell–derived precursor cells are able to develop into functioning neurons and glial cells. In some animal models of human disease, ES cell–based cell replacement has been promising (Brustle et al., 1999; Bjorklund et al., 2002).

Their pluripotency, however, makes ES cells challenging to use in vivo, as ES cells have a tumorigenic potential and can generate dysontogenetic tumors, teratomas, or teratocarcinomas (Langa et al., 2000; Reubinoff et al., 2000; Asano et al., 2003). These tumors are characterized by the presence of more or less differentiated cell types of all three germ layers. To exploit the neurogenic potential of ES cells for theraupeutic purposes, it is thus necessary to predifferentiate the cells and thus reduce their potential. Even minimal ES cell contamination of cell suspensions to be implanted can cause tumor growth.

Ontogenetically, ES cells precede the more specified neural precursor cells. In ES cells the neurogenic potential is only one aspect of pluripotency. Neural precursor cells are restricted in their fate choices and are categorized as multipotent.

NEURAL PRECURSOR CELLS ARE MULTIPOTENT, BIPOTENT, OR UNIPOTENT

Stem cells within each germ layer are called "multipotent." Because neural stem cells are part of the neuroectoderm, they are by definition multipotent. The use of the term *multipotent* in this context is more concrete and restricted than when the same term is used to describe the principle that stem cells by definition can produce mature cells of two or more lineages (multipotency).

In many, especially popular, contexts, the terms *adult stem cells* and *somatic stem cells* are used synonymously for multipotent stem cells, which are in contrast to the pluripotent ES cells. In this sense, *adult* stem cells can be derived from an embryo, a fetus, or early postnatally. In contrast, in the scientific literature, *adult* stem cells normally implies that the cells in question are found in or isolated from the organism after general development has ceased.

Matters have become further complicated by the identification of adult precursor cells that seem to take a position between multipotency and pluripotency (see below; Rietze et al., 2001; Toma et al., 2001; Jiang et al., 2002). These cells are rare and thus far have only been identified in cell culture and after many passages. Apparently, they can generate differentiating cells across the limits of one germ layer. It is not known whether this makes them fully pluripotent in the sense in which embryonic stem cells are pluripotent.

For most purposes, it is sufficient to distinguish between the three levels of totipotency, pluripotency, and multipotency (Table 3–1). Within the realm of adult neurogenesis (and with the possible exception mentioned above) we only encounter multipotent precursor cells (Table 3–2). These cells could be stem or progenitor cells with respect to their degree of self-renewal and multipotency, but their exact identity in a specific situation is often not known.

Hierarchically below the multipotent cells we find more limited precursor cells that can generate only two cell lineages or even only one. These are referred to as "bipotent" and "unipotent." *Unipotent* progenitor cells are cells that can expand the population of immediate precursors of differentiated cells, the last proliferative stage before differentiation and a postmitotic stage is reached. Unipotent progenitor cells are sometimes called "blasts," but this term, widely used in the hematopoetic system, remains ambiguous in the context neural stem cells.

NEURAL STEM CELLS IN THE DEVELOPING BRAIN

Adult neurogenesis is neuronal development under the conditions of the adult brain. Therefore, adult neurogenesis is a function of both immanent

Table 3–1. Classification of Stem and Progenitor Cells

	Precursor Cells	
	Stem Cells	Progenitor Cells
Self-renewal	Unlimited	Limited
Symmetric division	Yield two identical stem cells	Yield either two identical progenitor cells *or* two identical cells that differ from the progenitor cell
Developmental potential (degree of multipotency)	Totipotent (fertilized egg only) *or* Pluripotent (prime example: embryonic stem cells) or Multipotent (tissue-specific stem cells)	Multipotent Bipotent Unipotent ("blast"; no multipotency)

Table 3–2. Different Precursor Cells and Their Degree of Multipotency

Degree of Potency	Example	Source of	In the Brain
Totipotent	Only fertilized egg (zygote)	Entire individual	n/a
Pluripotent	Embryonic stem cell	All body tissues	n/a
	Hypothetically more-than-multipotent cells in embryonic, fetal, and adult tissues	Many, potentially all body tissues	?
Multipotent	Tissue-specific stem or progenitor cells	Cells of one germ blade or less	Neurons, astrocytes, and oligodendrocytes
Bipotent	Tissue-specific stem or progenitor cells	Two types of differentiated cells via dividing intermediates	Region-specific neurons and astrocytes, possibly astrocytes and oligodendrocytes
Unipotent	Lineage-determined progenitor cell	Single types of differentiated cells without further dividing intermediates	Proliferative direct precursor of single types of neurons or glial cells

Stem cells

Progenitor cells

n/a, not applicable.

(stem) cell properties and their interaction with a cellular environment that is permissive for stem cell activity and neuronal development, the "neurogenic niche." To understand this fundamental interaction better, adult neurogenesis should be considered in relation to embryonic and fetal development. Development of the nervous system begins with the induction of neuroepithelial (NE) cells from ES cells in the blastocyst (Fig. 3–3). Neuroepithelial cells are the primary neural stem cells. The first stage of differentiation is induction of the primitive ectoderm from which all ectodermal cells arise. The primitive ectoderm gives way to the two ectodermal lineages, surface ectoderm and neuroectoderm.

These steps can be related to the activity of certain key genes. The pluripotent ES cells, for example, are, among other markers, characterized by their expression of *Oct4*, which is down-regulated when the cells loose their pluripotency (Scholer et al., 1990; Rathjen et al., 2002). The early neurectodermal tissue forms a layer along the anterior midline of the egg cylinder, the neural plate. During formation of the neural plate, genes such as *Sox1* and *Gbx2* are up-regulated (Wassarman et al., 1997; Pevny et al., 1998). When the neural plate invaginates lengthwise to first form a grove, *Gbx2* is down-regulated. The grove then closes to become the neural tube.

The earliest neuroepithelial cells are found along the forming neural axis. Later, the primary population of stem cells resides in the wall of the neural tube. These cells are multipotent and characterized by expression of markers such as Sox1 and Sox2, nestin, and neural cell adhesion molecule (NCAM). From these results the central nervous system is generated. A subpopulation of stem cells migrates laterally and forms the neural crest, which becomes the origin of the peripheral and autonomous nervous system.

The neural tube encloses a cavity that becomes the primordial ventricular system of the brain. Throughout life, the walls of the ventricles remain a location of cell division and precursor cell action. This also holds true for parts of the ventricular system that become obliterated in the adult. The rostral migratory stream, for example, which provides the route of migration during neurogenesis in the adult olfactory system, surrounds the remnants of the olfactory ventricle.

The primary germinative zone for forebrain development is the ventricular plate, the wall of this primordial ventricle. Here stem cells divide in symmetric and asymmetric divisions and give rise to progenitor cell populations that reside in the subventricular zone (SVZ), just below the ventricular zone. The subventricular progenitor cells proliferate massively and produce first neurons and later glia.

Among others, two cell populations play a particular role in forebrain development: radial glia and Cajal Retzius neurons. Both are closely linked to stem cell activity. Radial glia, which was long considered to provide only the guidance structure for neuronal cell migration, has been identified as being part of the precursor cell pool itself (Malatesta et al., 2000; Noctor et al., 2001, 2002; Kriegstein and Gotz, 2003). Radial glia might generate other precursor cells from which neurons that populate the cortex are derived or do so directly. The developing neurons use the processes of radial glia that span from the ventricular to the pial surface of the brain to migrate to their final destination in the cortex (Rakic, 1971, 1972, 1974). Later, radial glia cells generate astrocytes and finally turn into astrocytes (Schmechel and Rakic, 1979; Voigt, 1989). Radial glia-like cells with many astrocytic properties persist in the neurogenic zones of the adult brain, where they might serve the same dual function as during development—as precursor cells and as more classical astrocytes (Alvarez-Buylla et al., 2001).

Cajal Retzius cells are a population of neurons generated early and reside in the molecular layer, the outermost layer if seen from the ventricular zone. Cajal-Retzius neurons express reelin, which is involved in regulating the migration of cortical neurons from the ventricular zone outward along the radial glial fibers (D'Arcangelo et al., 1995; Rice and Curran, 2001). In the absence of reelin, no radial glia scaffolding forms in the hippocampus (Forster et al., 2002) and cortex (Hartfuss et al., 2003), suggesting a close interdependency between Cajal-Retzius neurons and precursor cells.

Precursor cells from the ventricular plate in the dorsal brain produce the principal neurons of the cortex and astrocytes (Fig. 3–4). Principal neurons are excitatory neurons, for example, the pyramidal cells. Precursor cells from the ventricular zone in the ventral brain (the so-called ganglionic eminences) generate neurons in the ventral brain (e.g., the basal ganglia), oligodendrocytes, and the complex diversity of inhibitory interneurons of both the ventral and dorsal brain. Mid- and hindbrain structures, as well as specialized structures such as the hypothalamus, neurophypophysis, and others, originate from yet other stem cell populations whose relationship to those of the ventricular plate and the ganglionic eminences is not yet exactly known. Primary sensory epithelia such as retina, hair cells of the inner ear, and olfactory epithelium are derived from the optic, auditory, or olfactory placodes. Initiation of their development precedes cortical development.

Brain development in mammals continues postnatally. Some neuronal populations, for example, the cerebellar and hippocampal granule cell neurons, are almost entirely produced after birth. Conceptually, postnatal neurogenesis is more closely linked to embryonic and fetal neurogenesis than to adult neurogenesis. In the dentate gyrus of the hippocampus a complex transition between embryonic, postnatal, and adult neurogenesis occurs (Altman and Bayer, 1990a, 1990b). There is no similar analysis of the early postnatal SVZ. Despite studies that have compared the gene expression profiles of embryonic and adult neural stem cells (D'Amour and Gage, 2003), very little is known about the exact molecular changes underlying these profound transitions.

Taken together, during development the term *neural stem cells* does not identify a homogenous population of cells. Rather, neural stem cells represent a heterogeneous sequence of cells that possibly encompass representatives of different and potentially even unrelated lineages.

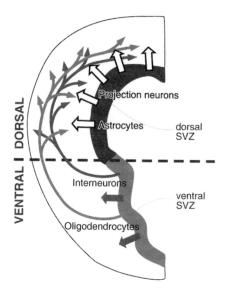

Figure 3–4. Regionalization of precursor cells. Brain development originates from precursor cells in the walls of the neural tube, which later become the walls of the ventricular system, the ventricular zone (VZ), and the cell layer below, the subventricular zone (SVZ). Different parts of the VZ and SVZ contribute differently to brain development. The precursor cells are regionalized. Here specification in ventral and dorsal precursor cells is depicted. In addition to ventral neurons, ventral precursor cells in the ganglionic eminences generate interneurons in the dorsal brain. The precursor cells in the adult brain appear to maintain this developmental regionalization, but few details are known about this (see also Fig. 4–5).

RADIAL GLIA AS STEM CELLS

Radial glia is the conventional name for a characteristic type of cell that plays several important roles during brain development. Radial glia function is essentially dual: radial glia acts as a precursor cell in the developing brain and serves as a guidance structure that leads new neurons from the site of division near the ventricular surface to their final position in the cortex (Fig. 3–5). Accordingly, radial glia is most abundant during the peak time of neurogenesis. There is now ample direct evidence that radial glia cells are the origin of cortical neurons (Cameron and Rakic, 1991; Malatesta et al., 2000, 2003; Hartfuss et al., 2001; Noctor et al., 2001, 2002; Gaiano and Fishell, 2002; Tramontin et al., 2003). The mother cells guide their daughter cells along their processes into their appropriate target region (Noctor et al., 2001).

Radial glia originates from the neuroepithelial cells of the walls of the neural tube. The main distinction between the two cell types is the development of glia features, such as the expression of glial filaments, marker proteins such as tenascin C, GLAST, and brain lipid binding protein (BLBP),

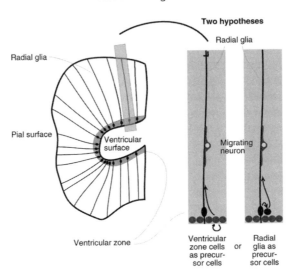

Figure 3–5. Dual functions of radial glia during development. Radial glia serves as precursor cells and as a guidance structure for the migration of newly generated neurons to their appropriate position in the cortex. The precursor cell function of radial glia does not imply that cells with a radial glial morphology are the only precursor cells in the brain. Expansion of the precursor pool appears to occur mainly on the level of intermediate progenitor cells that lack the characteristic morphology. In both neurogenic regions of the adult brain, cells with radial glia-like properties persist and seem to function as the highest-ranking precursor cells of these regions.

and the occurrence of glycogen inclusions (Kriegstein and Gotz, 2003). Radial glia expresses nestin throughout development (Hartfuss et al., 2001).

Most brain regions contain radial glia, but despite obvious similarities, radial glia might be a heterogeneous class of cells (Malatesta et al., 2003; Hack et al., 2004). Conclusions drawn from one brain region in one species and one point of development cannot be generalized. Also, radial glia is not the only cell type with stem cell properties in neurogenesis. It is assumed that radial glia cells generate intermediate precursor cells, but the existence of an independent population of precursor cells capable of neurogenesis cannot be excluded. In fact, the existence of several lineages of glial and neuronal precursor cells is widely acknowledged (McCarthy et al., 2001; Malatesta et al., 2003). In the neurogenic regions, morphologically characteristic radial glia persists into adulthood (Alvarez-Buylla et al., 2001; Alvarez-Buylla and Garcia-Verdugo, 2002). In other areas, radial glia transforms into astrocytes after the end of neurogenesis (Rakic, 1971; Eckenhoff and Rakic, 1988; Voigt, 1989; Misson et al., 1991).

In both the adult subgranular zone (SGZ) and SVZ astrocyte-like, radial glia–like cells retain stem cell properties and are thought to link adult neurogenesis with embryonic brain development (Alvarez-Buylla et al., 2001). In the hippocampus, radial glia cells of the adult dentate gyrus are a secondary population displaced from the original ventricular location and that no longer extends between the ventricular wall and the pial surface of the brain (Rickmann et al., 1987). But these cells show many characteristics of astrocytes. In the SVZ the original location near the ventricular surface is maintained.

Radial glia from different regions of the developing brain differs in the expression of distinct sets of neurogenic transcription factors known to control patterning of the developing brain (Stoykova et al., 1996; Corbin et al., 2000; Yun et al., 2001). Radial glia might thus be involved in defining regional specificity of neuronal development.

Radial glia of the dorsal forebrain, for example, expresses *Pax6*. Hippocampal radial glia–like cells in the adult, however, are Pax6 negative. In the adult SVZ, which is of dorsal origin, the radial glia–derived B cells are Pax6 negative as well. But migratory progeny of these cells, producing periglomerular interneurons in the olfactory bulb, express Pax6. Consequently, the pattern of Pax6 and thus its presumed functional role will differ between the fetal and adult period and between the two neurogenic regions. In Pax6-deficient mice, however, radial glia from the dorsal forebrain acts like radial glia of the ventral forebrain and instead of cortical projection neurons generates mainly glia and few neurons (Gotz et al., 1998). Intriguingly, these neurons were interneurons of the olfactory bulb. Radial glia in the lateral ganglionic eminence expresses Gsh2 and normally gives rise to interneurons in the olfactory bulb (Stenman et al., 2003); radial glia in the medial ganglionic eminence expresses *Olig2*, probably generating cortical interneurons and oligodendrocytes (Malatesta et al., 2003).

Most radial glia cells turn into astrocytes at the end of neurogenesis. However, the transformation of a subset of radial glia into radial glia–like precursor cells of the adult neurogenic regions is in line with other types of specialized development, such as into Bergmann glia of the cerebellum or Müller cells of the retina. The transition into a precursor cell function (or in some sense the persistence of such a function) might thus be a particularly intriguing example of a characteristic property of radial glia.

NEURAL STEM CELLS IN THE ADULT BRAIN

Only in the early 1990s was it discovered that neural stem cells could be isolated from both the developing and adult mammalian brain. Most experimental data on *adult* precursor cells reflect the situation in early adulthood. In rodents, which are used in most studies, sexual maturity and thus adulthood begin at approximately 4 weeks of age, the time (or just a few weeks thereafter) when cells are isolated in most studies (see also Chapter 10 on practical definitions of adulthood). Like human teenagers, who despite their self-perception and awakened sexuality do not behave mature by all (especially parental) standards, one can question how adult these animals are by other standards of maturity. Here the yield is very low; stem cells in the adult are rare. But they have been found in the oldest brain tissue. In a few studies neural stem cells have been isolated from old animals and even from the postmortem human brain (Palmer et al., 2001; Schwartz et al., 2003; Maslov et al., 2004); the latter, however to date only from infants.

The initial reports on precursor cells isolated from the adult brain focused on the two neurogenic regions, the hippocampus and olfactory bulb. The in vivo and ex vivo lines of research became mutually reinforcing. The existence of stem cells in the regions of supposed neurogenesis made this proposition all the more realistic, while adult neurogenesis gave meaning to the presence of stem cells in the adult brain. In somewhat neuronocentric terminology, the precursor cells of the neurogenic regions in the adult brain are sometimes referred to as "neuronal precursor cells." The term is equivalent, however, to *neural precursor cells*.

During development, cell proliferation in the ventricular zone and the SVZ can be distinguished. The first populations of stem cells during development are found in the ventricular zone, the multilayered wall of the premordial ventricles. From these first stem cells the SVZ forms (Boulder Committee, 1970). The massive expansion of cortical precursor cells that drive forebrain development originates from the SVZ. After embryonic and fetal brain development have ceased, however, the SVZ thins out. Cell divisions continue to be found in both the ependymal layer, the remainder of the ventricular zone, and in the SVZ. Which of these two contains the neural stem cells of the adult? Do archaic stem cells persist in the successor of the ventricular zone, the ependymal layer of the adult brain? Or does all stem cell activity in the adult originate from the SVZ?

Under normal conditions, the adult brain outside the SGZ and the SVZ appears to be non-neurogenic. Reports about physiological neurogenesis in other brain regions have remained unconfirmed or controversial at best, mostly because of technical issues (Chapters 7 and 8).

Intriguingly, however, neural stem and progenitor cells can be isolated from many non-neurogenic brain regions, including white matter tracts (Palmer et al., 1995). As in the fetal brain, it seems that adult neural precursor cells are heterogeneous; the degree of this heterogeneity is only beginning to become fully appreciated. The question arises as to whether it is only the microenvironment that differs between neurogenic and non-neurogenic regions or if the locally resident stem cells also differ. From a developmental perspective, the latter appears to be the case. There is no evidence that the adult brain would contain neuroepithelial cells as found in the walls of the neural tube. Adult precursor cells are regionalized.

Jeffrey Macklis and coworkers from Harvard University have shown that under the condition of a highly targeted, induced cell death in the neocortex of mice, new neurons can be generated in these regions (Magavi et al., 2000). Under pathological conditions, most notably local ischemia and cell death, reactive neurogenesis seems to be possible in at least some non-neurogenic regions (Arvidsson et al., 2002; Parent et al., 2002). Whether such reactive neurogenesis plays any functional role after exposure to real-life lesions is not clear, but precursor cell activity after an insult might be part of an abortive attempt for regeneration. On the other hand, we have no idea what the functional outcome would be in the absence of any precursor cell contribution to brain plasticity after damage. Similarly, it is not known how the stem and progenitor cells of non-neurogenic regions contribute to normal brain functions.

Even if precursor cells are not routinely generating neurons they might underlie the substantial production of new glial cells in the adult brain. Both astrocytes and oligodendrocytes are produced in considerable numbers in the adult brain. Microglia is also made in the adult brain but supposedly originates from blood monocytes that enter the brain. Their origins notwithstanding, microglia can proliferate in situ, under both normal and pathological conditions. The minority opinion that microglia and macroglia (astrocytes and oligodendrocytes) might share a common precursor has lost ground because microglia has never been found in neural stem cell cultures.

The rise of neural stem cell biology has made investigators wonder whether mature macroglia—astrocytes and oligodendrocytes—can divide at all or whether all their apparent proliferation in fact reflects precursor cell activity. Along these lines, new concepts in neuro-oncology hypothesize that gliomas, that is, brain tumors with characteristics of glia, in fact originate from precursor cells (Chapter 12). Similarly, in the reactive gliosis that occurs after brain injury, a phenomenon long considered to originate from mature astrocytes, local precursor cells might generate the activated astrocytes.

There are hundreds of known types of neurons in the adult brain. To date it is not known whether all neural and glial cell types can be generated from the stem cells present in the adult brain. Nor do we know whether the cellular environment in the adult brain could support new neurons or glial cells of any desirable phenotype. This seems unlikely, given the high specialization of adult neurogenesis. However, it remains to be shown to what degree this specificity is a function of precursor cell properties or of the permissive microenvironment (Chapter 8).

Based on the expression of different marker sets and the lack of an overlap between other markers, cell lineages can be identified in vivo. We will look at these in more detail in Chapters 5 and 6. That these proliferatively active cells are precursor cells, however, is usually a conclusion by analogy. When isolated from the brain and propagated in cell culture, many cells with antigen profiles equivalent to those of the putative precursor cells in vivo are self-renewing and multipotent. It has not yet been possible, however, to recapitulate the in vivo hypothesized precursor cell hierarchy in vitro and vice versa. In principal, multipotency can be studied in vivo by clonal retroviral labeling (Walsh and Cepko, 1992), but no successful attempt in the adult brain has been reported so far.

NEURAL PRECURSOR CELLS CAN BE STUDIED IN VITRO

The developmental potential and many other aspects of neural stem cell biology cannot be studied in vivo; they have to be isolated and investigated in cell cultures. Neural stem cells can be cultured in two different ways: as floating aggregates, called "neurospheres," or as adherent cultures (Fig. 3–6, Table 3–3). Both approaches share the use of growth factors and strictly serum-free conditions. Clive Svendsen, from the University of Madison, Wisconsin, has compared the two ways of culturing neural stem cells on two computer platforms, PC and Macintosh. This work nicely illustrates the combination of generally identical possibilities with at times still limited compatibility. The hope is to develop a kind of Linux of stem cell research, an open and stable code to produce neurons from defined stem cells.

Currently, the neurosphere method is the most widely used technique. It was originally described by Reynolds and Weiss in 1992 and further characterized by Angelo Viscovi and Derek van der Kooy and colleagues (Morshead et al., 1994, 1998; Craig et al., 1996; Gritti et al., 1996, 1999). In cell suspension with no adherent substrates but containing growth factors, the putative stem cells form floating clusters of cells, the neurospheres. These neurospheres are not identical to stem cells, and the detection of sphere-forming cells is not equivalent to that of stem cells. At best, neurospheres contain a few percent stem cells.

The second strategy, described by Palmer et al. (1999), employs the specific buoyancy of stem and progenitor cells in a Percoll gradient to enrich

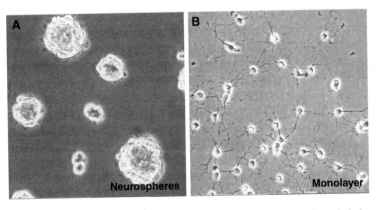

Figure 3–6. The two forms of precursor cell cultures from the adult brain. Neural precursor cells can be cultured as suspension or aggregate cultures, called "neurospheres," or as adherent monolayers. The two strategies do not yield exactly identical results. Note that neurospheres might contain stem cells but are not identical to stem cells. Only clonal analysis (Fig. 3–9) can ultimately determine whether a cell culture truly contains stem cells. See Table 3–3 for a comparison of the two cell culture strategies, and Figure 3–8 (Color Plate 3). Images by Harish Babu, Berlin.

Table 3–3. Neural Precursor Cell Cultures from the Adult Brain

	Neurospheres	Monolayers
Synonym	Aggregate cultures Cell cultures on nonadherent surface as floating cells	Adherent cultures Grown on surfaces with adhesive substrates such as laminin, fibronectin
Growth factors		
Mouse	EGF and/or FGF-2	
Rat	EGF or FGF-2	FGF-2
Human	EGF and/or FGF2 and/or LIF	EGF, FGF-2, LIF
References	Reynolds and Weiss, 1992 Morshead et al., 1994 Gritti et al., 1996, 1999 Pincus et al., 1998	Palmer et al., 1999, 2001 Schwartz et al., 2003

EGF, epidermal growth factor; FGF, fibroblast growth factor; LIF, lenkocyte inhibitory factor.

putative stem cells. The cells are then grown in the presence of mitogens on coated surfaces as adherent cultures. Enrichment by centrifugation gradients is not mandatory but increases the yield.

At present it is not clear how similar or different the two isolation strategies really are. But their mere existence excludes the possibility that the attribution of *stemness* could be based just on the method of isolation. Ways in which more stringent stem cell properties can be determined will be discussed below, but suffice it to say that stem cell behavior can be demonstrated in both systems and they both deliver similar results.

Many researchers prefer use of neurosphere cultures to that of adherent cultures because the former allows production of a greater number of cells and easier preparation of single-cell suspensions, which are needed for clonal analysis. However, this apparently greater ease of use might be deceptive. Again: *neurospheres* and *stem cells* are not the same. Clonal analysis is a means of establishing the self-renewal of putative stem cells. The aggregates resemble the embryoid bodies found when ES cells are propagated in vitro. Within the spheres the cells form three-dimensional structures; there are often inside-out gradients for certain characteristics. For example, most proliferating cells might be found on the outside, whereas the differentiating cells are found within. Adherent cultures, in contrast, allow better visualization of single-cell morphology, cell migration, differentiation, and maturation, although the yield is lower. Given the low abundance of stem cells in neurospheres, this impression might be misleading, however. A quantitative comparison between the two methods is still lacking. Cell-to-cell contacts are less prominent in adherent cultures, which presumably influences survival and differentiation. The potential for neuronal differentiation varies greatly across cultures from different isolations and among different research groups, even within one system.

Together both isolation strategies differ fundamentally from the culturing of hematopoetic stem cells. In the hematopoetic system, different precursor cells can be unambiguously identified by a distinct set of surface antigens that can be used for prospective isolation based on the binding of specific antibodies. This can be done, for example, through fluorescence-activated cell sorting (FACS): in a fine stream of single cells, the fluorescent antibody that has bound to the surface antigen of the precursor cells is recognized and an electric field is applied to direct each individual identified cell into a receptacle that takes up the cells of the desired antigen pattern. For smaller volumes one can alternatively (and more cheaply) couple iron beads to antibodies against precursor cell antigens and pull the binding cells from the solution by means of magnetic force.

For these prospective isolation methods, stem cells are operationally defined as cells with a particular antigen profile. This prospective definition per se does not reveal anything about the two cardinal stemness criteria of self-renewal and multipotency!

Today's neural stem cell cultures do not yet adequately reflect the situation that seems to prevail in vivo. Many regional identities are lost when the cells are brought into culture (Santa-Olalla et al., 2003; Hack et al., 2004). Neither self-renewal nor multipotency, however, can be feasibly (if at all) addressed in vivo, so an ex vivo approach to assess these aspects of stem cell identity and nature appears to be inevitable. But to put cells in vitro means that they will undergo a radical and complete change in their environment. The spatiotemporal signaling cues to which these cells are exposed in vivo change into a highly controlled environment brought in by the researcher. The precursor cells show a certain and relatively specific, intrinsically determined behavior in vitro that allows one to distinguish them from other cell populations brought into the same culture conditions and that would not show self-renewal and multipotency. The degree to which the culture conditions induce or disinhibit this behavior in the isolated cells is not known, however. Consequently, the potential of precursor cells ex vivo is not necessarily identical to their realized potential in vivo. In vitro conditions do not exactly replicate in vivo conditions, although progress has been made toward a better understanding of this issue. Several studies that have identified transcription factors, such as Dlx2 or Tlx, involved in the regulation of precursor cell activity at specific identifiable stages in vivo have also opened the way to using these markers as selection criteria in vitro and thus reduce heterogeneity in vitro (Doetsch et al., 2002; Shi et al., 2004). Precursor cells can also be isolated on the basis of surface antigens (Johansson et al., 1999; Roy et al., 1999, 2000; Rietze et al., 2001; Capela and Temple, 2002), but their relation to cells obtained by other means is not clear. The results have been both encouraging and disturbing because ex vivo the cells often tend to show a greater potential than that assumed from the in vivo data. Essentially, precursor cells ex vivo show a greater capacity for self-renewal and multipotency than that expected from their putative in vivo counterparts.

THE IDENTITY OF NEURAL PRECURSOR CELLS

One central, unresolved question of neural stem cell biology is the nature and identity of precursor cells in the adult brain. Through the neurosphere assay it was found that precursor cells from different brain regions do not behave identically under identical culture conditions (Hitoshi et al., 2002a, 2002b; Ostenfeld et al., 2002; Parmar et al., 2002). The differences, however, did not entirely reflect the origins of the precursor cells, for example, in terms of the neuronal subtypes that could be derived. While this can be partially explained by the limited specificity of the readout, the culture conditions themselves may impose certain homogenizing influences (Gabay et al., 2003; Santa-Olalla et al., 2003).

Thus regional differences in vivo will be underestimated by in vitro assays. The homogenizing effect of cell culture conditions might also explain the otherwise surprisingly few differences in gene expression patterns between embryonic and adult neural precursor cells (Ramalho-Santos et al., 2002). Again, choosing a different approach to isolate the cells of interest for comparison led to a different outcome and revealed that a number of plausible genetic differences between pluripotent and multipotent stem cell populations exist (D'Amour and Gage, 2003).

In addition to an unsatisfying reflection of regional precursor cell heterogeneity in vivo, in vitro assays show difficulties in differentiating between transiently amplifying progenitor cells and stem cells and therefore do not allow unambiguous conclusions about the position the cultured cells would have in the stem cell hierarchy in vivo. Culture conditions profoundly influence cells.

Most transcription factors are down-regulated in the growth phase of the neurosphere assay as well as in adherent cultures, with the notable exception of the *olig* genes (Hack et al., 2004). Culture conditions thus select for or induce the generation of *olig2*-expressing precursor cells. In vivo, *olig2* is not expressed by the astrocyte- or radial glia–like cells thought to represent the multipotent stem cells but by the highly proliferative intermediate progenitor cells (Hack et al., 2004).

Exposure to epidermal growth factor (EGF) transformed *Dlx2*-expressing, transiently amplifying cells into multipotent stem cells, on the one hand challenging use of the neurosphere assay as a simple indicator of the in vivo situation, but on the other impressively showing that precursor cells can in fact move along lineages, depending on limited instructive signals (Doetsch et al., 2002). This and similar results have led to the acknowledgment of a problematic divergence: in vitro and in vivo concepts do not exactly match. Ex vivo, multipotency can be detected in cell populations that in vivo do not seem to show it. There are several options to explain this phenomenon:

(1) either all of these cells are indeed multipotent in vivo and the in vivo assays are still too crude to detect this; (2) their multipotency is actively suppressed by the environment at some of the lineage stages in vivo; (3) the apparent multipotency reflects a dedifferentiation and thus a non-physiological or even pathological state, with no valid relationship to the in vivo situation; or (4) the in vitro assay does not adequately reflect the in vivo situation because in vitro and in vivo environments have different inductive effects on precursor cells. At present, no definitive answer to this important question has been found. Because in vivo experiments and de-velopmental considerations indicate heterogeneity among precursor cells and ex vivo experiments might suggest false homogeneity, the identity of precursor cells in the adult brain also remains unresolved.

ASTROCYTES AS STEM CELLS IN THE ADULT BRAIN AND STEM CELLS WITH ASTROCYTIC FEATURES

The issue of identity has a second aspect, related to the identification of pre-cursor cells in the adult brain. The finding of adult neurogenesis in the SVZ and olfactory bulb and the possibility of isolating precursor cells from these regions has raised the question of determining which cells seen in microscopic images of these regions in vivo are neural stem cells. Are stem cells "dis-guised" as other, more familiar cells (Morshead and van der Kooy, 2004)?

In the adult brain, neural precursor cells are not restricted to the SVZ but are also found in the SGZ and elsewhere in the brain parenchyma. The ter-tiary germinative matrix in the SGZ is of ventricular zone origin (see also Chapter 4), but in the adult does not show an anatomical connection to the SVZ.

Arturo Alvarez-Buylla and coworkers have found evidence that glial fibrillary acidic protein (GFAP)-positive cells of the subependymal layer (for the olfactory system) and the SGZ (for the hippocampus) could be the stem cells of these neurogenic regions. After temporary ablation of all prolifer-ating cells with cytostatic agent cytosine-β-D-arabinofuronoside (Ara-C), GFAP-expressing cells were the first to reappear (Doetsch et al., 1999a; Seri et al., 2001). Also, a reporter gene transmitted by a virus that could only infect (genetically engineered) GFAP-expressing cells was later found in neurons, evidence that neurons could originate from GFAP-positive cells in this re-gion (Doetsch et al., 1999b). From these data a unified theory has been de-ducted (Alvarez-Buylla et al., 2001). Astrocytes with stem cell qualities are supposedly derived from radial glia and radial glia ultimately originates from the early ventricular zone. Radial glia cells are self-renewing multi-potent cells during embryogenesis and early postnatally (Kriegstein and Gotz, 2003). Alvarez-Buylla proposed that "neural stem cells are contained within the developmental lineage that proceeds from neuroepithelial cells, through radial glia, to astrocytes" (Alvarez-Buylla et al., 2001). In this con-cept it is only a question of time during development whether the stem

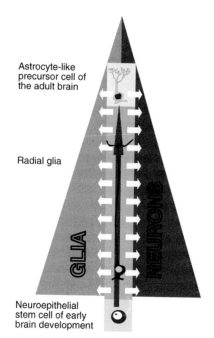

Figure 3–7. Proposed origin of adult precursor cells from radial glia. Arturo Alvarez-Buylla proposed a unifying hypothesis on the role of astrocyte-like precursor cells in the adult brain and their relationship to radial glia acting as precursor cells during development (Alvarez-Buylla et al., 2001). This pine tree model proposes continuity between the role of radial glia during embryonic brain development and the corresponding role of specialized astrocytes in neurogenic regions of the adult brain. These astrocytes are direct descendents of radial glia and maintain radial glia–like properties.

cells will display neuroepithelial, radial glial, or astrocytic characteristics (Fig. 3–7). Consequently, the exact nature of stem cells during neural development shifts. Experimental findings by Jonas Frisén's group (Johansson et al., 1999) and the prospective isolation of SVZ precursor cells by Parry Bartlett and coworkers (Rietze et al., 2001) argue against this theory. Frisén showed that sorting based on both DiI incorporation or Notch expression allowed the isolation of multipotent cells from the adult ventricular wall, suggesting that ependymal cells can act as stem cells in the adult brain (Johansson et al., 1999). This issue is discussed in greater detail in Chapter 5. By killing GFAP-expressing cells with a genetic construct that made them sensitive to ganciclovir, there was a 20-fold reduction in the number of self-renewing and multipotent precursor cells that could be isolated from the brain, further supporting the idea that GFAP-positive cells are the stem cells of the adult brain (Morshead et al., 2003). In a later study using a transgenic approach, a similar result was obtained. This study even suggested that morphologically the neurogenic astrocytes might differ from non-neurogenic astrocytes by having fewer processes (Garcia et al., 2004).

Despite the detection of GFAP in precursor cells, it might not be wise to bluntly apply the term *astrocytes*, which is associated with a differentiated, albeit heterogeneous, type of glial cell, to precursor cells. Within the hierarchy of stem cell biology, this kind of "astrocyte" would be found on a level that is conceptually super-ordinate to astrocytes in the classical sense. Also, not all astrocytes are stem cells. If the "unified theory" holds, however, it helps to explain the invisibility of stem cells in the adult brain. They might be disguised as astrocytes. On the other hand, this evidence suggests that GFAP immunoreactivity alone is not a sufficient criterion to identify either differentiated "true" astrocytes or stem cells. Hence the description of precursor cells as astrocyte-like or radial glia–like is useful. To make matters even more complicated, putative stem cells of the SGZ share further features with astrocytes, such as vascular endfeet and distinct electrophysiological characteristics (Filippov et al., 2003). For some glial biologists this issue serves as one further argument to abandon the idea of astrocytes as being one single cell type; rather, *astrocytes* might be an umbrella term for all neuroepithelial brain cells that are not neurons, or oligodendrocytes. In this sense, stem cells might be astrocytes, but the reverse will still not be true (Morshead and van der Kooy, 2004).

NEURAL PRECURSOR CELL MARKERS

Despite extensive searches, no unambiguous, positive neural stem cell markers have been found. This result even applies to strategies based on the assumed identity of stem cells with astrocytes or radial glia. GFAP alone is obviously insufficient, because many GFAP-positive astrocytes are not stem cells. However, conversely, elimination of GFAP-expressing cells efficiently eliminated multipotent precursor cells in several assays (Morshead et al., 2003; Garcia et al., 2004).

Radial glial precursor cells in the developing brain also express BLBP, GLAST, and RC2 (Hartfuss et al., 2001). In adult neurogenesis of canary birds, BLBP expression has been noted (Rousselot et al., 1997), but in mammalian neurogenic zones not all radial cells showed BLPB expression (Sundholm-Peters et al., 2004). It should be possible to isolate precursor cells prospectively on the basis of their BLPB expression, but this has not yet been demonstrated. GLAST and RC2 do not seem to be expressed in adult neurogenic zones.

Despite the usefulness of the concept of distinguishing between stem and progenitor cells, it is extremely difficult if not impossible to practically distinguish the two classes, particularly in vivo. Experiments can be designed that allow the classification in vitro (Seaberg and van der Kooy, 2002, 2003; Kim and Morshead, 2003), but culture conditions influence the outcome. The sphere-forming assay alone, if not combined with other analyses, has its limitations (Seaberg and van der Kooy, 2003; Morshead and van der Kooy, 2004).

The data discussed above also indicate that the identifications of stem and progenitor cells in vivo and in vitro do not necessarily match. Ex vivo, more cells appear multipotent than they should from their in vivo properties. Strictly speaking, all known neural stem cell markers thus identify precursor cells, that is, cells with a degree of stemness that remains to be determined. Ex vivo data might reveal a potential in cells that does not reflect the in vivo situation.

The failure to identify unique markers, even if the distinction of stem and progenitor cells is left aside, leads to several possible conclusions: (1) no such markers exist; (2) these markers have not been found yet; or (3) no marker has been found because adult precursor cells are not a real, distinguishable entity. The difficulties in finding unifying markers might indeed reflect the simple fact that we are faced with a very heterogeneous population of cells when we talk of stem cells. There might be common features across precursor cells but no obvious antigen properties reveal these shared traits. This heterogeneity might (but does not necessarily have to) reflect the distinction between stem and progenitor cells.

Neural stem cell biologists look with some envy to hematology where on the basis of a known combination of key surface antigens, a prospective isolation of hematopoetic precursor cells is possible. For example, hematopoetic precursor cells express CD34, and further subspecification can be achieved by the combination with other markers or the lack of their expression.

In principle, a prospective strategy can also be applied to identifying stem cells in the brain. Rodney L. Rietze and Perry F. Bartlett from Melbourne have described a method for isolating SVZ stem cells in which sorting by size is combined with enrichment for the absence of two types of surface molecules (Rietze et al., 2001). Cells that had low binding for antibodies against heat-stable antigen (HSA, mCD24a) and peanut agglutin (PSA) showed stem cell features in vitro. However, these essentially negative criteria do not allow unambiguous identification under other circumstances, particularly in vivo. The cells identified by Rietze et al. also lacked cilia and GFAP expression, two characteristics that had been described for SVZ precursor cells isolated by other methods.

In hematology, the analysis of so-called side populations has become an important tool. Cells differ in their ability to bind dyes with affinity to their DNA. During FACS one can identify a side population characterized by low binding to the fluorescent dye and high outflux of the dye from the cells. Kim and Morshead have applied this method to neural stem cell biology and found that the main and side populations differed in their level of stemness; nearly all cells with a sphere-forming capacity in their type of the assay were found in the side population (Kim and Morshead, 2003). GFAP, however, was found in both populations. Combining the side population criteria with positivity for the marker LewisX (LeX) further enriched for sphere-forming cells, although LeX is expressed in both GFAP-expressing and non-expressing putatitve precursor cells (Capela and Temple, 2002). LeX is identical to SSEA1, a marker expressed in many embryonic precursor cell populations.

CD133, also called prominin, is a membrane protein associated with neuroepithelial cells, where it plays an important role during asymmetric division (Koblar et al., 1998). CD133 is also expressed in several other precursor cell populations, most notably hematopoetic precursor cells, so it cannot serve as a neurally specific marker. Although nestin-expressing cells isolated from the fetal mouse brain expressed CD133 (Sawamoto et al., 2001) and CD133 has been used to prospectively isolate neural precursor cells from the fetal human brain (Uchida et al., 2002), CD133 expression by precursor cell populations of the adult brain is questionable.

Sox2 has been used to identify putative precursor cells in vivo, and a surprising overlap with GFAP expression was found. Isolating precursor cells on the basis of their expression of Sox2, D'Amour and Gage (2003) used gene expression profiling to compare the genetic profile of multipotent precursor cells with that of pluripotent stem cells from the embryo. They found that 158 genes from the chip were expressed only in neural stem cells but not in embryonic stem cells. These genes included a number of plausible and useful candidates: *Mash1, Hes5, Dlx1, Jun, Fgfr2, Notch1, Jak2, cyclinD2, doublecortin, Dab1,* and others. However, these cells again seem to represent those that in vivo are thought to reflect transiently amplifying progenitor cells, which ex vivo, but not in vivo, are multipotent. GFAP was not among these candidates. Similarly, cells in the SVZ that are in the G1 phase of the cell cycle and thus presumably represent the quiescent stem cells were found to be both nestin and GFAP negative, but did express Musashi (Maslov et al., 2004), a neural mRNA-binding protein that is highly enriched in neural precursor cells during embryogenesis but absent from mature neurons and glia (Sakakibara et al., 1996).

This raises the question of how to reconcile the different lines of evidence, because GFAP-positive cells show signs of multipotency *in vitro* and the concept of a radial glia–like cell as the origin of a precursor cell lineages *in vivo* is strong. The stem cells that are highest in the hierarchy remain elusive: most knowledge obtained ex vivo seems to apply to transiently amplifying progenitor cells.

For many practical purposes, the intermediate filament nestin (Lendahl et al., 1990) is a useful precursor cell marker (Fig. 3–8, Color Plate 3). However, neither sensitivity nor specificity of nestin is particularly high. In vivo, for example, blood vessels in the neurogenic zones can express nestin (Palmer et al., 2000). On the other hand, relatively quiescent cells of the SVZ were found to be nestin negtive (Maslov et al., 2004). In vitro a population of nestin-negative precursor cells gave rise to neurons and glia (Kukekov et al., 1997). These unresolved issues notwithstanding, nestin has proved to be a useful marker, especially when used in reporter gene mice, in which even the prospective isolation of precursor cells from the adult brain and the visualization of precursor cells in vivo has been possible (Yamaguchi et al., 2000; Sawamoto et al., 2001).

In vivo, the populations of the putative transiently amplifying progenitor cells in the neurogenic regions are negative for GFAP, but many of them are positive for doublecortin (DCX) and the polysialilated form of the neural cell adhesion molecule (PSA-NCAM). When adult hippocampal neurogenesis is stimulated, expansion occurs in these intermediate populations, and the same is probably true for the SVZ (Kronenberg et al., 2003). An

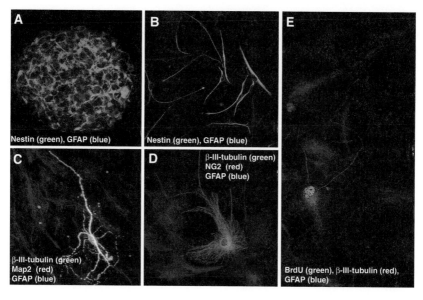

Figure 3–8 (Color Plate 3). Neural precursor cell markers in vitro. Neural precursor cells express precursor cell markers in both types of precursor cell cultures—neurospheres (*A*) and monolayers (*B*). Neurospheres from the adult hippocampus (A) espress both nestin and GFAP. Even under proliferation conditions, precursor cell cultures show hererogeneity. This is particularly obvious in neurospheres. Upon transition to differentiation conditions (C–E), precursor cells differentiate into cells with characteristics of the three neural lineages—neurons (here shown by immoreactivity against β-III-tubulin), astrocytes (GFAP), and oligodendrocytes (NG2). Note that the specificity of these markers is not undisputed (see Chapter 8). In *E*, a BrdU-labeled cell has acquired a neuronal phenotype, evidence of neurogenesis in vitro. Images by Harish Babu, Berlin.

analogous intermediate progenitor cell seems to exist in the glial lineage, but here no distinguishing markers are known (Steiner et al., 2004). The intermediate precursor cells of the SVZ express Dlx2 and this maker can be used to isolate this subpopulation (Doetsch et al., 2002). There are, however, Dlx2-negative, nonglial precursor cells that contribute to adult neurogenesis in the olfactory bulb (Hack et al., 2004).

Outside the neurogenic regions, many putative precursor cells express the proteoglycan NG2. Most of these cells are nestin positive. They represent either an inhomogeneous cell population or one cell type with heterogeneous function. Originally considered to be only a lineage-determined progenitor cell for oligodendrocytes (and possibly a subtype of astrocytes), NG2 cells are now regarded as somewhat mysterious cells between the domains of glia and neurons, most likely including a precursor cell potential (Berry et al., 2002; Horner et al., 2002; Stallcup, 2002). Within the adult

SGZ, NG2 cells are rare (Steiner et al., 2004), but they appear to correspond to a subpopulation of C cells in the SVZ (Aguirre et al., 2004). In addition they are almost evenly distributed throughout the brain. They respond to damage with proliferation and ex vivo might be multipotent (Belachew et al., 2003). NG2 cells, however, likely represent a very heterogeneous population of cells. We will return to NG2 cells in more detail in Chapter 8.

HOW CAN STEMNESS BE ASSESSED PRACTICALLY?

In the absence of sensitive and specific precursor cell markers, the question remains as to how precursor cells can be identified and, consequently, how candidate stemness markers can be validated. Stem cells are defined by (unlimited) self-renewal and multipotency. In vitro, both criteria can be assessed with reasonable accuracy but the conceptual and practical limitations discussed above exist. It is also important to remember that the ability to form neurospheres alone does not prove the stemness of the cells; rather, self-renewal *and* multipotency must be demonstrated (Fig. 3–9). Because this is not always done, in many contexts of brain research the deliberate use of the term *stem cell* is somewhat misleading, because an analysis of stemness has actually not been performed.

Self-renewal is tested by a clonal analysis, in which single cells isolated from such spheres can clonally generate new secondary spheres. A suspension of putative precursor cells is diluted to such a degree that when pipetted onto a microtiter plate, only one single cell is found in each individual well. This can be confirmed under the microscope. It is then examined whether the single cells can again form neurospheres or clusters of adherent cells, that under differentiation conditions show signs of multipotency. By this standard, the yield of stem cells in both types of precursor cell cultures (neurospheres and monolayers) is low and usually does not surpass a few percent. Although this result probably also reflects methodological issues, neither culture system contains pure stem cells.

Multipotency is routinely assessed after withdrawing growth factors EGF and fibroblast growth factor-2 (FGF-2) in stem cell cultures and adding serum and factors such as retinoic acid to the culture medium. The presence of cells from the three main neural lineages, neurons, astrocytes, and oligodendrocytes, is demonstrated by means of immunocytochemistry and taken as evidence of multipotency (Fig. 3–9). In most studies the identification of neurons, astrocytes, and oligodendrocytes is based on the detection of key antigens, such as β-III-tubulin, Map-2, or NeuN for neurons, O4 for oligodendrocytes, and GFAP for astrocytes. Microglia has never been found in these cultures.

One important general concern in addition to the issues of marker sensitivity and specificity is the possibility that culture conditions themselves might induce multipotency in the precursor cells. Consequently, there is no true evidence that neural stem cells in vivo are multipotent as long as this

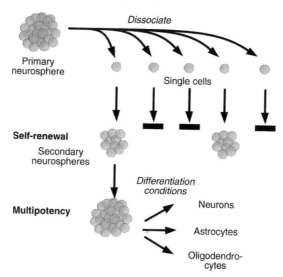

Figure 3–9. Stemness assay. To determine whether neurospheres in fact contains stem cells, it is dissociated and plated as single cells (clonal density). A varying percentage of the individualized cells form secondary neurospheres. This step can be repeated to support the conclusion that cells from the primary neurosphere are indeed self-renewing and thus fulfill the cardinal criterion of stem cells. The secondary sphere can also be transferred into differentiation conditions to assess its ability to form different cell types. Multipotency is the second stem cell criterion. In the eyes of some experts this criterion is not necessary if true self-renewal has been demonstrated. Assessment of multipotency on the level of primary neurospheres is almost meaningless because it cannot be determined whether the primary sphere indeed originated from one single stem cell.

conclusion is based only on an analogy drawn from in vitro studies, which might induce the multipotency in the first place.

In 1992, when Reynolds and Weiss first published data on EGF-dependent neural progenitor cells from the adult mouse brain (Reynolds et al., 1992; Reynolds and Weiss, 1992), the debate on culture conditions was further stimulated by the fact that the first results from rat hippocampi indicated that the precursor cells depended on FGF-2 (Palmer et al., 1995). On the one hand this result could have reflected differences in populations of cells or among species, but on the other concerns were raised that supposedly biological differences may have been introduced by the experimental conditions. Cells might respond differently because different treatments were applied to them. Although in this case it turned out that there were real differences between species and within populations regarding growth factor dependencies, the problem cannot be ruled out in general. It remains a valid concern that criteria used to define aspects of stemness in truth mirror the conditions we apply to the cells. An important example of this problem is the finding that cell growth in progenitor cell cultures can be enhanced when cells are grown under lower levels of oxygen that are closer to the partial pressure in brain tissue than in the atmosphere (Studer et al., 2000).

Implantation of neural stem cells in the developing or adult brain has confirmed the potential of these cells to integrate and differentiate and has shown that it is the local microenvironment that regulates these processes. For example, hippocampal progenitor cells implanted in the adult olfactory system developed into neuronal phenotypes typical of this area, but not like those of their hippocampal origin (Suhonen et al., 1996). Analogous results were found after implantation of spinal progenitors into the hippocampus (Shihabuddin et al., 2000) and even of hippocampal progenitors into the retina (Takahashi et al., 1998). These data also show how limited actual knowledge is about mimicking the neurogenic microenvironment in vitro. Few distinct neuronal (and glial) phenotypes have been clearly inducible in vitro thus far, dopaminergic neurons being a notable exception (Sakurada et al., 1999; Lee et al., 2000; Hall et al., 2003). Neurons with a dopaminergic phenotype also develop from the progeny of embryonic stem cells after implantation in a rat model of Parkinson disease (Bjorklund et al., 2002), a result further emphasizing the importance of microenvironmental clues for cellular differentiation. Other results have confirmed such regionally specific differentiation in the postnatal or adult brain (Lie et al., 2002; Aguirre et al., 2004). However, in neither case has it become obvious which regulatory signals conveyed the local induction and whether differentiation into phenotypes not predominant in the respective region might generally be possible.

Because precursor cells in the adult brain cannot yet be identified prospectively, the precursor cell nature *in vivo* is only inferred post hoc. The fact that precursor cells are dividing cells allows to use proliferation markers to identify precursor cells in vivo. However, this strategy is obviously not specific. Proliferating cells are labeled with a nucleotide analog, classically a radioactively marked thymidine or the thymidine analog bromodeoxyuridine (BrdU), which competes for integration into the newly synthesized strand of DNA during S phase of mitosis. Tritiated thymidine can be detected by autoradiography. BrdU can be detected by immunohistochemistry and therefore allows immunofluorescent double and triple labelings and analysis by confocal laser scanning microscopy. If upon investigation at a certain time after division the BrdU-containing cells display not only the proliferation marker but also a marker for differentiated neurons or glial cells, the retrospective conclusion is made that the cell in question was a precursor cell at the time when BrdU was present in the body. Constitutive proliferation markers such as cell cycle–associated antigens, for example, PCNA or mKi67, can be combined with markers such as nestin, Sox2, and BLPB to find further evidence of putative precursor cells in vivo. Their biological properties are then inferred from other studies having shown precursor cell properties in cells with particular antigen profiles.

GLIAL PROGENITOR CELLS

Glial progenitor cells are neural precursor cells that produce only glia. Historically, research on glial precursor cell biology has preceded the rise of neural stem cell biology by more than a decade. The O2A progenitor cell, first described by Martin Raff and Marc Noble in 1983 as a precursor giving rise to oligodendrocytes and one type of astrocytes (type 2 astrocyte) in vitro (Raff et al., 1983), has over the years been characterized in great detail. However, the O2A precursor cell has never been unambiguously identified in vivo. It is currently thought that O2A progenitor cells might be found among the NG2 cells of the brain (Nishiyama et al., 1996). In vitro, detailed lineage relationships have been revealed. Oligodendrocyte precursor biology had already achieved an intriguing level of sophistication when neural stem cells were not yet on the agenda. In glial precursor cell biology of the spinal cord, culture conditions have been identified that allow the growth of neuronal-restricted precursor cells and glial-restricted precursor cells (Herrera et al., 2001; Gregori et al., 2002; Liu et al., 2002).

Neural stem cell biology evolved to a large degree independent of glial precursor biology (Fig. 3–10), thus the terminology, concepts, and conclusions can differ considerably between the two fields (compare, for example, Liu and Rao, 2004; Rao, 2004). Many studies on glial precursor cell biology have been done on the spinal cord, whereas most studies in neural stem cell biology have favored the SVZ of the forebrain. Consequently, it is not clear, for example, whether the glial-restricted precursor cells (GRPs) that have been studied extensively (Noble et al., 2004) are identical to the glial progenitor cells of neural stem cell biology. In some sense the migratory doublecortin-expressing progenitor cells of the adult hippocampus and SVZ might be considered neural-restricted precursor cells (NRP), described as the neuronal counterpart to the GRPs. Such equalizations make intuitive sense, but no experimental data exist to really bridge the two parallel universes. Although the wording seems similar, the evidence to support the similarity of these differently evolved concepts is still lacking. This is not a trivial matter, because stem cells of the adult brain might actually represent a type of astrocyte, blurring the boundaries of seemingly well-defined cell populations on several conceptual levels. Because the neurogenic zones of the adult brain have not been studied from the perspective of classical glial precursor biology, we will not pursue this issue further in this book.

CAN STEM CELLS CROSS GERM LAYER LIMITS?

The issue of precursor cell identity can be taken one step further. The traditional concept of stem cell biology is that stem cells of the adult organism are tissue-specific—that is, they are only able to generate cell types of the tissue they are found in. From an evolutionary perspective this seems beneficial,

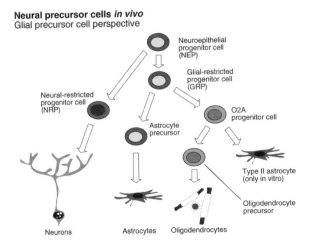

Neural precursor cells *in vivo*
Glial precursor cell perspective

Figure 3–10. Hierarchy of glial precursor cells. Historically, the rise of glial precursor cell biology preceded neural precursor cell biology by almost a decade. Most data in this field have been obtained in fetal spinal cord. The resulting schema is similar to the pedigree depicted in Figure 3–1 (middle left) but the nomenclature is different. The precursor cell function of radial glia and astrocyte-like cells is not yet reflected in this scheme (see Fig. 3–1, bottom, and 3–7).

because for regenerating the intestinal epithelium, for example,oligodendrocytes or pancreatic islet cells are not only not needed but also not wanted. The lineage restriction reduces the risk of malformation tumors, such as teratomas or teratocarcinomas. Surprisingly, however, a number of studies seem to suggest that stem or progenitor cells from one organ could cross limits of tissue specificity and generate differentiated cells in other organs (Fig. 3–11).

For example, studies have shown the generation of blood from neural stem or progenitor cells and of neurons and glia from hematopoeitic stem cells (Brazelton et al., 2000). Most surprisingly, 1 year after bone marrow transplantation, Purkinje neurons carrying the markers of the implanted bone marrow were found in the cerebellum (Priller et al., 2001; Weimann et al., 2003). Similarly, in the brains of female patients who had received a bone marrow graft from male donors, brain autopsy results revealed neurons carrying the Y chromosome (Mezey et al., 2000; Cogle et al., 2004). Because females do not have Y chromosomes, these neurons had to originate from the donor bone marrow cells.

Similar reports have demonstrated the generation of hepatocytes (Lagasse et al., 2000) and skeletal muscle from bone marrow cells (Ferrari et al., 1998; Gussoni et al., 1999). Conversely, bone marrow repopulation by neural precursor cells has been reported (Bjornson et al., 1999), and neural precursor cells were found to have a myogenic potential as well (Galli et al., 2000).

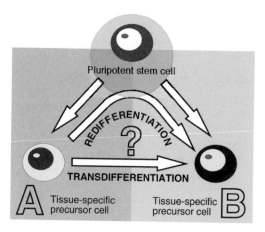

Figure 3–11. Can stem cells cross tissue boundaries? To explain the phenomenon that in some experiments tissue-specific precursor cells apparently generate progeny belonging to a different germ layer, the two concepts transdifferentiation and redifferentiation were developed, the latter involving a more-than-multipotent intermediate stage. Most supposed cases of transdifferentiation or redifferentiation have turned out to be caused by cell fusion, but this does not rule out the possibility that transdifferentiation or redifferentiation might actually exist.

These data have been regarded as evidence of transdifferentiation, the idea that under certain conditions cells differentiating from precursor cells of one germ layer can develop into cells from another. The underlying molecular principle lies in the possibility that the developmental program of isolated stem cells can be reprogrammed to form cells from another tissue. As yet unidentified cues *in vitro* or from the local microenvironment after implantation appear to be responsible for this process. Plausible candidate mechanisms include changes in DNA methylation and acetylation altering the accessibility of genes for regulatory cues. The results suggestive of transdifferentiation were startling because they put into question the validity of many statements made on the potential of stem cells.

However, a number of serious concerns have been raised against the plausibility of transdifferentiation (Anderson et al., 2001; Wagers et al., 2002). Most notably, cell fusion could underlie these findings (Terada et al., 2002; Ying et al., 2002). Cell fusion means that the grafted cell would not reprogram its developmental program but fuse with a host neuron, thus generating a cell with both donor and neuron markers. One way to detect cell fusion is very straightforward: fused cells should have more than the two chromosome sets of normal cells—they should be tetraploid, not diploid. Indeed, tetraploid cells can be found in some but not all circumstances of supposed transdifferentiation; both hepatocytes and Purkinje cells, two of the supposedly transdifferentiated cell types, are known to be aneuploid.

Nevertheless, in vitro, fusion has been found to be a very rare event (Terada et al., 2002; Ying et al., 2002).

Arguably, detection of aneuploidy in vivo is technically challenging. But the Purkinje neurons and hepatocytes supposedly derived from bone marrow could indeed be explained by cell fusion (Alvarez-Dolado et al., 2003; Wang et al., 2003), as suggested by studies in transgenic reporter gene mice. If cell fusion occurs, the fused cells would be tetraploid, unless there was an unprecedented merge and consecutive reduction of the genome (for which there is no evidence) or a fusion after which the invading nucleus threw out the host nucleus. Thus tetraploidy can be visualized with relative ease when the two fusing cells each contain a reporter gene that allows their unambiguous identification (Alvarez-Dolado et al., 2003). In the case of the "bone marrow–derived" Purkinje cell neurons and hepatocytes, exactly this was found. The reporter gene of the transplanted bone marrow was expressed in the same cell as the host reporter gene. If real transdifferentiation had occurred, only the graft reporter gene would have been detectable. Purkinje cells and hepatocytes might have a particular propensity to fuse.

If fusion has been established as a serious confounding factor in the theory of transdifferentiation, does this rule out the possibility of transdifferentiation? Proof of definite absence is generally difficult to establish. In fact, transdifferentiation of neural precursor cells into endothelial cells induced by cell–cell contact with other endothelial cells was shown not to depend on cell fusion (Wurmser et al., 2004). It is not clear to what degree this finding can be applied in principle to other examples of transdifferentiation. But the hope that the phenomenon is so common and robust that it can be used as basis for novel stem cell–based therapeutic approaches is not justified, given the available evidence.

A concept related to transdifferentiation is redifferentiation. Whereas in transdifferentiation the differentiating cells develop directly into a cell type from another germ layer, it is thought that in redifferentiation an intermediate step exists at which the cells revert to a more immature cell type common to the two germ layers. At present it is not known whether redifferentiation can occur. Most of the evidence put forth against transdifferentiation applies to redifferentiation as well.

The most problematic variant of this idea, a confounding explanation for apparent evidence of transdifferentiation or redifferentiation, might lie in the possibility of tumorigenic transformation. In cell culture, precursor cells may have lost their lineage determination and may have acquired a dedifferentiated state. The developmental potential of these transformed cells would indeed represent some sort of transdifferentiation or redifferentiation, but at the price of pathological phenotype and a tumorigenic potential.

Finally, the findings interpreted as evidence of transdifferentiation or redifferentiation could also be explained by the existence of a more-than-multipotent precursor cell, essentially equivalent to the hypothesized intermediate step during redifferentiation. CatherineVerfaillie and coworkers have identified in bone marrow a rare precursor cell that can differentiate into cells across germ layer boundaries (Jiang et al., 2002). Confusingly for many, this possibly pluripotent cell has been named "multipotent adult precursor cell" (MAPC). Similar findings have been reported for rare cells from skin (Toma et al., 2001) and brain (Rietze et al., 2001). However, the same problems that preclude establishment of the existence of multipotency in vivo also hamper the evaluation of whether cells with more-than-multipotent potential exist in situ. Although they may be a product of culture conditions, their rareness might indicate the differential susceptibility of various cells in the cultures to such inducing conditions and thus support the idea of precursor cell heterogeneity.

Culture conditions can thus determine the properties of precursor cells, with different sets of culture conditions yielding incommensurable results. This does not mean that precursor cell identities are culture artifacts but that precursor cell properties can be determined by external cues. This is in contrast to the view that stemness is an intrinsic property. However, there are differences in sensitivity of various types of cells to particular sets of environmental cues. The determinants of such differences in susceptibility might be interpreted as signs of stemness as well.

On the other hand, all cells of an individual share the same genetic information. Genetically, any cell is a potential stem cell. Whether this potential is realized depends on temporospatial contexts. If environment is everything, except for genes, epigenetic and environmental conditions must exist that determine stemness. The question is not whether these conditions exist at all, but whether it is possible to change conditions adequately in time and space to obtain the desired types of cells.

On the basis of findings suggestive of transdifferentiation, Helen Blau at Stanford University proposed that stem cells might not be a distinct type of cell but rather reflect a functional state that can be acquired by different types of cells under different circumstances (Blau et al., 2001). Cells susceptible to such local stemness-inducing cues would circulate throughout the body and context-dependently perform different stem cell functions. This radical interpretation is at minimum "great food for thought," because it turned the previous concept on its head. As a provable scientific hypothesis it faces considerable difficulties, because in this view stemness is inherently transient—to prove the cellular identity over time and through different states of stemness and differentiation will be difficult. One argument against this concept is that stem cells can in fact be prospectively isolated according to fixed sets of criteria. However, one could still argue that these criteria define a transient state that can at times be fulfilled by different cells. The question then is whether such a condition could still be aptly named a functional state only.

NEUROGENIC POTENTIAL OF MESENCHYMAL STEM CELLS

Independent of the mechanism hypothesized to underlie transdifferentiation, redifferentiation, or the existence of a more-than-multipotent potential of the precursor cell, many investigators consider mesenchymal stem cells to be a promising cellular source for neuronal replacement therapies. Mesenchymal stem cells are found in the bone marrow, where they are part of the stroma. Their lineage is thus independent of hematopoetic lineage. However, stromal stem cells of the bone marrow are part of the stem cell niche of the bone marrow, contributing to the microenvironment sustaining precursor cell activity in the hematopoetic system. In addition to bone marrow, mesenchymal stem cells are found in the adipose tissue and cartilage. This raises the question of possible heterogeneity among mesenchymal stem cells. However, like hematopoetic stem cells, mesenchymal stem cells can be identified prospectively by marker combinations, and under appropriate conditions, the cells differentiate into the osteoblast, adipocyte, and chondrocyte lineages (Lee et al., 2004). The controversial issue is to what degree mesenchymal stem cells can show neuronal differentiation. There is little doubt that, under appropriate culture conditions, mesenchymal stem cells can express markers associated with neuronal lineage (Levy et al., 2003). These conditions include, for example, exposure to DMSO (Woodbury et al., 2002) or conditioned media (Fu et al., 2004). The bone marrow–derived cells lose their mesenchymal markers, grow in agglomerates resembling neurospheres, and can be induced to differentiate into cells expressing neuronal, astrocytic, and oligodendrocytic markers in vitro (Hermann et al., 2004).

In most studies, no clonal analyses have been done to prove the multipotency of single mesenchymal precursor cells. A cautious interpretation is that under specific conditions mesenchymal precursor cells can show signs of incomplete neuronal development. At present it is not clear whether mesenchymal precursor cells can truly produce fully functional neurons and thus serve as a source for neuronal replacement strategies, as some studies have suggested (Kang et al., 2003). The caveats expressed in the context of other examples of transdifferentiation apply to these studies as well. However, because mesenchymal stem cells are a definable population of cells that can be prospectively isolated, they are in a class by themselves.

Most studies on the neurogenic potential of mesenchymal stem cells are in vitro studies, so the end point of neuronal maturation and functionality is difficult to determine; as discussed in Chapter 10, function on a single cell level is different from that on a system level in vivo. Studies showing signs of neuronal differentiation in mesenchymal stem cell cultures were not able to show appropriate electrophysiological responses (Padovan et al., 2003). However, cells did respond to NMDA and showed voltage-gated channels.

DMSO has been found to induce an incomplete morphological change toward a neuronal shape associated with the expression of some but not other neuronal markers (Neuhuber et al., 2004). Similar morphological alterations were also induced in fibroblasts. The incompleteness of neuronal marker profiles in the presumed neuronally differentiated mesenchymal cells is a recurrent finding in many studies (Neuhuber et al., 2004; Yang et al., 2004).

CONFLICTS OF CONCEPTS

Stem cells are at the center of a scientific revolution that profoundly changes the principles on which medicine is based. Not unlike the parallel genomic revolution, stem cell biology forces humanity to start looking at biology from within rather than, deductively from afar. Stem cells are characterized by a potential, and this potential is almost by definition inherently open. The world seen from the perspective of the stem cell (or the genome) is less deterministic than most deductive concepts of classical biology. This openness stimulates fantasy, and far-reaching consequences of stem cell biology for the treatment of incurable disease have been prophesied. At the same time, seemingly boundless potential raises fears because of the impending dangers to what people consider to be essentially human. This brings forth the old nature-versus-nurture debate in new clothing. How much of us is in our stem cells?

There is an obvious discrepancy between the public perception of stem cell biology and the science itself. This gap is the extension of what David Anderson has aptly named the "possible versus the actual" in stem cell research. In an influential review, Anderson placed the two fundamentally different types of stem cell research in opposition to each other, depending on whether the underlying biology or the potential application was the focus of interest (Anderson, 2001). He found only limited transfer of knowledge between the two groups and suspected a further divergence of evolving concepts. Applied science sees stem cell biology essentially as a toolbox for developing new cell-based therapies. It often uses nomenclature taken from the different context of basic research. Basic research tries to understand the fundamentals of cellular development and the parameters defining stemness. The term *lineage restriction*, for example, has solely descriptive and neutral meaning in basic stem cell biology, whereas in the field of applied stem cell research it is viewed as either an imposed limitation or a desired goal.

But both fields could and should benefit from each other. And while they are occasionally in the hand of one and the same researcher, both the public and the scientific debates have suffered from a lack of clear definitions. The excitement over the large therapeutic potential of stem cells has often occluded the simple fact that it is not at all clear what is meant by stem cell.

Neurologists and psychiatrists long for new stem cell–based therapies. The discovery of neural (or neuronal) stem cells has initiated the movement of stem cell biology from the realms of classical embryology and hematology to mainstream biology. An independent new field of neural stem cell biology has also developed. The discovery of adult neurogenesis has fundamentally altered the perception of the brain and the relationship between structure and function.

There is currently no single sufficiently precise definition of stem cells. In a 1997 review on neural stem cells, Morrison, Shah, and Anderson coined an often quoted aphorism, comparing the difficulties in defining stem cells to the remark made by U.S. Supreme Court Justice Byron White on pornography: "It is hard to define, but I know it when I see it" (Morrison et al., 1997). The analogy stuck not only because of its wit but also because of its metaphorical power to encapsulate the fundamental problem without using wordy explanations. It reveals the important fact that despite the lack of an articulated definition, subconscious, operational definitions of stem cells are very much in place. The consequence is twofold. On the positive side the tacit understanding that stem cells are somehow sufficiently definable enables everyday research. On the negative side the lack of a matured concept obviously breeds errors and missed opportunities. This is particularly important when it comes to political and legal decisions affecting stem cell biology and its application in medicine.

REFERENCES

Aguirre AA, Chittajallu R, Belachew S, Gallo V (2004) NG2-expressing cells in the subventricular zone are type C–like cells and contribute to interneuron generation in the postnatal hippocampus. J Cell Biol 165:575–589.

Altman J, Bayer SA (1990a) Migration and distribution of two populations of hippocampal progenitors during the perinatal and postnatal periods. J Comp Neurol 301:365–381.

Altman J, Bayer SA (1990b) Mosaic organization of the hippocampal neuroepithelium and the multiple germinal sources of dentate granule cells. J Comp Neurol 301:325–342.

Altman J, Das GD (1965) Autoradiographic and histologic evidence of postnatal neurogenesis in rats. J Comp Neurol 124:319–335.

Alvarez-Buylla A, Garcia-Verdugo JM (2002) Neurogenesis in adult subventricular zone. J Neurosci 22:629–634.

Alvarez-Buylla A, Garcia-Verdugo JM, Tramontin AD (2001) A unified hypothesis on the lineage of neural stem cells. Nat Rev Neurosci 2:287–293.

Alvarez-Dolado M, Pardal R, Garcia-Verdugo JM, Fike JR, Lee HO, Pfeffer K, Lois C, Morrison SJ, Alvarez-Buylla A (2003) Fusion of bone-marrow-derived cells with Purkinje neurons, cardiomyocytes and hepatocytes. Nature 425:968–973.

Anderson DJ (2001) Stem cells and pattern formation in the nervous system: the possible versus the actual. Neuron 30:19–35.

Anderson DJ, Gage FH, Weissman IL (2001) Can stem cells cross lineage boundaries? Nat Med 7:393–395.

Arvidsson A, Collin T, Kirik D, Kokaia Z, Lindvall O (2002) Neuronal replacement from endogenous precursors in the adult brain after stroke. Nat Med 8:963–970.

Asano T, Ageyama N, Takeuchi K, Momoeda M, Kitano Y, Sasaki K, Ueda Y, Suzuki Y, Kondo Y, Torii R, Hasegawa M, Ookawara S, Harii K, Terao K, Ozawa K, Hanazono Y (2003) Engraftment and tumor formation after allogeneic in utero transplantation of primate embryonic stem cells. Transplantation 76:1061–1067.

Aubert J, Dunstan H, Chambers I, Smith A (2002) Functional gene screening in embryonic stem cells implicates Wnt antagonism in neural differentiation. Nat Biotechnol 20:1240–1245.

Belachew S, Chittajallu R, Aguirre AA, Yuan X, Kirby M, Anderson S, Gallo V (2003) Postnatal NG2 proteoglycan-expressing progenitor cells are intrinsically multipotent and generate functional neurons. J Cell Biol 161:169–186.

Berry M, Hubbard P, Butt AM (2002) Cytology and lineage of NG2–positive glia. J Neurocytol 31:457–467.

Bjorklund LM, Sanchez-Pernaute R, Chung S, Andersson T, Chen IY, McNaught KS, Brownell AL, Jenkins BG, Wahlestedt C, Kim KS, Isacson O (2002) Embryonic stem cells develop into functional dopaminergic neurons after transplantation in a Parkinson rat model. Proc Natl Acad Sci USA 8:8.

Bjornson CR, Rietze RL, Reynolds BA, Magli MC, Vescovi AL (1999) Turning brain into blood: a hematopoietic fate adopted by adult neural stem cells in vivo. Science 283:534–537.

Blau HM, Brazelton TR, Weimann JM (2001) The evolving concept of a stem cell: entity or function? Cell 105:829–841.

Boulder Committee (1970) Embryonic vertebrate central nervous system: revised terminology. The Boulder Committee. Anat Rec 166:257–261.

Brazelton TR, Rossi FMV, Keshet GI, Blau HM (2000) From marrow to brain: expression of neuronal phenotypes in adult mice. Science 290:1775–1779.

Brustle O, Jones KN, Learish RD, Karram K, Choudhary K, Wiestler OD, Duncan ID, McKay RD (1999) Embryonic stem cell–derived glial precursors: a source of myelinating transplants. Science 285:754–756.

Cai L, Hayes NL, Takahashi T, Caviness VS Jr., Nowakowski RS (2002) Size distribution of retrovirally marked lineages matches prediction from population measurements of cell cycle behavior. J Neurosci Res 69:731–744.

Cameron RS, Rakic P (1991) Glial cell lineage in the cerebral cortex: a review and synthesis. Glia 4:124–137.

Capela A, Temple S (2002) LeX/ssea-1 is expressed by adult mouse CNS stem cells, identifying them as nonependymal. Neuron 35:865–875.

Castelo-Branco G, Wagner J, Rodriguez FJ, Kele J, Sousa K, Rawal N, Pasolli HA, Fuchs E, Kitajewski J, Arenas E (2003) Differential regulation of midbrain dopaminergic neuron development by Wnt-1, Wnt-3a, and Wnt-5a. Proc Natl Acad Sci USA 100:12747–12752.

Cogle CR, Yachnis AT, Laywell ED, Zander DS, Wingard JR, Steindler DA, Scott EW (2004) Bone marrow transdifferentiation in brain after transplantation: a retrospective study. Lancet 363:1432–1437.

Corbin JG, Gaiano N, Machold RP, Langston A, Fishell G (2000) The *Gsh2* homeodomain gene controls multiple aspects of telencephalic development. Development 127:5007–5020.

Craig CG, Tropepe V, Morshead CM, Reynolds BA, Weiss S, van der Kooy D (1996) In vivo growth factor expansion of endogenous subependymal neural precursor cell populations in the adult mouse brain. J Neurosci 16:2649–2658.

D'Amour KA, Gage FH (2003) Genetic and functional differences between multipotent neural and pluripotent embryonic stem cells. Proc Natl Acad Sci USA 100(Suppl 1):11866–11872.

D'Arcangelo G, Miao GG, Chen SC, Soares HD, Morgan JI, Curran T (1995) A protein related to extracellular matrix proteins deleted in the mouse mutant reeler. Nature 374:719–723.

Doetsch F, Caille I, Lim DA, Garcia-Verdugo JM, Alvarez-Buylla A (1999b) Subventricular zone astrocytes are neural stem cells in the adult mammalian brain. Cell 97:703–716.

Doetsch F, Garcia-Verdugo JM, Alvarez-Buylla A (1999a) Regeneration of a germinal layer in the adult mammalian brain. Proc Natl Acad Sci USA 96:11619–11624.

Doetsch F, Petreanu L, Caille I, Garcia-Verdugo JM, Alvarez-Buylla A (2002) EGF converts transit-amplifying neurogenic precursors in the adult brain into multipotent stem cells. Neuron 36:1021–1034.

Eckenhoff MF, Rakic P (1988) Nature and fate of proliferative cells in the hippocampal dentate gyrus during the lifespan of the rhesus monkey. J Neurosci 8:2729–2747.

Ferrari G, Cusella-De Angelis G, Coletta M, Paolucci E, Stornaiuolo A, Cossu G, Mavilio F (1998) Muscle regeneration by bone marrow–derived myogenic progenitors. Science 279:1528–1530.

Filippov V, Kronenberg G, Pivneva T, Reuter K, Steiner B, Wang LP, Yamaguchi M, Kettenmann H, Kempermann G (2003) Subpopulation of nestin-expressing progenitor cells in the adult murine hippocampus shows electrophysiological and morphological characteristics of astrocytes. Mol Cell Neurosci 23:373–382.

Forster E, Tielsch A, Saum B, Weiss KH, Johanssen C, Graus-Porta D, Muller U, Frotscher M (2002) Reelin, Disabled 1, and beta 1 integrins are required for the formation of the radial glial scaffold in the hippocampus. Proc Natl Acad Sci USA 99:13178–13183.

Fu YS, Shih YT, Cheng YC, Min MY (2004) Transformation of human umbilical mesenchymal cells into neurons in vitro. J Biomed Sci 11:652–660.

Gabay L, Lowell S, Rubin LL, Anderson DJ (2003) Deregulation of dorsoventral patterning by FGF confers trilineage differentiation capacity on CNS stem cells in vitro. Neuron 40:485–499.

Gaiano N, Fishell G (2002) The role of notch in promoting glial and neural stem cell fates. Annu Rev Neurosci 25:471–490.

Galli R, Borello U, Gritti A, Minasi MG, Bjornson C, Coletta M, Mora M, De Angelis MG, Fiocco R, Cossu G, Vescovi AL (2000) Skeletal myogenic potential of human and mouse neural stem cells. Nat Neurosci 3:986–991.

Garcia AD, Doan NB, Imura T, Bush TG, Sofroniew MV (2004) GFAP-expressing progenitors are the principal source of constitutive neurogenesis in adult mouse forebrain. Nat Neurosci 7:1233–1241.

Gotz M, Stoykova A, Gruss P (1998) Pax6 controls radial glia differentiation in the cerebral cortex. Neuron 21:1031–1044.

Gregori N, Proschel C, Noble M, Mayer-Proschel M (2002) The tripotential glial-restricted precursor (GRP) cell and glial development in the spinal cord: generation of bipotential oligodendrocyte-type-2 astrocyte progenitor cells and dorsal–ventral differences in GRP cell function. J Neurosci 22:248–256.

Gritti A, Frolichsthal-Schoeller P, Galli R, Parati EA, Cova L, Pagano SF, Bjornson CR, Vescovi AL (1999) Epidermal and fibroblast growth factors behave as mitogenic regulators for a single multipotent stem cell–like population from the subventricular region of the adult mouse forebrain. J Neurosci 19:3287–3297.

Gritti A, Parati EA, Cova L, Frolichsthal P, Galli R, Wanke E, Faravelli L, Morassutti DJ, Roisen F, Nickel DD, Vescovi AL (1996) Multipotential stem cells from the adult mouse brain proliferate and self-renew in response to basic fibroblast growth factor. J Neurosci 16:1091–1100.

Gussoni E, Soneoka Y, Strickland CD, Buzney EA, Khan MK, Flint AF, Kunkel LM, Mulligan RC (1999) Dystrophin expression in the *mdx* mouse restored by stem cell transplantation. Nature 401:390–394.

Hack MA, Sugimori M, Lundberg C, Nakafuku M, Gotz M (2004) Regionalization and fate specification in neurospheres: the role of Olig2 and Pax6. Mol Cell Neurosci 25:664–678.

Hall AC, Mira H, Wagner J, Arenas E (2003) Region-specific effects of glia on neuronal induction and differentiation with a focus on dopaminergic neurons. Glia 43:47–51.

Hartfuss E, Forster E, Bock HH, Hack MA, Leprince P, Luque JM, Herz J, Frotscher M, Gotz M (2003) Reelin signaling directly affects radial glia morphology and biochemical maturation. Development 130:4597–4609.

Hartfuss E, Galli R, Heins N, Gotz M (2001) Characterization of CNS precursor subtypes and radial glia. Dev Biol 229:15–30.

Hermann A, Gastl R, Liebau S, Popa MO, Fiedler J, Boehm BO, Maisel M, Lerche H, Schwarz J, Brenner R, Storch A (2004) Efficient generation of neural stem cell–like cells from adult human bone marrow stromal cells. J Cell Sci 117:4411–4422.

Herrera J, Yang H, Zhang SC, Proschel C, Tresco P, Duncan ID, Luskin M, Mayer-Proschel M (2001) Embryonic-derived glial-restricted precursor cells (GRP cells) can differentiate into astrocytes and oligodendrocytes in vivo. Exp Neurol 171:11–21.

Hitoshi S, Alexson T, Tropepe V, Donoviel D, Elia AJ, Nye JS, Conlon RA, Mak TW, Bernstein A, van der Kooy D (2002b) Notch pathway molecules are essential for the maintenance, but not the generation, of mammalian neural stem cells. Genes Dev 16:846–858.

Hitoshi S, Tropepe V, Ekker M, van der Kooy D (2002a) Neural stem cell lineages are regionally specified, but not committed, within distinct compartments of the developing brain. Development 129:233–244.

Horner PJ, Thallmair M, Gage FH (2002) Defining the NG2-expressing cell of the adult CNS. J Neurocytol 31:469–480.

Jiang Y, Jahagirdar BN, Reinhardt RL, Schwartz RE, Keene CD, Ortiz-Gonzalez XR, Reyes M, Lenvik T, Lund T, Blackstad M, Du J, Aldrich S, Lisberg A, Low WC, Largaespada DA, Verfaillie CM (2002) Pluripotency of mesenchymal stem cells derived from adult marrow. Nature 418:41–49.

Johansson CB, Momma S, Clarke DL, Risling M, Lendahl U, Frisen J (1999) Identification of a neural stem cell in the adult mammalian central nervous system. Cell 96:25–34.

Kang SK, Lee DH, Bae YC, Kim HK, Baik SY, Jung JS (2003) Improvement of neurological deficits by intracerebral transplantation of human adipose tissue–derived stromal cells after cerebral ischemia in rats. Exp Neurol 183:355–366.

Kaplan MS (1983) Proliferation of subependymal cells in the adult primate CNS: differential uptake of DNA labelled precursors. J Hirnforsch 24:23–33.

Kilpatrick TJ, Bartlett PF (1993) Cloning and growth of multipotential neural precursors: requirements for proliferation and differentiation. Neuron 10:255–265.

Kilpatrick TJ, Bartlett PF (1995) Cloned multipotential precursors from the mouse cerebrum require FGF-2, whereas glial restricted precursors are stimulated with either FGF-2 or EGF. J Neurosci 15:3653–3661.

Kim M, Morshead CM (2003) Distinct populations of forebrain neural stem and progenitor cells can be isolated using side-population analysis. J Neurosci 23:10703–10709.

Koblar SA, Turnley AM, Classon BJ, Reid KL, Ware CB, Cheema SS, Murphy M, Bartlett PF (1998) Neural precursor differentiation into astrocytes requires signaling through the leukemia inhibitory factor. Proc Natl Acad Sci USA 95:3178–3181.

Kosodo Y, Roper K, Haubensak W, Marzesco AM, Corbeil D, Huttner WB (2004) Asymmetric distribution of the apical plasma membrane during neurogenic divisions of mammalian neuroepithelial cells. EMBO J 23:2314–2324.

Kriegstein AR, Gotz M (2003) Radial glia diversity: a matter of cell fate. Glia 43:37–43.

Kronenberg G, Reuter K, Steiner B, Brandt MD, Jessberger S, Yamaguchi M, Kempermann G (2003) Subpopulations of proliferating cells of the adult hippocampus respond differently to physiologic neurogenic stimuli. J Comp Neurol 467:455–463.

Kukekov VG, Laywell ED, Thomas LB, Steindler DA (1997) A nestin-negative precursor cell from the adult mouse brain gives rise to neurons and glia. Glia 21:399–407.

Lagasse E, Connors H, Al-Dhalimy M, Reitsma M, Dohse M, Osborne L, Wang X, Finegold M, Weissman IL, Grompe M (2000) Purified hematopoietic stem cells can differentiate into hepatocytes in vivo. Nat Med 6:1229–1234.

Langa F, Kress C, Colucci-Guyon E, Khun H, Vandormael-Pournin S, Huerre M, Babinet C (2000) Teratocarcinomas induced by embryonic stem (ES) cells lacking vimentin: an approach to study the role of vimentin in tumorigenesis. J Cell Sci 113 (Pt 19):3463–3472.

Lee RH, Kim B, Choi I, Kim H, Choi HS, Suh K, Bae YC, Jung JS (2004) Characterization and expression analysis of mesenchymal stem cells from human bone marrow and adipose tissue. Cell Physiol Biochem 14:311–324.

Lee SH, Lumelsky N, Studer L, Auerbach JM, McKay RD (2000) Efficient generation of midbrain and hindbrain neurons from mouse embryonic stem cells. Nat Biotechnol 18:675–679.

Lendahl U, Zimmerman LB, McKay RDG (1990) CNS stem cells express a new class of intermediate filament protein. Cell 60:585–595.

Levy YS, Merims D, Panet H, Barhum Y, Melamed E, Offen D (2003) Induction of neuron-specific enolase promoter and neuronal markers in differentiated mouse bone marrow stromal cells. J Mol Neurosci 21:121–132.

Lie DC, Dziewczapolski G, Willhoite AR, Kaspar BK, Shults CW, Gage FH (2002) The adult substantia nigra contains progenitor cells with neurogenic potential. J Neurosci 22:6639–6649.

Liu Y, Rao MS (2004) Glial progenitors in the CNS and possible lineage relationships among them. Biol Cell 96:279–290.

Liu Y, Wu Y, Lee JC, Xue H, Pevny LH, Kaprielian Z, Rao MS (2002) Oligodendrocyte and astrocyte development in rodents: an in situ and immunohistological analysis during embryonic development. Glia 40:25–43.

Magavi S, Leavitt B, Macklis J (2000) Induction of neurogenesis in the neocortex of adult mice. Nature 405:951–955.

Malatesta P, Hack MA, Hartfuss E, Kettenmann H, Klinkert W, Kirchhoff F, Gotz M (2003) Neuronal or glial progeny: regional differences in radial glia fate. Neuron 37:751–764.

Malatesta P, Hartfuss E, Gotz M (2000) Isolation of radial glial cells by fluorescent-activated cell sorting reveals a neuronal lineage. Development 127:5253–5263.

Maslov AY, Barone TA, Plunkett RJ, Pruitt SC (2004) Neural stem cell detection, characterization, and age-related changes in the subventricular zone of mice. J Neurosci 24:1726–1733.

McCarthy M, Turnbull DH, Walsh CA, Fishell G (2001) Telencephalic neural progenitors appear to be restricted to regional and glial fates before the onset of neurogenesis. J Neurosci 21:6772–6781.

McKay R (1997) Stem cells in the central nervous system. Science 276:66–71.

Mezey E, Chandross KJ, Harta G, Maki RA, McKercher SR (2000) Turning blood into brain: cells bearing neuronal antigens generated in vivo from bone marrow. Science 290:1779–1782.

Misson JP, Austin CP, Takahashi T, Cepko CL, Caviness VS, Jr. (1991) The alignment of migrating neural cells in relation to the murine neopallial radial glial fiber system. Cereb Cortex 1:221–229.

Morrison SJ, Shah NM, Anderson DJ (1997) Regulatory mechanisms in stem cell biology. Cell 88:287–298.

Morshead CM, Craig CG, van der Kooy D (1998) In vivo clonal analyses reveal the properties of endogenous neural stem cell proliferation in the adult mammalian forebrain. Development 125:2251–2261.

Morshead CM, Garcia AD, Sofroniew MV, van Der Kooy D (2003) The ablation of glial fibrillary acidic protein-positive cells from the adult central nervous system results in the loss of forebrain neural stem cells but not retinal stem cells. Eur J Neurosci 18:76–84.

Morshead CM, Reynolds BA, Craig CG, McBurney MW, Staines WA, Morassutti D, Weiss S, van der Kooy D (1994) Neural stem cells in the adult mammalian forebrain: a relatively quiescent subpopulation of subependymal cells. Neuron 13:1071–1082.

Morshead CM, van der Kooy D (2004) Disguising adult neural stem cells. Curr Opin Neurobiol 14:125–131.

Mujtaba T, Piper DR, Kalyani A, Groves AK, Lucero MT, Rao MS (1999) Lineage-restricted neural precursors can be isolated from both the mouse neural tube and cultured ES cells. Dev Biol 214:113–127.

Neuhuber B, Gallo G, Howard L, Kostura L, Mackay A, Fischer I (2004) Reevaluation of in vitro differentiation protocols for bone marrow stromal cells: disruption of actin cytoskeleton induces rapid morphological changes and mimics neuronal phenotype. J Neurosci Res 77:192–204.

Nishiyama A, Lin XH, Giese N, Heldin CH, Stallcup WB (1996) Co-localization of NG2 proteoglycan and PDGF alpha-receptor on O2A progenitor cells in the developing rat brain. J Neurosci Res 43:299–314.

Noble M, Proschel C, Mayer-Proschel M (2004) Getting a GR(i)P on oligodendrocyte development. Dev Biol 265:33–52.

Noctor SC, Flint AC, Weissman TA, Dammerman RS, Kriegstein AR (2001) Neurons derived from radial glial cells establish radial units in neocortex. Nature 409:714–720.

Noctor SC, Flint AC, Weissman TA, Wong WS, Clinton BK, Kriegstein AR (2002) Dividing precursor cells of the embryonic cortical ventricular zone have morphological and molecular characteristics of radial glia. J Neurosci 22:3161–3173.

Ostenfeld T, Joly E, Tai YT, Peters A, Caldwell M, Jauniaux E, Svendsen CN (2002) Regional specification of rodent and human neurospheres. Brain Res Dev Brain Res 134:43–55.

Padovan CS, Jahn K, Birnbaum T, Reich P, Sostak P, Strupp M, Straube A (2003) Expression of neuronal markers in differentiated marrow stromal cells and CD133+ stem-like cells. Cell Transplant 12:839–848.

Palmer TD, Markakis EA, Willhoite AR, Safar F, Gage FH (1999) Fibroblast growth factor-2 activates a latent neurogenic program in neural stem cells from diverse regions of the adult CNS. J Neurosci 19:8487–8497.

Palmer TD, Ray J, Gage FH (1995) FGF-2-responsive neuronal progenitors reside in proliferative and quiescent regions of the adult rodent brain. Mol Cell Neurosci 6:474–486.

Palmer TD, Schwartz PH, Taupin P, Kaspar B, Stein SA, Gage FH (2001) Cell culture. Progenitor cells from human brain after death. Nature 411:42–43.

Palmer TD, Willhoite AR, Gage FH (2000) Vascular niche for adult hippocampal neurogenesis. J Comp Neurol 425:479–494.

Parent JM, Vexler ZS, Gong C, Derugin N, Ferriero DM (2002) Rat forebrain neurogenesis and striatal neuron replacement after focal stroke. Ann Neurol 52:802–813.

Parmar M, Skogh C, Bjorklund A, Campbell K (2002) Regional specification of neurosphere cultures derived from subregions of the embryonic telencephalon. Mol Cell Neurosci 21:645–656.

Perrier AL, Studer L (2003) Making and repairing the mammalian brain—in vitro production of dopaminergic neurons. Semin Cell Dev Biol 14:181–189.

Pevny LH, Sockanathan S, Placzek M, Lovell-Badge R (1998) A role for *SOX1* in neural determination. Development 125:1967–1978.

Pincus DW, Keyoung HM, Harrison-Restelli C, Goodman RR, Fraser RA, Edgar M, Sakakibara S, Okano H, Nedergaard M, Goldman SA (1998) Fibroblast growth factor-2/brain-derived neurotrophic factor-associated maturation of new neurons generated from adult human subependymal cells. Ann Neurol 43:576–585.

Priller J, Persons DA, Klett FF, Kempermann G, Kreutzberg GW, Dirnagl U (2001) Neogenesis of cerebellar Purkinje neurons from gene-marked bone marrow cells in vivo. J Cell Biol 155:733–738.

Raff MC, Miller RH, Noble M (1983) A glial progenitor cell that develops in vitro into an astrocyte or an oligodendrocyte depending on culture medium. Nature 303:390–396.

Rakic P (1971) Neuron–glia relationship during granule cell migration in developing cerebellar cortex. A Golgi and electron microscopic study in *Macacus rhesus*. J Comp Neurol 141:283–312.

Rakic P (1972) Mode of cell migration to the superficial layers of fetal monkey neocortex. J Comp Neurol 145:61–83.

Rakic P (1974) Neurons in rhesus monkey visual cortex: systematic relation between time of origin and eventual disposition. Science 183:425–427.

Ramalho-Santos M, Yoon S, Matsuzaki Y, Mulligan RC, Melton DA (2002) "Stemness": transcriptional profiling of embryonic and adult stem cells. Science 298:597–600.

Rao M (2004) Stem and precursor cells in the nervous system. J Neurotrauma 21:415–427.

Rathjen J, Haines BP, Hudson KM, Nesci A, Dunn S, Rathjen PD (2002) Directed differentiation of pluripotent cells to neural lineages: homogeneous formation and differentiation of a neurectoderm population. Development 129:2649–2661.

Ray J, Raymon HK, Gage FH (1995) Generation and culturing of precursor cells and neuroblasts from embryonic and adult central nervous system. Methods Enzymol 254:20–37.

Reubinoff BE, Pera MF, Fong CY, Trounson A, Bongso A (2000) Embryonic stem cell lines from human blastocysts: somatic differentiation in vitro. Nat Biotechnol 18:399–404.

Reynolds BA, Tetzlaff W, Weiss S (1992) A multipotent EGF-responsive striatal embryonic progenitor cell produces neurons and astrocytes. J Neurosci 12:4565–4574.

Reynolds BA, Weiss S (1992) Generation of neurons and astrocytes from isolated cells of the adult mammalian central nervous system. Science 255:1707–1710.

Rice DS, Curran T (2001) Role of the reelin signaling pathway in central nervous system development. Annu Rev Neurosci 24:1005–1039.

Richards LJ, Kilpatrick TJ, Bartlett PF (1992) De novo generation of neuronal cells from the adult mouse brain. Proc Natl Acad Sci USA 89:8591–8595.

Rickmann M, Amaral DG, Cowan WM (1987) Organization of radial glial cells during the development of the rat dentate gyrus. J Comp Neurol 264:449–479.

Rietze RL, Valcanis H, Brooker GF, Thomas T, Voss AK, Bartlett PF (2001) Purification of a pluripotent neural stem cell from the adult mouse brain. Nature 412:736–739.

Rousselot P, Heintz N, Nottebohm F (1997) Expression of brain lipid binding protein in the brain of the adult canary and its implications for adult neurogenesis. J Comp Neurol 385:415–426.

Roy NS, Benraiss A, Wang S, Fraser RA, Goodman R, Couldwell WT, Nedergaard M, Kawaguchi A, Okano H, Goldman SA (2000) Promoter-targeted selection and isolation of neural progenitor cells from the adult human ventricular zone. J Neurosci Res 59:321–331.

Roy NS, Wang S, Harrison-Restelli C, Benraiss A, Fraser RA, Gravel M, Braun PE, Goldman SA (1999) Identification, isolation, and promoter-defined separation of mitotic oligodendrocyte progenitor cells from the adult human subcortical white matter. J Neurosci 19:9986–9995.

Sakakibara S, Imai T, Hamaguchi K, Okabe M, Aruga J, Nakajima K, Yasutomi D, Nagata T, Kurihara Y, Uesugi S, Miyata T, Ogawa M, Mikoshiba K, Okano H (1996) Mouse-Musashi-1, a neural RNA-binding protein highly enriched in the mammalian CNS stem cell. Dev Biol 176:230–242.

Sakurada K, Ohshima-Sakurada M, Palmer TD, Gage FH (1999) Nurr1, an orphan nuclear receptor, is a transcriptional activator of endogenous tyrosine hydroxylase in neural progenitor cells derived from the adult brain. Development 126:4017–4026.

Santa-Olalla J, Baizabal JM, Fregoso M, del Carmen Cardenas M, Covarrubias L (2003) The in vivo positional identity gene expression code is not preserved in neural stem cells grown in culture. Eur J Neurosci 18:1073–1084.

Sawamoto K, Yamamoto A, Kawaguchi A, Yamaguchi M, Mori K, Goldman SA, Okano H (2001) Direct isolation of committed neuronal progenitor cells from transgenic mice coexpressing spectrally distinct fluorescent proteins regulated by stage-specific neural promoters. J Neurosci Res 65:220–227.

Schmechel DE, Rakic P (1979) A Golgi study of radial glial cells in developing monkey telencephalon: morphogenesis and transformation into astrocytes. Anat Embryol (Berl) 156:115–152.

Scholer HR, Ruppert S, Suzuki N, Chowdhury K, Gruss P (1990) New type of POU domain in germ line–specific protein Oct-4. Nature 344:435–439.

Schwartz PH, Bryant PJ, Fuja TJ, Su H, O'Dowd DK, Klassen H (2003) Isolation and characterization of neural progenitor cells from post-mortem human cortex. J Neurosci Res 74:838–851.

Seaberg RM, van der Kooy D (2002) Adult rodent neurogenic regions: the ventricular subependyma contains neural stem cells, but the dentate gyrus contains restricted progenitors. J Neurosci 22:1784–1793.

Seaberg RM, van der Kooy D (2003) Stem and progenitor cells: the premature desertion of rigorous definitions. Trends Neurosci 26:125–131.

Seri B, Garcia-Verdugo JM, McEwen BS, Alvarez-Buylla A (2001) Astrocytes give rise to new neurons in the adult mammalian hippocampus. J Neurosci 21:7153–7160.

Shi Y, Chichung Lie D, Taupin P, Nakashima K, Ray J, Yu RT, Gage FH, Evans RM (2004) Expression and function of orphan nuclear receptor TLX in adult neural stem cells. Nature 427:78–83.

Shihabuddin LS, Horner PJ, Ray J, Gage FH (2000) Adult spinal cord stem cells generate neurons after transplantation in the adult dentate gyrus. J Neurosci 20:8727–8735.

Stallcup WB (2002) The NG2 proteoglycan: past insights and future prospects. J Neurocytol 31:423–435.

Steiner B, Kronenberg G, Jessberger S, Brandt MD, Reuter K, Kempermann G (2004) Differential regulation of gliogenesis in the context of adult hippocampal neurogenesis in mice. Glia 46:41–52.

Stenman J, Toresson H, Campbell K (2003) Identification of two distinct progenitor populations in the lateral ganglionic eminence: implications for striatal and olfactory bulb neurogenesis. J Neurosci 23:167–174.

Stoykova A, Fritsch R, Walther C, Gruss P (1996) Forebrain patterning defects in *Small eye* mutant mice. Development 122:3453–3465.

Studer L, Csete M, Lee SH, Kabbani N, Walikonis J, Wold B, McKay R (2000) Enhanced proliferation, survival, and dopaminergic differentiation of CNS precursors in lowered oxygen. J Neurosci 20:7377–7383.

Suhonen JO, Peterson DA, Ray J, Gage FH (1996) Differentiation of adult hippocampus-derived progenitors into olfactory neurons in vivo. Nature 383:624–627.

Sundholm-Peters NL, Yang HK, Goings GE, Walker AS, Szele FG (2004) Radial glia–like cells at the base of the lateral ventricles in adult mice. J Neurocytol 33:153–164.

Takahashi M, Palmer TD, Takahashi J, Gage FH (1998) Widespread integration and survival of adult-derived neural progenitor cells in the developing optic retina. Mol Cell Neurosci 12:340–348.

Takahashi T, Nowakowski RS, Caviness VS Jr. (1996) The leaving or Q fraction of the murine cerebral proliferative epithelium: a general model of neocortical neuronogenesis. J Neurosci 16:6183–6196.

Terada N, Hamazaki T, Oka M, Hoki M, Mastalerz DM, Nakano Y, Meyer EM, Morel L, Petersen BE, Scott EW (2002) Bone marrow cells adopt the phenotype of other cells by spontaneous cell fusion. Nature 416:542–545.

Thomson JA, Marshall VS, Trojanowski JQ (1998) Neural differentiation of rhesus embryonic stem cells. APMIS 106:149–156; discussion 156–147.

Toma JG, Akhavan M, Fernandes KJ, Barnabe-Heider F, Sadikot A, Kaplan DR, Miller FD (2001) Isolation of multipotent adult stem cells from the dermis of mammalian skin. Nat Cell Biol 3:778–784.

Tramontin AD, Garcia-Verdugo JM, Lim DA, Alvarez-Buylla A (2003) Postnatal development of radial glia and the ventricular zone (VZ): a continuum of the neural stem cell compartment. Cereb Cortex 13:580–587.

Uchida K, Kumihashi K, Kurosawa S, Kobayashi T, Itoi K, Machida T (2002) Stimulatory effects of prostaglandin E2 on neurogenesis in the dentate gyrus of the adult rat. Zoolog Sci 19:1211–1216.

van der Kooy D, Weiss S (2000) Why stem cells? Science 287:1439–1441.

Voigt T (1989) Development of glial cells in the cerebral wall of ferrets: direct tracing of their transformation from radial glia into astrocytes. J Comp Neurol 289:74–88.

Wagers AJ, Sherwood RI, Christensen JL, Weissman IL (2002) Little evidence for developmental plasticity of adult hematopoietic stem cells. Science 297:2256–2259.

Walsh C, Cepko CL (1992) Widespread dispersion of neuronal clones across functional regions of the cerebral cortex. Science 255:434–440.

Wang X, Willenbring H, Akkari Y, Torimaru Y, Foster M, Al-Dhalimy M, Lagasse E, Finegold M, Olson S, Grompe M (2003) Cell fusion is the principal source of bone-marrow-derived hepatocytes. Nature 422:897–901.

Wassarman KM, Lewandoski M, Campbell K, Joyner AL, Rubenstein JL, Martinez S, Martin GR (1997) Specification of the anterior hindbrain and establishment of a normal mid/hindbrain organizer is dependent on *Gbx2* gene function. Development 124:2923–2934.

Weimann JM, Charlton CA, Brazelton TR, Hackman RC, Blau HM (2003) Contribution of transplanted bone marrow cells to Purkinje neurons in human adult brains. Proc Natl Acad Sci USA 100:2088–2093.

Weissman IL, Anderson DJ, Gage F (2001) Stem and progenitor cells: origins, phenotypes, lineage commitments, and transdifferentiations. Annu Rev Cell Dev Biol 17:387–403.

Westmoreland JJ, Hancock CR, Condie BG (2001) Neuronal development of embryonic stem cells: a model of GABAergic neuron differentiation. Biochem Biophys Res Commun 284:674–680.

Woodbury D, Reynolds K, Black IB (2002) Adult bone marrow stromal stem cells express germline, ectodermal, endodermal, and mesodermal genes prior to neurogenesis. J Neurosci Res 69:908–917.

Wurmser AE, Nakashima K, Summers RG, Toni N, D'Amour KA, Lie DC, Gage FH (2004) Cell fusion–independent differentiation of neural stem cells to the endothelial lineage. Nature 430:350–356.

Yamaguchi M, Saito H, Suzuki M, Mori K (2000) Visualization of neurogenesis in the central nervous system using nestin promoter-GFP transgenic mice. Neuroreport 11:1991–1996.

Yang LY, Liu XM, Sun B, Hui GZ, Fei J, Guo LH (2004) Adipose tissue–derived stromal cells express neuronal phenotypes. Chin Med J (Engl) 117:425–429.

Ying QL, Nichols J, Evans EP, Smith AG (2002) Changing potency by spontaneous fusion. Nature 416:545–548.

Yun K, Potter S, Rubenstein JL (2001) Gsh2 and Pax6 play complementary roles in dorsoventral patterning of the mammalian telencephalon. Development 128:193–205.

Zhang SC, Wernig M, Duncan ID, Brustle O, Thomson JA (2001) In vitro differentiation of transplantable neural precursors from human embryonic stem cells. Nat Biotechnol 19:1129–1133.

4

Neuronal Development

Neural stem cell biology of the adult organism and the study of adult neurogenesis are essentially neural developmental biology under the conditions of the adult brain. To understand the particularities of adult neurogenesis it is necessary to see it in the context of neural development in general. In this chapter we will take up some of the thoughts about precursor cells in the developing brain that were discussed in the previous chapter. We will take a closer look at development of the brain and the different roles that precursor cells play within it. Although the overview provided in this chapter is limited and selective in terms of key concepts relevant to adult neurogenesis, it is important that adult neurogenesis be seen against the backdrop of neurogenesis in a general sense.

If neural stem cell biology is developmental biology, the reverse is also true: brain development is to a large degree a matter of stem cells. All development originates from stem cells, which are those cells in which the genome is in its most accessible form. Development is the realization of the potentials the genome harbors.

From the very first moment when the egg becomes fertilized, its further development is governed by an interaction between the DNA and the environment, or everything that is not the DNA. One might even argue that for any given gene, *environment* could mean other genes as well.

The most direct molecular interactors with DNA are transcription factors, which are regulatory molecules that have a DNA binding motif. Alone but often together with cofactors a transcription factor can bind to regulatory regions of a specific gene and induce or inhibit its transcription. Because transcription factors interact directly with the genome and its potentials they are at the center of studies on mechanisms of development and stem cell biology. Networks of intracellular signaling cascades converge on transcription factors and lead to their activation or inhibition. Transcription factors are thus like the home stretch in a complex cascade of regulation.

The human organism is built from a mere 30,000 genes. This efficiency is only possible because genes have different meanings in different contexts. Many structural proteins and even RNA can double as enzymes, for example. Different organs contain the same basic structural elements but use them toward different ends. The same principle applies to transcription factors and other intracellular signaling molecules. During brain development the same repertoire of regulatory molecules and transcription factors is active at different stages of development. The exact function, however, differs with location and time and is thus context-sensitive. Development is a temporally unidirectional shift of such contexts. As a consequence, transcription factors ultimately induce the shifts in their own meaning. Very few factors are specific for only one developmental situation. An understanding of the molecular bases of adult neurogenesis requires not only identification of the factors involved but also their position in a regulatory network.

ASYMMETRIC DIVISION AS A FUNDAMENTAL MECHANISM OF STEM CELL BIOLOGY

Fundamental insight into the molecular bases of neuronal development came from work on the flatworm *Caenorhabiditis elegans*, the dew fly *Drosophila melanogaster*, and the zebrafish *Danio rerio*. In these species many genes and mechanisms regulating neurogenesis are highly conserved. The homologues in the different animals can play different roles, however, and mammals often have more and other isoforms of a given factor than nematodes, insects, or lower vertebrates. The contributions of individual molecules to identifiable steps of neuronal development can nonetheless be successfully studied in these less complex organisms.

The divisions of neuroblasts in *Drosophila* contain some essential concepts of neural stem cell biology in nucleo. We have seen in Chapter 3 that asymmetric divisions are a hallmark of stem cells. In theory, only through asymmetric divisions can self-renewal be combined with the ability to differentiate. Asymmetric divisions generate cells with different fates. It is still possible that in some contexts, asymmetric division might not be a characteristic of individual precursor cells but its consequence (daughter cells with different fates) could be achieved in a stochastic manner within a population of differentiating precursor cells. But asymmetric divisions of neuroepithelial cells and neuroblasts have been directly visualized with time-lapse videomicroscopy (Haubensak et al., 2004). Asymmetric divisions of radial glia, which have neural stem cell properties, have been observed in a similar way (Miyata et al., 2001; Noctor et al., 2001).

In *Drosophila* larvae, the neuroblasts individually move from their initial position in the band of neuroepithelial cells into they embryo. The neuroblasts divide asymmetrically, producing one neuroblast and one so-called ganglion mother cell. This ganglion mother cell divides exactly one more time, resulting in the presence of two glial or neuronal cells (plus the neuroblast from the first, asymmetric division). As shown in Figure 4–1 (Color Plate 4), this asymmetrical division occurs in a highly organized spatial pattern. The neuroblasts are polarized cells, just like most other epithelial (surface) cells. Polarity means, for example, that with reference to the apical surface, cellular contents are not randomly distributed within the cell but show a spatial preference. In *Drosophila* neuroblasts a number of transcription factors, such as Numb, Prospero, Miranda, Staufen, Inscutable, and Bazooka, show a polar distribution. Inscutable and Bazooka are located

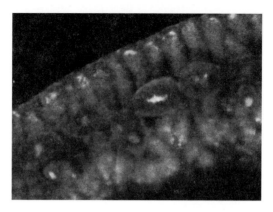

Figure 4–1 (Color Plate 4). Asymmetric cell division in *Drosophila* larvae. Embryonic *Drosophila* neuroblasts delaminate from the single-layered neuroectodermal epithelium (top) and subsequently divide repeatedly in an asymmetric fashion. Both the epithelium and the neuroblasts show a pronounced apical–basal polarity. In both cell types, the Bazooka/PAR-3 protein (red) is localized in the apical cytocortex. In contrast, the Miranda protein (blue), which functions as an adaptor protein for the cell fate determinant Prospero, is restricted to the basal cortex of dividing neuroblasts and segregates exclusively into the budding ganglion mother cell. DNA is stained in green. Apical is the top of the figure. Image by Andreas Wodarz, Göttingen.

apically; Numb, Prospero, and Miranda are located basally. This distribution is an active, cytosceleton-dependent process.

The neuroblasts divide along a horizontal plane parallel to the apical surface (Fig. 4–2). The metaphase plane of the mitotic spindle separates the cell into two compartments, one apical, one basal, that differ in their contents of transcription factors. Consequently, when the division is completed, the two daughter cells carry different transcriptional signals within them. For example, Prospero, which is located in the basal compartment of the neuroblast and is thus later found in the ganglion mother cell, ultimately induces the exit from the cell cycle and is involved in determining that a ganglion mother cell divides only one more time. The mammalian homologue to Prospero is Prox1, which seems to play an important and potentially similar role in adult hippocampal neurogenesis. Numb, on the other hand, which co-segregates with Prospero to the basal compartment of the neuroblast, can again be distributed asymmetrically before the second division, allowing the development of cells with two different fates (two neuronal phenotypes) from one ganglion mother cell.

In *Drosophila*, symmetric divisions are associated with a vertical cleavage plane; asymmetric divisions with a horizontal cleavage plane. In mammals, no such strict spatial orientation of the mitotic plane with a mandatory 90° turn of the cleavage plane between symmetric and asymmetric division is found. In some cases, most notably the initiation of cortical development

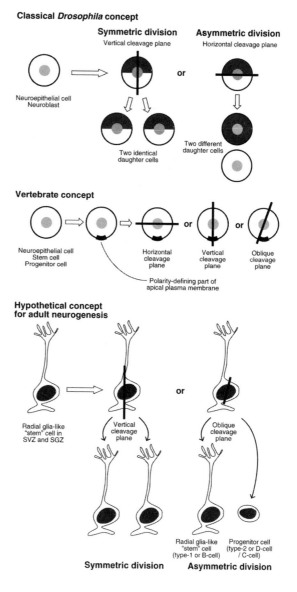

Classical *Drosophila* concept

Symmetric division
Vertical cleavage plane

Asymmetric division
Horizontal cleavage plane

Neuroepithelial cell
Neuroblast

Two identical
daughter cells

Two different
daughter cells

Vertebrate concept

Neuroepithelial cell
Stem cell
Progenitor cell

Horizontal
cleavage
plane

Vertical
cleavage
plane

Oblique
cleavage
plane

Polarity-defining part of
apical plasma membrane

**Hypothetical concept
for adult neurogenesis**

Radial glia-like
"stem" cell in
SVZ and SGZ

Vertical
cleavage
plane

Oblique
cleavage
plane

Radial glia-like
"stem" cell
(type-1 or B-cell)

Progenitor cell
(type-2 or D-cell)
/ C-cell)

Symmetric division   **Asymmetric division**

Figure 4–2. Asymmetric cell division in the mammalian brain. Mammalian stem cells show asymmetric cell divisions but depart from the pattern seen in *Drosophila* (see Fig. 4–1, Color Plate 4). In neuroepithelial cells, orientation of a small, highly specialized membrane region, characterized by expression of prominin/CD133, in relation to the cleavage plane determines whether the division is symmetric or asymmetric. The application of this concept to adult neurogenesis, as shown in the lower half of the figure, is pure speculation at present. There is no evidence of CD133 expression in the adult neurogenic regions. The concept is based on the work of Wieland Huttner and colleagues (Wodarz and Huttner, 2003; Kosodo et al., 2004).

and on a descriptive level, the pattern was initially thought to be suggestively similar to the situation in *Drosophila* (Chenn and McConnell, 1995), but this impression turned out to be not generalizable. Rather, it seems that in neuroepithelial cells and their progeny both symmetric and asymmetric divisions involve a vertical cleavage plane (Kosodo et al., 2004). However, inclusion or exclusion of a small but highly specialized portion of the apical cell membrane, characterized by the expression of prominin/CD133, is sufficient to distinguish symmetric from asymmetric divisions. The "horizontal" division thus differs only by a few degrees from a true vertical division, which would cut exactly through this small apical spot (Kosodo et al., 2004).

Despite the obvious differences, the fundamental principle is conserved in mammals that a cleavage plane, which is different from an intracellular axis formed by transcription factors involved in fate determination, causes the asymmetric distribution of these transcription factors and thereby results in different fates of the daughter cells (see Fishell and Kriegstein, 2003, for review of this concepts in relation to radial glia as precursor cells in neurogenesis). Also, many of the transcription factor associated with asymmetric divisions in *Drosophila* are conserved in mammals. The mammalian numb homologue, for example, has been shown to be connected with asymmetric division in mouse cortical development (Shen et al., 2002). Its function, however, appears to be more complex than in the fly. Notch1 is another example of a key regulatory transcription factor that is distributed asymmetrically during early mammalian neurogenesis (Chenn and McConnell, 1995). In general, however, much less is known about the molecular mechanisms underlying asymmetric stem cell divisions in vertebrates (and mammals in particular) than in flies (Wodarz and Huttner, 2003).

Irrespective of their fundamental role in stem cell biology, not all asymmetric divisions will necessarily obey the same principles. In the context of adult neurogenesis, both symmetric and asymmetric divisions occur, but details about their regulation and the asymmetric distribution of transcription factors are still lacking. The prominin/CD133-dependent mechanism characteristic of the neuroepithelial cells of embryonic brain development has not yet been detected in the neurogenic zones of the adult brain.

GENERAL PATTERNS OF MAMMALIAN BRAIN DEVELOPMENT

Brain development in mammals is characterized by three major stages. The first phase is an expansion phase, during which stem cells produce growth by massive symmetric divisions. It is followed by the phases of first neurogenesis and then gliogenesis, during which the expanded precursor cells give rise to differentiating cells. At birth, neurogenesis has ceased in most parts of the brain. Neurogenesis and gliogenesis are characterized by asymmetric divisions of the precursor cells and the co-occurrence of cell death, by which a surplus of newly generated cells is eliminated. Gliogenesis again occurs in two waves. First, astrocytes are produced after neurogenesis has begun to cease. Then, oligodendrocytes are generated, most of them postnatally. Within neurogenesis, excitatory principal or projecting neurons and inhibitory interneurons are derived from different sources and at different times.

One key topic of developmental neurobiology is the investigation of how the immense cellular diversification occurs. Symmetric and asymmetric divisions in the single layer of proliferating neuroepithelial cells in the developing mouse brain have been visualized by time-lapse microscopy *in vitro* (Qian et al., 1998, 2000; Haubensak et al., 2004). Similarly, radial glia was observed to divide asymmetrically, giving rise to another radial glia cell and one cell entering neuronal differentiation (Miyata et al., 2001; Noctor et al., 2001; Fishell and Kriegstein, 2003). It seems that neurons can thus be either derived directly from radial glia or from intermediate precursor cells (Noctor et al., 2001). Despite gross similarities in the patterns of division, however, the precursor cells in different regions of the developing brain have different potentials.

The fact that transcriptional regulation is context-sensitive gives precursor cells a positional identity, that is, a spatially and temporally determined nature depending on transcription factor patterns. This determination is more flexible in terms of space than in terms of time. Precursor cells from the spinal cord can be transplanted into the hippocampus and behave region-specifically. Precursor cells from the hippocampus can participate in the production of retinal cells. Embryonic precursor cells also readily integrate after implantation into later developmental stages. But the reverse is not necessarily true: adult precursor cells cannot generally regain functions of earlier developmental stages because development is essentially unidirectional and characterized by an increasing restriction of developmental potentials. This does not mean that this pattern could under no circumstances be overcome. As discussed in Chapter 3, the more-than-multipotent precursor cells identified in adult-generated cell cultures only after very many passages might be examples of such effective reprogramming. However, the time scales of these experiments also show that reprogramming will probably be the exception, not the rule. In vivo, indications for a reprogramming of temporal identity are scarce.

The shifting potential of precursor cells over time can be recapitulated in vitro when precursor cells are isolated at different time points of development (Qian et al., 2000). Acutely isolated cells will tend to differentiate into neurons during the peak of neurogenesis in vivo; into astrocytes when cells are taken, while astrogenesis is high; and into oligodendrocytes, if they are isolated, when the generation of oligodendrocytes dominates in vivo. The acutely isolated cells reflect the stage of brain development in vivo. More surprisingly, the temporal specification also becomes apparent when precursors isolated at early embryonic stages (embryonic day 12 [E12] of a mouse) are followed longitudinally in culture (Qian et al., 2000). These cells sequentially go through phases of predominant neurogenesis, astrogenesis, and oligodendrogenesis. The earlier cells are still multipotent, the later cells are destined to a glial fate. This implies that there must be a precursor cell–immanent program that determines the changes in developmental potential. Positional identity is thus not entirely separable from temporal identity. To some degree, a certain time is equivalent to a specific place, and vice versa.

Besides determining positional identity, two other key regulations have to occur. First, within a precursor cell's positional identity it must be instructed as to whether it should expand by symmetric or asymmetric divisions, be quiescent, or die. Second, and finally, cellular differentiation must be initiated.

Adult neurogenesis is in continuity with embryonic brain development. There is no evidence that completely different principles govern embryonic and adult neurogenesis. However, precursor cells in adult neurogenesis have a strong temporal and positional identity with a limited developmental potential in vivo. The roots for this specification lie in embryonic development. Precursor cells in the neurogenic regions of the adult brain have intrinsic properties that are region-dependent. On the other hand, as demonstrated by ex vivo experiments and manipulation of the in vivo conditions, the realization of their potential is highly dependent on the cellular microenvironment, the stem cell niche that provides neurogenic permissiveness.

FROM FERTILIZED EGG TO INITIATION OF BRAIN DEVELOPMENT

Development of the nervous system begins at the blastocyst stage of the embryo (Fig. 4–3). It is conceivable that at one brief period all embryonic stem cells are equal in their potential. Even this assumption can be questioned, however. The zygote, because of its totipotency considered the ultimate stem cell, violates one key principle for stem cells: it does not show unlimited self-renewal. After two or three divisions totipotency is lost. Many researchers are thus convinced that early development goes through a series

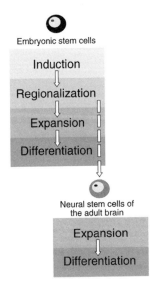

Figure 4–3. Sequence of events in brain development. Adult neurogenesis is in continuity with embryonic brain development. The neurogenic zones of the adult brain are formed during brain development (see also Fig. 3–8). Adult neurogenesis recapitulates only parts of embryonic and fetal neurogenesis.

of symmetric divisions followed by an immediate step of differentiation that makes the two daughter cells different from the mother cell. Interaction among these rapidly expanding cells would at once introduce further differences, through the simple fact that some cells find themselves in the center of the cell cluster and are thus surrounded by many others of their kind, whereas other cells are exposed to the outer environment.

Within the ectoderm neural induction leads to specification of the neuroectoderm. Induced by so-called organizer regions, the neural plate next invaginates along the midline. Known factors involved in this neural induction are noggin, chordin, and follistatin. The longitudinal groove closes on the top and thereby forms the neural tube, whose walls contain neuroepithelial precursor cells. The first neural specification of stem cells occurs here. For embryonic stem cells, development into neuroepithelial precursor cells appears to be something like a default state. Neurons also quite readily develop from embryonic stem cell cultures. The non-neuronal differentiation into epidermis, in contrast, requires active signaling through the bone morphogenic proteins (BMPs). For example, BMP 4, antagonizes chordin activity and thus suppresses neural induction.

POSITIONAL IDENTITY OF PRECURSOR CELLS

While the neural tube develops, the precursor cells become *regionalized*, that is, they acquire their positional potential. It is believed that the originally very similar precursor cells begin to distinguish themselves from their neighbors by further divisions, analogously to the model situation in the neuroblasts of *Drosophila*. The first patterning of this kind occurs along the anterior–posterior axis of the embryo. From the posterior regions, the spinal cord develops; the anterior part generates the brain. One key molecule relevant for the transition to neural patterning is retinoic acid (RA). In the developing nervous system, a posterior–anterior gradient of RA expression forms, which in turn leads to a graded induction of a class of genes called *Hox* genes in the posterior part of the neural tube that will later become spinal cord and hindbrain. Making use of this role, RA is added in vitro when growth factors are withdrawn to induce differentiation in neural precursor cell cultures.

The different *Hox* genes regulate further subdivisions of the future spinal cord. In the more anterior regions, multiple other so-called homeodomain genes are involved in specification of the precursor cells from which the telencephalic structures will develop. A particularly clear boundary is the midbrain–hindbrain border, which is characterized by a sharply defined expression of two transcription factors, Wnt1 and engrailed-1 (En1), and the growth factor FGF-8. Overexpression of FGF-8 moves the midbrain–hindbrain border posteriorly (Brodski et al., 2003).

In the anterior parts of the brain, the anterior–posterior axis is defined by growth factors FGF-2, -4, and -8, Wnt 3A and 8, ligands of nuclear RA receptors, and other so-called morphogens (Altmann and Brivanlou, 2001).

Transcription factor Emx1 defines the anterior half of the hemisphere in the telencephalon, and Emx2 defines the posterior half. *Emx2* is required for the development of a normally proportioned neocortex (Bishop et al., 2000; Mallamaci et al., 2000). The *Pax* gene family consists of nine members with numerous effects on brain development. *Pax6* in particular plays key roles at several restriction points. One of these is that Pax6 is expressed in a gradient that is the reverse of Emx2 expression. Such opposing gradients are a frequent mechanism of determining positional identity. Between the two sources of the regulatory molecules, individual positions are characterized by two coordinates defined by graded expression of each of the two factors. Moving from one source toward the other is reflected in decreasing expression of the first factor while the other increases. Higher dimensional systems with more than two gradients likely exist. Although it is not clear how a cell can sense subtle gradients and respond specifically, the spatial resolution of such a system is extremely high. The only theoretical alternative would be a system in which every single position is defined by individual molecules.

Emx2 is most strongly expressed in the posterior part of the hemispheres, Pax6 in the anterior part. In the mature cortex, various specialized areas are found along the anterior-posterior axis—the frontal, cingular, somatosensory, motor, insular, and visual cortices, to name just the largest. In a *Pax6* mutant, the posterior areas, the visual cortex, become enlarged because Emx2 activity dominates. In an *Emx2* mutant, by contrast, the more anterior areas, such as the motor cortex, are bigger because the anterior Pax6 effects dominate (Bishop et al., 2000; Mallamaci et al., 2000). FGF-8 seems to up-regulate Emx2 expression, and thus FGF-8 overexpression has a similar effect than a *Pax6* knockout.

Parallel to anterior–posterior regionalization, dorsal–ventral specification occurs. In the neural tube, the most dorsal cells (the roof plate) specialize in secreting bone morphogenic proteins (BMPs) whereas the most ventral cells (the floor plate) secrete sonic hedgehog (Shh), thereby forming another reciprocal gradients. BMP signaling is also involved in the most dorsal part of the neural tube when a population of precursor cells sequester and migrate laterally to form the neural crest, the origin of the autonomous nervous system.

Adult neurogenesis occurs only in the anterior part of the CNS not posteriorly (in the spinal cord). Neurogenesis in the adult olfactory system is ultimately derived from a ventral source; neurogenesis in the adult hippocampus is developmentally of dorsal origin.

EXPANSION THROUGH PRECURSOR CELL PROLIFERATION

The morphogens stage, responsible for positional identity, is followed by the mitogen phase. Positioned precursor cell populations are adequately expanded. Interestingly, many of the morphogens also serve as inducers of proliferation. This additional function might be a consequence of positional identity with its specific patterns of gene expression. Retinoic acid, for example, is required to maintain sufficient levels of FGF-8 and Shh expression. FGF-8 in turn appears to maintain proliferative activity. In the dorsal–ventral gradient of Wnt signaling, Wnt causes precursor cell self-renewal near the roof plate (the source of Wnt) but induces exit from the cell cycle at greater distances (Megason and McMahon, 2002). Consequently, the Wnt gradient is inversely related to neuronal differentiation, which begins ventrally. As a final example, *Emx2* and *Pax6*, both involved in patterning of the cortex, are also necessary to maintain a sufficient level of cell proliferation in the cortical germinative zones.

Some classical growth factors are probably examples of the reverse case—their primary function appears to lie in mitogenic activity (hence their name). Both EGF and FGF-2 are potent inducers of precursor cell proliferation in vitro. But at least for FGF-2, additional functions in defining positional identity have also been discussed.

With these stages the preneurogenesis phase comes to an end. The ventricular zone precursor cells undergo dramatic changes in morphology and acquire characteristics of radial glia (Gotz, 2003). The current hypothesis is that during neurogenesis radial glia act as precursor cells (Fishell and Kriegstein, 2003; Anthony et al., 2004).

In adult neurogenesis the precursor cells are thought to be direct progeny of the embryonic precursor cells (Alvarez-Buylla et al., 2001). Both neurogenic regions contain precursor cells that have certain radial glial properties but at the same time show distinguishing features. The detailed lineage relationship and developmental path are not yet known.

INDUCTION OF NEURONAL DIFFERENTIATION

Whereas differentiation of embryonic stem cells into neural precursor cells might be a default state, differentiation into neurons from these neural precursors requires active induction. The genes involved in this induction, called "proneural genes," all seem to belong to the family of basic helix-loop-helix (bHLH) genes. There seems to be a core program of bHLH activity that is involved in neurogenesis, no matter when and where the given neurons develop (Kintner, 2002). This principle is highly relevant for adult neurogenesis, although our present knowledge of bHLH genes in adult neurogenesis is limited. Some bHLH genes are primarily involved in neural determination, which is a reversible stage and different from terminal differentiation. Activity of proneural genes leads to a state of a predetermined neuroblast. Other bHLH genes are involved in inducing terminal neuronal differentiation. The activity of the latter is a consequence of the activity of the first.

Examples of determinative bHLH genes are *Mash1* and *NeuroD*, the first of which relate to the *achaete-scute* system in *Drosophila*, whereas *NeuroD* relates to *Atonal,* as do the *Neurogenins* (Brunet and Ghysen, 1999). In the fly, *achaete-scute* genes are required for the segregation of the neuroblasts by a mechanism called "lateral inhibition." They are determinative; *Neurogenin* genes, in contrast, are involved in terminal differentiation. Consequently, there is a cascade of different bHLH genes that consecutively regulates neuronal determination and differentiation. An important question is whether such a cascade of bHLH activity is relevant to adult neurogenesis and serves the same functions there.

The classic example for lateral inhibition is the function of Notch, a receptor molecule that makes cells maintain an epidermal fate. When *notch* is knocked out in *Drosophila,* essentially all ectodermal precursor cells become neuroblasts. *Achaete-scute* induces the expression of delta, one of the ligands to notch. Even within a group of neighboring identical ectodermal cells, the expression levels of individual proteins, including delta, varies slightly in a stochastic manner. An increased level of delta in one cell, call it *A,* will lead to increased binding of delta to notch on the neighboring cell, call it *B,* and the notch activation will down-regulate *achaete-scute* and consequently delta in *B.* Consequently, the neighboring cells *A* and *B* are developmentally driven apart. Lowered delta expression in *B* will mean less notch activation on *A,* further supporting neuroblast differentiation of *A.* Vertebrates have *achaete-scute* homologs such as *Mash1* and have at least four *Notch* genes plus four notch ligands (two *delta* genes and two *jagged* genes, which are homologs to the second *Drosophila* notch-ligand besides delta, serrate). Unfortunately, the intuitive system of lateral inhibition is not found in the same form in vertebrates. However, Notch inhibits the activity of proneural genes in vetebrate neurogenesis and leads to the development of astrocytes (Tanigaki et al., 2001).

Mash1, NeuroD, Neurogenin 1 and *2,* and *Math 1* and *2* are all involved in determining positional identity (at least in the dorsoventral axis of the spinal cord) and generic neuronal identity. They all prevent gliogenesis. However, their expression is largely not overlapping, indicating that they have further functions in initiating the specification of neuronal subtypes (Farah et al., 2000; Tomita et al., 2000; Mizuguchi et al., 2001; Nieto et al., 2001).

Besides the proneural genes, other factors are involved in inducing the shift from proliferation to differentiation. Again, some of the usual suspects reappear with different functions. BMP activity, for example, induces not only proliferation via activation of the BMP-1A receptor but also expression of another receptor, the BMP-1B receptor, which has an entirely different function. Activation of BMP-1B up-regulates $p21^{kip1}$, an inhibitor of the cell cycle (Panchision et al., 2001). After dorsalized cells have been primed by BMP-1A activation, BMP-1B signaling leads to neuronal differentiation. Consequently, there will be a point in development at which there is competition between the activity of the two receptors and the balance can shift either way. There are other examples of such competitive actions, and stochastic mechanisms might be an important principle to manage the transition between two developmental stages.

In those tissues of the dorsal brain that expand late, such as the cerebellum and the cortex, Shh acts as a mitogen counteracting BMP signals that induce differentiation. Again, a balance of two antagonistic factors, here two ligands at different receptors, in contrast to the situation with one ligand at two receptors discussed above, controls expansion of cell numbers and exit from the cell cycle.

Proneural genes are expressed in adult neurogenesis as well. BMP, for example, counteracts neurogenesis in the subventricular zone (SVZ) and is antagonized by locally secreted noggin to achieve neurogenic permissiveness. NeuroD is expressed early in the presumably lineage-determined precursor cells in the adult hippocampus, whereas Mash1 is expressed in the adult SVZ.

MIGRATION AND CORTICAL LAYER FORMATION

The neocortex is characterized by a highly ordered, six-layered structure parallel to the ventricular and outer surface, and a subdivision in cortical areas in the tangential dimension. The hippocampus is also a cortical region but belongs to the evolutionary older archicortex and has a simplified layered structure with only three strata. Neuronal function is specified within these spatial coordinates. Areas differ in their input and output pathways and in details of their network structure. Layers contain different neuronal populations. The two major classes are principal or projection neurons, the large pyramidal neurons of layer 2 being prime examples, and numerous types of interneurons. The cortical projection neurons are derived from the (dorsal) ventricular zone (VZ). Most interneurons, however, originate from a ventral part of the ventricular zone, called the "ganglionic eminences," and thus have to migrate in from a greater distance and cross the paths of radially migrating neurons from the VZ. All neurons have to find their place within the enfolding structure of the developing cortex (Fig. 4–4).

Molecularly, areas and layers are not defined by the expression of unique genes. Rather, positional information is derived from distinguishing expression patterns of many different genes, most notably transcription factors, that are not unique to any layer or region. The expression of the same gene can differ in different layers and different areas. Therefore, in the early VZ, where no layers yet exist, no strict molecular spatial prespecification that would represent the later areas *and* layers is possible. Arealization and layer formation are intricately linked and interdependent over development. The degree to which cortical specification of areas and layers occurs is dependent on intrinsic versus extrinsic influences, and the subject of the debate between the "protomap" theory (which favors intrinsic regulation) and the "protocortex" theory (which favors dependence on extrinsic cues).

When cell proliferation in the VZ generates the first postmitotic neurons, these accumulate on top of the VZ. The layer that forms, called the "preplate"

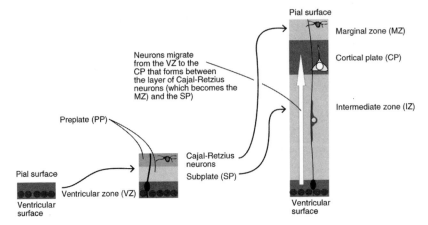

Figure 4–4. Layer formation during cortex development. The six-layered neo-cortex of the mammalian brain is built up from expanded progenitor cell pools in the ventricular and subventricular zones. See text for details. Cajal Retzius neu-rons are pioneer neurons in the outermost layer. Radial glia serves as a guidance structure for the positioning of new neurons. Adult hippocampal neurogenesis takes place in an archicortical region and reflects some of the characteristics of this pattern. These are absent in adult olfactory bulb neurogenesis.

(PP), contains a population of highly specialized neurons, the Cajal Retzius neurons. These cells with characteristic horizontal processes secrete reelin, a factor necessary for building the forming glial scaffold along which the cortical neurons find their final positions and for regulating neuronal mi-gration itself (Forster et al., 2002). Except for the Cajal Retzius neurons that remain near the pial surface of the brain throughout development, the neu-ronal populations that form first are those of the deep layers. Cortical matu-ration occurs in an inside-out fashion. The later cells have to pass those that were generated previously (Angevine and Sidman, 1961; Rakic, 1974).

At the time of PP formation, radial glia cells build up in the VZ and with their radial processes establish contact with the pial surface on top of the PP. Neurons are generated from two cellular sources: from radial glia in the VZ and from intermediate precursor cells in the SVZ (Noctor et al., 2004). New neurons use the radial processes to migrate toward the pial surface and thereby pass those that were produced earlier (Rakic, 1974). During this process they show a complex pattern of movements including an initial retrograde migration toward the ventricle, followed by a reversal of their bipolar shape and migration toward the pial surface (Noctor et al., 2004). The migrating cells accumulate within the PP and split it into an outer marginal zone (MZ), which contains the Cajal Retzius neurons and an inner "deep subplate" (SP). The new zone in between is called the "cortical plate" (CP). The CP widens while more cells migrate in and over time form the cortical layers in an inside-out fashion. The MZ transforms into layer 1; the

VZ resolves in the ependymal layer and the underlying SVZ, which remains a germinative zone throughout life. The SVZ is called a "secondary germinative matrix," because it is derived from the primary germinative zone of the VZ.

Intrinsic and extrinsic mechanisms interact in the formation of cortical area and layer specification. The general basis of neural development is that there is a permanent interaction between intrinsic (genetic) and extrinsic (activity) regulatory principles.

The SP is very homogenous across the entire cortex. The earliest developing projection neurons within the SP form very extensive and excessive immature connections. Parallel to layer formation, this far-reaching connectivity is later trimmed back to the appropriate distribution patterns. Just as neurons are generated in excess and then selected for function, the same happens with neurites of the new neurons. These selection and trimming processes are activity-dependent. The major input to the neocortex arises from the dorsal thalamus and mediates the somatic, auditory, and visual sensory input. The sensory input provides the strongest structure-forming signals at a time when the sensory experience of the outer world is limited to the uterus. In vitro data suggest that this input might already affect very early, proliferative stages of neurogenesis (Dehay et al., 2001). However, thalamocortical input of the various modalities becomes instrumental in defining the formation of areas within the CP. Increasing specification of neurons within the CP is thereby tightly linked to the growing complexity of thalamocortical projections during development. The CP becomes regionalized in an input-dependent manner.

Transcription factors can be linked to layer formation. Similar to the anterior–posterior gradient build by Emx2 and Pax6 expression, the orphan nuclear receptor COUP-TF1 is expressed low anteriorly and high posteriorly. This gradient is probably dependent on the Emx2/Pax6 gradient, because in contrast to other factors the distribution of Emx2 and Pax6 expression is normal in COUP-TF1 knockouts (Zhou et al., 2001). COUP-TF1 mutants, however, do not live long enough to determine how COUP-TF1 deficiency affects the full realization of cortical structuring. But COUP-TF1 mice lack SP and layer 4 neurons (Zhou et al., 1999). Because normally, COUP-TF1 is highly expressed in the dorsal thalamus, it might well be that these losses are due to a disturbance in thalamocortical input (Liu et al., 2000).

There are molecular mechanisms of arealization that are to some degree independent of thalamocortical input. Mice that lack the homeodomain gene *Gbx2* or bHLH gene *Mash1* fail to develop a normal prenatal thalamocortical input but have normal expression patterns for many genes in the hemispheres, a finding suggesting that these are independent of thalamocortical projections (Miyashita-Lin et al., 1999; Tuttle et al., 1999). In general, however, thalamocortical afferents are a key regulator of cortical development as much as the development of proper thalamocortical input is dependent on preceding intrinsic molecular patterns.

The hippocampus is a cortical brain structure belonging to the three-layered archicortex, and during hippocampal development a similar program to that in the neocortex unfolds. Details about the exact similarities and differences are still lacking, however. But adult hippocampal neurogenesis is likely to share more principles with embryonic neocortical development than neurogenesis in the adult olfactory bulb, which is a noncortical brain region and ultimately of ventral origin.

NEURITE EXTENSION

Neurons are polar structures with two types of neurites: the (usually) one axon and multiple dendrites differ structurally and functionally. Dendrites receive signals from other (presynaptic) neurons, and axons transmit signals to other (postsynaptic) neurons. Whereas the axon does not allow much room for individuality, the dendritic tree of a given neuronal population is something like its morphological fingerprint. Primarily by virtue of its dendritic tree, every neuron has this distinct structural identity. To achieve neurite development, neurons must first establish polarity and then translate this into determining the origins of the axon and dendrites on the soma. They must physically extend the neurites in an organized way and in tune with neighboring cells.

The complex of signaling molecules Par3, Par6, and atypical protein kinase (aPKC), which is highly conserved throughout evolution, is involved in determining polarity in epithelial cells. To some degree neurons inherit their polarity from precursor cells in asymmetric divisions, and a signal transduction cascade involving the Par3–Par6–aPKC complex takes part in establishing early neuronal polarity. If the complex is blocked in neuronal cell cultures, no axon forms among the earliest undetermined neurites (Shi et al., 2003). Beyond this internal switch, changes in cytoskeleton assembly (Inagaki et al., 2001) as well as extracellular cues determine axon selection (Esch et al., 1999). However, in vivo, axonal growth might precede dendritic growth, so that a sequential instruction rather than a selection among undetermined neurites leads to axonal growth.

Despite their fundamental differences, axons and dendrites share many similarities and many factors affect their development (Goldberg, 2003). In particular, some extracellular factors such as semaphorin 3A and slit affect both axon and dendrites. Slit and its receptors robo, for example, promote both dendrite and axon growth (Wang et al., 1999; Whitford et al., 2002). Semaphorin 3A, in contrast, attracts dendrites and repulses axons and thus has a differential effect requiring a different action on the receptor side (Song et al., 1998; Polleux et al., 2000). One hypothesis that attempts to make sense of the seemingly limited specificity of factors regulating axon and dendrite development is that neurons switch between a dendritic and axonal growth mode (Goldberg et al., 2002). In addition, neurotrophins nerve growth factor (NGF), brain-derived neurotrophic factor (BDNF), and NT3, for example, influence dendritic growth, but different types of neurons respond with a different growth and branching pattern (McAllister et al., 1997). Taken together, this implies that there are intrinsic differences both between different types of neurons and within a given neuron over time that allow specification of dendritic and axonal morphology.

Neurite development has two aspects: one is the description of the physical act of extension, the other is the molecular mechanism underlying this process. Neurites grow by sending out a highly plastic and sensitive structure called a "growth cone" that travels toward the target and trails behind the elongating neurite. Most neurons have only one axon, which can be extremely long; motoneurons in the lumbar spinal cord of humans are more than 1 meter in length. The growth cone does not have to cover this entire distance because the correctly positioned axon grows with the organism.

Axonal growth cones have to choose a path to follow and they have to decide the direction to go on this path. The pathways are defined by cell–cell interactions and extracellular matrix molecules (Hynes and Lander, 1992; Tessier-Lavigne and Goodman, 1996) and diffusible repulsive cues.

Slit, for example, first discovered in *Drosophila*, is expressed in the midline and acts as a repulsant (Simpson et al., 2000b). The different receptors for slit—robo, robo2, and robo3—mediate this effect. Axons from different cells express different combinations of robo receptors. Ectopic expression of robo2 and robo3 causes medial axons to go laterally; deletion of robo and robo2 makes lateral axons to divert medially (Rajagopalan et al., 2000; Simpson et al., 2000a).

Semaphorin 3 also acts as a repellent of axonal growth and leads to a concentration of axonal projections. When Sema3A or its receptors are knocked out, axons tend to have wider, more diffuse target fields (Kitsukawa et al., 1997; Taniguchi et al., 1997).

Directional information and polarity of axonal growth are mediated by long-range-acting diffusible cues, which can act as chemoattractants or repellents. Some axons (the commissural fibers) have to cross the midline to reach their target structure, which poses a particular problem because axons somehow have to "know" on which side of the midline they are in order to draw opposite conclusions from the cues (Tessier-Lavigne et al., 1988). In spinal cord development, chemoattractants secreted by the floor plate direct commissural growth (Placzek et al., 1990). Extracellular matrix molecules called "netrins" are candidates for being mediators of this effect (Kennedy et al., 1994; Shirasaki et al., 1995, 1996; Serafini et al., 1996).

The floor plate (and presumably its equivalent in rostral brain parts) is also thought to secrete a repellent factor that prevents those axons that should not cross the midline from doing so (Colamarino and Tessier-Lavigne, 1995; Tamada et al., 1995). Interestingly, one of these cues might be identical to one of the chemoattractants. Netrin 1 seems to act as a chemorepellent on the axons (Varela-Echavarria et al., 1997). It thus seems that, depending on the type of neurons, growth cones can draw different, even opposite conclusions from the same available cues.

Because dendrites are so numerous and cover such large territories, dendritic growth is even more complex than axon development and much less understood. Different classes of neurons have signature architectures of the dendritic trees but within this framework dendritic development is highly individual. How is this balance between shared pattern and individual form achieved? How do the dendrites know where to branch? Some factors with other functions during neuronal development play a role in the shaping of dendrites—BMPs, for example (Lein et al., 1995), and the neurotrophins (McAllister et al., 1997) are involved in this step. The slit–robo system also takes part in shaping dendritic morphology (Wang et al., 1999; Whitford et al., 2002).

In *Drosophila*, one particular class of neurons consists of four members with very distinct dendritic arborization patterns. Mutation or overexpression of homeodomain transcription factor *cut*, which also plays an earlier role in neuronal development, causes cell class–specific changes in dendritic morphology (Grueber et al., 2003). Other transcription factors have special functions in dendritic arborization. For example, studies in *Drosophila* have shown that a loss-of-function mutation of the gene *hamlet* causes cells with normally unbranched dendrites to develop elaborate dendritic trees, whereas its overexpression reduces branching in neurons with normally arborized dendrites (Moore et al., 2002).

These few examples should make sufficiently clear that neuronal development does not stop after fate determination and reaching the target position. The diverse functions of some classes of transcription factors reach well into this stage and some new genes participate in this immensely complex part of development. Like essentially all other parts of neuronal development, neurite extension is based on the interaction of innate genetic programs and environmental cues. Neurite formation is activity-dependent, and some factors such as CPG15, whose expression responds to activity, take part in mediating this aspect of development (Nedivi et al., 1998).

At present, no specific information is available about the mechanisms underlying neurite extension during adult neurogenesis. Adult hippocampal neurogenesis produces excitatory granule cells with a large dendritic field in the molecular layer of the dentate gyrus and a relatively long axon along the mossy fiber tract to hippocampal region CA3. Neurogenesis in the adult olfactory bulb, in contrast, produces two classes of interneurons with only local connections. The profoundly different patterns of connectivity of new neurons in the two neurogenic regions make it likely that various developmental mechanisms will make different contributions to the process.

ACTIVITY-DEPENDENT DEVELOPMENT OF NEURONAL CIRCUITS

One key property of brain development is that it is to a large degree activity-dependent. Developing neurons respond to electrical activity and fine-tune their development accordingly. Embryonic development proper, that is, development up to the existence of the brain anlage, appears to be relatively independent of electrical activity. In the adult, precursor cells can respond to electrical activity and such activity may be one of the factors determining the course of precursor cell proliferation and neuronal differentiation (Deisseroth et al., 2004).

For the developing brain, most data on activity-dependent regulation relate to postmitotic stages and the formation of synapses and circuits. It was long thought that axon and dendrite elongation were independent of electrical activity and only guided by chemical cues. However, electrical activity is, for example, necessary for the establishment of thalamocortical projections (Catalano and Shatz, 1998). In vitro, electrical stimulation of *Xenopus* neurons leads to an increase in cAMP, which modulates the response of growth cones to guidance cues from being repulsed to being attracted (Ming et al., 2001). In general, the response of axonal growth cones to electrical activity is cell type-dependent, making it difficult to generalize how activity influences neurite extension. Synapse formation and the establishment of neuronal networks, however, are clearly activity-dependent. Activity has influences even before synapses are present and activity determines where synapses form. Thus the presence of spots of membrane specialization that allow the exchange of information between neurons precedes the existence of morphologically definable synapses. After the axon has reached the target zone, the filopodia of the arriving growth cone seek contact. Immediately before synapses are established, filopodia on both the future pre- and postsynaptic side become highly mobile. Their contact marks the initiation of synapse formation (Alsina et al., 2001). The presynaptic side goes well prepared into this encounter and contains preassembled packages of structural elements such as receptors that will be used in the building of the synapse (Washbourne et al., 2002). At least in hippocampal neurons, presynaptic development occurs before postsynaptic differentiation (Okabe et al., 2001). The filopodia on the dendritic side are soon replaced by spines, or thorn-like protrusions on the dendrite, on which the synapses sit. The spines first appear as immature protospines and over time develop into mature spines. Even in established networks, however, spines and synapses remain in some flux; in the brain, connections are not welded together. Maintenance is activity-dependent as well.

In the developing brain, two forms of activity shape the evolving structure. First, spontaneous activity is generated by the tissue itself in the absence of external stimuli (Katz and Shatz, 1996). This activity spreads through excitatory synapses but also through gap junctions. Second, postnatal and adult refinement of networks is heavily dependent on sensory stimuli and is mediated by synaptic activity.

Intracellularly, calcium ions mediate activity-dependent effects by acting on various intracellular messenger systems. Calcium oscillations can be found in many developing neuronal circuits and affect fiber outgrowth and differentiation (Spitzer et al., 2000). N-methyl-D-aspartate (NMDA) receptors are involved in this response. When NMDA receptors were blocked in *Xenopus*, dendritic branching was inhibited (Rajan et al., 1999). There is thus a link between axon and dendrite formation and synapse development. Young synapses might be silent until they are depolarized for the first time; their maturation depends on NMDA receptor activation together with strong and concurrent afferent inputs. This situation is similar if not identical to that of long-term potentiation (LTP), the electrophysiological and structural substrate of learning. In fact, one can imagine the entire process of network formation as learning. Activity within the network determines which connections are maintained and which are eliminated. Many more synapses are initiated than will be maintained. Neurons that fail to make useful connections in this process are removed.

During network formation the building and dismantling of synapses is a very fast process that takes only a few hours for a single synapse (Alsina et al., 2001). After a synapse is removed, the branch of the axon will retract. In this sense, the activity-dependent shaping of neuronal networks is a highly dynamic process that occurs on the level of single axons and dendrites by means of a rapid fine-tuning of the synaptic connections (Antonini and Stryker, 1993; Cline, 2001; Trachtenberg and Stryker, 2001).

However, activity-dependent effects go beyond the individual synapse. Long-term potentiation is quite specific and might only spread to adjacent synapses. However, LTP might also have effects on local filopodia motility and dendritic sprouting, resulting in new spines and possibly new synapses (Engert and Bonhoeffer, 1999).

Electrical activity triggers the expression of many plasticity-related genes. Calcium influx increases cAMP levels, which induce the phosphorylation of cAMP response element binding protein (CREB). CREB in turn is not only involved in mediating the structural changes underlying synapse maturation but also many other intracellular correlates of plasticity. In adult neurogenesis, for example, CREB phosphorylation is associated with cell survival. The activity-dependent up-regulation of CPG15 discussed above, underscores the relationship between neurite and synapse formation. Prominent among the genes induced by electrical activity are the neurotrophins, which are produced and secreted in response to electrical activity (Schinder and Poo, 2000). Neurotrophins have many effects on synapse formation, maturation, and maintenance (Poo, 2001) as well as on neurite and spine stability (McAllister et al., 1999). For example, BDNF can be released from axons (Hartmann et al., 2001) and affects dendrites (Aakalu et al., 2001). Thus neurotrophins seem to play an important role in the activity-dependent shaping and maintenance of neuronal networks.

NEUROTROPHIC FACTORS PROMOTE CELL SURVIVAL OR DEATH

In embryonic and adult neurogenesis a wave of cell death occurs shortly after the new neurons have begun to make functional connections. The usefulness of the connection they make appears to be the selection principle. The neuronal network is not built up neuron by neuron; instead, a vast number of neurons are generated, of which only a small functional subset survives. It has been estimated that five times as many projection neurons are generated than will survive (Oppenheim, 1991). This subtractive method is somewhat similar to a sculptor who chisels Venus of Milo out of a block of marble. The central difference is that in the brain the sculpturor is the sculpture itself; the network liberates itself from excess parts in an activity-dependent way. The first victims are synapses and branches of neurites, but if activity in a given cell falls below a particular threshold the cell is eliminated. This occurs via programmed cell death, or apoptosis. Development is thus inseparably interwoven with cell death. Paradoxically, apoptosis is a principle of maturation. Activity-dependent fate is determined by secreted factors that promote either survival or cell death.

The neurotrophic hypothesis developed by Rita Levi-Montalcini states that neuronal survival is dependent on trophic support from the target zones. In a classic experiment, she showed that administration of antibodies against NGF when the developing neurons innervated their targets would lead to death of the neurons, whereas exogenous NGF would rescue neurons that otherwise would have died (Levi-Montalcini, 1987). When NGF or its receptor TrkA is lacking, cell survival similarly decreases (Lewin and Barde, 1996). These initial findings have been extended to the large family of neurotrophic factors, including the neurotrophins proper (NGF, BDNF, NT3, NT4), neurotrophic cytokines (CNTF, LIF-1, interleukin-6, and others), and the families of Glia-derived neurotrophic factor (GDNF)- and hepatocyte growth factor (HGF)-related proteins (Davis and Murphey, 1994; Lewin and Barde, 1996; Airaksinen and Saarma, 2002). Different factors act differently on different populations of neurons. Neurons read and integrate over a spectrum of neurotrophic signals. Among other parameters, this pattern depends on the distribution of the different receptors that mediate neurotrophic factor action. Receptor expression not only differs between different cells but also over time in the same cell (Buchman and Davies, 1993; Ninkina et al., 1996).

Neurotrophic trophic support can be provided retrogradely from the postsynaptic neuron, anterogradely from the presynaptic neuron, in an autocrine manner from the neuron itself, or from the surrounding glia in particular astrocytes and microglia. In the course of development, neurons become dependent on neurotrophic factors. Neurotrophic factors have many functions during neuronal development, but it appears to be relatively late that neurotrophic signals become a matter of life and death. The acquired responsiveness to BDNF, for example, is mirrored in the delayed expression of the BDNF receptor Trk-B (Vogel and Davies, 1991; Robinson et al., 1996). BDNF is also transported anterogradely. It is not only involved in stimulating dendritic growth but also affects the survival of the postmitotic neuron (Altar et al., 1997; Caleo et al., 2000). An activity-dependent autocrine signaling by neurotrophins has been shown for hippocampal pyramidal cells in vitro (Boukhaddaoui et al., 2001). In some populations of sensory neurons the preference of different growth factors can change over time (Buchman and Davies, 1993; Enokido et al., 1999), and sometimes extracellular signals are required to mediate this switch (Paul and Davies, 1995). It is likely that similar activity-dependent switches (albeit perhaps very subtle) are more the rule than the exception and are found in other neuronal cell types as well. The means by which sequential expression of receptors is regulated is not yet known. Some brain regions are patterned independent of complete input signals, which implies that there must be an intrinsic program that makes them independent of external neurotrophic cues (Lopez-Mascaraque and de Castro, 2002).

Neurotrophins bind not only to the Trk receptors but also to the p75 receptor, which, among many other functions (which include survival-promoting effects), can also induce cell death via an intracellular cell death domain (Coulson et al., 2004). The co-activation of the antagonistically acting receptors is modulated by context and activity. When Trk receptors are absent, the pro-apoptotic action of p75 activation tips the balance toward cell death (Barrett and Bartlett, 1994). Active Trk-A, in contrast, stimulates signaling along the PI3K/Akt pathway, which suppresses apoptotic signals mediated by p75. p53, a central molecule in the induction of cell death, is inhibited and the expression of trk-A itself is increased (Kaplan and Miller, 2000).

The best studied neurotrophin in adult neurogenesis is BDNF, which promotes neurogenesis in the SVZ and olfactory bulb in vivo (Pencea et al., 2001). Also, BDNF heterozygous null mutants had reduced adult hippocampal neurogenesis (Lee et al., 2002). Because BDNF expression is regulated in an activity-dependent way, BDNF is a likely candidate for providing trophic stimuli to the developing new neurons in the adult brain.

SEROTONIN AND NEURONAL DEVELOPMENT

Serotonin plays a particular role in brain development and the regulation of adult neurogenesis. Serotonin function is multifaceted and is mediated through several receptors with different downstream effects (Gaspar et al., 2003). Serotonergic innervation is extremely widespread and reaches the entire brain. All serotonergic input to the brain arises from the raphe nuclei and the reticular formation of the brain stem. The number of serotonergic neurons is rather small (about 20,000 in a rat). Serotonergic neurons are generated very early during development. They are born between E10 to E12 in a mouse, thus preceding cortical (and hippocampal) development. These features make the serotonergic system an ideal candidate for providing relatively general and coordinating stimuli to brain development. In the mature brain, for example, the serotonergic system has effects on levels of wakefulness, attention, and alertness, on aggression, and on exploratory behavior. One could imagine the serotonergic system also as a sensor and announcer of activity in a very general sense. Because both brain development and brain plasticity (and thus adult neurogenesis) are strongly influenced by activity, a central role of serotonin in these processes makes intuitive sense.

Surprisingly, however, the patterns of serotonin effects on development are so complex but also redundant that many mutants of the serotonergic system have an almost normal phenotype. Nevertheless, even if changes in this system are not obvious they might be highly relevant to brain functions. Such changes have been connected with minute developmental changes hypothesized to underlie psychiatric disorders such as depression, schizophrenia, autism, and drug abuse. In the context of these disorders disturbed plasticity of the adult brain, including adult neurogenesis, has been discussed as well.

In addition to brain-stem serotonergic neurons, some developing neurons, mostly glutamatergic neurons in sensory systems, go through a transient stage of an incomplete serotonergic phenotype. They appear to borrow serotonin as a neurotransmitter; they can take up serotonin from their environment but cannot synthesize it. The exact functional consequences of this process are not yet understood, but it might be relevant to adult neurogenesis, because both the serotonin transporter (SERT) and Vmat2 (which packages serotonin into synaptic vesicles) remain expressed in the two neurogenic regions of the adult brain (Hansson et al., 1998; Lebrand et al., 1998; Gaspar et al., 2003).

Elevated serotonin levels appear to be associated with reduced developmental cell death in some brain areas (Persico et al., 2003). The consequence of elevated serotonin levels in early postnatal life is a lack of segregation between the territories that axons cover in their projection area, particularly in the visual and somatosensory cortex (Vitalis et al., 1998; Rebsam et al., 2002; Upton et al., 2002). Additional elimination of one of the serotonin receptors, 1B, leads to rescue of this phenotype (Salichon et al., 2001). This and other examples show that differential effects of serotonin are mediated by the various serotonin receptors, whose expression is dynamically regulated across time, across neuronal cell types, and across different domains within the same cell. Different receptors on dendrites and axons lead to specific effects (Jolimay et al., 2000). Many effects on granule cell development and adult neurogenesis seem to be mediated by the 1A receptor (Yan et al., 1997; Brezun and Daszuta, 1999; Santarelli et al., 2003; Banasr et al., 2004). These include an effect of serotonin on cell proliferation, which in the developing heart is mediated by the 2B receptor (Nebigil et al., 2000).

Serotonin is also involved in controlling the later developmental steps of neuronal maturation, including fine-tuning of the neurites and cell survival. Particularly the 2B receptor is responsible for these effects in early development, and the 2A and 2C receptors take over at least part of this role later. Serotonin 2B receptor activation can modulate BDNF (Vaidya et al., 1997) and can thus act antiapoptotically, probably through the PI3K/Akt pathway (Nebigil et al., 2003). The 2C receptor plays a role in synaptic plasticity, both during development and in the adult (Gu and Singer, 1995; Tecott et al., 1995; Kojic et al., 2000; Edagawa et al., 2001).

DEVELOPMENT OF NEUROGENIC ZONES OF THE ADULT BRAIN

The Subventricular Zone

As outlined above, brain development originates from the neuroepithelial cells lining the primordial ventricles. This layer, which becomes the ventricular zone, gives rise to a secondary proliferative matrix that forms just below the ventricular zone and expands rapidly: the subventricular zone (SVZ). In mice, the SVZ first appears in the ventral brain around E11 (Sturrock and Smart, 1980). During embryonic development an SVZ can be found in all ventricles, but not below the fourth ventricle. The dividing SVZ cells do not show the characteristic nuclear movements during the cell cycle described for the ventricular zone (Takahashi et al., 1995). In mice, at E15 cell divisions in the SVZ have surpassed proliferation in the VZ and lead to a massive thickening of the SVZ. Around birth the VZ is no longer recognizable as a germinative layer (Bayer and Altman, 1991).

The embryonic SVZ can be divided into two distinct regions, each of which gives rise to specific neuronal populations (Fig. 4–5, Table 4–1). As part of the dorsal forebrain the neocortical SVZ gives rise to the layered cortex, including the principal neurons of the hippocampus; as part of the ventral forebrain the ganglionic eminences produce interneurons, astrocytes, and oligodendrocytes in many brain regions in the ventral and dorsal brain (Pleasure et al., 2000a; He et al., 2001; Marshall and Goldman, 2002). The ganglionic eminences got their name from the protrusions they form in the ventricular wall and can be divided into the medial ganglionic eminence (MGE), the lateral ganglionic eminence (LGE), and, as described more recently, the caudal ganglionic eminence (CGE). They are distinguished by the expression of marker transcription factors. The expression of homeobox genes *Nkx2.1*, *Dlx1*, and *Dlx2* distinguishes the ganglionic eminences from the dorsal SVZ and the SVZ from the VZ (Parnavelas, 2000). Most notably, *Dlx* identifies progeny from the ganglionic eminences but is not expressed in progeny of dorsal precursor cells. However, Dlx is not expressed in all ventral precursor cells, which suggests that Dlx-negative cells might give rise to Dlx-positive cells (He et al., 2001). A recent paradigm shift in developmental neurobiology was the insight that radial glia constitutes the majority of precursor cells in the VZ, giving rise to intermediates in the SVZ, not vice versa (Gotz, 2003). Whereas in the dorsal brain, radial glial processes span from the ventricular to the pial surface, in the ganglionic eminences they only reach into the anlage of the basal ganglia (Edwards et al., 1990).

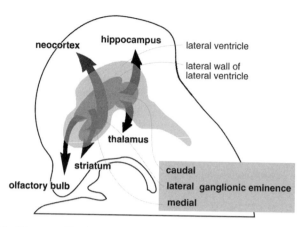

Figure 4–5. The ganglionic eminences. The ganglionic eminences contribute cell neuronal (and glial) cell populations throughout the brain (see also Fig. 3–1 and 3–4; Table 4–1). Hippocampal projection neurons, including granule cells, are derived from the dorsal subventricular zone but hippocampal interneurons originate from the medial ganglionic eminces. Olfactory bulb interneurons are derived from the lateral ganglionic eminence. It thus appears that adult hippocampal neurogenesis is dorsal, whereas adult neurogenesis in the olfactory bulb is ventral.

Migration from the MGE precedes migration from the LGE. Cells from the MGE produce interneurons in the neocortex and hippocampus. It is not clear whether the pioneer interneurons, the Cajal-Retzius cells, which are found in the marginal zone of the cortex and hippocampus, are derived from the MGE (Anderson et al., 1999; Wichterle et al., 2001). The cells from the ganglionic eminences migrate tangential to the radially migrating cells in the neocortical SVZ and thus have to cross their path. The LGE might contribute to cortical interneurogenesis as well, but this scenario is not yet fully resolved (Tamamaki et al., 1997; Anderson et al., 1999). However, with some contributions from the MGE the LGE produces many neurons of the striatum, including the DARPP32-positive spiny interneurons (Deacon et al., 1994), as well as neurons in many other regions, such as the septum and thalamus (Wichterle et al., 1999, 2001). The anterior part of the LGE produces interneurons in the olfactory bulb, the posterior part in the striatum (Stenman et al., 2003). Throughout adulthood astrocyte-like stem cells (B cells) of the adult SVZ are thought to produce new interneurons for the olfactory bulb. Additionally, after ischemia new striatal interneurons, including DARPP32-positive cells (which are of ventral origin), can be generated from SVZ precursor cells (Arvidsson et al., 2002). B cells of the adult SVZ that are Dlx negative are derived from Gsh2-expressing cells of the LGE but do not express transcription factor Er81, which is found in the anterior LGE, in migrating cells of the adult SVZ and in olfactory bulb interneurons. Like the situation during embryonic development, it thus seems that Dlx-negative

Table 4-1. Origins of Some Neuronal Populations

Germinative Zone	Transcription Factor 1	Brain Region	Neuronal Population	Transcription Factor 2	Reference
Dorsal (Ventricular Zone)	Pax6, Ngn, Emx	Neocortex	Glutamatergic projection neurons Deep layers	Otx1	Frantz and McConnell, 1996
		Hippocampus	Principal neurons	Otx1	Acampora et al., 1996
			Granule cells	NeuroD, Mash1	Pleasure et al., 2000a
(Subventricular Zone)			Glutamatergic projection neurons Superficial layers	Svet1	Tarabykin et al., 2001
Ventral Lateral	Dlx1/2	Olfactory bulb	Interneurons	Gsh2, Er81	Corbin et al., 2000; Stenman et al., 2003
		Striatum	Interneurons		Deacon et al., 1994; Anderson et al., 1997; Stenman et al., 2003
		? Neocortex	Interneurons		He et al., 2001

		Nkx2.1 Mash1 (Ascl1)	Casarosa et al., 1999, Sussel, 1999;
Medial	Hippocampus	Interneurons (primary source)	Pleasure et al., 2000b
	Neocortex	Interneurons	He et al., 2001
	Neocortex	Cholinergic neurons	Wichterle et al., 1999; Marin et al., 2000
	Septum	Cholinergic neurons	
	Striatum	Cholinergic neurons	Nkx2.1
Caudal	Cortex (posterior)	(Oligodendrocytes astrocytes)	Mash1 (Ascl1) Nery et al., 2002
	Hippocampus	Interneurons Mossy cells (?Few principal neurons)	
	Striatum (posterior)	Medium spiny interneurons	
	Globus pallidus (posterior)	Medium spiny interneurons	

Table compiled from Parnavelas, (2000), Brazel et al. (2003), Gotz (2003), and others. The neurogenic regions of the adult brain are shaded.

precursor cells generate Dlx-positive intermediates which then give rise to adult-born interneurons. Consequently, the currently available data suggest that the system of adult neurogenesis in the adult olfactory bulb is of ventral origin. In contrast, dorsal SVZ precursor cells give rise to precursor cells of the adult SGZ and glutamatergic projection neurons including the dentate gyrus granule cells. After ischemia and growth factor infusion, a repopulation of hippocampal area CA1 with new glutamatergic neurons has been described, which originated from the posterior part of the adult SVZ below the corpus callosum (Nakatomi et al., 2002). This pattern suggests that the adult SVZ contains precursor cells that, under appropriate stimulation, can produce excitatory hippocampal neurons. The exact lineage relationship of these precursor cells to precursor cells of the adult dentate gyrus is not known, however.

The lateral wall of the SVZ can be divided into two parts: a cell-rich spandril below the corpus callosum, and the ventricular wall adjacent to the striatum (Fig. 4–6). It has been proposed that the latter are the remnants of the ganglionic eminences (Brazel et al., 2003). In this theory, the roof of the lateral ventricles represents the remnants of the dorsal SVZ. What is called SVZ in the context of adult neurogenesis is essentially a ventral structure, although the presence of "dorsal" factors such as Pax6 might indicate a mixed cellular composition. The function of the dorsally derived SVZ in the adult brain has not yet been studied in much detail. However, it has been suggested that after ischemia and induction by growth factors EGF and FGF, new CA1 projection neurons arise in the hippocampus, presumably originating from a dorsal SVZ population (Nakatomi et al., 2002). The medial walls of the lateral ventricles show a SVZ as well, but their function is in the developing and adult brain is not known. It might well be that they form a continuity with the SVZ in the lateral wall.

In the postnatal SVZ, Dlx identifies the transiently amplifying progenitor cells (C cells) and the migratory A cells ("neuroblasts") (Doetsch et al., 2002). The expression pattern shows a large overlap with polysialated neural cell adhesion molecule (PSA-NCAM) and doublecortin. The surrounding cells are astrocyte-like cells, including the local radial glia–like precursor cells (B cells), classical astrocytes without precursor cell function, and ependyma. Consequently, in the adult SVZ, the Dlx-positive cells are interspersed with other cell types; anterior–ventrally they concentrate and form a core in the spandril leading into the rostral migratory stream. This pattern gives the impression of a different cellular composition than that in the SVZ proper (Rothstein and Levison, 2002; Brazel et al., 2003).

Some authors divide the SVZ of the postnatal brain into an anterior part (designated "aSVZ"; Luskin et al., 1997) as the source of the cells migrating into the rostral migratory stream to the olfactory bulb, and the dorsolateral part as a main source of glia. However, migrating SVZ cells, forming a network of crisscrossing chains, can be found throughout the lateral ventricular walls of the lateral ventricles in rodents (Doetsch et al., 1997) and thus

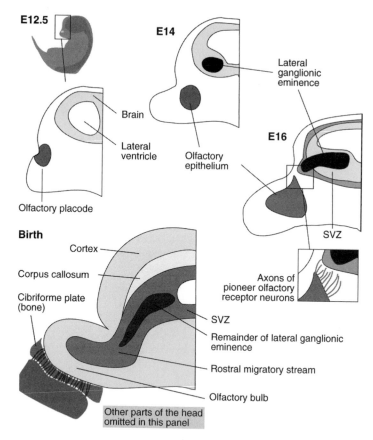

Figure 4–6. Development of the olfactory bulb. The olfactory epithelium is derived from the olfactory placode, whereas the olfactory bulb is of ventral subventricular zone (SVZ) origin. Early input from axons of pioneer olfactory receptor neurons influence development of the olfactory bulb.

the distinction of an aSVZ is not generally made. Migrating precursor cells from many parts of the SVZ converging toward the entrance to the rostral migratory stream might give the impression of an increased neurogenic potential by resident precursor cells of this region.

Development of the Olfactory Bulb

The olfactory bulb contains the first central neuron of the olfactory system, to which the olfactory receptor neurons of the olfactory epithelium in the nasal cavity project. The olfactory bulb shows a rather simple layered structure and is otherwise organized in glomeruli, consisting of the principal projecting neurons, mitral cells, tufted cells, and several types of interneurons within the glomeruli and in the periglomerular layer (Fig. 4–7).

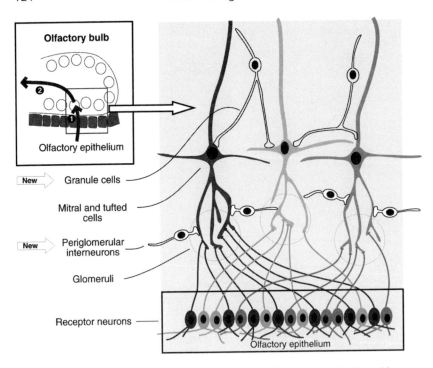

Figure 4–7. Principal network structure of the olfactory bulb. The olfactory receptor neurons are the first neurons of the olfactory tract. The mitral/tufted cells, located in the glomeruli of the olfactory bulb are the second neuron, which project to the olfactory tubercle and other structures of the rhinencephalon. Adult neurogenesis generates interneurons in the granule cell layer and in the periglomerular region. No mitral or tufted cells are produced in adulthood. The olfactory bulb is not topologically structured like the visual system. Rather, olfactory neurons of the same type project to the same glomeruli in the olfactory bulb.

Development of the olfactory system begins with formation of the olfactory epithelium from the olfactory placode, and the olfactory bulb from the olfactory primordium in the rostral telencephalon. This specific part of the ventricular wall later becomes the (obliterated) olfactory ventricle. Even in the adult, the olfactory bulb contains neural precursor cells. It is not clear whether these cells are direct descendants of this primordium or represent the precursor cells migrating in from the adult SVZ. From the ventricular primordium the projecting neurons, the mitral cells, and the tufted cells are generated. The interneurons are derived from the LGE (Corbin et al., 2000; Stenman et al., 2003).

The first pioneer axons arriving from the olfactory epithelium (the peripheral receptor field in the olfactory system) reach the ventricular wall and induce an increased number of cells to exit from the cell cycle (Gong and

Shipley, 1995). This causes a bulging of the olfactory bulb (De Carlos et al., 1995, 1996). Although induction by the pioneer axons seems important, even the Pax6 null-mutant, which lacks an olfactory epithelium and consequently olfactory axons, develops a rudimentary olfactory bulb (Jimenez et al., 2000).

Like the hypotheses for cortical development, a protomap hypothesis (the patterning occurs before migration and the migrating cells are heterogeneous and follow intrinsic control) and a protocortex hypothesis (the cells are homogeneous and are patterned according to specific local stimuli at later time points) have been formulated. As in the cortex, it seems that both hypotheses are true and neither is sufficient for a full explanation of olfactory bulb development. Development of the olfactory bulb is influenced by the olfactory epithelium but not entirely dependent on it. Particularly the late stages of neuronal maturation in the olfactory bulb might be influenced by input from the olfactory epithelium (Stout and Graziadei, 1980; Matsutani and Yamamoto, 2000). But olfactory bulb neurons can survive without input from the olfactory epithelium (see Chapter 5).

The earliest projection neurons form before the bulb itself becomes recognizable. Development of the olfactory bulb follows a rather rigid sequence (Hinds, 1968a, 1968b). Neurogenesis in the accessory olfactory bulb precedes the main bulb. The projection neurons arise first, followed by the mitral cells; the various types of interneurons are generated last. At the time the interneurons are migrating in a morphologically recognizable olfactory bulb has formed. The interneurons have to migrate over increasing distances from the lateral ganglionic eminence (and later the SVZ) into the bulb. Their migratory route becomes ensheathed by glial cells and turns into the rostral migratory stream that persists into adulthood. Only neurogenesis of interneurons originates from precursor cells in the adult SVZ and can be found throughout life.

The olfactory bulb principal neurons project to the olfactory cortex, olfactory tubercle, anterior olfactory nucleus, piriform cortex, entorhinal cortex, and amygdala (reviewed in Lopez-Mascaraque and de Castro, 2002). The earliest cells project to the most posterior target structures, the later-born neurons to the more anterior nuclei (Derer et al., 1977; Bayer, 1983). The projections of the olfactory bulb are not topographic because projection neurons from all over the bulb can project to the same neuronal populations in the olfactory cortex and amygdala (Scott et al., 1980). Afferents from the olfactory epithelium originating from the same type of odor receptor converge on very few olfactory glomeruli (Treloar et al., 2002), which in turn project to clusters of target neurons in the olfactory cortex (Fig. 4–7). The pattern of glomeruli representing specific receptors is highly characteristic (Ressler et al., 1994; Vassar et al., 1994; Mombaerts et al., 1996). Thus, although the olfactory bulb is not a topographical map of the olfactory epithelium, it is, much more astonishingly, an anatomical map of the approximately 1500 receptor types. This complex and specific patterning seems to be dependent on the olfactory receptor proteins themselves. The individual olfactory proteins are characteristic of the different receptor types. If one region of the receptor protein is genetically replaced by another this causes a targeting of the projection to other glomeruli (Bozza et al., 2002).

Development of the olfactory bulb projections involves several candidate guidance mechanisms. PSA-NCAM as well as other NCAM forms are associated with development of the lateral olfactory tract, the main output structure of the olfactory bulb (Seki and Arai, 1991; Stoeckli and Landmesser, 1995). The slit–robo system is also prominently involved in the formation of the projections (Li et al., 1999). Interestingly, both systems also seem to play a role in guiding adult-generated neurons into the olfactory bulb—in the opposite direction to that of the axons during development.

DEVELOPMENT OF HIPPOCAMPAL DENTATE GYRUS AND SUBGRANULAR ZONE

The hippocampus is part of the archicortex. Despite the simple network structure of archicortex, with three layers instead of six, the sequence of gross development in the dentate gyrus is more complicated than in the rest of the hippocampus and in neocortex. Whereas development of the CA fields follows the general pattern of other cortical regions, in the dentate gyrus three germinative matrices follow each other. During embryonic development, the hippocampus becomes displaced by the much stronger growing cortical regions and is rolled into the characteristic shape that provoked its name, *hippocampus*, meaning sea horse. The sequence of germinative centers distinguishes neurogenesis in the dentate gyrus from the olfactory system, where the germinative zone found in the adult SVZ is at least locally the more or less direct successor of the matrix active during embryonic brain development. Development of the dentate gyrus thus originates from an ectopic precursor cell pool.

Like the other cortical regions, development of the hippocampus originates from the VZ in the dorsal forebrain. The hippocampus is part of the medial cortex. Patterning signals for this regions are provided by a small region called the "cortical hem," which is rich in the expression of BMPs (Furuta et al., 1997) and Wnt factors (Grove et al., 1998). The hippocampus originates from the region dorsal to the cortical hem. This region is characterized by the expression of Wnt receptor Frizzled (Kim et al., 2001). From E10 on, Wnt3a is the only Wnt whose expression is exclusive to the cortical hem. Wnt3a null mutants lack the hippocampus (Lee et al., 2000). In contrast, mutants for Lef1, which is a transcription factor in the Wnt signaling pathway, lack the dentate gyrus only (Galceran et al., 2000).

Initially, the region from which the dentate gyrus will develop is not clearly demarcated, but by E18 (in the rat) cell proliferation in this zone decreases, while the neighboring regions that give rise to ammon's horn and the fimbrial structures maintain their proliferation. A subventricular proliferative zone, the secondary germinative matrix, builds up during this time. From this matrix cells migrate to the future site of the dentate gyrus (Altman and Bayer, 1990a, 1990b). Cells from the secondary matrix later form the outer shell of the dentate gyrus (Fig. 4–8). Early postnatally (again in the rat), the secondary matrix is almost resolved and a tertiary matrix that is most active during early postnatal development, postnatal day 3 (P3) to P10, takes over. The tertiary matrix is derived from the secondary matrix, which splits around E22. One part in a first migration gives rise to the outer granule cells, the other to the tertiary matrix in what later will be referred to as the hilus, or plexiform layer, of the dentate gyrus. The tertiary matrix produces the inner shell of the granule cell layer and thereby the greater part of the total granule cell number. In the granule cell layer, the oldest granule cells are on the outside, the youngest are on the inside. The tertiary germinative matrix becomes increasingly confined to the SGZ, from which the new neurons of adult hippocampal neurogenesis are generated. At present it is not clear whether this process is only an increasing spatial confinement or represents a transition to a qualitatively distinct fourth germinative matrix. Hippocampal interneurons, like other interneurons in the cortex, originate from the ganglionic eminence (Pleasure et al., 2000a).

Dentate gyrus development is dependent on Cajal-Retzius neurons and radial glia, as in the neocortical regions. Radial glia has a dual function in this process. In addition to the long-known function of guiding migration of newborn neurons to their final location in the layered cortex, radial glia–like cells also serve precursor cell functions in this region (Seri et al., 2001, 2004). The link between the two functions has not yet been fully elucidated and thus it is not clear whether all radial glial cells do in fact serve both functions and whether all radial glial cells have the potential to do so. In any case, radial glia formation in the dentate anlage around E13 precedes granule cell development, and in all of the subsequent germinative matrices radial glia is discernible. In mice with a defect in Wnt signaling, radial glia scaffolding was disorganized and the precursor pool did not develop properly (Zhou et al., 2004).

The original radial glia, which spans between the ventricular and the pial surfaces as in other cortical regions, becomes separated into two bundles. One is the supragranular bundle, which runs parallel to the hippocampal fissure, the other is the fimbrial bundle, which co-localizes with the secondary germinative matrix. Radial glia in the secondary matrix first runs tangential to what later becomes the granule cell layer, but a subset leads to the future hilus. Consequently, radial glia of the tertiary matrix (in the hilus) is then found to be almost perpendicular to the supragranular glia and crosses the granule cell layer in a radial fashion (Rickmann et al., 1987; Sievers et al., 1992). This development parallels the pattern described by Altman and Bayer for proliferative matrices.

Late postnatally, the cell bodies of the radial glia become restricted to the SGZ; their processes end in the molecular layer. This condition persists

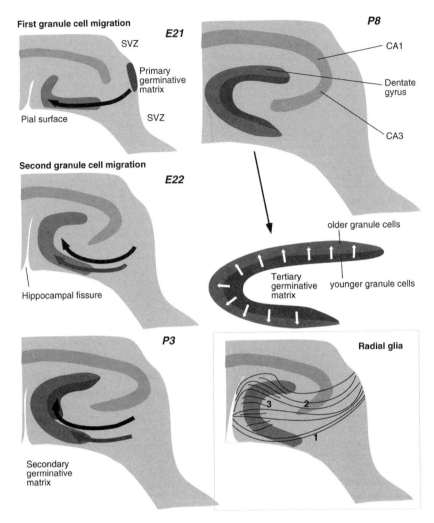

First granule cell migration

E21

SVZ

Primary germinative matrix

Pial surface

SVZ

Second granule cell migration

E22

Hippocampal fissure

P3

Secondary germinative matrix

P8

CA1

Dentate gyrus

CA3

older granule cells

Tertiary germinative matrix

younger granule cells

Radial glia

3 2

1

Figure 4–8. Development of the dentate gyrus. In the course of dentate gyrus development, two waves of migration of precursor cells follow each other. From a primary germinative region in the wall of the lateral ventricle, these cells found a secondary matrix that gives way to a third matrix, which persists into adulthood as the precursor cell population in the subgranular zone. The granule cell layer is built in an outside–inside fashion. The first granule cell migration forms the outer shell, the second migration and the secondary and tertiary germinative matrices produce the inner layers. Alterations in the radial gial structures parallel this development. This simplified compilation is based on works by Rickmann et al. (1987) and Altman and Bayer (1990a, 1990b).

into adulthood. A subset of these radial glial cells functions as precursor cells in the adult dentate gyrus. It is therefore possible that each germinative matrix in the developing dentate gyrus has its own distinctive set of radial glia. The first set would have the typical orientation of a base at the ventricular surface and apical contact at the pia. The secondary, tertiary, and quaternary radial glia would lack these contacts and only maintain an end foot on the basal membrane of a blood vessel (just as in the SVZ the B cell touches the ventricular surface). The radial process would be independent of surface contact. Alternatively, other blood vessels could provide the second contact as they seem to do in the SVZ. This hypothetical structure has to be confirmed in detailed anatomical studies. It seems, however, that radial glia-like cells of the adult SGZ terminate in the molecular layer without mandatory contact with blood vessels.

NEURONAL DEVELOPMENT IN THE ADULT

Theoretically, there is no reason to assume that neuronal development in the adult is an exact replication of embryonic development. Conditions, starting points, time course, the cells involved, and the purpose the entire process serves in the larger picture are too different. On the other hand, evolution tends to reuse established systems, which are then modified according the new function. In any case, adult neurogenesis does not recapitulate all aspects of brain development. Positional information and patterning remain fixed; the developmental potential in vivo is highly limited to one or two neuronal populations. Ex vivo data suggest that in adult neurogenesis, many developmental options are actively suppressed. In cell culture, precursor cells are multipotent and can generate neurons, astrocytes, and oligodendrocytes. In vivo, they seem to produce primarily neurons. As discussed in Chapter 3, cell culture conditions might well be instructive for multipotency, but the susceptibility of the cells to such stimuli remains a property of the precursor cells. Among the possible factors that restrict neurogenesis in vivo, BMPs are strong candidates (Lim et al., 2000). Notch is another likely antineurogenic factor in vivo, but no detailed functional study for adult neurogenesis exists yet.

The conclusion from this discussion is that, ironically, a large part of regulation in the neurogenic zones of the adult brain is antineurogenic and actually limits neurogenesis in order to achieve it within a physiologically desirable range.

REFERENCES

Aakalu G, Smith WB, Nguyen N, Jiang C, Schuman EM (2001) Dynamic visualization of local protein synthesis in hippocampal neurons. Neuron 30:489–502.
Acampora D, Mazan S, Avantaggiato V, Barone P, Tuorto F, Lallemand Y, Brulet P, Simeone A (1996) Epilepsy and brain abnormalities in mice lacking the *Otx1* gene. Nat Genet 14:218–222.

Airaksinen MS, Saarma M (2002) The GDNF family: signalling, biological functions and therapeutic value. Nat Rev Neurosci 3:383–394.

Alsina B, Vu T, Cohen-Cory S (2001) Visualizing synapse formation in arborizing optic axons in vivo: dynamics and modulation by BDNF. Nat Neurosci 4:1093–1101.

Altar CA, Cai N, Bliven T, Juhasz M, Conner JM, Acheson AL, Lindsay RM, Wiegand SJ (1997) Anterograde transport of brain-derived neurotrophic factor and its role in the brain. Nature 389:856–860.

Altman J, Bayer SA (1990a) Migration and distribution of two populations of hippocampal progenitors during the perinatal and postnatal periods. J Comp Neurol 301:365–381.

Altman J, Bayer SA (1990b) Mosaic organization of the hippocampal neuroepithelium and the multiple germinal sources of dentate granule cells. J Comp Neurol 301:325–342.

Altmann CR, Brivanlou AH (2001) Neural patterning in the vertebrate embryo. Int Rev Cytol 203:447–482.

Alvarez-Buylla A, Garcia-Verdugo JM, Tramontin AD (2001) A unified hypothesis on the lineage of neural stem cells. Nat Rev Neurosci 2:287–293.

Anderson S, Mione M, Yun K, Rubenstein JL (1999) Differential origins of neocortical projection and local circuit neurons: role of *Dlx* genes in neocortical interneuronogenesis. Cereb Cortex 9:646–654.

Anderson SA, Eisenstat DD, Shi L, Rubenstein JL (1997) Interneuron migration from basal forebrain to neocortex: dependence on *Dlx* genes. Science 278:474–476.

Angevine J, Sidman R (1961) Autoradiographic study of cell migration during histogenesis of the cerebral cortex of the mouse. Nature 192:266–268.

Anthony TE, Klein C, Fishell G, Heintz N (2004) Radial glia serve as neuronal progenitors in all regions of the central nervous system. Neuron 41:881–890.

Antonini A, Stryker MP (1993) Rapid remodeling of axonal arbors in the visual cortex. Science 260:1819–1821.

Arvidsson A, Collin T, Kirik D, Kokaia Z, Lindvall O (2002) Neuronal replacement from endogenous precursors in the adult brain after stroke. Nat Med 8:963–970.

Banasr M, Hery M, Printemps R, Daszuta A (2004) Serotonin-induced increases in adult cell proliferation and neurogenesis are mediated through different and common 5-HT receptor subtypes in the dentate gyrus and the subventricular zone. Neuropsychopharmacology 29:450–460.

Barrett GL, Bartlett PF (1994) The p75 nerve growth factor receptor mediates survival or death depending on the stage of sensory neuron development. Proc Natl Acad Sci USA 91:6501–6505.

Bayer SA (1983) 3H-thymidine-radiographic studies of neurogenesis in the rat olfactory bulb. Exp Brain Res 50:329–340.

Bayer SA, Altman J (1991) Neocortical Development. New York: Raven Press.

Bishop KM, Goudreau G, O'Leary DD (2000) Regulation of area identity in the mammalian neocortex by Emx2 and Pax6. Science 288:344–349.

Boukhaddaoui H, Sieso V, Scamps F, Valmier J (2001) An activity-dependent neurotrophin-3 autocrine loop regulates the phenotype of developing hippocampal pyramidal neurons before target contact. J Neurosci 21:8789–8797.

Bozza T, Feinstein P, Zheng C, Mombaerts P (2002) Odorant receptor expression defines functional units in the mouse olfactory system. J Neurosci 22:3033–3043.

Brazel CY, Romanko MJ, Rothstein RP, Levison SW (2003) Roles of the mammalian subventricular zone in brain development. Prog Neurobiol 69:49–69.

Brezun JM, Daszuta A (1999) Depletion in serotonin decreases neurogenesis in the dentate gyrus and the subventricular zone of adult rats. Neuroscience 89:999–1002.

Brodski C, Weisenhorn DM, Signore M, Sillaber I, Oesterheld M, Broccoli V, Acampora D, Simeone A, Wurst W (2003) Location and size of dopaminergic and serotonergic cell populations are controlled by the position of the midbrain–hindbrain organizer. J Neurosci 23:4199–4207.

Brunet JF, Ghysen A (1999) Deconstructing cell determination: proneural genes and neuronal identity. Bioessays 21:313–318.

Buchman VL, Davies AM (1993) Different neurotrophins are expressed and act in a developmental sequence to promote the survival of embryonic sensory neurons. Development 118:989–1001.

Caleo M, Menna E, Chierzi S, Cenni MC, Maffei L (2000) Brain-derived neurotrophic factor is an anterograde survival factor in the rat visual system. Curr Biol 10:1155–1161.

Casarosa S, Fode C, Guillemot F (1999) Mash1 regulates neurogenesis in the ventral telencephalon. Development 126:525–534.

Catalano SM, Shatz CJ (1998) Activity-dependent cortical target selection by thalamic axons. Science 281:559–562.

Chenn A, McConnell S (1995) Cleavage orientation and the asymmetric inheritance of Notch1 immunoreactivity in mammalian neurogenesis. Cell 82:631–641.

Cline HT (2001) Dendritic arbor development and synaptogenesis. Curr Opin Neurobiol 11:118–126.

Colamarino SA, Tessier-Lavigne M (1995) The axonal chemoattractant netrin-1 is also a chemorepellent for trochlear motor axons. Cell 81:621–629.

Corbin JG, Gaiano N, Machold RP, Langston A, Fishell G (2000) The Gsh2 homeodomain gene controls multiple aspects of telencephalic development. Development 127:5007–5020.

Coulson EJ, Reid K, Shipham KM, Morley S, Kilpatrick TJ, Bartlett PF (2004) The role of neurotransmission and the Chopper domain in p75 neurotrophin receptor death signaling. Prog Brain Res 146:41–62.

Davis GW, Murphey RK (1994) Long-term regulation of short-term transmitter release properties: retrograde signaling and synaptic development. Trends Neurosci 17:9–13.

Deacon TW, Pakzaban P, Isacson O (1994) The lateral ganglionic eminence is the origin of cells committed to striatal phenotypes: neural transplantation and developmental evidence. Brain Res 668:211–219.

De Carlos JA, Lopez-Mascaraque L, Valverde F (1995) The telencephalic vesicles are innervated by olfactory placode-derived cells: a possible mechanism to induce neocortical development. Neuroscience 68:1167–1178.

De Carlos JA, Lopez-Mascaraque L, Valverde F (1996) Early olfactory fiber projections and cell migration into the rat telencephalon. Int J Dev Neurosci 14:853–866.

Dehay C, Savatier P, Cortay V, Kennedy H (2001) Cell-cycle kinetics of neocortical precursors are influenced by embryonic thalamic axons. J Neurosci 21:201–214.

Deisseroth K, Singla S, Toda H, Monje M, Palmer TD, Malenka RC (2004) Excitation-neurogenesis coupling in adult neural stem/progenitor cells. Neuron 42:535–552.

Derer P, Caviness VS Jr., Sidman RL (1977) Early cortical histogenesis in the primary olfactory cortex of the mouse. Brain Res 123:27–40.

Doetsch F, Garcia-Verdugo JM, Alvarez-Buylla A (1997) Cellular composition and three-dimensional organization of the subventricular germinal zone in the adult mammalian brain. J Neurosci 17:5046–5061.

Doetsch F, Petreanu L, Caille I, Garcia-Verdugo JM, Alvarez-Buylla A (2002) EGF converts transit-amplifying neurogenic precursors in the adult brain into multipotent stem cells. Neuron 36:1021–1034.

Edagawa Y, Saito H, Abe K (2001) Endogenous serotonin contributes to a developmental decrease in long-term potentiation in the rat visual cortex. J Neurosci 21:1532–1537.

Edwards MA, Yamamoto M, Caviness VS Jr. (1990) Organization of radial glia and related cells in the developing murine CNS. An analysis based upon a new monoclonal antibody marker. Neuroscience 36:121–144.

Engert F, Bonhoeffer T (1999) Dendritic spine changes associated with hippocampal long-term synaptic plasticity. Nature 399:66–70.

Enokido Y, Wyatt S, Davies AM (1999) Developmental changes in the response of trigeminal neurons to neurotrophins: influence of birthdate and the ganglion environment. Development 126:4365–4373.

Esch T, Lemmon V, Banker G (1999) Local presentation of substrate molecules directs axon specification by cultured hippocampal neurons. J Neurosci 19:6417–6426.

Farah MH, Olson JM, Sucic HB, Hume RI, Tapscott SJ, Turner DL (2000) Generation of neurons by transient expression of neural bHLH proteins in mammalian cells. Development 127:693–702.

Fishell G, Kriegstein AR (2003) Neurons from radial glia: the consequences of asymmetric inheritance. Curr Opin Neurobiol 13:34–41.

Forster E, Tielsch A, Saum B, Weiss KH, Johanssen C, Graus-Porta D, Muller U, Frotscher M (2002) Reelin, Disabled 1, and beta 1 integrins are required for the formation of the radial glial scaffold in the hippocampus. Proc Natl Acad Sci USA 99:13178–13183.

Frantz GD, McConnell SK (1996) Restriction of late cerebral cortical progenitors to an upper-layer fate. Neuron 17:55–61.

Furuta Y, Piston DW, Hogan BL (1997) Bone morphogenetic proteins (BMPs) as regulators of dorsal forebrain development. Development 124:2203–2212.

Galceran J, Miyashita-Lin EM, Devaney E, Rubenstein JL, Grosschedl R (2000) Hippocampus development and generation of dentate gyrus granule cells is regulated by LEF1. Development 127:469–482.

Gaspar P, Cases O, Maroteaux L (2003) The developmental role of serotonin: news from mouse molecular genetics. Nat Rev Neurosci 4:1002–1012.

Goldberg JL (2003) How does an axon grow? Genes Dev 17:941–958.

Goldberg JL, Klassen MP, Hua Y, Barres BA (2002) Amacrine-signaled loss of intrinsic axon growth ability by retinal ganglion cells. Science 296:1860–1864.

Gong Q, Shipley MT (1995) Evidence that pioneer olfactory axons regulate telencephalon cell cycle kinetics to induce the formation of the olfactory bulb. Neuron 14:91–101.

Gotz M (2003) Glial cells generate neurons—master control within CNS regions: developmental perspectives on neural stem cells. Neuroscientist 9:379–397.

Grove EA, Tole S, Limon J, Yip L, Ragsdale CW (1998) The hem of the embryonic cerebral cortex is defined by the expression of multiple *Wnt* genes and is compromised in Gli3-deficient mice. Development 125:2315–2325.

Grueber WB, Jan LY, Jan YN (2003) Different levels of the homeodomain protein cut regulate distinct dendrite branching patterns of *Drosophila* multidendritic neurons. Cell 112:805–818.

Gu Q, Singer W (1995) Involvement of serotonin in developmental plasticity of kitten visual cortex. Eur J Neurosci 7:1146–1153.

Hansson SR, Cabrera-Vera TM, Hoffman BJ (1998) Infraorbital nerve transection alters serotonin transporter expression in sensory pathways in early postnatal rat development. Brain Res Dev Brain Res 111:305–314.

Hartmann M, Heumann R, Lessmann V (2001) Synaptic secretion of BDNF after high-frequency stimulation of glutamatergic synapses. EMBO J 20:5887–5897.

Haubensak W, Attardo A, Denk W, Huttner WB (2004) Neurons arise in the basal neuroepithelium of the early mammalian telencephalon: a major site of neurogenesis. Proc Natl Acad Sci USA 101:3196–3201.

He W, Ingraham C, Rising L, Goderie S, Temple S (2001) Multipotent stem cells from the mouse basal forebrain contribute GABAergic neurons and oligodendrocytes to the cerebral cortex during embryogenesis. J Neurosci 21:8854–8862.

Hinds JW (1968a) Autoradiographic study of histogenesis in the mouse olfactory bulb. II. Cell proliferation and migration. J Comp Neurol 134:305–322.

Hinds JW (1968b) Autoradiographic study of histogenesis in the mouse olfactory bulb. I. Time of origin of neurons and neuroglia. J Comp Neurol 134:287–304.

Hynes RO, Lander AD (1992) Contact and adhesive specificities in the associations, migrations, and targeting of cells and axons. Cell 68:303–322.

Inagaki N, Chihara K, Arimura N, Menager C, Kawano Y, Matsuo N, Nishimura T, Amano M, Kaibuchi K (2001) CRMP-2 induces axons in cultured hippocampal neurons. Nat Neurosci 4:781–782.

Jimenez D, Garcia C, de Castro F, Chedotal A, Sotelo C, de Carlos JA, Valverde F, Lopez-Mascaraque L (2000) Evidence for intrinsic development of olfactory structures in Pax-6 mutant mice. J Comp Neurol 428:511–526.

Jolimay N, Franck L, Langlois X, Hamon M, Darmon M (2000) Dominant role of the cytosolic C-terminal domain of the rat 5-HT1B receptor in axonal-apical targeting. J Neurosci 20:9111–9118.

Kaplan DR, Miller FD (2000) Neurotrophin signal transduction in the nervous system. Curr Opin Neurobiol 10:381–391.

Katz LC, Shatz CJ (1996) Synaptic activity and the construction of cortical circuits. Science 274:1133–1138.

Kennedy TE, Serafini T, de la Torre JR, Tessier-Lavigne M (1994) Netrins are diffusible chemotropic factors for commissural axons in the embryonic spinal cord. Cell 78:425–435.

Kim AS, Lowenstein DH, Pleasure SJ (2001) Wnt receptors and Wnt inhibitors are expressed in gradients in the developing telencephalon. Mech Dev 103:167–172.

Kintner C (2002) Neurogenesis in embryos and in adult neural stem cells. J Neurosci 22:639–643.

Kitsukawa T, Shimizu M, Sanbo M, Hirata T, Taniguchi M, Bekku Y, Yagi T, Fujisawa H (1997) Neuropilin-semaphorin III/D-mediated chemorepulsive signals play a crucial role in peripheral nerve projection in mice. Neuron 19:995–1005.

Kojic L, Dyck RH, Gu Q, Douglas RM, Matsubara J, Cynader MS (2000) Columnar distribution of serotonin-dependent plasticity within kitten striate cortex. Proc Natl Acad Sci USA 97:1841–1844.

Kosodo Y, Roper K, Haubensak W, Marzesco AM, Corbeil D, Huttner WB (2004) Asymmetric distribution of the apical plasma membrane during neurogenic divisions of mammalian neuroepithelial cells. EMBO J 23:2314–2324.

Lebrand C, Cases O, Wehrle R, Blakely RD, Edwards RH, Gaspar P (1998) Transient developmental expression of monoamine transporters in the rodent forebrain. J Comp Neurol 401:506–524.

Lee J, Duan W, Mattson MP (2002) Evidence that brain-derived neurotrophic factor is required for basal neurogenesis and mediates, in part, the enhancement of neurogenesis by dietary restriction in the hippocampus of adult mice. J Neurochem 82:1367–1375.

Lee SM, Tole S, Grove E, McMahon AP (2000) A local Wnt-3a signal is required for development of the mammalian hippocampus. Development 127:457–467.

Lein P, Johnson M, Guo X, Rueger D, Higgins D (1995) Osteogenic protein-1 induces dendritic growth in rat sympathetic neurons. Neuron 15:597–605.

Levi-Montalcini R (1987) The nerve growth factor 35 years later. Science 237:1154–1162.

Lewin GR, Barde YA (1996) Physiology of the neurotrophins. Annu Rev Neurosci 19:289–317.

Li HS, Chen JH, Wu W, Fagaly T, Zhou L, Yuan W, Dupuis S, Jiang ZH, Nash W, Gick C, Ornitz DM, Wu JY, Rao Y (1999) Vertebrate slit, a secreted ligand for the transmembrane protein roundabout, is a repellent for olfactory bulb axons. Cell 96:807–818.

Lim DA, Tramontin AD, Trevejo JM, Herrera DG, Garcia-Verdugo JM, Alvarez-Buylla A (2000) Noggin antagonizes BMP signaling to create a niche for adult neurogenesis. Neuron 28:713–726.

Liu Q, Dwyer ND, O'Leary DD (2000) Differential expression of COUP-TFI, CHL1, and two novel genes in developing neocortex identified by differential display PCR. J Neurosci 20:7682–7690.

Lopez-Mascaraque L, de Castro F (2002) The olfactory bulb as an independent developmental domain. Cell Death Differ 9:1279–1286.

Luskin MB, Zigova T, Soteres BJ, Stewart RR (1997) Neuronal progenitor cells derived from the anterior subventricular zone of the neonatal rat forebrain continue to proliferate in vitro and express a neuronal phenotype. Mol Cell Neurosci 8:351–366.

Mallamaci A, Muzio L, Chan CH, Parnavelas J, Boncinelli E (2000) Area identity shifts in the early cerebral cortex of *Emx2–/–* mutant mice. Nat Neurosci 3:679–686.

Marin O, Anderson SA, Rubenstein JL (2000) Origin and molecular specification of striatal interneurons. J Neurosci 20:6063–6076.

Marshall CA, Goldman JE (2002) Subpallial dlx2–expressing cells give rise to astrocytes and oligodendrocytes in the cerebral cortex and white matter. J Neurosci 22:9821–9830.

Matsutani S, Yamamoto N (2000) Differentiation of mitral cell dendrites in the developing main olfactory bulbs of normal and naris-occluded rats. J Comp Neurol 418:402–410.

McAllister AK, Katz LC, Lo DC (1997) Opposing roles for endogenous BDNF and NT-3 in regulating cortical dendritic growth. Neuron 18:767–778.

McAllister AK, Katz LC, Lo DC (1999) Neurotrophins and synaptic plasticity. Annu Rev Neurosci 22:295–318.

Megason SG, McMahon AP (2002) A mitogen gradient of dorsal midline Wnts organizes growth in the CNS. Development 129:2087–2098.

Ming G, Henley J, Tessier-Lavigne M, Song H, Poo M (2001) Electrical activity modulates growth cone guidance by diffusible factors. Neuron 29:441–452.

Miyashita-Lin EM, Hevner R, Wassarman KM, Martinez S, Rubenstein JL (1999) Early neocortical regionalization in the absence of thalamic innervation. Science 285:906–909.

Miyata T, Kawaguchi A, Okano H, Ogawa M (2001) Asymmetric inheritance of radial glial fibers by cortical neurons. Neuron 31:727–741.

Mizuguchi R, Sugimori M, Takebayashi H, Kosako H, Nagao M, Yoshida S, Nabeshima Y, Shimamura K, Nakafuku M (2001) Combinatorial roles of olig2 and neurogenin2 in the coordinated induction of pan-neuronal and subtype-specific properties of motoneurons. Neuron 31:757–771.

Mombaerts P, Wang F, Dulac C, Chao SK, Nemes A, Mendelsohn M, Edmondson J, Axel R (1996) Visualizing an olfactory sensory map. Cell 87:675–686.

Moore AW, Jan LY, Jan YN (2002) hamlet, a binary genetic switch between single- and multiple-dendrite neuron morphology. Science 297:1355–1358.

Nakatomi H, Kuriu T, Okabe S, Yamamoto S, Hatano O, Kawahara N, Tamura A, Kirino T, Nakafuku M (2002) Regeneration of hippocampal pyramidal neurons after ischemic brain injury by recruitment of endogenous neural progenitors. Cell 110:429–441.

Nebigil CG, Choi DS, Dierich A, Hickel P, Le Meur M, Messaddeq N, Launay JM, Maroteaux L (2000) Serotonin 2B receptor is required for heart development. Proc Natl Acad Sci USA 97:9508–9513.

Nebigil CG, Etienne N, Messaddeq N, Maroteaux L (2003) Serotonin is a novel survival factor of cardiomyocytes: mitochondria as a target of 5-HT2B receptor signaling. FASEB J 17:1373–1375.

Nedivi E, Wu GY, Cline HT (1998) Promotion of dendritic growth by CPG15, an activity-induced signaling molecule. Science 281:1863–1866.

Nery S, Fishell G, Corbin JG (2002) The caudal ganglionic eminence is a source of distinct cortical and subcortical cell populations. Nat Neurosci 5:1279–1287.

Nieto M, Schuurmans C, Britz O, Guillemot F (2001) Neural bHLH genes control the neuronal versus glial fate decision in cortical progenitors. Neuron 29:401–413.

Ninkina N, Adu J, Fischer A, Pinon LG, Buchman VL, Davies AM (1996) Expression and function of TrkB variants in developing sensory neurons. EMBO J 15:6385–6393.

Noctor SC, Flint AC, Weissman TA, Dammerman RS, Kriegstein AR (2001) Neurons derived from radial glial cells establish radial units in neocortex. Nature 409:714–720.

Noctor SC, Martinez-Cerdeno V, Ivic L, Kriegstein AR (2004) Cortical neurons arise in symmetric and asymmetric division zones and migrate through specific phases. Nat Neurosci 7:136–144.

Okabe S, Miwa A, Okado H (2001) Spine formation and correlated assembly of presynaptic and postsynaptic molecules. J Neurosci 21:6105–6114.

Oppenheim RW (1991) Cell death during development of the nervous system. Annu Rev Neurosci 14:453–501.

Panchision DM, Pickel JM, Studer L, Lee SH, Turner PA, Hazel TG, McKay RD (2001) Sequential actions of BMP receptors control neural precursor cell production and fate. Genes Dev 15:2094–2110.

Parnavelas JG (2000) The origin and migration of cortical neurones: new vistas. Trends Neurosci 23:126–131.

Paul G, Davies AM (1995) Trigeminal sensory neurons require extrinsic signals to switch neurotrophin dependence during the early stages of target field innervation. Dev Biol 171:590–605.

Pencea V, Bingaman KD, Wiegand SJ, Luskin MB (2001) Infusion of brain-derived neurotrophic factor into the lateral ventricle of the adult rat leads to new neurons in the parenchyma of the striatum, septum, thalamus, and hypothalamus. J Neurosci 21:6706–6717.

Persico AM, Baldi A, Dell'Acqua ML, Moessner R, Murphy DL, Lesch KP, Keller F (2003) Reduced programmed cell death in brains of serotonin transporter knockout mice. Neuroreport 14:341–344.

Placzek M, Tessier-Lavigne M, Jessell T, Dodd J (1990) Orientation of commissural axons in vitro in response to a floor plate-derived chemoattractant. Development 110:19–30.

Pleasure SJ, Anderson S, Hevner R, Bagri A, Marin O, Lowenstein DH, Rubenstein JL (2000a) Cell migration from the ganglionic eminences is required for the development of hippocampal GABAergic interneurons. Neuron 28:727–740.

Pleasure SJ, Collins AE, Lowenstein DH (2000b) Unique expression patterns of cell fate molecules delineate sequential stages of dentate gyrus development. J Neurosci 20:6095–6105.

Polleux F, Morrow T, Ghosh A (2000) Semaphorin 3A is a chemoattractant for cortical apical dendrites. Nature 404:567–573.

Poo MM (2001) Neurotrophins as synaptic modulators. Nat Rev Neurosci 2:24–32.

Qian X, Goderie SK, Shen Q, Stern JH, Temple S (1998) Intrinsic programs of patterned cell lineages in isolated vertebrate CNS ventricular zone cells. Development 125:3143–3152.

Qian X, Shen Q, Goderie SK, He W, Capela A, Davis AA, Temple S (2000) Timing of CNS cell generation: a programmed sequence of neuron and glial cell production from isolated murine cortical stem cells. Neuron 28:69–80.

Rajagopalan S, Vivancos V, Nicolas E, Dickson BJ (2000) Selecting a longitudinal pathway: Robo receptors specify the lateral position of axons in the Drosophila CNS. Cell 103:1033–1045.

Rajan I, Witte S, Cline HT (1999) NMDA receptor activity stabilizes presynaptic retinotectal axons and postsynaptic optic tectal cell dendrites in vivo. J Neurobiol 38:357–368.

Rakic P (1974) Neurons in rhesus monkey visual cortex: systematic relation between time of origin and eventual disposition. Science 183:425–427.

Rebsam A, Seif I, Gaspar P (2002) Refinement of thalamocortical arbors and emergence of barrel domains in the primary somatosensory cortex: a study of normal and monoamine oxidase a knock-out mice. J Neurosci 22:8541–8552.

Ressler KJ, Sullivan SL, Buck LB (1994) Information coding in the olfactory system: evidence for a stereotyped and highly organized epitope map in the olfactory bulb. Cell 79:1245–1255.

Rickmann M, Amaral DG, Cowan WM (1987) Organization of radial glial cells during the development of the rat dentate gyrus. J Comp Neurol 264:449–479.

Robinson M, Adu J, Davies AM (1996) Timing and regulation of trkB and BDNF mRNA expression in placode-derived sensory neurons and their targets. Eur J Neurosci 8:2399–2406.

Rothstein RP, Levison SW (2002) Damage to the choroid plexus, ependyma and subependyma as a consequence of perinatal hypoxia/ischemia. Dev Neurosci 24:426–436.

Salichon N, Gaspar P, Upton AL, Picaud S, Hanoun N, Hamon M, De Maeyer E, Murphy DL, Mossner R, Lesch KP, Hen R, Seif I (2001) Excessive activation of serotonin (5-HT) 1B receptors disrupts the formation of sensory maps in monoamine oxidase A and 5-HT transporter knock-out mice. J Neurosci 21:884–896.

Santarelli L, Saxe M, Gross C, Surget A, Battaglia F, Dulawa S, Weisstaub N, Lee J, Duman R, Arancio O, Belzung C, Hen R (2003) Requirement of hippocampal neurogenesis for the behavioral effects of antidepressants. Science 301:805–809.

Schinder AF, Poo M (2000) The neurotrophin hypothesis for synaptic plasticity. Trends Neurosci 23:639–645.

Scott JW, McBride RL, Schneider SP (1980) The organization of projections from the olfactory bulb to the piriform cortex and olfactory tubercle in the rat. J Comp Neurol 194:519–534.

Seki T, Arai Y (1991) Expression of highly polysialylated NCAM in the neocortex and piriform cortex of the developing and the adult rat. Anat Embryol 184:395–401.

Serafini T, Colamarino SA, Leonardo ED, Wang H, Beddington R, Skarnes WC, Tessier-Lavigne M (1996) Netrin-1 is required for commissural axon guidance in the developing vertebrate nervous system. Cell 87:1001–1014.

Seri B, Garcia-Verdugo JM, Collado-Morente L, McEwen BS, Alvarez-Buylla A (2004) Cell types, lineage, and architecture of the germinal zone in the adult dentate gyrus. J Comp Neurol 478:359.

Seri B, Garcia-Verdugo JM, McEwen BS, Alvarez-Buylla A (2001) Astrocytes give rise to new neurons in the adult mammalian hippocampus. J Neurosci 21:7153–7160.

Shen Q, Zhong W, Jan YN, Temple S (2002) Asymmetric Numb distribution is critical for asymmetric cell division of mouse cerebral cortical stem cells and neuroblasts. Development 129:4843–4853.

Shi SH, Jan LY, Jan YN (2003) Hippocampal neuronal polarity specified by spatially localized mPar3/mPar6 and PI 3-kinase activity. Cell 112:63–75.

Shirasaki R, Mirzayan C, Tessier-Lavigne M, Murakami F (1996) Guidance of circumferentially growing axons by netrin-dependent and -independent floor plate chemotropism in the vertebrate brain. Neuron 17:1079–1088.

Shirasaki R, Tamada A, Katsumata R, Murakami F (1995) Guidance of cerebellofugal axons in the rat embryo: directed growth toward the floor plate and subsequent elongation along the longitudinal axis. Neuron 14:961–972.

Sievers J, Hartmann D, Pehlemann FW, Berry M (1992) Development of astroglial cells in the proliferative matrices, the granule cell layer, and the hippocampal fissure of the hamster dentate gyrus. J Comp Neurol 320:1–32.

Simpson JH, Bland KS, Fetter RD, Goodman CS (2000a) Short-range and long-range guidance by Slit and its Robo receptors: a combinatorial code of Robo receptors controls lateral position. Cell 103:1019–1032.

Simpson JH, Kidd T, Bland KS, Goodman CS (2000b) Short-range and long-range guidance by slit and its Robo receptors. Robo and Robo2 play distinct roles in midline guidance. Neuron 28:753–766.

Song H, Ming G, He Z, Lehmann M, McKerracher L, Tessier-Lavigne M, Poo M (1998) Conversion of neuronal growth cone responses from repulsion to attraction by cyclic nucleotides. Science 281:1515–1518.

Spitzer NC, Lautermilch NJ, Smith RD, Gomez TM (2000) Coding of neuronal differentiation by calcium transients. Bioessays 22:811–817.

Stenman J, Toresson H, Campbell K (2003) Identification of two distinct progenitor populations in the lateral ganglionic eminence: implications for striatal and olfactory bulb neurogenesis. J Neurosci 23:167–174.

Stoeckli ET, Landmesser LT (1995) Axonin-1, Nr-CAM, and Ng-CAM play different roles in the in vivo guidance of chick commissural neurons. Neuron 14:1165–1179.

Stout RP, Graziadei PP (1980) Influence of the olfactory placode on the development of the brain in *Xenopus laevis* (Daudin). I. Axonal growth and connections of the transplanted olfactory placode. Neuroscience 5:2175–2186.

Sturrock RR, Smart IH (1980) A morphological study of the mouse subependymal layer from embryonic life to old age. J Anat 130:391–415.

Sussel L, Marin O, Kimura S, Rubenstein JL (1999) Loss of Nkx2.1 homeobox gene function results in a ventral to dorsal molecular respecification within the basal telencephalon: evidence for a transformation of the pallidum into the striatum. Development 126:3359–3370.

Takahashi T, Nowakowski RS, Caviness VS, Jr. (1995) The cell cycle of the pseudostratified ventricular epithelium of the embryonic murine cerebral wall. J Neurosci 15:6046–6057.

Tamada A, Shirasaki R, Murakami F (1995) Floor plate chemoattracts crossed axons and chemorepels uncrossed axons in the vertebrate brain. Neuron 14:1083–1093.

Tamamaki N, Fujimori KE, Takauji R (1997) Origin and route of tangentially migrating neurons in the developing neocortical intermediate zone. J Neurosci 17:8313–8323.

Tanigaki K, Nogaki F, Takahashi J, Tashiro K, Kurooka H, Honjo T (2001) Notch1 and Notch3 instructively restrict bFGF-responsive multipotent neural progenitor cells to an astroglial fate. Neuron 29:45–55.

Taniguchi M, Yuasa S, Fujisawa H, Naruse I, Saga S, Mishina M, Yagi T (1997) Disruption of semaphorin III/D gene causes severe abnormality in peripheral nerve projection. Neuron 19:519–530.

Tarabykin V, Stoykova A, Usman N, Gruss P (2001) Cortical upper layer neurons derive from the subventricular zone as indicated by Svet1 gene expression. Development 128:1983–1993.

Tecott LH, Sun LM, Akana SF, Strack AM, Lowenstein DH, Dallman MF, Julius D (1995) Eating disorder and epilepsy in mice lacking 5-HT2c serotonin receptors. Nature 374:542–546.

Tessier-Lavigne M, Goodman CS (1996) The molecular biology of axon guidance. Science 274:1123–1133.

Tessier-Lavigne M, Placzek M, Lumsden AG, Dodd J, Jessell TM (1988) Chemotropic guidance of developing axons in the mammalian central nervous system. Nature 336:775–778.

Tomita K, Moriyoshi K, Nakanishi S, Guillemot F, Kageyama R (2000) Mammalian achaete-scute and atonal homologs regulate neuronal versus glial fate determination in the central nervous system. EMBO J 19:5460–5472.

Trachtenberg JT, Stryker MP (2001) Rapid anatomical plasticity of horizontal connections in the developing visual cortex. J Neurosci 21:3476–3482.

Treloar HB, Feinstein P, Mombaerts P, Greer CA (2002) Specificity of glomerular targeting by olfactory sensory axons. J Neurosci 22:2469–2477.

Tuttle R, Nakagawa Y, Johnson JE, O'Leary DD (1999) Defects in thalamocortical axon pathfinding correlate with altered cell domains in Mash-1-deficient mice. Development 126:1903–1916.

Upton AL, Ravary A, Salichon N, Moessner R, Lesch KP, Hen R, Seif I, Gaspar P (2002) Lack of 5-HT(1B) receptor and of serotonin transporter have different effects on the segregation of retinal axons in the lateral geniculate nucleus compared to the superior colliculus. Neuroscience 111:597–610.

Vaidya VA, Marek GJ, Aghajanian GK, Duman RS (1997) 5-HT2A receptor-mediated regulation of brain-derived neurotrophic factor mRNA in the hippocampus and the neocortex. J Neurosci 17:2785–2795.

Varela-Echavarria A, Tucker A, Puschel AW, Guthrie S (1997) Motor axon subpopulations respond differentially to the chemorepellents netrin-1 and semaphorin D. Neuron 18:193–207.

Vassar R, Chao SK, Sitcheran R, Nunez JM, Vosshall LB, Axel R (1994) Topographic organization of sensory projections to the olfactory bulb. Cell 79:981–991.

Vitalis T, Cases O, Callebert J, Launay JM, Price DJ, Seif I, Gaspar P (1998) Effects of monoamine oxidase A inhibition on barrel formation in the mouse somatosensory cortex: determination of a sensitive developmental period. J Comp Neurol 393:169–184.

Vogel KS, Davies AM (1991) The duration of neurotrophic factor independence in early sensory neurons is matched to the time course of target field innervation. Neuron 7:819–830.

Wang KH, Brose K, Arnott D, Kidd T, Goodman CS, Henzel W, Tessier-Lavigne M (1999) Biochemical purification of a mammalian slit protein as a positive regulator of sensory axon elongation and branching. Cell 96:771–784.

Washbourne P, Bennett JE, McAllister AK (2002) Rapid recruitment of NMDA receptor transport packets to nascent synapses. Nat Neurosci 5:751–759.

Whitford KL, Marillat V, Stein E, Goodman CS, Tessier-Lavigne M, Chedotal A, Ghosh A (2002) Regulation of cortical dendrite development by Slit-Robo interactions. Neuron 33:47–61.

Wichterle H, Garcia-Verdugo JM, Herrera DG, Alvarez-Buylla A (1999) Young neurons from medial ganglionic eminence disperse in adult and embryonic brain. Nat Neurosci 2:461–466.

Wichterle H, Turnbull DH, Nery S, Fishell G, Alvarez-Buylla A (2001) In utero fate mapping reveals distinct migratory pathways and fates of neurons born in the mammalian basal forebrain. Development 128:3759–3771.

Wodarz A, Huttner WB (2003) Asymmetric cell division during neurogenesis in *Drosophila* and vertebrates. Mech Dev 120:1297–1309.

Yan W, Wilson CC, Haring JH (1997) 5-HT1a receptors mediate the neurotrophic effect of serotonin on developing dentate granule cells. Brain Res Dev Brain Res 98:185–190.

Zhou C, Qiu Y, Pereira FA, Crair MC, Tsai SY, Tsai MJ (1999) The nuclear orphan receptor COUP-TFI is required for differentiation of subplate neurons and guidance of thalamocortical axons. Neuron 24:847–859.

Zhou C, Tsai SY, Tsai MJ (2001) COUP-TFI: an intrinsic factor for early regionalization of the neocortex. Genes Dev 15:2054–2059.

Zhou CJ, Zhao C, Pleasure SJ (2004) Wnt signaling mutants have decreased dentate granule cell production and radial glial scaffolding abnormalities. J Neurosci 24:121–126.

5

Neurogenesis in the Adult Olfactory System

The olfactory system contains not one but two neurogenic regions of the adult nervous system: a turnover of olfactory receptor neurons, which occurs in the olfactory epithelium and thus originates from a population of precursor cells outside the central nervous system (CNS), and adult neurogenesis in the olfactory bulb, which is part of the CNS and in which two types of interneurons are generated from a population of precursor cells in the lateral walls of the ventricles. Historically, the exploration of both processes was done parallel to and to a large degree independent of each other. However, despite the separate precursor populations, both forms of adult neurogenesis are intricately linked. Many features are shared between neurogenesis in the olfactory epithelium and within the CNS.

Smelling is our sense for chemicals. Our olfactory system can distinguish an estimated 10,000 smells and thus thousands of chemical compounds. This task is accomplished by the integration of signals from about ten million olfactory receptor neurons specialized in the detection of individual chemical compounds. Roughly 2% of the human genome are needed to encode for the variety of hundreds of odor receptors.

It is not necessary to name the chemical compounds underlying a particular smell to react appropriately. Smelling is a powerful alarm system that not only warns of impending dangers but also attracts animals to food and mates. Rodents and canines rely on the olfactory system as much as humans rely on the visual system to form an inner representation of the world. The olfactory memory is one of the strongest forms of memory we have. We cannot consciously revoke olfactory memory; a tiny olfactory cue is sufficient to kick off a wealth of associations and profound memories, often closely associated with emotions.

Olfactory receptor neurons are not nearly as long-lasting as the memories they help to generate. These neurons are continuously exchanged through neurogenesis in the adult olfactory epithelium. Olfactory receptor neurons project to the olfactory bulb where they form connections to the mitral and tufted cells within distinct clusters called glomeruli. The mitral and tufted cells project out of the olfactory bulb to the olfactory tubercle. Adult neurogenesis in the olfactory bulb replaces two types of interneurons interacting with mitral and tufted cells. Whereas the receptor neurons are constantly replaced, the mitral and tufted cells, the second neuron in the olfactory system, are stable and only interneurons relating between them are replaced or added.

ADULT NEUROGENESIS IN THE OLFACTORY EPITHELIUM

Neuronal Development in the Olfactory Epithelium

Neurogenesis in the adult olfactory epithelium generates new olfactory receptor neurons. The first description of neurogenesis in the adult mammalian olfactory epithelium was reported by Nagahara in 1940. Adult neurogenesis in the olfactory epithelium was rediscovered in the early 1970s (Graziadei, 1973; Graziadei and DeHan, 1973; Graziadei and Graziadei, 1979a, 1979b). Since then it has been described for humans and nonhuman primates (Graziadei et al., 1980) and is conserved in rodents into old age (Loo et al., 1996). Olfactory receptor neurons reside within the olfactory epithelium in the roof of the nasal cavity. In mice the dividing cells are located primarily along the margins of the epithelium, in rats more proliferative cells are found in the center (Martinez-Marcos et al., 2000). Whether this location is of functional relevance is not known.

The amount of neurogenesis in the adult olfactory epithelium is the highest of all known neurogenic regions. It has been speculated that one of the possible reasons for this high neuronal turnover in the olfactory epithelium is that olfactory receptor neurons are exposed to and particularly sensitive to chemical noxious agents. By virtue of the necessity to recognize chemical molecules, supposedly they are particularly vulnerable to the neurotoxic effects of these substances and thus need to be replaced constantly.

Neuronal development proceeds from the precursor cells, which are at the most basal level of the olfactory epithelium. Differentiating cells migrate vertically to more superficial layers while they mature. It seems that horizontal migration occurs only before neuronal differentiation begins on the level of precursor cells. This causes a columnar organization of neuronal development. The developing neurons begin to express a sequence of neuronal markers, from immature to mature. Immature neuronal markers are, for example, transcription factor NeuroD, expressed on the level just above the basal globose cells, and β-III-tubulin. Mature markers are the olfactory-specific G-protein subunit (Golf) and olfactory marker protein (OMP).

The new neurons have to send their axons to the olfactory bulb. Early during their rise the new neurons also express GAP43, a protein associated with axon elongation. The distance between olfactory epithelium and the olfactory bulb is therefore a region of extremely high axonal growth in the adult. A specialized local population of glia cells, called "olfactory ensheathing glia," promotes axonal growth.

Neuronal Precursor Cells in the Adult Olfactory Epithelium

The precursor cell population for adult neurogenesis in the olfactory epithelium resides in the olfactory epithelium itself (Fig. 5–1). They are found in the basal layer, express keratin, and are called "globose basal cells." Although widely equated with the stem cells in this system, it is not quite clear whether the globose cells actually are the most stem-like cells in the olfactory epithelium. They certainly account for most of the ongoing cell divisions (Huard and Schwob, 1995).

Intermediate filament nestin is expressed in many CNS precursor cells. In the olfactory epithelium, however, it appears that the nestin-expressing cells are not the basal globose cells but the neigboring sustentacular cells. Sustentacular cells, in turn, might have a function similar to that of radial

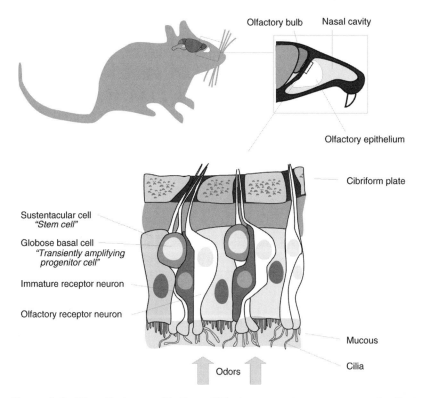

Figure 5–1. The olfactory epithelium. Olfactory receptor neurons are the first neurons of the olfactory system. They show lifelong turnover. The highest-ranking stem cells of the olfactory epithelium appear to be the sustentacular cells, which correspond to radial glial cells of the central nervous system. The globose basal cells are the transiently amplifying progenitor cells of this system. They give rise to immature receptor neurons. Differentiated receptor neurons carry cilia, which are embedded in a layer of mucous in which odorants dissolve.

glia in the CNS. As we have seen in Chapter 3, radial glia–like cells play a dual role in adult neurogenesis. They serve as stem cells and scaffold for the ensuing neuronal migration and differentiation. A similar function of sustentacular cells has not yet been demonstrated for the olfactory epithelium. But the sustentacular cells express transcription factor Pax6 (Davis and Reed, 1996). *Pax6* is one of the master genes in neurogenesis and affects lineage choices between glial and neuronal differentiation. It might well be that the neurogenic system of the olfactory epithelium mirrors the situation in the neurogenic regions of the adult CNS with respect to the basic cellular structure as well.

Anne Calof from the University of California, Irvine, has described a progression through three different stages of progenitor cells. The "stem cell" of this system gives rise to a transiently amplifying progenitor cell, which can be identified by its expression of transcription factor Mash1 (Davis and Reed, 1996). The stem cell as well as differentiated neurons do not express Mash1. The Mash1-negative stem cell might be identical to the sustentacular cell but currently this is only a hypothesis. The transiently amplifying progenitor cell in turn generates an "immediate neuronal precursor," in the terminology of Calof and colleagues, from which the new olfactory receptor neurons arise. Independent of this and like the intermediate progenitor cells in the other neurogenic systems, globose basal cells show multipotency ex vivo and after reimplantation (Chen et al., 2004).

Regulation of Neurogenesis in the Adult Olfactory Epithelium

As one might expect, neurogenesis in the adult olfactory epithelium can be influenced by numerous manipulations. It is helpful to sort out the potential regulators according to their conceptual level. A change in behavior leads to changes on a systems level that in turn affect communication between cells, leading to effects on the transcriptional control of genes responsible for neurogenesis. For example, exploratory behavior might set the stage for alertness in the olfactory system, which leads to an increase in neurotrophin 3 (NT3) that in turn stimulates the PI3K/Akt pathway promoting neuronal survival. In reality, such interactions are far more complex and we will come back to such networks again.

The means by which neurogenesis in the olfactory epithelium is regulated in response to behavior is not well studied. It is believed that an increase in olfactory behavior will lead to greater exposure to chemical noxae and thus to more damage to olfactory epithelium, which in turn should provoke increased cellular turnover. The latter stage has in fact been demonstrated; what is missing is evidence that this is the physiological way to regulate neurogenesis in the olfactory epithelium. Is damage the main stimulus, or are there other, essentially positive or instructive mechanisms as well?

Tampering with the olfactory system induces neurogenesis of the olfactory epithelium. Already some of the earliest reports on adult olfactory receptor neurogenesis identified damage as a neurogenic stimulus. In 1979, Graziadei reported that damage to the axons of the olfactory receptor neurons causes severe retrograde degeneration that essentially depletes the olfactory epithelium of receptor neurons (Graziadei and Graziadei, 1979a). Macrophages clear the area of damage. Macrophages also up-regulate leukocyte inhibitory factor (LIF), which can stimulate neurogenesis at early stages of progenitor cell proliferation (Getchell et al., 2002). This fits with the hypothesis that inflammatory cells and mediators are important regulators of adult neurogenesis (see Chapter 9).

About 1 week after the damage, a strong proliferative response of basal cells can be detected and after roughly 1 month the olfactory epithelium is reconstituted to normal strengths. A detailed description of developmental stages in olfactory receptor neurogenesis is given in the Graziadeis' admirable 1979 study, in which the basal cells are identified as the stem cells driving adult neurogenesis (Graziadei and Graziadei, 1979a, 1979b). Many studies have elaborated on these initial findings. For example, it was found that the receptors of the reconstituted epithelium indeed become functional and can respond to odors (Costanzo, 1985).

Closing one naris is a less invasive way to deprive olfactory receptor neurons. Naris occlusion on postnatal day 1 in rats acutely depressed cell proliferation in the olfactory epithelium. Reopening of the naris 20 days later resulted in a sharp rebound and reconstitution of the normal thickness of the epithelium within days (Farbman et al., 1988; Mirich and Brunjes, 2001). Anne Calof has hypothesized that the precursor cells of the olfactory epithelium "sense" the neuronal density in the epithelium and that a local regulatory mechanism thus allows maintainence of the olfactory epithelium at a defined receptor density.

On the level of growth factors, the regulators of neurogenesis in the adult olfactory epithelium include fibroblast growth factor-2 (FGF-2), epidermal growth factor (EGF), insulia–like growth factor-1 (IGF-1), brain-derived neurotrophic factor (BDNF), platelet-derived growth factor (PDGF), NT3, transforming growth factor-β (TGF-β), and LIF. All of these have been shown to be able to influence neurogenesis. In vitro, FGF-2 acted as strong mitogen on the globose basal cells, TGF-β induced neuronal differentiation, and PDGF acted as a survival promoting factor (Newman et al., 2000). This might be indicative of a sequential role of these factors. In explant cultures, however, only FGF-2 had an effect on neuronal outgrowth and differentiation (MacDonald et al., 1996). In vivo, LIF was the only factor that was measurably induced before the onset of precursor cell proliferation when ablation of the olfactory bulb was used to trigger neurogenesis in the olfactory epithelium (Bauer et al., 2003). Generally, the finding that a given factor can influence neurogenesis in vitro (or in vivo) does not necessarily mean that it actually does so in the physiologic regulation of adult neurogenesis.

In vitro, mechanical stress to rodent olfactory epithelial cell cultures resulted in increased neurogenesis even in the absence of any added growth factors (Feron et al., 1999a). However, these cultures were not clonal precursor cell cultures, thus still allowing for the possibility that endogenous growth factors participate in the proneurogenic talk between different cell types of cultures. These examples show how difficult it is to characterize the regulatory role of a single communication molecule in the regulation of adult neurogenesis.

Another common thread in the regulation of neuronal development is that the effects of a large variety of external cues, be they growth factors, hormones, or neurotransmitters, merge on a much smaller number of transcription factors. These factors control restriction points of neuronal development. One of the great mysteries of biology is how integration over all the different signals occurs and specificity of the response is maintained.

Mash1 is one of the transcription factors known to be important in this system. Mash1 is expressed in the highly proliferative progenitor cells of the olfactory epithelium, which are likely identical to the globose cell. During development, Mash1 is also required to establish the precursor cell population of the medial ganglionic eminence. Accordingly, Mash1-mutant mice show neuronal losses in the olfactory epithelium and the autonomous system, both of which arise from the medial ganglionic eminence (Casarosa et al., 1999).

Olfactory progenitor cells exposed to bone morphogenic proteins (BMPs), known from embryology as strong inhibitors of neurogenesis, lose Mash1 expression (Shou et al., 1999). This finding is more evidence that the transcription factors controlling embryonic neurogenesis might also be involved in the adult.

For Hes1 and Hes5, too, only developmental data are available (Cau et al., 2000). They indicate that Hes1 regulates Mash1 transcription, first to define regional domains in which neurogenesis is to occur in the olfactory placode, and second to control the number of precursor cells within this domain. Hes1 is a suppressor of transcription, thus acting as a negative regulator. In double mutants for *Hes1* and *Hes5*, *Neurogenin1*, a gene downstream of Mash1 signaling, is up-regulated, inducing neurogenesis. It is not yet clear whether Hes1 has this same role during adult neurogenesis.

The selection of transcription factors discussed above reflects the patchy knowledge of them we have at present. But it should become clear how hypotheses on transcriptional regulation in the adult can be derived from embryonic development and that adult neurogenesis cannot be understood without reference to embryonic development.

Adult Neurogenesis in the Olfactory Epithelium as a Window to the Central Nervous System

In the general scientific view, neurogenesis in the olfactory epithelium might be somewhat undervalued. What makes adult olfactory neurogenesis particularly appealing is that it can serve as an accessible system in which to study neuronal development in adult humans. All the various steps, from precursor cell proliferation over migration to axon elongation and synaptogenesis, occur within a small area that lies outside the skull. Rett syndrome, for example, is an inherited neurodevelopmental disorder due to a mutation in the gene that encodes methyl CpG binding protein 2 (*mecp2*), which in turn is a repressor of gene transcription primarily in neurons. Most neuronal populations are inaccessible even for more invasive routine diagnostics. But Rett syndrome has been successfully diagnosed from biopsies of olfactory epithelium (Ronnett et al., 2003)—probably not with good enough validity for clinical use, but nevertheless impressive. Many more disturbances of neuronal development could be diagnosed from the olfactory epithelium, provided the problem affects the olfactory cells as much as the central neurons.

This potential clinical applicability makes further comparative studies worthwhile. An understanding of adult neurogenesis in the olfactory epithelium and its relationship to neurogenesis in the olfactory bulb might help us to learn about neurogenesis within the CNS generally. Some researchers have even attempted to study the cellular basis of psychiatric disorders such as schizophrenia from the olfactory epithelium (Arnold et al., 1998; Smutzer et al., 1998; Feron et al., 1999b). Although the immense complexity of schizophrenia and the vast number of unknowns in this disorder require that caution be used in this approach, the strategy is intriguing and might lead to novel ways of diagnosing deficits in plasticity underlying neuropsychiatric disorders. The degree to which plasticity in the olfactory epithelium reflects plasticity within the CNS must first be established.

Beyond experimental and diagnostic aspects, some researchers are convinced that adult neurogenesis in the olfactory epithelium might provide a resource for cell therapy. Autologous neural precursor cells in the olfactory epithelium could be harvested through biopsy from the nasal cavity. The open issue of precursor cell heterogeneity in the adult CNS, however, will have even greater relevance if stem cells from the periphery are included. Whether neural precursor cells from the olfactory epithelium could be used as a source to replace lost neurons in the CNS is not known at present.

Olfactory ensheathing glia, the specialized glia of the olfactory epithelium that promotes axonal growth, is also of special interest with regard to reconstitutive efforts after axonal damage. For example, in spinal cord injury, local glial cells prevent regenerative axonal growth, thus one could try to transplant permissive olfactory ensheathing glia to enable the regrowing axons to bridge the area of damage (Bunge and Pearse, 2003; Barnett and Riddell, 2004).

ADULT NEUROGENESIS IN THE OLFACTORY BULB

The second form of adult neurogenesis in the olfactory system occurs within the boundaries of the CNS and generates interneurons in the olfactory bulb

—one type in the granule cell layer and two types in the periglomerular region. This form of adult neurogenesis is usually referred to as adult olfactory bulb neurogenesis because in the olfactory bulb the terminally differentiated new neurons are found. However, the entire process of neuronal development spreads out over a much larger brain area between the ventricle walls and the olfactory bulb (Fig. 4–6 and 5–2).

The Adult Subventricular Zone

The precursor cell population feeding neurogenesis in the adult olfactory bulb resides in the subventricular zone (SVZ) of the lateral wall of the lateral ventricles. The SVZ is defined as a one- or two-cell body–wide zone below the ependyma. The term *subependymal layer* is sometimes used synonymously, but most groups prefer *subventricular zone* (Boulder Committee, 1970). From the SVZ the developing new neurons migrate over a relatively long distance into the olfactory bulb. They do so in a particular form of migration called "chain migration." The anatomical structure along which this migration occurs is called the "rostral migratory stream" (RMS) or sometimes "rostral migratory path" (RMP).

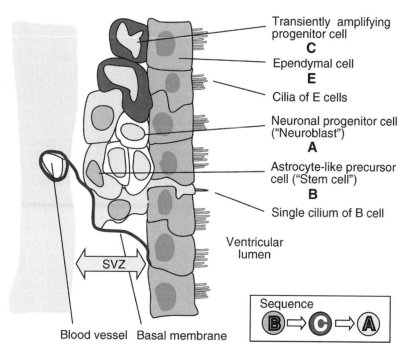

Figure 5–2. Cellular composition of the adult subventricular zone (SVZ). Concept and nomenclature are based on the work of Fiona Doetsch, Arturo Alvarez-Buylla, and colleagues (Doetsch et al., 1999a, 1999b). See also Figure 5–3.

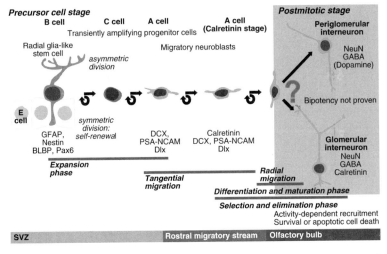

Figure 5–3. Developmental stages in adult olfactory bulb neurogenesis. Neuronal development in the subventricular zone (SVZ), rostral migratory stream (RMS), and olfactory bulb proceeds through a series of stages that can be identified immunohistochemically. This pattern shows similarities to but also important differences from the situation in the hippocampus (Fig. 6–4). BLBP, brain lipid binding protein; DCX, doublecortin; Dlx and Pax6, homeobox genes; GFAP, glial fibrillary acidic protein; PSA–NCAM, polysialylated neural cell adhesion molecule.

The SVZ is a remnant of the SVZ of the embryonic forebrain. During embryonic development, precursor cell activity in the ventricular zone precedes proliferation in the SVZ. Neuroepithelial cells directly lining the ventricle expand, first thickening the ventricular layer, then building up a distinct SVZ. In mice the SVZ becomes first visible in the ganglionic eminences around embryonic day 11 (E11) (Smart, 1976). By E15, proliferation in the SVZ surpasses cell divisions in the ventricular zone. Radial glia not only provides guidance structure to newly generated cells but also acts as precursor cells. Postnatally, radial glia transforms into a type of astrocyte located in the SVZ while still retaining some characteristics of radial glia (Alvarez-Buylla et al., 2001). These radial glia–like astrocytes no longer span the entire cortical thickness but reach from the ventricular surface to Virchow-Robin spaces around the deep blood vessels of the cortex, thereby still maintaining contact with the pial surface (Fig. 5–2). In the postnatal and adult brain, the ventricular zone has transformed into the ependyma, the epithelial lining of the ventricles. In this process, the pseudostratified epithelium of the ventricular zone turns into a simple, columnar epithelium (Sturrock and Smart, 1980). The ependymal cells carry cilia in large numbers. Through gaps between the ependymal cells, the astrocyte-like precursor cells of the adult SVZ reach the ventricular surface. The close contact between ependyma and astrocyte-like precursor cells might have important regulatory functions. The ependymal cells secrete noggin, which antagonizes the action of BMPs in the neurogenic niche of the SVZ and thus inhibits gliogenesis and promotes neurogenesis (Lim et al., 2000).

B Cells Are the Astrocyte-Like Stem Cells of the Subventricular Zone

In 1997, Fiona Doetsch, Arturo Alvarez-Buylla, and colleagues showed that glial fibrillary acidic protein (GFAP)-expressing astrocytic cells act as the primary stem cells in the adult SVZ (Doetsch et al., 1997). They named these astrocytes "B cells" and identified in vivo, a transiently amplifying progenitor cell (C cell) originating from the B cell and in turn giving rise to immature neurons or neuroblasts (A cell, Figs. 5–2 and 5–4). Ultrastructurally, two types of SVZ astrocytes could be distinguished; B1 cells close to the ependyma, and B2 cells toward the striatum. B2 cells ensheathe migratory A cells (Doetsch et al., 1997). It is not known whether this distinction relates to differences in precursor cell properties as well.

The particular anatomical situation in the SVZ became the topic of a scientific debate over whether the stem cells of the ventricular wall region were subventricular astrocytes or ependymal cells. Jonas Frisén from the Karolinska Institutet in Stockholm argued for an ependymal source because he was able to demonstrate that stem cells derived from the ventricle wall would pick up dyes and retroviruses injected into the ventricles, confirming their contact with the ventricular surface (Johansson et al., 1999). Also, cells with multiple cilia, a characteristic of ependymal cells, behaved like precursor cells ex vivo. In contrast, Arturo Alvarez-Buylla and colleagues favored the idea that astrocytes with cell bodies below the ependyma were the stem cells of the adult SVZ.

Selective elimination of dividing cells in the SVZ with cytostatic agent cytosine arabinoside (Ara-C) resulted in a complete loss of all signs of adult neurogenesis (Fig. 5–4). In particular, the rapidly dividing progenitor cells (C cells) disappeared. Over time, after the treatment neurogenesis reappeared (Doetsch et al., 1999b). Cells that expressed glial fibrillary acidic protein (GFAP) reappeared first. Other proliferative cells followed, and this sequence of events was interpreted as a genealogy: later cells originated from the early GFAP-positive cells.

In addition, a large proportion of SVZ precursor cells in vitro express GFAP. An isolation protocol based on the expression of GFAP allowed the prospective culture of cells with stem cell properties from this region (Laywell et al., 2000). Laywell and colleagues examined the precursor cell properties of astrocytes from various brain regions and found that astrocyte monolayers including those derived from the SVZ showed self-renewal and multipotency, whereas ependymal cells showed growth in agglomerates but were unipotent only (Laywell et al., 2000).

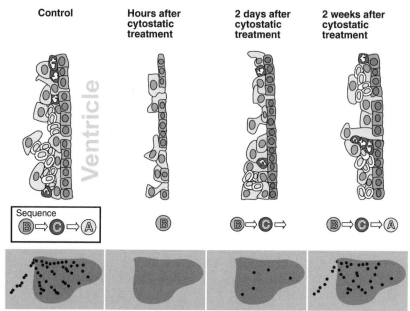

PSA-NCAM-positive chains in the lateral wall of the lateral ventricle

Figure 5–4. Cytostatic drugs disrupt integrity of the subventricular zone. Cytostatic drugs wipe out the highly proliferative progenitor cell populations (C and A) but spare some B cells. These repopulate the germinative matrix over time after the chemic assault. These findings have provided evidence of the hypothesis that astrocyte-like B cells are the stem cells of this region. Note, however, the B cells within the band of ependymal cells early after drug administration. The question of whether ependymal cells might transform into B cells remains open. Schematic drawing is based on a figure in Doetsch et al. (1999a).

Derek van der Kooy's group at the University of Toronto addressed this issue by microdissecting the SVZ and the ependymal layer. They found that ependymal cells were unipotent and produced only glial cells in the neurosphere assay. Cells in the SVZ, by contrast, turned out to be multipotent ex vivo (Chiasson et al., 1999).

However, because ependymal cells can in principle express GFAP, although they do not do so under normal conditions, the possibility that ependymal cells are stem cells cannot be excluded. The process of isolating cells from the tissue might induce GFAP expression in ependymal cells.

Doetsch and colleagues thus made use of a transgenic mouse (GFAP-TVA, which was developed by Eric Holland and Harold Varmus) in which the receptor for an avian virus not infectious for mammalian cells is expressed under the GFAP promoter. The avian virus was coupled to β-galactosidase as reporter gene and injected into the ventricle. Because the GFAP promoter drives the receptor expression, only GFAP-positive cells could be infected by the virus and thus acquire the reporter gene. Because the reporter gene itself was expressed under a ubiquitous promoter, the expression of the reporter gene product was maintained after infection and after the GFAP promoter had become inactive. Thus, cells that at later time points expressed β-galactosidase could be identified as originating from a cell that must have expressed GFAP (and therefore the avian virus receptor) when the virus was injected. This method confirmed that lineage-restricted precursor cells and new neurons were derived from an originally GFAP-positive cell in vivo (Doetsch et al., 1999a). Similarly, elimination of all proliferating GFAP-positive cells by expressing tymidine kinase under the GFAP promoter, which made them sensitive to the deadly action of the drug ganclicovir, resulted in a loss of stem cells that could be isolated from the adult SVZ (Imura et al., 2003). This stem cell depletion was specific to the SVZ (and probably the hippocampus) but did not affect the retina, a region that does contain neural precursor cells but undergoes no adult neurogenesis (Morshead et al., 2003).

Consequently, the stem cell (that is, the precursor cell highest in the local precursor cell hierarchy) of the adult ventricular wall appears to be a cell with astrocytic features whose cell body resides in the SVZ but extends a cellular process between the ependymal cells and thus maintains direct contact with the ventricular surface (Fig. 5–2). Unlike ependymal cells, which carry a number of long cilia, B cells carry one single cilium on this ventricular surface, similar to the one cilium of neural precursor cells during embryonic development. B cells thus share with ependymal cells (E cells) contact with the ventricular surface and the presence of cilia in general. To some degree, the debate about the ependymal or subependymal nature of SVZ stem cells was thus semantic. However, it is not clear whether the distinction and relationship between E and B cells are fixed or whether an exchange between the two populations can occur. The transformation of E cells into B cells is theoretically imaginable, but at present no concrete data support this idea.

C Cells are the Transiently Amplifying Progenitor Cells of the Subventricular Zone, A Cells, the Migrating Neuroblasts

In addition to the GFAP-positive B cells and ependymal E cells, Doetsch and Alvarez-Buylla identified by light and electron microscopy the transiently amplifying progenitor cell they called "C cell" (Doetsch, 2003). After injection of proliferation markers such as bromodeoxyuridine (BrdU) or tritiated thymidine, C cells are most frequently labeled; they represent the largest pool of dividing cells in the SVZ. C cells maintain close proximity to the radial elements provided by B cells, leading to highly proliferative clusters of C cells. From the transiently amplifying progenitor cells the young migrating neurons, or A cells, are derived. Most of the A cells express the polysialylated form of the neural cell adhesion molecule (PSA-NCAM) and doublecortin (DCX), two molecules associated with neuronal migration.

The sequence of developmental stages in the adult SVZ, RMS, and olfactory bulb is B–C–A, with the E cells standing outside this order (Fig. 5–4). There are no D cells in the SVZ. The pattern is similar to that proposed for the olfactory epithelium: stem cell (B cells, corresponding to sustentacular cells), transiently amplifying progenitor cell (C cells, corresponding to globose basal cells), neuroblast (A cells). In this in vivo model, all three cell types are considered to be self-renewing, although possibly to a different degree (Doetsch et al., 2002b).

The expression patterns of key transcription factors have shed some light on the potential heterogeneity and lineage relationship of precursor cells in the adult SVZ. C cells express transcription factor Dlx2 and can be isolated on the basis of this expression (Doetsch et al., 2002a). In the developing brain, progenitor cells in the medial and lateral ganglionic eminences that express Dlx2 generate interneurons and oligodendrocytes throughout the brain (Pleasure et al., 2000; He et al., 2001), including the hippocampus and the olfactory bulb. In addition, Dlx transcription factors play a specific role in dopaminergic development (Saino-Saito et al., 2003). In the periglomerular layers of the adult olfactory bulb, a small number of new interneurons is found that, in addition to GABA, employ dopamine as a neurotransmitter (Gall et al., 1987).

Many C cells also express Pax6 (Hack et al., 2004). During development, Pax6 is expressed in radial glia of the dorsal brain and null mutants of Pax6 lack normal radial glia in the developing cortex and consequently show abortive cortex development (Gotz et al., 1998). Pax6, however, is not expressed in radial glia of the lateral ganglionic eminence that gives rise to olfactory bulb interneurons. Because the Pax6 mutant is embryonically lethal, the role of Pax6 in adult neurogenesis in the olfactory bulb cannot be studied by targeted mutagenesis.

A large proportion of the proliferating cells in the adult SVZ express Olig2 (Hack et al., 2004), which suggests that these cells are in the oligodendrocytic lineage. Their lineage relationship to the precursor cells producing neurons and astrocytes is not yet clear. SVZ precursor cells contribute to the production of oligodendrocytes in the postnatal brain (Levison and Goldman, 1993; Marshall and Goldman, 2002). After experimentally induced demyelination, new oligodendrocytes of SVZ origin have been described, but the identity of their precursor has not yet been identified (Nait-Oumesmar et al., 1999). Olig2-positive cells might not participate in cell genesis in the olfactory bulb but leave the SVZ or the RMS toward the corpus callosum and cortex, where they become oligodendrocytes. During development, however, cells from the ganglionic eminences give rise to interneurons in the olfactory bulb *and* oligodendrocytes, a result implying that a common precursor cell for both populations exists (He et al., 2001; Yung et al., 2002). Olig2-positive cells are negative for PSA-NCAM, but some of them express the LeX/SSEA1 antigen that is expressed by both astrocytic and nonastrocytic cells in the SVZ (Capela and Temple, 2002). This would imply that if B cells are multipotent in vivo and generate neurons, astrocytes, and oligodendrocytes, lineage separation would have to occur between B and C cells.

Oligodendrocytic lineage in the SVZ is likely to originate from cells expressing the chondroitin sulfate proteoglycan NG2 (see also Chapter 8). NG2 is expressed in glial progenitor cells that generate oligodendrocytes and one type of astrocytes (O2A progenitor cells). Adan Aguirre, Vittorio Gallo, and coworkers at the Children's National Medical Center in Washington, D.C., reported that these cells (in their experiment identified by the expression of CNPase, however) behaved like C cells in vitro, expressed an identical pattern of marker proteins such as Dlx, Mash1, and LeX, and were multipotent. However, C cells of the adult SVZ do not express NG2. Thus, the exact lineage relationship to the C cells of the adult brain is not yet clear (Aguirre et al., 2004). Interestingly, however, upon implantation in the developing hippocampus, the NG2-positive cells also developed into interneurons.

Consistent with the role of being amplifying progenitor cells, C cells have also been characterized by their expression of the receptor to mitogen EGF (Hoglinger et al., 2004). The sensitivity of this property when used as a marker is not yet known, however.

At present it is not clear how the cell types that can be distinguished in vivo relate to cells that after isolation from the adult SVZ show stem cell properties in vitro. Data from Derek van der Kooy's group in Toronto indicate that both stem cells (with unlimited self-renewal) and lineage-restricted progenitor cells can be isolated from the SVZ (Morshead et al., 1994, 1998; Craig et al., 1996). Astrocytes from the SVZ can be cultured in vitro and can produce FGF- and EGF-dependent neurospheres (Laywell et al., 2000). At the same time, most precursor cells isolated from the SVZ by means of any protocol seem to correspond to C cells in vivo, indicating that upon exposure to EGF, C cells reveal a latent potential for true stem cell behavior, self-renewal, and within-tissue multipotency (Doetsch et al., 2002a). Prospective isolation of an SVZ precursor cell with strong sphere-forming capacity has been based on the expression of nestin and the absence of GFAP, heat-stable antigen, and peanut agglutinin (two surface molecules) (Rietze et al., 2001), presumably also corresponding to C cells.

The SVZ astrocytes provide neurogenic cues to precursor cells isolated from the adult SVZ, which suggests that the close spatial interaction of B cells with C and A cells in vivo reflects cell-to-cell communication in the control of adult neurogenesis (Lim and Alvarez-Buylla, 1999). An analogous pattern is found in the adult dentate gyrus (Song et al., 2002; Seri et al., 2004).

Cell cycle length is an important parameter in controlling the rate of cell division. Regulation of cell cycle length occurs mainly by varying the duration of the G1 phase, bringing dividing cells in a state of transient cell cycle arrest. This state is also called "G1 transition" and is associated with the expression of p27kip1. P27kip1 binds to cell cycle–dependent kinases (cdk) whose enzymatic activity controls the length of the cell cycle and specifically causes a lengthening of the G1 phase. Accordingly, both dividing and terminally postmitotic cells are p27kip1 negative. Increased p27kip1 activity provides a mechanism to arrest proliferative cells in the cell cycle and thereby effectively control the expansion of the population. Loss of p27kip1 function in null-mutant mice resulted in an increase in BrdU incorporation in the SVZ by increasing the population of C cells and consequently A cells. The number of B cells, in contrast, was unaffected (Doetsch et al., 2002b). A second cdk inhibitor, p19ink4d, shows only low expression in the SVZ but high expression in the RMS. This finding raises the possibility that different progenitor cells use different mechanisms to control their expansion (Coskun and Luskin, 2001).

Chain Migration of Neuroblasts to the Olfactory Bulb

Precursor cells can be found in the entire lateral wall of the lateral ventricle. Neural precursor cells and A cells in particular can be isolated from distant caudal parts of the SVZ—in rats, millimeters away from the beginning of the RMS. The RMS itself is several millimeters long in rats, but many centimeters long in primates. Migration over these distances occurs in a unique pattern, or chain migration (Lois and Alvarez-Buylla, 1994; Lois et al., 1996).

During development, immature neurons generally migrate in two distinct forms (Fig. 5–5). Movement of newly generated neurons from the ventricular plate out to their terminal position within the layers of the cortex is *radial* migration. This type of migration depends on radial glia as a guiding structure. The second form of migration is *tangential* migration, which is typical for the integration of interneurons from the ganglionic eminences. It occurs parallel to the germinative matrix and does not rely on radial glia as a guiding structure.

Chain migration has features of both radial and tangential migration. In rodents, as the route along which the developing neurons migrate, the RMS is shielded against the rest of the brain by glial cells, which form a tube-like structure. These astrocytes are slowly dividing and have been equaled to the B cells of the SVZ. They may perform precursor cell functions in the RMS and olfactory bulb as well (Gritti et al., 2002). Otherwise the exact function of this glial tube is unknown, because chain migration can occur in the absence of astrocytes. In rabbits, for example, migration toward the olfactory bulb occurs in chains but independent of a glial ensheathing (Luzzati et al., 2003). In humans, neither the anatomical structure of an RMS nor migratory chains have been detected, thus it is questionable whether neuroblast migration between the SVZ and olfactory bulb occurs in humans at all (Sanai et al., 2004). This migration has been found in monkeys, however (Kornack and Rakic, 2001; see Chapter 11 and Fig. 11–3, Color Plate 13). Removal of the rodent olfactory bulb causes an almost complete disappearance of the glia ensheathing the RMS but only a reduction in the migration toward the site of the olfactory bulb, which also does not occur in a disorderly fashion (Jankovski et al., 1998).

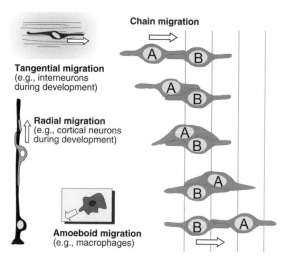

Figure 5–5. Chain migration. Migrating neuronally determined progenitor cells (A cells) travel between the subventricular zone and olfactory bulb in a particular form of migration that is independent of a glial guidance structure. In chain migration, the migrating cells guide each other in what is called "homotypic" migration. This mechanism is distinct from the radial and tangential migration found during brain development. In the brain, amoeboid (free) migration is found in microglia and macrophages.

In the rodent RMS, the new neurons do not rely entirely on surrounding glia either, because they do not migrate individually along guiding glial cells; rather, they use each other as guide for the next step. Because they slide along other cells of their own kind, this type of migration is called "homotypic." Small groups (chains) of cells lead each other on the way. One cell will extend a prominent growth cone that serves as a guidance structure for the migration of a few following cells. These in turn leave behind a process that the first cell of the next chain can use to direct its migration.

Pathways of this kind can be found as a network crisscrossing the lateral walls of the ventricles, becoming denser rostrally and merging toward the characteristic dorsoanterior spandril under the corpus callosum. All of these paths feed into the RMS, which essentially represents a tissue volume immediately around the obliterated olfactory ventricle connecting the lateral ventricle with the olfactory bulb. In this way, there is continuity between the SVZ, the RMS, and the core tissue of the olfactory bulb, where the arriving new cells disperse and migrate toward the granule cell layer and the periglomerular layers.

During migration, A cells continue to divide and initiate neuronal maturation (Menezes et al., 1995). Proliferation, however, is much slower than in the SVZ and the cell cycle time is lengthened (Smith and Luskin, 1998). Migrating A cells express immature neuronal markers such as DCX, PSA-NCAM, and β-III-tubulin. DCX is a protein that is associated with neuronal migration (Gleeson et al., 1999). Like in the adult hippocampus, DCX expression in the SVZ and RMS is associated with the most critical period of neuronal development, ranging from a progenitor cell stage to the existence of a differentiated neuron that is integrated into the circuitry (Brown et al., 2003; Ambrogini et al., 2004; Rao and Shetty, 2004).

The network of migratory chains crisscrossing the SVZ have a predominant orientation toward the RMS. Migration is generally unidirectional toward the olfactory bulb, although many individual pieces of the paths can have other directions (compare Fig. 5–5). Because as no clear anatomical guidance structure exists, differentially expressed guidance molecules might be responsible for steering migration. PSA-NCAM enables migration but it is neither specific nor sufficient (Hu et al., 1996; Chazal et al., 2000).

The different SVZ cells express both Ephrin receptor tyrosine kinases and their ligands in varying patterns. In the nervous system, Ephrin activity is involved in axon guidance (Drescher, 1997; Orioli and Klein, 1997). Interference with Ephrin signaling in the adult brain in vivo inhibits the migration of A cells toward the olfactory bulb and increases cell proliferation in the SVZ (Conover et al., 2000).

The receptor tyrosine kinase ErbB4 and its ligands, the neurogenins, are expressed in the SVZ and RMS. Conditional ErbB4 mutants targeted to nestin- or GFAP-expressing cells show impaired chain migration of A cells and disturbed neuronal differentiation (Anton et al., 2004).

An attractant factor in the olfactory bulb might direct migrating A cells toward the bulb. Surprisingly, however, the cells migrated in the right direction even when the olfactory bulb was ablated (Jankovski et al., 1998; Kirschenbaum et al., 1999). Others have proposed that it is less an attractant in the olfactory bulb and more a repellent from the more caudal parts of the SVZ that directs cell migration.

Part of this driving force is Slit, a repulsant factor that is present in the adult striatum and choroid plexus and repels neural precursor cells both in vitro (Wu et al., 1999). In slit mutants, migration in the SVZ and RMS is reduced and occurs laterally and backwards, so slit might normally prevent migrating SVZ cells from wandering into other brain regions, somewhat like putting a fence around the SVZ. Migrating neuroblasts (A cells) express the receptor for slit, robo. It came as a surprise that the migrating cells also express slit itself. The repulsant theory of migration in the RMS had already been dismissed because slit is effective over a distance of a millimeter at most. If slit were secreted in an autocrine or paracrine fashion, however, the migrating neuroblasts themselves would help to distribute the factor necessary for migration. If slit acted solely as a repulsant, this would not make sense; the cells would prevent their own migration and that of the following cells. It is thus believed that slit has other functions in migration as well, with the repulsive action playing actually a subordinate role in vivo.

Guofa Liu and Yi Rao from Washington University in St. Louis revisited the chemoattractant hypothesis and found that when the olfactory bulb was removed, migration toward the olfactory bulb strongly decreased but was not completely stopped (Liu and Rao, 2003). This decrease could be averted by transplanting a piece of olfactory bulb. The same result did not occur when a piece of neocortex was implanted or when some known chemoattractants were applied. These results argue in favor of a novel chemoattractant in the olfactory bulb. This chemoattractant remains to be identified, but because directed migration does not completely disappear in the absence of an olfactory bulb, there must be another, equally unknown mechanism that is independent of the olfactory bulb.

If the olfactory bulb is removed, cell proliferation in the SVZ decreases over time and migration to the site of the bulb is reduced but does not completely cease. New postmitotic neurons accumulate at the lesion where they might leave remnants of the RMS and direct their further migration specifically toward the frontal cortex and the anterior olfactory nucleus. The promotion of cell migration was also maintained for implanted SVZ precursor cells (Jankovski et al., 1998), which suggests that the olfactory bulb is not required for many aspects of neuronal migration and differentiation.

Neuronal Maturation in the Adult Olfactory Bulb

In migrating A cells, expression of signs of a more mature neuronal phenotype is delayed until the cells have reached the olfactory bulb. Only here do they become positive for their neurotransmitter and show electrophysiological signs of neuronal maturity (Carleton et al., 2003). A few migrating cells start expressing calretinin during their migration (Jankovski and Sotelo, 1996). Calretinin identifies interneurons in the glomeruli and the granule cell layer of the olfactory bulb but is not found in the tyrosine hydroxylase–positive periglomerular interneurons (Jacobowitz and Winsky, 1991; Rogers and Resibois, 1992; Li et al., 2002).

The RMS terminates in the core of the olfactory bulb. Through an unknown mechanism, the incoming immature neurons switch the direction of their migration and start to move radially into the granule cell layer and toward the periglomerular layer. Details of how this radial migration is accomplished are not yet available. In fact, this migration is not classically radial because no radial glia is present in the adult olfactory bulb.

A large proportion of new cells arriving in the olfactory bulb die (Biebl et al., 2000). Consequently, a surplus of neurons reaches the olfactory bulb and is eliminated thereafter (Fig. 5–6). There is a high density of cell death in the SVZ and RMS as well, but in absolute terms, most of the elimination occurs in the olfactory bulb. The fact that cell death is largely delayed to this late point of development suggests that functional connections are required to decide whether a new cell will survive or not. Survival would depend on a Hebbian mechanism of recruiting new cells into function.

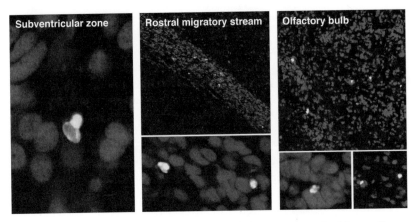

Figure 5–6. Apoptotic cell death during adult neurogenesis. New cells are generated in excess and most of them are eliminated by programmed cell death. Eighty percent of cell death within the neurogenic region of the olfactory bulb occurs in the olfactory bulb, but the density of cell death is highest in the rostral migratory system. Apoptotic cell death is visualized with the (terminal deoxynucleotidyl transferase–mediated dUPT nick end labeling) (TUNEL) method. Images by H. Georg Kuhn and Christiana Cooper-Kuhn, Gothenburg.

The receptor neurons in the olfactory epithelium project to the olfactory bulb, where they form synapses with the second neuron of the olfactory pathway, the mitral and tufted cells. The synapses cluster in distinctive structures, the glomeruli of the olfactory bulb. It is not the mitral and tufted cells that are produced by adult olfactory bulb neurogenesis, but three types of interneurons, one within the granule cell layer and two in the periglomerular region (see Fig. 4–7 for the network map). The projection neurons are generated prenatally. The new granule cells account for about 95% of the new neurons and are GABAergic (Fig. 5–7, Color Plate 5). The second population of newly generated interneurons is found in the periglomerular layer and accounts for 5% of the total number of new neurons. These neurons are GABAergic as well, but 10% of them (0.5% of the total population of new neurons) also have dopamine as neurotransmitter (Gall et al., 1987; Kosaka et al., 1987; Winner et al., 2002). These dopaminergic neurons can be recognized by their expression of tyrosine hydroxylase (TH). Very rarely, new neurons are seen in the external plexiform layer of the olfactory bulb.

The first signs of mRNA for TH, one of the key enzymes of dopaminergic differentiation, are found in migrating cells in the RMS; TH protein, however, is only in the mature new cells in the olfactory bulb (Baker et al., 2001).

Retroviral labeling of SVZ precursor cells has confirmed that both populations are of SVZ origin (see also Fig. 5–8, Color Plate 5), although it has also been proposed that those progenitor cells that divide latest during migration in the SVZ produce the periglomerular neurons (Betarbet et al.,

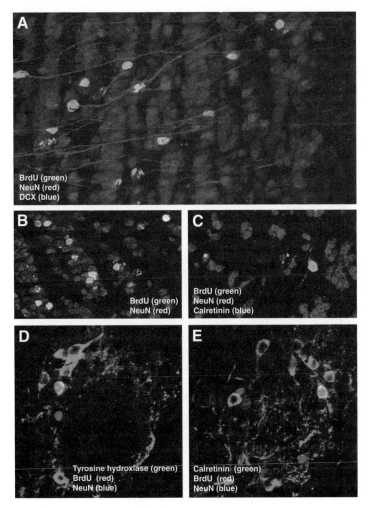

Figure 5–7 (Color Plate 5). Adult-generated neurons in the olfactory bulb. Confocal-microscopic depiction of key antigens is used to identify newly generated cells in the course of adult neurogenesis in the olfactory bulb. A and B: Demonstration of neurogenesis by BrdU/NeuN colocalization. C and E: New neurons in the granule cell layer are calretinin positive, whereas periglomerular interneurons are not. D: A small percentage of the new periglomerular interneurons expresses tyrosine hydroxylase, the key enzyme of the dopamine synthesis pathway. Images by H. Georg Kuhn and Christiana Cooper-Kuhn, Gothenburg.

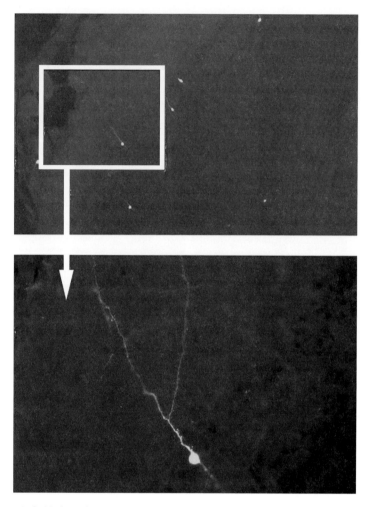

Figure 5–8 (Color Plate 6). Retroviral labeling of adult-generated neurons in the olfactory bulb. Through labeling of dividing cells in the subventricular zone with a retrovirus expressing green fluorescent protein as reporter gene, the extended morphology of new neurons in the olfactory bulb can be visualized. Image by Rainer Glass, Berlin.

1996). After complete transection of the RMS immediately followed by BrdU-labeling of dividing cells, neurogenesis was reduced because migration of labeled precursor cells from the SVZ precursor cells was inhibited (Fuku-shima et al., 2002). The limited neurogenesis, however, that persisted in the bulb affected both the granule cell layer and the periglomerular zone, suggesting that proliferative cells within the bulb can generate both types of interneurons. Despite these parallel developments involving continued division in the course of migration for both populations, there are some hints that different precursor cell types in the SVZ might generate the interneurons in the granule cell layer and the periglomerular region.

In a study that used an inducible transgenic model that allowed the specific targeting of nestin-expressing cells, only the newly generated periglomerular neurons were labeled but not new interneurons in the granule cell layer. This result suggests a specified developmental path, possibly originating from a separate population of precursor cells (Beech et al., 2004). Interestingly, the different types of new interneurons in the periglomerular zone, TH-positive or calretinin-positive, appeared to originate from the same precursor cell pool separate from those cells that produce new interneurons in the granule cell layer. At the same time, all new interneurons appear ultimately to be derived from Dlx- and Er81-positive cells from the lateral embryonic eminence in the fetal brain (Stenman et al., 2003). The connection between these two findings and to B cells as the putative common stem cell of the adult SVZ is unknown. It is also not clear why the regulatable transgene differentiated between the presumed two lineages. Consequently, the question of exact lineage relationships and precursor cell hierarchies in the adult SVZ, RMS, and olfactory bulb requires further research and might be more complex than initially thought.

Neural precursor cells can be isolated from the olfactory bulb. After killing dividing cells with a cytostatic agent, large numbers of new C cells appeared in the olfactory bulb as early as 2 days after the treatment—too soon for migration from the SVZ (Gritti et al., 2002). C cells are normally rare in the olfactory bulb. In this experiment, however, no new TH-expressing cells were found during the recovery of adult neurogenesis in the olfactory bulb after cytostatic treatment.

In the adult olfactory bulb of young adult rodents, several ten thousand new neurons are generated each day. Many of these cells die, but over the life span of a mouse or rat there might be a modest increase in the size of the olfactory bulb. This net growth, however, has not yet been firmly established by stereological means. In 1977, Hinds and McNelly wrote that the rodent olfactory bulb does not grow over the rodent life span and in rats shows a stable size until 2 years of age, after which there is a decrease in size. The study focused, however, on the principal neurons of the olfactory bulb, the mitral and tufted cells. Kaplan and Hinds later reported that the number of granule cells in the rat olfactory bulb almost doubled between 4 and 31 months of age (Kaplan et al., 1985). New neurons in the olfactory bulb have long survival periods after an initial peak at about 2 weeks after cell division (Kato et al., 2000). After labeling dividing cells with BrdU, the number of new neurons in the olfactory bulb did not change between 4 weeks and 2 years after labeling (Winner et al., 2002). This finding argues in favor of the idea that adult neurogenesis in the olfactory bulb is partially cumulative and partially leads to a neuronal turnover. This is in contrast to the cellular turnover in the olfactory epithelium, where adult neurogenesis maintains a constant receptor cell number under the pressure of constant damage to the olfactory neurons.

REFERENCES

Aguirre AA, Chittajallu R, Belachew S, Gallo V (2004) NG2-expressing cells in the subventricular zone are type C–like cells and contribute to interneuron generation in the postnatal hippocampus. J Cell Biol 165:575–589.

Alvarez-Buylla A, Garcia-Verdugo JM, Tramontin AD (2001) A unified hypothesis on the lineage of neural stem cells. Nat Rev Neurosci 2:287–293.

Ambrogini P, Lattanzi D, Ciuffoli S, Agostini D, Bertini L, Stocchi V, Santi S, Cuppini R (2004) Morpho-functional characterization of neuronal cells at different stages of maturation in granule cell layer of adult rat dentate gyrus. Brain Res 1017:21–31.

Anton ES, Ghashghaei HT, Weber JL, McCann C, Fischer TM, Cheung ID, Gassmann M, Messing A, Klein R, Schwab MH, Lloyd KC, Lai C (2004) Receptor tyrosine kinase ErbB4 modulates neuroblast migration and placement in the adult forebrain. Nat Neurosci 7:1319–1328.

Arnold SE, Smutzer GS, Trojanowski JQ, Moberg PJ (1998) Cellular and molecular neuropathology of the olfactory epithelium and central olfactory pathways in Alzheimer's disease and schizophrenia. Ann NY Acad Sci 855:762–775.

Baker H, Liu N, Chun HS, Saino S, Berlin R, Volpe B, Son JH (2001) Phenotypic differentiation during migration of dopaminergic progenitor cells to the olfactory bulb. J Neurosci 21:8505–8513.

Barnett SC, Riddell JS (2004) Olfactory ensheathing cells (OECs) and the treatment of CNS injury: advantages and possible caveats. J Anat 204:57–67.

Bauer S, Rasika S, Han J, Mauduit C, Raccurt M, Morel G, Jourdan F, Benahmed M, Moyse E, Patterson PH (2003) Leukemia inhibitory factor is a key signal for injury-induced neurogenesis in the adult mouse olfactory epithelium. J Neurosci 23:1792–1803.

Beech RD, Cleary MA, Treloar HB, Eisch AJ, Harrist AV, Zhong W, Greer CA, Duman RS, Picciotto MR (2004) Nestin promoter/enhancer directs transgene expression to precursors of adult generated periglomerular neurons. J Comp Neurol 475:128–141.

Betarbet R, Zigova T, Bakay RA, Luskin MB (1996) Dopaminergic and GABAergic interneurons of the olfactory bulb are derived from the neonatal subventricular zone. Int J Dev Neurosci 14:921–930.

Biebl M, Cooper CM, Winkler J, Kuhn HG (2000) Analysis of neurogenesis and programmed cell death reveals a self-renewing capacity in the adult rat brain. Neurosci Lett 291:17–20.

Boulder Committee (1970) Embryonic vertebrate central nervous system: revised terminology. The Boulder Committee. Anat Rec 166:257–261.

Brown JP, Couillard-Despres S, Cooper-Kuhn CM, Winkler J, Aigner L, Kuhn HG (2003) Transient expression of doublecortin during adult neurogenesis. J Comp Neurol 467:1–10.

Bunge MB, Pearse DD (2003) Transplantation strategies to promote repair of the injured spinal cord. J Rehabil Res Dev 40:55–62.

Capela A, Temple S (2002) LeX/ssea-1 is expressed by adult mouse CNS stem cells, identifying them as nonependymal. Neuron 35:865–875.

Carleton A, Petreanu LT, Lansford R, Alvarez-Buylla A, Lledo PM (2003) Becoming a new neuron in the adult olfactory bulb. Nat Neurosci 6:507–518.

Casarosa S, Fode C, Guillemot F (1999) Mash1 regulates neurogenesis in the ventral telencephalon. Development 126:525–534.

Cau E, Gradwohl G, Casarosa S, Kageyama R, Guillemot F (2000) *Hes* genes regulate sequential stages of neurogenesis in the olfactory epithelium. Development 127:2323–2332.

Chazal G, Durbec P, Jankovski A, Rougon G, Cremer H (2000) Consequences of neural cell adhesion molecule deficiency on cell migration in the rostral migratory stream of the mouse. J Neurosci 20:1446–1457.

Chen X, Fang H, Schwob JE (2004) Multipotency of purified, transplanted globose basal cells in olfactory epithelium. J Comp Neurol 469:457–474.

Chiasson BJ, Tropepe V, Morshead CM, van der Kooy D (1999) Adult mammalian forebrain ependymal and subependymal cells demonstrate proliferative potential, but only subependymal cells have neural stem cell characteristics. J Neurosci 19:4462–4471.

Conover JC, Doetsch F, Garcia-Verdugo JM, Gale NW, Yancopoulos GD, Alvarez-Buylla A (2000) Disruption of Eph/ephrin signaling affects migration and proliferation in the adult subventricular zone. Nat Neurosci 3:1091–1097.

Coskun V, Luskin MB (2001) The expression pattern of the cell cycle inhibitor p19(INK4d) by progenitor cells of the rat embryonic telencephalon and neonatal anterior subventricular zone. J Neurosci 21:3092–3103.

Costanzo RM (1985) Neural regeneration and functional reconnection following olfactory nerve transection in hamster. Brain Res 361:258–266.

Craig CG, Tropepe V, Morshead CM, Reynolds BA, Weiss S, van der Kooy D (1996) In vivo growth factor expansion of endogenous subependymal neural precursor cell populations in the adult mouse brain. J Neurosci 16:2649–2658.

Davis JA, Reed RR (1996) Role of Olf-1 and Pax-6 transcription factors in neurodevelopment. J Neurosci 16:5082–5094.

Doetsch F (2003) The glial identity of neural stem cells. Nat Neurosci 6:1127–1134.

Doetsch F, Caille I, Lim DA, Garcia-Verdugo JM, Alvarez-Buylla A (1999a) Subventricular zone astrocytes are neural stem cells in the adult mammalian brain. Cell 97:703–716.

Doetsch F, Garcia-Verdugo JM, Alvarez-Buylla A (1997) Cellular composition and three-dimensional organization of the subventricular germinal zone in the adult mammalian brain. J Neurosci 17:5046–5061.

Doetsch F, Garcia-Verdugo JM, Alvarez-Buylla A (1999b) Regeneration of a germinal layer in the adult mammalian brain. Proc Natl Acad Sci USA 96:11619–11624.

Doetsch F, Petreanu L, Caille I, Garcia-Verdugo JM, Alvarez-Buylla A (2002a) EGF converts transit-amplifying neurogenic precursors in the adult brain into multipotent stem cells. Neuron 36:1021–1034.

Doetsch F, Verdugo JM, Caille I, Alvarez-Buylla A, Chao MV, Casaccia-Bonnefil P (2002b) Lack of the cell-cycle inhibitor p27Kip1 results in selective increase of transit-amplifying cells for adult neurogenesis. J Neurosci 22:2255–2264.

Drescher U (1997) The Eph family in the patterning of neural development. Curr Biol 7:R799–807.

Farbman AI, Brunjes PC, Rentfro L, Michas J, Ritz S (1988) The effect of unilateral naris occlusion on cell dynamics in the developing rat olfactory epithelium. J Neurosci 8:3290–3295.

Feron F, Mackay-Sim A, Andrieu JL, Matthaei KI, Holley A, Sicard G (1999a) Stress induces neurogenesis in non-neuronal cell cultures of adult olfactory epithelium. Neuroscience 88:571–583.

Feron F, Perry C, Hirning MH, McGrath J, Mackay-Sim A (1999b) Altered adhesion, proliferation and death in neural cultures from adults with schizophrenia. Schizophr Res 40:211–218.

Fukushima N, Yokouchi K, Kawagishi K, Moriizumi T (2002) Differential neurogenesis and gliogenesis by local and migrating neural stem cells in the olfactory bulb. Neurosci Res 44:467–473.

Gall CM, Hendry SH, Seroogy KB, Jones EG, Haycock JW (1987) Evidence for co-existence of GABA and dopamine in neurons of the rat olfactory bulb. J Comp Neurol 266:307–318.

Getchell TV, Shah DS, Partin JV, Subhedar NK, Getchell ML (2002) Leukemia inhibitory factor mRNA expression is upregulated in macrophages and olfactory receptor neurons after target ablation. J Neurosci Res 67:246–254.

Gleeson JG, Lin PT, Flanagan LA, Walsh CA (1999) Doublecortin is a microtubule-associated protein and is expressed widely by migrating neurons. Neuron 23:257–271.

Gotz M, Stoykova A, Gruss P (1998) Pax6 controls radial glia differentiation in the cerebral cortex. Neuron 21:1031–1044.

Graziadei G, Graziadei P (1979a) Neurogenesis and neuron regeneration in the olfactory system of mammals. II. Degeneration and reconstitution of the olfactory neurons after axotomy. J Neurocytol 8:197–213.

Graziadei PP (1973) Cell dynamics in the olfactory mucosa. Tissue Cell 5:113–131.

Graziadei PP, DeHan RS (1973) Neuronal regeneration in frog olfactory system. J Cell Biol 59:525–530.

Graziadei PP, Graziadei GA (1979b) Neurogenesis and neuron regeneration in the olfactory system of mammals. I. Morphological aspects of differentiation and structural organization of the olfactory sensory neurons. J Neurocytol 8:1–18.

Graziadei PP, Karlan MS, Graziadei GA, Bernstein JJ (1980) Neurogenesis of sensory neurons in the primate olfactory system after section of the fila olfactoria. Brain Res 186:289–300.

Gritti A, Bonfanti L, Doetsch F, Caille I, Alvarez-Buylla A, Lim DA, Galli R, Verdugo JM, Herrera DG, Vescovi AL (2002) Multipotent neural stem cells reside into the rostral extension and olfactory bulb of adult rodents. J Neurosci 22:437–445.

Hack MA, Sugimori M, Lundberg C, Nakafuku M, Gotz M (2004) Regionalization and fate specification in neurospheres: the role of Olig2 and Pax6. Mol Cell Neurosci 25:664–678.

He W, Ingraham C, Rising L, Goderie S, Temple S (2001) Multipotent stem cells from the mouse basal forebrain contribute GABAergic neurons and oligodendrocytes to the cerebral cortex during embryogenesis. J Neurosci 21:8854–8862.

Hinds JW, McNelly NA (1977) Aging of the rat olfactory bulb: growth and atrophy of constituent layers and changes in size and number of mitral cells. J Comp Neurol 72:345–367.

Hoglinger GU, Rizk P, Muriel MP, Duyckaerts C, Oertel WH, Caille I, Hirsch EC (2004) Dopamine depletion impairs precursor cell proliferation in Parkinson disease. Nat Neurosci 7:726–735.

Hu H, Tomasiewicz H, Magnuson T, Rutishauser U (1996) The role of polysialic acid in migration of olfactory bulb interneuron precursors in the subventricular zone. Neuron 16:735–743.

Huard JM, Schwob JE (1995) Cell cycle of globose basal cells in rat olfactory epithelium. Dev Dyn 203:17–26.

Imura T, Kornblum HI, Sofroniew MV (2003) The predominant neural stem cell isolated from postnatal and adult forebrain but not early embryonic forebrain expresses GFAP. J Neurosci 23:2824–2832.

Jacobowitz DM, Winsky L (1991) Immunocytochemical localization of calretinin in the forebrain of the rat. J Comp Neurol 304:198–218.

Jankovski A, Garcia C, Soriano E, Sotelo C (1998) Proliferation, migration and differentiation of neuronal progenitor cells in the adult mouse subventricular zone surgically separated from its olfactory bulb. Eur J Neurosci 10:3853–3868.

Jankovski A, Sotelo C (1996) Subventricular zone–olfactory bulb migratory pathway in the adult mouse: cellular composition and specificity as determined by heterochronic and heterotopic transplantation. J Comp Neurol 371:376–396.

Johansson CB, Momma S, Clarke DL, Risling M, Lendahl U, Frisen J (1999) Identification of a neural stem cell in the adult mammalian central nervous system. Cell 96:25–34.

Kaplan MS, McNelly NA, Hinds JW (1985) Population dynamics of adult-formed granule neurons of the rat olfactory bulb. J Comp Neurol 239:117–125.

Kato T, Yokouchi K, Kawagishi K, Fukushima N, Miwa T, Moriizumi T (2000) Fate of newly formed periglomerular cells in the olfactory bulb. Acta Otolaryngol 120:876–879.

Kirschenbaum B, Doetsch F, Lois C, Alvarez-Buylla A (1999) Adult subventricular zone neuronal precursors continue to proliferate and migrate in the absence of the olfactory bulb. J Neurosci 19:2171–2180.

Kornack DR, Rakic P (2001) The generation, migration, and differentiation of olfactory neurons in the adult primate brain. Proc Natl Acad Sci USA 98:4752–4757.

Kosaka T, Kosaka K, Heizmann CW, Nagatsu I, Wu JY, Yanaihara N, Hama K (1987) An aspect of the organization of the GABAergic system in the rat main olfactory bulb: laminar distribution of immunohistochemically defined subpopulations of GABAergic neurons. Brain Res 411:373–378.

Laywell ED, Rakic P, Kukekov VG, Holland EC, Steindler DA (2000) Identification of a multipotent astrocytic stem cell in the immature and adult mouse brain. Proc Natl Acad Sci USA 97:13883–13888.

Levison SW, Goldman JE (1993) Both oligodendrocytes and astrocytes develop from progenitors in the subventricular zone of postnatal rat forebrain. Neuron 10:201–212.

Li Z, Kato T, Kawagishi K, Fukushima N, Yokouchi K, Moriizumi T (2002) Cell dynamics of calretinin-immunoreactive neurons in the rostral migratory stream after ibotenate-induced lesions in the forebrain. Neurosci Res 42:123–132.

Lim DA, Alvarez-Buylla A (1999) Interaction between astrocytes and adult subventricular zone precursors stimulates neurogenesis. Proc Natl Acad Sci USA 96:7526–7531.

Lim DA, Tramontin AD, Trevejo JM, Herrera DG, Garcia-Verdugo JM, Alvarez-Buylla A (2000) Noggin antagonizes BMP signaling to create a niche for adult neurogenesis. Neuron 28:713–726.

Liu G, Rao Y (2003) Neuronal migration from the forebrain to the olfactory bulb requires a new attractant persistent in the olfactory bulb. J Neurosci 23:6651–6659.

Lois C, Alvarez-Buylla A (1994) Long-distance neuronal migration in the adult mammalian brain. Science 264:1145–1148.

Lois C, Garcia-Verdugo J-M, Alvarez-Buylla A (1996) Chain migration of neuronal precursors. Science 271:978–981.

Loo AT, Youngentob SL, Kent PF, Schwob JE (1996) The aging olfactory epithelium: neurogenesis, response to damage, and odorant-induced activity. Int J Dev Neurosci 14:881–900.

Luzzati F, Peretto P, Aimar P, Ponti G, Fasolo A, Bonfanti L (2003) Glia-independent chains of neuroblasts through the subcortical parenchyma of the adult rabbit brain. Proc Natl Acad Sci USA 100:13036–13041.

MacDonald KP, Murrell WG, Bartlett PF, Bushell GR, Mackay-Sim A (1996) FGF2 promotes neuronal differentiation in explant cultures of adult and embryonic mouse olfactory epithelium. J Neurosci Res 44:27–39.

Marshall CA, Goldman JE (2002) Subpallial dlx2-expressing cells give rise to astrocytes and oligodendrocytes in the cerebral cortex and white matter. J Neurosci 22:9821–9830.

Martinez-Marcos A, Ubeda-Banon I, Deng L, Halpern M (2000) Neurogenesis in the vomeronasal epithelium of adult rats: evidence for different mechanisms for growth and neuronal turnover. J Neurobiol 44:423–435.

Menezes JRL, Smith CM, Nelson KC, Luskin MB (1995) The division of neuronal progenitor cells during migration in the neonatal mammalian forebrain. Mol Cell Neurosci 6:496–508.

Mirich JM, Brunjes PC (2001) Activity modulates neuronal proliferation in the developing olfactory epithelium. Brain Res Dev Brain Res 127:77–80.

Morshead CM, Craig CG, van der Kooy D (1998) In vivo clonal analyses reveal the properties of endogenous neural stem cell proliferation in the adult mammalian forebrain. Development 125:2251–2261.

Morshead CM, Garcia AD, Sofroniew MV, van Der Kooy D (2003) The ablation of glial fibrillary acidic protein–positive cells from the adult central nervous system results in the loss of forebrain neural stem cells but not retinal stem cells. Eur J Neurosci 18:76–84.

Morshead CM, Reynolds BA, Craig CG, McBurney MW, Staines WA, Morassutti D, Weiss S, van der Kooy D (1994) Neural stem cells in the adult mammalian forebrain: a relatively quiescent subpopulation of subependymal cells. Neuron 13:1071–1082.

Nagahara Y (1940) Experimentelle Studien über die histologischen Veränderungen des Geruchsorgans nach der Olfactoriusdurchschneidung. Beitrage zur Kenntnis des feineren Baus der Geruchsorgans. Jpn J Med Sci Pathol 5:165–199.

Nait-Oumesmar B, Decker L, Lachapelle F, Avellana-Adalid V, Bachelin C, Van Evercooren AB (1999) Progenitor cells of the adult mouse subventricular zone proliferate, migrate and differentiate into oligodendrocytes after demyelination. Eur J Neurosci 11:4357–4366.

Newman MP, Feron F, Mackay-Sim A (2000) Growth factor regulation of neurogenesis in adult olfactory epithelium. Neuroscience 99:343–350.

Orioli D, Klein R (1997) The Eph receptor family: axonal guidance by contact repulsion. Trends Genet 13:354–359.

Pleasure SJ, Anderson S, Hevner R, Bagri A, Marin O, Lowenstein DH, Rubenstein JL (2000) Cell migration from the ganglionic eminences is required for the development of hippocampal GABAergic interneurons. Neuron 28:727–740.

Rao MS, Shetty AK (2004) Efficacy of doublecortin as a marker to analyse the absolute number and dendritic growth of newly generated neurons in the adult dentate gyrus. Eur J Neurosci 19:234–246.

Rietze RL, Valcanis H, Brooker GF, Thomas T, Voss AK, Bartlett PF (2001) Purification of a pluripotent neural stem cell from the adult mouse brain. Nature 412:736–739.

Rogers JH, Resibois A (1992) Calretinin and calbindin-D28k in rat brain: patterns of partial co-localization. Neuroscience 51:843–865.

Ronnett GV, Leopold D, Cai X, Hoffbuhr KC, Moses L, Hoffman EP, Naidu S (2003) Olfactory biopsies demonstrate a defect in neuronal development in Rett's syndrome. Ann Neurol 54:206–218.

Saino-Saito S, Berlin R, Baker H (2003) Dlx-1 and Dlx-2 expression in the adult mouse brain: relationship to dopaminergic phenotypic regulation. J Comp Neurol 461:18–30.

Sanai N, Tramontin AD, Quinones-Hinojosa A, Barbaro NM, Gupta N, Kunwar S, Lawton MT, McDermott MW, Parsa AT, Manuel-Garcia Verdugo J, Berger MS, Alvarez-Buylla A (2004) Unique astrocyte ribbon in adult human brain contains neural stem cells but lacks chain migration. Nature 427:740–744.

Seri B, Garcia-Verdugo JM, Collado-Morente L, McEwen BS, Alvarez-Buylla A (2004) Cell types, lineage, and architecture of the germinal zone in the adult dentate gyrus. J Comp Neurol 478:359.

Shou J, Rim PC, Calof AL (1999) BMPs inhibit neurogenesis by a mechanism involving degradation of a transcription factor. Nat Neurosci 2:339–345.

Smart IH (1976) A pilot study of cell production by the ganglionic eminences of the developing mouse brain. J Anat 121:71–84.

Smith CM, Luskin MB (1998) Cell cycle length of olfactory bulb neuronal progenitors in the rostral migratory stream. Dev Dyn 213:220–227.

Smutzer G, Lee VM, Trojanowski JQ, Arnold SE (1998) Human olfactory mucosa in schizophrenia. Ann Otol Rhinol Laryngol 107:349–355.

Song H, Stevens CF, Gage FH (2002) Astroglia induce neurogenesis from adult neural stem cells. Nature 417:39–44.

Stenman J, Toresson H, Campbell K (2003) Identification of two distinct progenitor populations in the lateral ganglionic eminence: implications for striatal and olfactory bulb neurogenesis. J Neurosci 23:167–174.

Sturrock RR, Smart IH (1980) A morphological study of the mouse subependymal layer from embryonic life to old age. J Anat 130:391–415.

Winner B, Cooper-Kuhn CM, Aigner R, Winkler J, Kuhn HG (2002) Long-term survival and cell death of newly generated neurons in the adult rat olfactory bulb. Eur J Neurosci 16:1681–1689.

Wu W, Wong K, Chen J, Jiang Z, Dupuis S, Wu JY, Rao Y (1999) Directional guidance of neuronal migration in the olfactory system by the protein Slit. Nature 400:331–336.

Yung SY, Gokhan S, Jurcsak J, Molero AE, Abrajano JJ, Mehler MF (2002) Differential modulation of BMP signaling promotes the elaboration of cerebral cortical GABAergic neurons or oligodendrocytes from a common sonic hedgehog–responsive ventral forebrain progenitor species. Proc Natl Acad Sci USA 99:16273–16278.

6

Adult Hippocampal Neurogenesis

Adult hippocampal neurogenesis produces new granule cells in the dentate gyrus, the first relay station of the trisynaptic network of the hippocampus. The axons of the new granule cells add to the mossy fiber connection between the dentate gyrus and CA3. Neurogenesis in the adult hippocampus is locally much more confined than in the subventricular zone (SVZ) and olfactory bulb. In mice, proliferation of the precursor cells, migration, and differentiation into mature neurons occurs within a radius of about 100µ. Quantitatively the two neurogenic regions differ dramatically: against the thousands of neurons generated for the rodent olfactory bulb, hippocampal neurogenesis produces only few new cells.

Extreme local restriction and scarceness of the new cells does not prevent adult hippocampal neurogenesis from enjoying a particular fascination. The scientific studies on adult hippocampal neurogenesis by far outnumber those on adult olfactory bulb neurogenesis; in 2003 they were roughly twice as numerous. One reason for this preference is that from an anthropocentric point of view, the potential functional relevance of new hippocampal neurons appears greater than in the olfactory system. Dogs and rodents, no doubt, would have an opposite opinion. But the hippocampus plays a central role in current concepts of how the human brain and mind work. The hippocampus is called the "gateway to memory" and although this does apply to rodents as well, adult neurogenesis might here be linked to those processes that we consider essentially human. All animals learn and all mammals require their hippocampus for certain types of learning. The hippocampus prepares and evaluates information before long-term storage takes place in neocortical regions. The hippocampus is thus not the primary storage area itself but processes and consolidates so-called declarative information, the knowledge of facts and events. One aspect of how the hippocampus processes declarative contents is by relating items in space and time. The hippocampus enables the positioning of information in coordinate systems, thus making memory episodic. Human long-term memory of declarative and episodic contents is considered an essential prerequisite for consciousness, self-awareness, and a sense of personal history that can be experienced and communicated.

Thus it is not the hippocampus itself that makes us human, rather, its function contributes to preparing the foundation for those cognitive abilities that set us apart from other animals. Adult hippocampal neurogenesis cannot be the factor that explains these important differences because we share it with all mammals. Adult neurogenesis certainly is in no sense uniquely human; quite the contrary, it seems that we have rather less of it than other mammals. The new neurons in the hippocampus will not directly solve the puzzle of human cognition and consciousness, but if we attempt to really understand the hippocampus, it will not be possible to leave out adult hippocampal neurogenesis.

ANATOMY

The hippocampus is a bilateral structure found within the temporal lobes of the hemispheres. *Hippocampus* stands for the Latin word for seahorse, and a prepared human hippocampus indeed resembles the elegantly curved appearance of a seahorse. The area dentata of the hippocampus even mirrors the characteristic serrated back of the seahorse. The rodent hippocampus, on which most of our observations are based, lack this imaginative resemblance.

The hippocampus is part of the evolutionary "old" part of the cortex, the allocortex with its subdivision called archicortex. This region of the cortex is also called the "limbic cortex"; the hippocampus is part of the limbic system and is thereby involved in the processing of emotions. In contrast to the six-layered neocortex, the allocortex has a three-layered structure with a deep plexiforme layer, a band of principal neurons, and a superficial fiber layer.

The hippocampus consists of four parts: the dentate gyrus (also area dentata, or fascia dentata), the cornu ammonis (ammon's horn), the presubiculum, and the subiculum. In all modern descriptions of the hippocampus we encounter the term *CA*, which originally stood for *cornu ammonis* but has taken on a life of its own. In 1933 the anatomist Lorente de Nò subdivided the cornu ammonis into four parts, which have been numbered CA1, CA2, CA3, and CA4. Both the patterns of fiber connections and the expression patterns of marker genes have confirmed this anatomical description.

Dentate gyrus and CA fields constitute the essentially trisynaptic core circuit of the hippocampus (Figs. 6–1 and 10–5). Afferents from the entorhinal cortex reach the dendrites of the granule cells in the dentate gyrus, where they form the first synapse. The axons of the granule cells build the mossy fiber tract that reaches the pyramidal neurons in CA3, where they terminate in unusually large and complex structures, the mossy fiber butons. These are interspersed with interneurons and contain the second synapse with the neurons of CA3. The pyramidal neurons of CA3 project via the Shaffer collateral pathway to CA1, where the third synapse is located. CA1 pyramidal neurons have an axon to the subiculum (from where a projection returns to the entorhinal cortex). This trisynaptic circuit is an important and useful concept, but it is a simplification.

Under physiological conditions, adult hippocampal neurogenesis is found only in the dentate gyrus, where it generates new granule cells. There is no

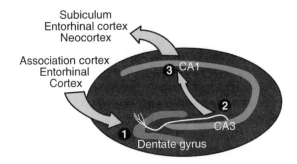

Figure 6–1. The trisynaptic backbone of hippocampal circuitry. Adult hippocampal neurogenesis generates only new granule cells in the dentate gyrus and thus only modifies the mossy fiber connection between the dentate gyrus and CA3. All other subsystems do not incorporate new neurons.

conclusive evidence that new neurons are formed in other hippocampal regions, although single reports have proposed otherwise and await confirmation (Rietze et al., 2000). As in other reports of putative neurogenesis outside the dentate gyrus and the SVZ and olfactory bulb (see Chapter 8), the number of new neurons would have to be minute.

THE SUBGRANULAR ZONE

In vivo, the precursor cells of the dentate gyrus reside in a narrow band of tissue, the subgranular zone (SGZ). For earlier anatomists this zone was not recognized as a structure that required a name and was nothing more than the border between the granule cell layer and the hilus (or plexiforme layer, or CA4). Other than the SVZ, before 1965 the SGZ was not recognized as a germinative matrix. Descriptively, the SGZ is usually defined as a layer about three cell nuclei wide (20 to 25 μm), including the basal cell band of the granule cell layer and a two nucleus–wide zone into the hilus (Fig. 6–2, Color Plate 7).

The SGZ provides a neurogenic microenvironment that is permissive for neuronal development throughout life. The SGZ contains astrocytes resembling radial glial elements (Seri et al., 2001; Filippov et al., 2003; Fukuda et al., 2003), the putative stem cells of this region, several different types of neuronal and glial progenitor cells (Filippov et al., 2003; Fukuda et al., 2003; Kronenberg et al., 2003; Seri et al., 2004), and neurons in all stages of neuronal differentiation and maturation (Brandt et al., 2003; Ambrogini et al., 2004).

The dentate gyrus and the SGZ receive input from numerous neurotransmitter systems that link this region with essentially the entire brain (Fig. 6–3). The excitatory input that carries the contents to be processed in the hippocampus reaches the dentate gyrus through the perforant path from the

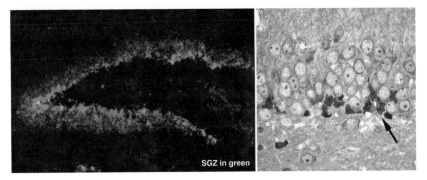

Figure 6–2 (Color Plate 7). The subgranular zone (SGZ). The SGZ contains the neurogenic niche in the adult dentate gyrus. The SGZ can be visualized with nuclear staining that contrasts it against the neurons of the granule cell layer (left). In the semi-thin section SGZ cells, including the radial glia–like structures, can be distinguished, even in the absence of immunohistochemical labeling (right). Note how the dark cells, the putative precursor cells, tightly surround a blood vessel (arrow). Compare also with Figures 6–4 and 6–6 (Color Plate 9).

entorhinal cortex. The other input systems are thought to primarily modulate the processing of information. Serotonergic input from the raphe nuclei, acetylcholinergic projections from the septum, noradrenergic fibers from the locus coeruleus, and dopaminergic fibers from the ventral tegmental area terminate in the dentate gyrus. In addition, at least seven types of interneurons contribute to the dentate gyrus (Freund and Buzsaki, 1996). Whereas interneurons are inhibitory, the hilus also contains mossy cells, a class of excitatory neurons that receive input from numerous sources including collaterals of the mossy fibers and project back to the molecular layer of the dentate gyrus. The different cells of the SGZ have not yet been fully characterized in terms of the many different types of neuronal input this region receives. Although the position of the different cells of the SGZ within the network of the hippocampus is not yet clear, the SGZ is a brain region with unusually complex and diverse innervation.

The SGZ is also a highly vascularized region. Theo Palmer of Stanford University has established the concept of the "vascular niche" as the enabling microenvironment for the precursor cells of the SGZ (Palmer et al., 2000). This theory assumes a close interaction between vascular structures and precursor cell activity (see also Chapter 8). The finding that vascular endothelial growth factor (VEGF) is a potent regulator of angiogenesis on the one hand and precursor cell activity and adult neurogenesis on the other supports this idea (Jin et al., 2002; Cao et al., 2004; Schanzer et al., 2004). In careful microanatomical analyses, Mercier, Kitasako, and Hatton (2002) described how the entire structural unit including precursor cells, blood

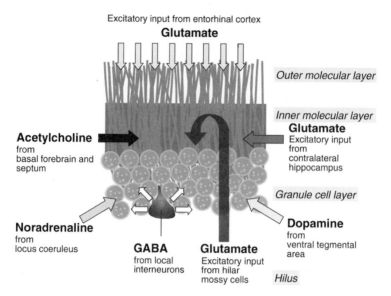

Figure 6–3. Input to the dentate gyrus. Several fiber systems, characterized by their neurotransmitter, reach the dentate gyrus and influence the regulation of adult neurogenesis.

vessels, and microglia is enclosed by a shared basal membrane. The close regulatory interaction between precursor cells and immune cells, most notably microglia but possibly also macrophages, is part of an important theory about the regulation of precursor cell activity under pathological but possibly also physiological conditions. The concept of the stem cell niche and of neurogenic permissiveness will be discussed in greater detail in Chapter 8.

Despite the contact between precursor cells and blood vessels in the SGZ, there is at present no support for the speculation that the hippocampal precursor cells might be actually blood-borne. In experiments with genetically marked bone marrow, no evidence of integration of bone marrow–derived precursor cells into the SGZ has been found (Priller et al., 2001). However, one study suggested that after ischemia, adventitia cells of local blood vessels could function as precursor cells (Yamashima et al., 2004).

PRECURSOR CELLS IN THE ADULT HIPPOCAMPUS

A central concept of stem cell biology is that different degrees of stemness can be distinguished with respect to both the extent of self-renewal and the degree of multipotency. A simplified version of this idea is the pattern of stem cell–progenitor cell–blast that can be found repeatedly in the context of many stem cell systems. We have seen that this pattern is applicable to the SVZ as well, where astrocyte-like B cells (the stem cells) give rise to

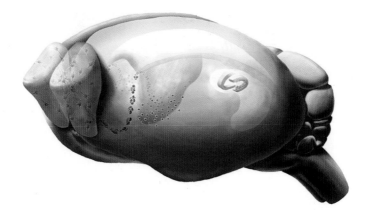

Color Plate 1. The two neurogenic regions in the adult brain. Only two regions of the adult mammalian brain appear to be neurogenic under physiological conditions. Precursor cells residing in the lateral walls of the lateral ventricle give rise to new interneurons in the olfactory bulb. Neurogenesis in the adult hippocampus generates new excitatory granule cells throughout life. Both forms of adult neurogenesis originate from different precursor cell populations, are independently regulated, and serve entirely different functions. See Chapter 8 for details on the distinction between neurogenic and non-neurogenic regions, the key criteria for this distinction, and also their limitations. Illustration by Jared Travnicek.

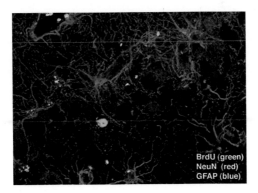

Color Plate 2. Neurogenesis in the adult human hippocampus. Peter Eriksson, neurologist in Gothenbury, Sweden, identified terminally ill patients who had received injections of bromodeoxyuridine (BrdU) for tumor staging purposes. He received their informed consent and after their death was able to examine their brains. He applied the same histologic methods that are routinely used to visualize adult neurogenesis in rodents. The confocal microscopic image shows the human dentate gyrus; BrdU is green, NeuN is red, astrocytic marker GFAP is blue. One granule cell is double-labeled for BrdU and NeuN and thereby identified as a new neuron (compare with Fig. 1–1). Reprinted from Eriksson et al. (1998), with permission of the authors and *Nature Medicine*.

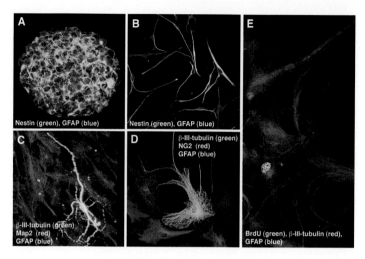

Color Plate 3. Neural precursor cell markers in vitro. Neural precursor cells express precursor cell markers in both types of precursor cell cultures—neurospheres (*A*) and monolayers (*B*). Neurospheres from the adult hippocampus (A) espress both nestin and GFAP. Even under proliferation conditions, precursor cell cultures show hererogeneity. This is particularly obvious in neurospheres. Upon transition to differentiation conditions (C–E), precursor cells differentiate into cells with characteristics of the three neural lineages—neurons (here shown by immoreactivity against β-III-tubulin), astrocytes (GFAP), and oligodendrocytes (NG2). Note that the specificity of these markers is not undisputed (see Chapter 8). In *E*, a BrdU-labeled cell has acquired a neuronal phenotype, evidence of neurogenesis in vitro. Images by Harish Babu, Berlin.

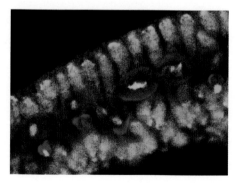

Color Plate 4. Asymmetric cell division in *Drosophila* larvae. Embryonic *Drosophila* neuroblasts delaminate from the single-layered neuroectodermal epithelium (top) and subsequently divide repeatedly in an asymmetric fashion. Both the epithelium and the neuroblasts show a pronounced apical–basal polarity. In both cell types, the Bazooka/ PAR-3 protein (red) is localized in the apical cytocortex. In contrast, the Miranda protein (blue), which functions as an adaptor protein for the cell fate determinant Prospero, is restricted to the basal cortex of dividing neuroblasts and segregates exclusively into the budding ganglion mother cell. DNA is stained in green. Apical is the top of the figure. Image by Andreas Wodarz, Göttingen.

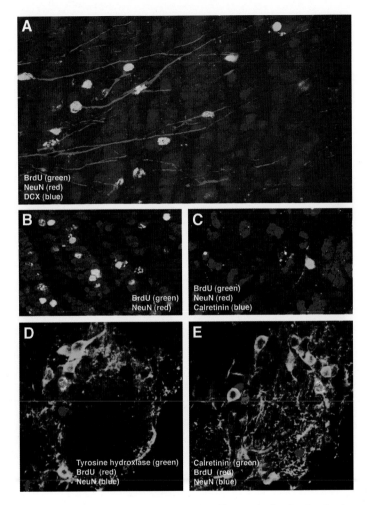

Color Plate 5. Adult-generated neurons in the olfactory bulb. Confocal-microscopic depiction of key antigens is used to identify newly generated cells in the course of adult neurogenesis in the olfactory bulb. A and B: Demonstration of neurogenesis by BrdU/ NeuN colocalization. C and E: New neurons in the granule cell layer are calretinin positive, whereas periglomerular interneurons are not. D: A small percentage of the new periglomerular interneurons expresses tyrosine hydroxylase, the key enzyme of the dopamine synthesis pathway. Images by H. Georg Kuhn and Christiana Cooper-Kuhn, Gothenburg.

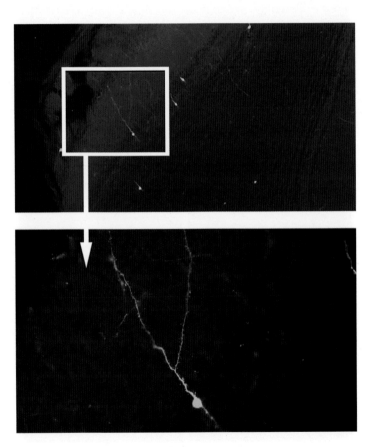

Color Plate 6. Retroviral labeling of adult-generated neurons in the olfactory bulb. Through labeling of dividing cells in the subventricular zone with a retrovirus expressing green fluorescent protein as reporter gene, the extended morphology of new neurons in the olfactory bulb can be visualized. Image by Rainer Glass, Berlin.

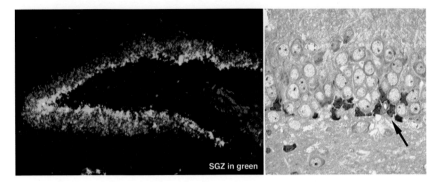

Color Plate 7. The subgranular zone (SGZ). The SGZ contains the neurogenic niche in the adult dentate gyrus. The SGZ can be visualized with nuclear staining that contrasts it against the neurons of the granule cell layer (left). In the semi-thin section SGZ cells, including the radial glia–like structures, can be distinguished, even in the absence of immunohistochemical labeling (right). Note how the dark cells, the putative precursor cells, tightly surround a blood vessel (arrow). Compare also with Figures 6–4 and 6–6 (Color Plate 9).

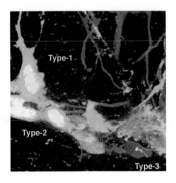

Color Plate 8. Precursor cell types in the adult subgranular zone. Radial glia–like type-1 cells give rise to transiently amplifying type-2 cells that in turn generate type-3 cells (left). See Figure 6–4 for details (nestin–GFP, green; DCX, blue; BrdU, red). Reprinted from Kempermann et al. (2004) with kind permission of Elsevier.

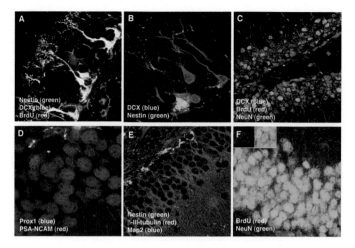

Color plate 9. Phenotypes of adult-generated cells in the dentate gyrus. Confocal-microscopic depiction of key antigens is used to identify newly generated cells in the course of adult neurogenesis in the hippocampus. A: Nestin-GFP-expressing radial type-1 cells and type-2 progenitor cells. B and C: DCX expression characterizes a range of cells from rounded proliferative cells to immature neurons with dendritic trees. D: Transcription factor Prox1 is expressed early in the course of development in the adult hippocampus and here coincides with the expression of PSA-NCAM. E: β-III tubulin and Map2 are neuronal markers expressed in the adult dentate gyrus, but because of their cytoplasmic expression they are more difficult to use than nuclear antigen to demonstrate co-localization. β-III-tubulin is expressed transiently in the SGZ; Map2 labels all neuronal processes. F: NeuN is the standard marker used to identify new neurons in the adult brain. Panel A from Filippov et al. (2003) with kind permission of Elsevier. Images by Barbara Steiner (A–E) and Golo Kronenberg (F), Berlin.

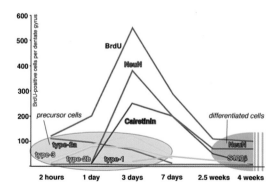

Color Plate 10. During adult hippocampal neurogenesis, a phase of expansion is followed by a phase of (presumably activity-dependent) survival or apoptotic elimination. After a single dose of BrdU, BrdU-positive cells progress through the stages explained in Figure 6–4. See also Figure 6–5. Reprinted from Kempermann et al. (2004) with kind permission of Elsevier.

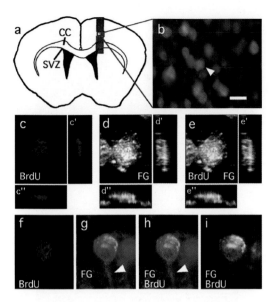

Color Plate 11. Targeted neurogenesis in the adult murine neocortex. In the experiment by Magavi et al. (2000) explained in Figure 8–2, new cortical neurons made appropriate target connections in the thalamus, here visualized with retrograde fluorogold tracing (FG) in BrdU-positive cells. *a* and *b*: Camera lucida drawing and photo of a BrdU-positive (red)/ FG (white) retrogradely labeled neuron. CC, corpus callosum; SVZ, subventricular zone. Arrowhead indicates labeled neuron. Scale bar: 20μm. *c–e*: Confocal three-dimensional reconstruction of the neuron. *f*: BrdU-positive (red) nucleus of a new FG-positive cortico-thalamic neuron. *g–i*: FG-positive (blue) cell body with labeled axon (arrowheads). Reprinted with kind permission by Jeffrey D. Macklis, Cambridge, Massachusetts, and *Nature* Publishing Group.

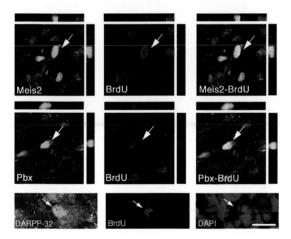

Color Plate 12. Regenerative neurogenesis after ischemia. During ischemia-induced regenerative neurogenesis in the adult striatum, the new neurons went through an intermediate transient stage, at which they expressed transcription factors Pbx and Meis2. Mature neurons expressed DARP-32. See text and Figure 9–6 for details. Figure from Arvidsson et al. (2002), reprinted with kind permission of Olle Lindvall, Lund, and *Nature Medicine*.

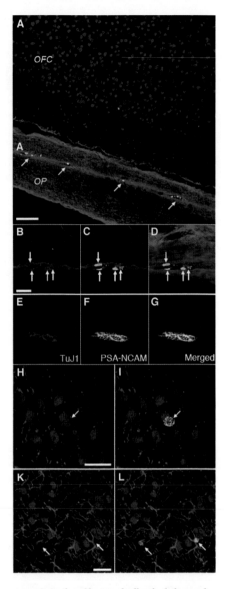

Color Plate 13. Neurogenesis in the olfactory bulb of adult monkeys. Kornack and Rakic (2001b) reported newly generated neurons in the olfactory bulb of macaque monkeys. *A*: Below the orbitofrontal cortex (OFC) the rostral migratory stream (arrows) is visible in the olfactory peduncle (OP). BrdU-labeled cells (green) ar found in the GFAP-positive (blue) pathway. *B–D*: b-III-tubulin-expressing cells are in the stream (*B*, red), a few of which are BrdU-labeled (*C*, green); *D* again shows the GFAP-positive environment (blue) *E* and *F*: β-III-tubulin-labeling coincides with expression of PSA-NCAM. *H* and *I*: A newly generated neuron in the olfactory bulb of a macaque monkey is shown, 97 days after the last injection of BrdU (NeuN, red; BrdU, green; GFAP, blue) *K* and *L*: An example of a newly generated, non-neuronal cell in the same region. Scale bars, 100 μm for *A*; 25 μm for *B–G*; 20 μm for *H–L*. Reprinted with kind permission of the authors and the Copyright 2001 National Academy of Sciences, U.S.A.

C cells (the transiently amplifying progenitor cells), which give rise to migrating A cells (the blasts). It is also found in the dentate gyrus.

In 1995, Jasodarah Ray, Theo D. Palmer, and Fred H. Gage from San Diego reported that fibroblast growth factor-2 (FGF-2) responsive precursor cells could be isolated from the rodent hippocampus (Ray et al., 1993; Palmer et al., 1995). Palmer and coworkers from the same group reported in 1997 that "primordial stem cells" existed in the adult rodent hippocampus (Palmer et al., 1997). The use of the term *primordial* underscored the finding that these cells fulfilled the criteria of true stem cells with unlimited self-renewal and multipotency. The study introduced a protocol for adherent precursor cell cultures, as described in Chapter 3 (Fig. 6–4).

In contrast to these data based on adherent cell cultures, one report based on the neurosphere assay questioned whether the hippocampus could indeed contain stem cells defined in the strictest sense (Seaberg and van der Kooy, 2002). Under the conditions of the neurosphere assay, no secondary spheres were found when single cells from the original spheres were plated out, and the cells did not show signs of multipotency in that no spheres displayed both glial and neuronal differentiation. According to the definition of stem cells, the hippocampus would thus contain only lineage-restricted progenitor cells with limited self-renewal (Seaberg and van der Kooy, 2002, 2003). It was hypothesized that the detection of stem cells in precursor cell cultures derived from the hippocampus could in fact be due

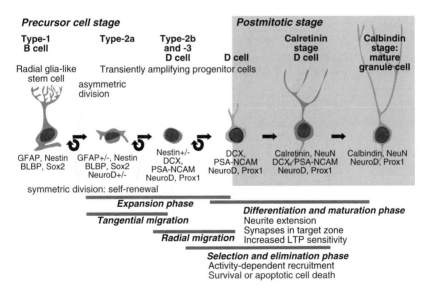

Figure 6–4. Developmental stages in adult hippocampal neurogenesis. Neuronal development in the dentate gyrus proceeds through a series of stages that can be identified immunohistochemically. This pattern shows similarities to but also relevant differences from the situation in the olfactory bulb (Fig. 5–3). See also Figure 6–6 (Color Plate 9).

to stem cell contamination from the ventricular wall. It seems more likely, however, that the discrepancy resulted from differences in cell culture and isolation protocols, leading to the enrichment of different cell populations. This explanation would further strengthen the theory that stem cell properties are not entirely intrinsic and can be modulated by environmental cues. Independent of potential technical issues, the problem of precursor cell heterogeneity between SVZ and SGZ persists. For example, hippocampal cells tend to be less proliferative than SVZ cells. It is not known whether this is primarily a function of culture conditions that have to be optimized for cells from the two regions (which might then turn out to be otherwise equivalent) or a difference in fundamental properties that could also be detected in situ.

On the basis of in vivo data, there is considerable precursor cell heterogeneity within the SGZ. The general pattern mirrors the situation in the SVZ, but a number of important differences have been noted.

Type 1 Cells Are the Radial Glia-Like Precursor Cells of the Subgranular Zone

As in the SVZ, the putative stem cells of the adult SGZ show a characteristic morphology resembling radial glia and have astrocytic properties (Seri et al., 2001). The cells have a triangular-shaped soma that is somewhat larger than the surrounding granule cells (Fig. 6–5, Color Plate 8). Their resemblance to radial glia is due to a long and strong apical process that reaches into the granule cell layer, where it branches sparsely into the outer third of the granule cell band (Filippov et al., 2003; Fukuda et al., 2003; Mignone et al., 2004). When the processes reach the inner molecular layer they spread out in numerous small branches, which gives the cells a tree-like appearance. The existence of radial glia-like cells in the developing and adult dentate gyrus has been known for a long time (Eckenhoff and Rakic, 1984; Kosaka and Hama, 1986; Rickmann et al., 1987). In the developing hippocampus, radial glia-like cells provide a scaffold is necessary for the normal formation of the dentate gyrus (Caviness, 1973; Stanfield and Cowan, 1979; Forster et al., 2002). The current opinion is that radial glia cells also function as precursor cells during development (Chapters 3 and 4). Hippocampus and dentate gyrus are of dorsal origin, but interneurons are derived from ventral sources. The detailed contributions of ventral and dorsal radial glia to dentate gyrus development and the structure of the postnatal and adult germinateive matrix in the SGZ are not known. In addition, in the context of the adult hippocampus, the term radia glia-like is mainly descriptive. The identity of these cells in the adult dentate gyrus with radial glia during brain development and the exact lineage relationship remain to be shown.

Those radial glia-like cells that express precursor cell marker nestin are called "type-1 cells" (Fig. 6–5, Color Plate 8). In contrast to the corresponding astrocytic cells of the SVZ (B cells), type-1 cells not only have astrocytic

Figure 6–5 (Color Plate 8). Precursor cell types in the adult subgranular zone. Radial glia–like type-1 cells give rise to transiently amplifying type-2 cells that in turn generate type-3 cells (left). See Figure 6–4 for details (nestin–GFP, green; DCX, blue; BrdU, red). Reprinted from Kempermann et al. (2004) with kind permission of Elsevier.

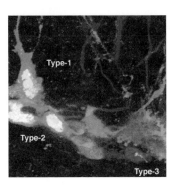

properties but also a suggestive radial glia–like morphology (Filippov et al., 2003; Fukuda et al., 2003). They consistently express astrocytic marker protein GFAP and are negative for S100β, another astrocytic protein (Seri et al., 2004; Steiner et al., 2004). Type-1 cells have vascular endfeet in the SGZ with a process broadly attached to the basal membrane of blood vessels (Filippov et al., 2003). Electrophysiologically, type-1 cells have classical astrocytic properties. They have passive membrane properties and potassium currents (Filippov et al., 2003; Fukuda et al., 2003). Their astrocytic nature is thus firmly established. Analogous to cells in the SVZ, the GFAP-positive cells with radial glia-like morphology in the dentate gyrus were first designated B cells by Bettina Seri and Arturo Alvarez-Buylla (Seri et al., 2001), but the nomenclature was abandoned in a later study (Seri et al., 2004). In mice, roughly half of the GFAP-positive radial glia–like processes are also nestin positive. It is not clear whether nestin expression marks an activational state of these cells or whether it identifies a constitutive subpopulation. Nestin expression is associated with precursor cell activity in vitro but its sensitivity and specificity in vivo are largely undetermined. On the basis of nestin-GFP expression, nestin-positive cells were extracted from the brain with fluorescence-activated cell sorting (FACS). These cells formed primary neurospheres in vitro but unfortunately, no clonal analysis nor generation of secondary spheres was performed in that experiment (Mignone et al., 2004).

The different terms used to connote the various cell types in adult hippocampus neurogenesis are presented in Table 6–1. Morphologically and with regard to spatial orientation in the tissue, the radial glia–like precursor cells of the SGZ differ from subventricular B cells, which apparently serve an analogous function. But whereas SVZ precursor cells generate inhibitory interneurons in the olfactory bulb, SGZ precursor cells produce one type of excitatory neuron. It thus seems that SGZ precursor cells are dorsal, whereas SVZ precursor cells are ventral, although some of them can express dorsal transcription factor Pax6 (Chapter 4). In addition, some regulators of hippocampal neurogenesis, such as environmental stimuli, have no effect on neurogenesis in the olfactory bulb (Brown et al., 2003) and vice versa

Table 6–1. Cell Types in Adult Hippocampus Neurogenesis

Stage of Development	Alternate Nomenclature	Mitotic Activity	Description	Key Antigens
Type-1	A vertical (B cell in Seri et al., 2001)	Proliferative	Vertical astrocyte or radial glia–like stem cell	GFAP, Nestin, Sox2, BLBP
Type-2a	?	Proliferative	Transiently amplifying precursor cell	Nestin, Sox2; some have NeuroD
Type-2b	(D1)	Proliferative	Transiently amplifying precursor cell (lineage-determined)	Nestin, NeuroD, DCX, PSA-NCAM
Type-3	D1/D2	Proliferative		DCX, PSA-NCAM; NeuroD
Calretinin stage	D2/D3	Postmitotic	Immature granule cell, neurite extension	DCX–PSA-NCAM, NeuroD, Prox1, NeuN, calretinin
Mature granule cell		Postmitotic		NeuroD, Prox1, NeuN, calbindin

BLBP, brain lipid binding protein; DCX, doublecortin; GFAP, glial fibrillary acidic protein; PSA-NCAM, polysialylated neural cell adhesion molecule.

(Rochefort et al., 2002). Through the use of relatively neutral yet distinct nomenclature to describe precursor cells in the SGZ we can avoid a premature conceptual equivalence with the situation in the SVZ, without conflicting with the data obtained by Seri and colleagues.

When Seri and colleagues eliminated cell proliferation through the application of cytostatic agents, they found that the first cells to reappear were glial fibrillary acidic protein (GFAP)-expressing cells (Seri et al., 2001). The other cell types and stages of neuronal development followed over time. Similarly, use of the GFAP-TVA transgenic mouse allowed timed and specific labeling of the progeny of GFAP-expressing cells. Several weeks after injecting the virus that could only infect GFAP-expressing cells, the reporter gene was found in neurons. From these findings it was concluded that GFAP-expressing cells were the stem cells of the hippocampus.

However, GFAP expression and radial glia morphology do not necessarily have to identify the same cell. Consequently, Alvarez-Buylla and colleagues (2001) use only the term *astrocytes* for the stem cells of the SGZ (and SVZ). Still, this terminology led to misunderstandings in some comments, because obviously not all astrocytes are stem cells. Similarly, in some contexts the label *radial glia* for the precursor cells in adult hippocampal neurogenesis might evoke a conceptual identity between embryonic and adult development that could turn out to be problematic.

Type-1 cells account for approximately two-thirds of the nestin-expressing cells in the SGZ of adult mice. In contrast, only 5% of the cell divisions among the nestin-expressing cells of the SGZ are in type-1 cells with radial glia morphology (Kronenberg et al., 2003). This low number does not completely match other estimates of astrocytic proliferation in the SGZ (Seri et al., 2004; Steiner et al., 2004). It might thus be that in addition to the radial glia–like cells, GFAP-expressing precursor cells exist, which account for part of the precursor cell activity in the SGZ. The hypothesis is that there might be a proliferative intermediate cell type combining features of astrocyte-like cells with a precursor cell type of nonradial appearance. This type of precursor cell might be found among the type-2 cells introduced below or define yet another subpopulation.

The number of type-1 cells identified as labeled after a single injection of proliferation marker bromodeoxyuridine (BrdU) remains very constant over long periods of time (Kronenberg et al., 2003). Under pathological conditions, however, such as the induction of experimental seizures, proliferation of radial glia-like cells has been reported (Huttmann et al., 2003). Generally, it might seem improbable that type-1 cells, with their tree-like morphology and extension between the blood vessels of the SGZ and fibers of the inner molecular layer, could undergo division at all. But type-1 cells would divide asymmetrically. Asymmetric division is another hallmark of stem cells and would further support the idea that type-1 cells are the highest-ranking precursor cells in the SGZ. The orientation in the granule cell layer and the gross morphology would be maintained during this division, and a daughter cell would bud off at the base of the type-1 cell (see also Fig. 4–2).

The daughter cells of type-1 cells express nestin as well and have been named "type-2 cells" (Filippov et al., 2003; Fukuda et al., 2003). In the nomenclature by Seri and Alvarez-Buylla, based on GFAP and not nestin–GFP expression, the progeny of the vertical astrocyte-like precursor cells are called "D cells" (Seri et al., 2001, 2004).

Type 2 and Type 3 Cells Are Transiently Amplifying Progenitor Cells

Type-2 cells are nestin-expressing cells that have plump, short processes oriented more or less parallel to the SGZ (Figs. 6–4 and 6–5, Color Plate 8). Immunohistochemical and light microscopy studies show that they do not express GFAP and are highly proliferative. Type-2 cells have an irregularly shaped nucleus with dense chromatin. GFAP negativity should be taken with a grain of salt, though, because this class of cell might likely include the nonradial glia–like precursor cells with astrocytic properties mentioned above.

In rats it is somewhat more obvious than in mice that cell division in the SGZ occurs in clusters. These clusters form around central blood vessels and contain the radial glia-like cells. Within days after the initial division, the newly generated cells spread out along the SGZ. The morphology of type-2 cells supports the possibility of tangential migration during this stage. This tangential migration is spatially very limited in comparison to migration in the SVZ and rostral migratory stream (RMS).

Expression of the avian leukosis virus under the Nestin promoter enabled targeted labeling of the progeny of nestin-expressing cells, analogous to use of the GFAP promoter to identify the progeny of GFAP-expressing cells (Seri et al., 2004). Both manipulations resulted in the presence of labeled granule cells, indicating that GFAP-positive and nestin-positive cells can contribute to adult hippocampal neurogenesis. In the study by Seri and colleagues, no nestin-positive astrocytes without radial morphology were found. Consequently, in their schema no equivalence to type-2 cells exists (Table 6–1). Presumably, the reporter gene product green fluorescent protein (GFP) will persist for a short time after the promoter driving the reporter gene has shut down, resulting in nestin–GFP detection in cells that are already nestin negative. Therefore, in this experimental strategy marker persistence gives some evidence of lineage relationships.

Type-2 cells come in two subtypes, one negative (type 2a) and one positive (type-2b) for immature neuronal marker doublecortin (DCX) (Kronenberg et al., 2003). Type-2b cells show signs of precursor cell identity (nestin–GFP) and neuronal lineage determination. These findings further support the hypothesis that nestin-expressing cells give rise to new neurons. DCX shows an almost complete overlap with the polysialylated form of the neural cell adhesion molecule (PSA-NCAM). Type-1 cells are always negative for DCX and

PSA-NCAM. DCX expression is associated with both the initiation of neuronal differentiation and migration (Francis et al., 1999). Developing granule cells go through a transient stage of DCX and PSA-NCAM expression (Seki and Arai, 1993; Brandt et al., 2003; Rao and Shetty, 2004). Although the signaling upstream of DCX expression is not yet known in detail, the DCX promoter contains a binding motif for NeuroD that is expressed in some type-2a cells. NeuroD expression precedes PSA-NCAM expression during adult hippocampal neurogenesis (Seki, 2002). The type-2 stage thus comprises the transition from a glia-like precursor cell to neuronal determination. At no later stage has an overlap between glial and neuronal markers or properties been found, which suggests that if the precursor cells of the SGZ are multipotent in vivo and can give rise to both neurons and glia, this fate choice should occur on the level of type-1 or type-2a cells. At least in the SGZ, DCX is strictly associated with neuronal lineage.

Type-3 cells are DCX positive, but nestin negative. These cells can also divide but only a few do so at any given time. It appears that this stage is one of great morphological changes. We find horizontally oriented type-3 cells similar to the orientation of type-2 cells, but often with longer horizontal processes. Other type-3 cells seem to be more vertically oriented. All possible orientations between these two extremes can be found. The nucleus of type-3 cells is rounded. Type-3 cells invariably express PSA-NCAM.

The type-3 stage is also the stage of radial migration into the granule cell layer. Few dividing cells can be found within the granule cell layer at any given time and these cells generally seem to be DCX positive (or astrocytes). Occasionally, however, these cells can be nestin positive as well. Therefore, radial migration, at least in some cases, might be initiated on the level of type-2b cells, but the migrating cells readily lose their nestin expression when they reach the granule cell layer. It is not clear whether radial migration needs to have ended before the cells terminally exit the cell cycle. It is also not clear whether the final exit from the cell cycle can only occur on the level of type-3 cells. The electrophysiological data and the expression of neuronal transcription factors such as NeuroD in type-2 cells suggest that signals for terminal neuronal differentiation can successfully reach the cells earlier. Type-2b and type-3 cells also express transcription factor Prox1, which remains expressed throughout granule cell development and is found in all adult granule cells (Kronenberg et al., 2003). The type-3 stage comprises a transition from a potentially proliferative state to the postmitotic immature neuron.

The distance of radial migration into the granule cell layer is limited. Most new cells remain in the SGZ and the inner third of the granule cell layer; few reach the outer third (Kempermann et al., 2003). The cells reach their final position early, presumably still during a progenitor cell stage. Afterwards the distribution of new cells does not substantially change.

Through electrophysiological investigation of non–process bearing, nestin-GFP-positive cells, different stages of neuronal differentiation were found. Whereas most cells had astrocytic membrane properties like those of type-1 cells, some had the intermediate complex phenotype, previously described for glial progenitor cells, and a few cells showed the first electrophysiological characteristics of neurons. These cells received GABAergic or glutamatergic input. One might hypothesize that the occurrence of the two transmitter phenotypes reflects a sequence of events. During brain development, in many neuronal populations GABAergic input precedes glutamatergic input. These findings suggest that neuronal differentiation can take place on the level of nestin-positive precursor cells. In DCX-expressing cells the electrophysiological transition from immature to mature neuronal properties occurs (Ambrogini et al., 2004). Fittingly, DCX- or PSA-NCAM-positive cells with a more mature dendritic morphology suggestive of receiving physiological input showed increased synaptic plasticity compared to that of older granule cells (see below; Wang et al., 2000; Schmidt-Hieber et al., 2004).

In summary, four cell types with the precursor cell properties of nestin expression and mitotic activity can be found in the adult SGZ (Kempermann et al., 2004). These cells differ in their morphology, proliferative activity, migratory behavior, and expression of key marker antigens. Applying the classical construct of stem cell biology to these cells, type-1 cells are the stem cells, type-2 cells are the transiently amplifying progenitor cells, and type-3 cells are the (migrating) neuroblasts that mark the transition to postmitotic immature neurons. All of these cells can divide, and after a single injection of BrdU, over time the distribution of BrdU-labeled cells progresses through these four types of cells. This unidirectional redistribution among the BrdU-labeled cells of the SGZ suggests sequential marker progression and therefore development. For example, no type-1 cell has been found to be DCX or Prox1 positive. No type-3 cell, in turn, has been found to express GFAP.

Type-2b and type-3 cells correspond to the D cell described by Seri and colleagues (2004). All D cells are DCX and PSA-NCAM positive. The category thus includes the early postmitotic stages of granule cell differentiation (Table 6–1), and D cells can be subdivided into three categories based on morphology. D1 cells seem to correspond to type-2a cells; D3 cells, to the immature granule cells. The D2 stage can be further subdivided into three subcategories and comprises the progression from horizontal to vertical orientation of the cells. D2 cells are proliferative and mature into D3 cells.

NEURONAL MATURATION IN THE ADULT DENTATE GYRUS

Type-3 cells (and possibly some type-2b cells) exit from the cell cycle and begin the terminal postmitotic differentiation of granule cells. This stage of neuronal development is characterized by the transient expression of calretinin, which is later exchanged for calbindin, present in the mature granule cells (Brandt et al., 2003). This switch of calcium-binding proteins occurs very rapidly and in mice takes place approximately 2 to 3 weeks after the cells have become postmitotic. During the calretinin-positive phase the cells also express Prox1 and postmitotic neuronal marker NeuN. After Prox1, NeuN is the second known mature marker that persists in the new neurons (Fig. 6–6, Color Plate 9). Accordingly, 1 day after a single injection of BrdU, a small number of BrdU/NeuN-positive cells can be found; after 3 days their number is already considerably high. The early presence of NeuN in BrdU-labeled cells cannot be taken as evidence of dividing neurons. To the contrary, NeuN-positive cells have never been found to express cell cycle markers (Ki67, PCNA, pH3, etc.) or to contain BrdU within minutes after the injection, confirming that NeuN-positive cells are postmitotic. However, because a NeuN-positive young neuron is derived from a predifferentiated type-3 cell, it might be detected by BrdU/NeuN-immunoreaction as early as 1 or 2 days

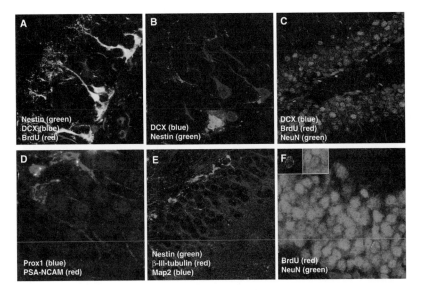

Figure 6–6 (Color Plate 9). Phenotypes of adult-generated cells in the dentate gyrus. Confocal-microscopic depiction of key antigens is used to identify newly generated cells in the course of adult neurogenesis in the hippocampus. A: Nestin-GFP-expressing radial type-1 cells and type-2 progenitor cells. B and C: DCX expression characterizes a range of cells from rounded proliferative cells to immature neurons with dendritic trees. D: Transcription factor Prox1 is expressed early in the course of development in the adult hippocampus and here coincides with the expression of PSA-NCAM. E: β-III tubulin and Map2 are neuronal markers expressed in the adult dentate gyrus, but because of their cytoplasmic expression they are more difficult to use than nuclear antigen to demonstrate co-localization. β-III-tubulin is expressed transiently in the SGZ; Map2 labels all neuronal processes. F: NeuN is the standard marker used to identify new neurons in the adult brain. Panel A from Filippov et al. (2003) with kind permission of Elsevier. Images by Barbara Steiner (A–E) and Golo Kronenberg (F), Berlin.

after the last division. The "mature" marker NeuN consequently also detects quite immature neurons.

The phase of DCX and calretinin expression is the period of dendrite and axon formation and functional maturation. The largest part of the dendritic tree is built during this period (Brandt et al., 2003; Ambrogini et al., 2004; Rao and Shetty, 2004), including the transient appearance of a basal dendrite (Ribak et al., 2004). Axon elongation occurs rapidly after the cells have become postmitotic (Hastings and Gould, 1999) and the appropriate axonal connections to CA3 are established (Stanfield and Trice, 1988; Hastings and Gould, 1999; Markakis and Gage, 1999). TUC4, associated with growth cone activity, is expressed in this phase (see Chapter 7). At the calretinin stage the cells keep the vertical morphology of the late type-3 cells. Their nucleus is rounded or slightly triangular, and an apical dendrite becomes clearly visible on DCX or PSA-NCAM staining. At the stage of calretinin expression, the dendrite has already acquired relatively mature morphology and reaches far up into the inner molecular layer. Within the granule cell layer proper it often has a close spatial relationship to the apical process of vertical astrocytes and type-1 cells. This might indicate that the radial glia–like process serves as a guidance structure for the forming dendrites.

About 2 weeks after having become postmitotic but still coexpressing PSA-NCAM, the newly generated cells can be visualized with enhanced green fluorescent protein (EGFP) as reporter gene under a truncated version of the promoter of proopiomelanocortin (POMC) (Overstreet et al., 2004). POMC is normally not expressed in the dentate gyrus, so the biological meaning of this promoter activity is not clear. The construct nonetheless allows researchers to examine the new neurons in an advanced immature state.

The first signs of neuronal function, in terms of the generation of action potentials and detectability of GABAergic synapses and glutamatergic input from the entorhinal cortex, can be found when the cells still express nestin–GFP and thus presumably are on the progenitor cell level. Using immunohistochemistry and reverse transcription polymerase chain reaction (RT-PCR) on cells filled with biocytin during patch-clamp examination, Patrizia Ambrogini and colleagues (2004) showed that GABAergic input precedes glutamatergic input in a pattern frequently found during embryonic development.

In 2002 Henriette van Praag and colleagues labeled newly generated cells with a retrovirus expressing GFP and showed that at 7 weeks after division the new granule cells showed electrophysiological responses very similar to those of surrounding older cells (van Praag et al., 2002). On the basis of PSA-NCAM expression in retrovirally labeled cells, Christoph Schmidt-Hieber, Peter Jonas, and Josef Bischofsberger of Freiburg University showed that the newly generated neurons have a lower threshold for the induction of long-term potentiation (LTP), the supposed electrophysiological correlate of learning (Schmidt-Hieber et al., 2004). This result confirmed an earlier observation by Sabrina Wang and Martin Wojtowicz from the University of Toronto, who reported the first evidence of an increased level of synaptic plasticity in newly generated cells (Wang et al., 2000).

That the new cells form appropriate connections has also been shown by infecting the entorhinal cortex with pseudorabies virus carrying a reporter gene. Pseudorabies infection is transmitted transsynaptically. The appearance of the reporter gene in new dentate gyrus granule cells confirmed the presence of synapses on their dendrites. Presence of reporter gene in CA3 fields demonstrated appropriate axonal connections (Carlen et al., 2002).

The entire cohort of new cells born at a given date of BrdU injection and destined to survive matures into responsiveness to synaptic stimulation between 2 weeks (when there is no response) and 7 weeks (when the same proportion of new cells responds than of older cells) after division (Jessberger and Kempermann, 2003). In this latter study, the response to synaptic activation was measured by assessing the activity-dependent up-regulation of immediate early genes.

CELL DEATH AND CELL NUMBERS

Like during embryonic, fetal, and postnatal neurogenesis and as in neurogenesis of the SVZ–olfactory bulb system, the precursor cells of the adult SGZ produce a vast surplus of progenitor cells of neuronal lineage and a surplus of immature neurons. The cells not recruited into function are eliminated by apoptotic cell death (Biebl et al., 2000).

The majority of dividing cells in the SGZ are type-2 cells. By 1 day later, the progeny of these divisions has doubled in the number of BrdU-labeled cells. This result is expected because every cell division generates two labeled daughter cells, and one cell cycle apparently lasts about 1 day. The maximum number of labeled cells is reached at 3 days after a single injection of BrdU (Kronenberg et al., 2003). It is estimated that many of the dividing cells go through two to three cell cycles. By this time, most of the BrdU-labeled cells have already turned into type-3 cells. The number of labeled cells is higher than at 1 day after BrdU injection, but not eight times as high (2^3), the hypothetical number of cells that could be reached if all new cells survived. The dilution of BrdU below the level of detection accounts for some false-negative cells (Hayes and Nowakowski, 2002), but if cell death did not account for the greatest part of the difference, the dentate gyrus would literally explode. This event does not take place because cell death eliminates most of the newly generated cells (Fig. 6–7, Color Plate 10).

Most cell death seems to occur once the cells have left the cell cycle, have become postmitotic, and express both DCX and calretinin. The elimination of cells is rapid. The number of fragmented nuclei, a morphological indication of cell death, is highest at 3 days after an injection with BrdU (Seki, 2002). It has been hypothesized that elimination is the default pathway, counteracted by activity-dependent, survival-promoting rescue effects. These are

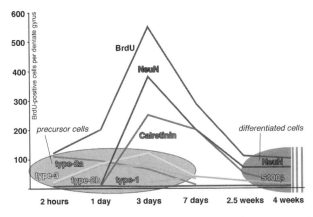

Figure 6–7 (Color Plate 10). During adult hippocampal neurogenesis, a phase of expansion is followed by a phase of (presumably activity-dependent) survival or apoptotic elimination. After a single dose of BrdU, BrdU-positive cells progress through the stages explained in Figure 6–4. See also Figure 6–5. Reprinted from Kempermann et al. (2004) with kind permission of Elsevier.

elicited by "cognitive" stimuli such as exposure to an enriched environment or more specific learning stimuli (Kempermann et al., 1997a, 1998; Gould et al., 1999). The survival-promoting effects are long-lasting (Kempermann and Gage, 1999). Two to 3 weeks after exit from the cell cycle the number of new cells remains very stable. Even at 1 year after the BrdU injection, the latest time point investigated in the mouse hippocampus, the number was unchanged (Kempermann et al., 2003).

A consequence of this developmental pattern is that proliferation is a poor predictor of net neurogenesis (Kempermann et al., 1997b; Kempermann and Gage, 2002). In some studies, especially older ones, proliferation was measured as the only parameter describing neurogenesis. Cell division in the SGZ is correlated with net neurogenesis but not identical to it. As depicted in Figure 6–7 (Color Plate 10), the number of newly generated cells that is produced during the proliferation (expansion) phase of adult hippocampal neurogenesis is massively reduced by an activity dependent selection process. Adult hippocampal neurogenesis is largely regulated on the level of cell survival and neuronal differentiation. In addition, assessment of proliferation is also influenced by the labeling paradigm (Hayes and Nowakowski, 2002).

When only young, immature cells are dying, adult neurogenesis must lead to a growing dentate gyrus. Rats have approximately 1.2 million granule cells per dentate gyrus, mice have 300,000, and humans have 15 million (West and Gundersen, 1990). Even in the earliest reports on adult hippocampal neurogenesis it was concluded that new neurons are added to the granule cell layer and do not replace dying older cells (Altman and Das, 1965; Bayer et al., 1982; Bayer, 1985; Crespo et al., 1986). In 1982, Shirley Bayer estimated a 35% to 43% net growth of the dentate gyrus in rats (Bayer et al., 1982; Bayer, 1985). According to stereological analysis, however, one later study did not find significant change in the total granule cell number of rats between 5 months and 24 months of age (Merrill et al., 2003), possibly because there was considerable interindividual and interstrain variation. In mice there was a 40% increase in the volume of the dentate gyrus in roughly the first year of life (Peirce et al., 2003). In the absence of specific stimuli—that is, more or less the genetically determined baseline level, the total increase in the number of granule cells in mice might range from 30% to 40% between ages 4 weeks and 1 year, after which it plateaus. At the age of 36 days, about 4800 new granule cells are generated per day in a C57BL/6 mouse. If extrapolated from this rate, over a lifespan adult neurogenesis would generate a dentate gyrus 10 times as large as that in reality. However, adult neurogenesis strongly decreases with increasing age, resulting in a lack of measurable growth of the dentate gyrus later in life (Fig. 6–8). Quantitatively, adult neurogenesis in the dentate gyrus occurs relatively early in life. However, adult neurogenesis persists into very old age, although at a very low rate (Kuhn et al., 1996; Kempermann et al., 1998; Cameron and McKay, 1999).

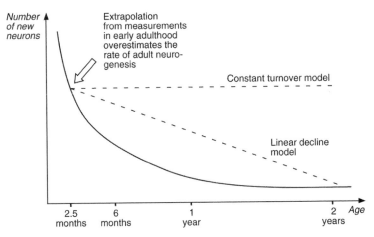

Figure 6–8. Age-dependent decrease in adult hippocampal neurogenesis. Schematic depiction of the inverse relationship between adult hippocampal neurogenesis and the net increase in the total granule cell number. Most of adult hippocampal neurogenesis occurs fairly early in life and many quantitative estimates of neurogenesis rates are too high, because they are based on samples from young animals. The depicted relationship also argues against a substantial neuronal turnover in the dentate gyrus.

NEW INTERNEURONS IN THE ADULT DENTATE GYRUS?

Adult hippocampal neurogenesis generates only granule cells in the dentate gyrus. Under physiologic conditions no exceptions from this rule have been detected. All postmitotic new neurons express transcription factor Prox1, specific to granule cells (Brandt et al., 2003). Nevertheless, one study claimed that a large number of basket cell interneurons are generated in the adult mouse, resulting in a complete turnover of the entire population of basket cells within roughly 1 month (Liu et al., 2003). In contrast to the excitatory granule cells, which are the principal neurons of the dentate gyrus project to CA3, interneurons form local inhibitory circuits. A total of seven different types of interneurons have been described for the dentate gyrus (Freund and Buzsaki, 1996). Basket cells are interneurons located in SGZ and hilus, have a very large cell body, and express the calcium-binding protein parvalbumin. In the report claiming newly generated basket cells, a complex experimental design was used in which neurons of BrdU-treated animals were transduced with a virus expressing the reporter gene GFP. The electrophysiological properties of infected neurons were determined, by determining post hoc whether the cells that by electrophysiological standards were interneurons contained BrdU. In studies based on the commonly used paradigm of examining the phenotype of BrdU-labeled cells several weeks after BrdU, no BrdU-labeled basket cells have been reported (Brandt et al., 2003; Seri et al., 2004). By modifying cell culture conditions, both excitatory and inhibitory neurons could be derived from hippocampal precursor cells ex vivo (Vicario-Abejon et al., 2000). However, granule cells that are glutamatergic neurons can also express GABA, particularly under stressing conditions (Schwarzer and Sperk, 1995; Sloviter et al., 1996). The functional correlate of this observation is not known.

As a general concern, if new interneurons could be produced in the adult dentate gyrus, they very likely would have to originate from ventral precursor cells, not the dorsal cells that produce granule cells. Implantion of NG2-positive cells from the SVZ that are supposedly of ventral origin into the postnatal hippocampus resulted in NG2 cell–derived hippocampal interneurons (Aguirre et al., 2004). Further research is necessary to elucidate the potential for interneurogenesis in the adult hippocampus.

GLIOGENESIS IN THE ADULT DENTATE GYRUS

Precursor cells isolated from the adult hippocampus are multipotent in vitro. In vivo, both neurogenesis and gliogenesis are found in the dentate gyrus. It is unknown, however, whether both lineages originate from an identical precursor cells in vivo. As stated above, beyond the type-1 and type-2a stage no overlap between neuronal and glial markers has been reported, which suggests that if a shared precursor cell exists in vivo, it should be found during these early stages. In the dentate gyrus, gliogenesis is largely equivalent to the generation of new astrocytes. With respect to the generation of new oligodendrocytes there are conflicting results, most likely reflecting strain and species differences. NG2-expressing cells, thought to be precursor cells in the oligodendrocytic lineage, can be found in the SGZ, but their rate of division appears to be extremely low (Steiner et al., 2004). However, Aguirre and coworkers (2004) have reported that NG2-cells from the developing SVZ have C-cell properties (see Chapter 5) and when implanted into the early postnatal hippocampus developed into local interneurons. Oligodendrocytes originate from the ganglionic eminences in the ventral SVZ, whereas the neural precursor cells of the adult SGZ are thought to derive from the dorsal ventricular wall. It is thus likely that in the adult dentate gyrus the lineages of neurons and astrocytes on the one hand and of oligodendrocytes on the other are separate and based on different populations of precursor cells. Ex vivo, however, precursor cells from the adult dentate gyrus are multipotent and produce all three lineages—neurons, astrocytes, and oligodendrocytes (Palmer et al., 1997).

Morphologically, many newly generated astrocytes in the adult dentate gyrus differ from astrocyte-like precursor cells. The radial glia–like type-1 cells have been called "vertical astrocytes," whereas the newly generated astrocytes of the adult SGZ are "horizontal astrocytes" (Seri et al., 2004; Steiner et al., 2004). Both types of astrocytes express GFAP, but in contrast to type-1 cells, horizontal astrocytes also express S100β. In the SGZ, S100β-positive cells have never been found in cell cycle (Steiner et al., 2004). Presumably, the S100β-positive horizontal astrocytes are postmitotic. Alternatively, they might down-regulate S100β before reentering the cell cycle. The immediate precursor of the S100β-positive astrocytes is a progenitor cell within the glial lineage. This glial-determined progenitor is characterized by GFAP expression and the absence of S100β, nestin, and radial glia morphology (Steiner et al., 2004). It seems likely that this intermediate cell also originates from the radial glia–like precursor, but the final proof of bipotentiality in vivo is lacking. Like neurogenesis, astrogenesis is regulated by numerous stimuli, with many stimuli affecting both lineages similarly. Nevertheless, regulation in both lineages appears to be independent (Steiner et al., 2004).

REFERENCES

Altman J, Das GD (1965) Autoradiographic and histologic evidence of postnatal neurogenesis in rats. J Comp Neurol 124:319–335.
Aguirre AA, Chittajallu R, Belachew S, Gallo V (2004) NG2–expressing cells in the subventricular zone are type C–like cells and contribute to interneuron generation in the postnatal hippocampus. J Cell Biol 165:575–589.
Alvarez-Buylla A, Garcia-Verdugo JM, Tramontin AD (2001) A unified hypothesis on the lineage of neural stem cells. Nat Rev Neurosci 2:287–293.
Ambrogini P, Lattanzi D, Ciuffoli S, Agostini D, Bertini L, Stocchi V, Santi S, Cuppini R (2004) Morpho-functional characterization of neuronal cells at different

stages of maturation in granule cell layer of adult rat dentate gyrus. Brain Res 1017:21–31.

Bayer SA (1985) Neuron production in the hippocampus and olfactory bulb of the adult rat brain: addition or replacement? Ann NY Acad Sci 457:163–172.

Bayer SA, Yackel JW, Puri PS (1982) Neurons in the rat dentate gyrus granular layer substantially increase during juvenile and adult life. Science 216:890–892.

Biebl M, Cooper CM, Winkler J, Kuhn HG (2000) Analysis of neurogenesis and programmed cell death reveals a self-renewing capacity in the adult rat brain. Neurosci Lett 291:17–20.

Brandt MD, Jessberger S, Steiner B, Kronenberg G, Reuter K, Bick-Sander A, Von der Behrens W, Kempermann G (2003) Transient calretinin-expression defines early postmitotic step of neuronal differentiation in adult hippocampal neurogenesis of mice. Mol Cell Neurosci 24:603–613.

Brown J, Cooper-Kuhn CM, Kempermann G, Van Praag H, Winkler J, Gage FH, Kuhn HG (2003) Enriched environment and physical activity stimulate hippocampal but not olfactory bulb neurogenesis. Eur J Neurosci 17:2042–2046.

Cameron HA, McKay RD (1999) Restoring production of hippocampal neurons in old age. Nat Neurosci 2:894–897.

Cao L, Jiao X, Zuzga DS, Liu Y, Fong DM, Young D, During MJ (2004) VEGF links hippocampal activity with neurogenesis, learning and memory. Nat Genet 36:827–835.

Carlen M, Cassidy RM, Brismar H, Smith GA, Enquist LW, Frisen J (2002) Functional integration of adult-born neurons. Curr Biol 12:606–608.

Caviness VS Jr. (1973) Time of neuron origin in the hippocampus and dentate gyrus of normal and reeler mutant mice: an autoradiographic analysis. J Comp Neurol 151:113–120.

Crespo D, Stanfield BB, Cowan WM (1986) Evidence that late-generated granule cells do not simply replace earlier formed neurons in the rat dentate gyrus. Exp Brain Res 62:541–548.

Eckenhoff MF, Rakic P (1984) Radial organization of the hippocampal dentate gyrus: a Golgi, ultrastructural, and immunocytochemical analysis in the developing rhesus monkey. J Comp Neurol 223:1–21.

Filippov V, Kronenberg G, Pivneva T, Reuter K, Steiner B, Wang LP, Yamaguchi M, Kettenmann H, Kempermann G (2003) Subpopulation of nestin-expressing progenitor cells in the adult murine hippocampus shows electrophysiological and morphological characteristics of astrocytes. Mol Cell Neurosci 23:373–382.

Forster E, Tielsch A, Saum B, Weiss KH, Johanssen C, Graus-Porta D, Muller U, Frotscher M (2002) Reelin, Disabled 1, and beta 1 integrins are required for the formation of the radial glial scaffold in the hippocampus. Proc Natl Acad Sci USA 99:13178–13183.

Francis F, Koulakoff A, Boucher D, Chafey P, Schaar B, Vinet MC, Friocourt G, McDonnell N, Reiner O, Kahn A, McConnell SK, Berwald-Netter Y, Denoulet P, Chelly J (1999) Doublecortin is a developmentally regulated, microtubule-associated protein expressed in migrating and differentiating neurons. Neuron 23:247–256.

Freund TF, Buzsaki G (1996) Interneurons of the hippocampus. Hippocampus 6:347–470.

Fukuda S, Kato F, Tozuka Y, Yamaguchi M, Miyamoto Y, Hisatsune T (2003) Two distinct subpopulations of nestin-positive cells in adult mouse dentate gyrus. J Neurosci 23:9357–9366.

Gould E, Beylin A, Tanapat P, Reeves A, Shors TJ (1999) Learning enhances adult neurogenesis in the hippoampal formation. Nat Neurosci 2:260–265.

Hastings NB, Gould E (1999) Rapid extension of axons into the CA3 region by adult-generated granule cells. J Comp Neurol 413:146–154.

Hayes NL, Nowakowski RS (2002) Dynamics of cell proliferation in the adult dentate gyrus of two inbred strains of mice. Brain Res Dev Brain Res 134:77–85.

Huttmann K, Sadgrove M, Wallraff A, Hinterkeuser S, Kirchhoff F, Steinhauser C, Gray WP (2003) Seizures preferentially stimulate proliferation of radial glia-like astrocytes in the adult dentate gyrus: functional and immunocytochemical analysis. Eur J Neurosci 18:2769–2778.

Jessberger S, Kempermann G (2003) Adult-born hippocampal neurons mature into activity-dependent responsiveness. Eur J Neurosci 18:2707–2712.

Jin K, Zhu Y, Sun Y, Mao XO, Xie L, Greenberg DA (2002) Vascular endothelial growth factor (VEGF) stimulates neurogenesis in vitro and in vivo. Proc Natl Acad Sci USA 99:11946–11950.

Kempermann G, Gage FH (1999) Experience-dependent regulation of adult hippocampal neurogenesis: effects of long-term stimulation and stimulus withdrawal. Hippocampus 9:321–332.

Kempermann G, Gage FH (2002) Genetic determinants of adult hippocampal neurogenesis correlate with acquistion, but not probe trial performance in the water maze task. Eur J Neurosci 16:129–136.

Kempermann G, Gast D, Kronenberg G, Yamaguchi M, Gage FH (2003) Early determination and long-term persistence of adult-generated new neurons in the hippocampus of mice. Development 130:391–399.

Kempermann G, Jessberger S, Steiner B, Kronenberg G (2004) Milestones of neuronal development in the adult hippocampus. Trends Neurosci 27:447–452.

Kempermann G, Kuhn HG, Gage FH (1997a) More hippocampal neurons in adult mice living in an enriched environment. Nature 386:493–495.

Kempermann G, Kuhn HG, Gage FH (1998) Experience-induced neurogenesis in the senescent dentate gyrus. J Neurosci 18:3206–3212.

Kempermann G, Kuhn HG, Gage FH (1997b) Genetic influence on neurogenesis in the dentate gyrus of adult mice. Proc Natl Acad Sci USA 94:10409–10414.

Kosaka T, Hama K (1986) Three-dimensional structure of astrocytes in the rat dentate gyrus. J Comp Neurol 249:242–260.

Kronenberg G, Reuter K, Steiner B, Brandt MD, Jessberger S, Yamaguchi M, Kempermann G (2003) Subpopulations of proliferating cells of the adult hippocampus respond differently to physiologic neurogenic stimuli. J Comp Neurol 467:455–463.

Kuhn HG, Dickinson-Anson H, Gage FH (1996) Neurogenesis in the dentate gyrus of the adult rat: age-related decrease of neuronal progenitor proliferation. J Neurosci 16:2027–2033.

Liu S, Wang J, Zhu D, Fu Y, Lukowiak K, Lu Y (2003) Generation of functional inhibitory neurons in the adult rat hippocampus. J Neurosci 23:732–736.

Markakis E, Gage FH (1999) Adult-generated neurons in the dentate gyrus send axonal projections to the field CA3 and are surrounded by synaptic vesicles. J Comp Neurol 406:449–460.

Mercier F, Kitasako JT, Hatton GI (2002) Anatomy of the brain neurogenic zones revisited: fractones and the fibroblast/macrophage network. J Comp Neurol 451:170–188.

Merrill DA, Karim R, Darraq M, Chiba AA, Tuszynski MH (2003) Hippocampal cell genesis does not correlate with spatial learning ability in aged rats. J Comp Neurol 459:201–207.

Mignone JL, Kukekov V, Chiang AS, Steindler D, Enikolopov G (2004) Neural stem and progenitor cells in nestin-GFP transgenic mice. J Comp Neurol 469:311–324.

Overstreet LS, Hentges ST, Bumaschny VF, de Souza FS, Smart JL, Santangelo AM,

Low MJ, Westbrook GL, Rubinstein M (2004) A transgenic marker for newly born granule cells in dentate gyrus. J Neurosci 24:3251–3259.

Palmer TD, Ray J, Gage FH (1995) FGF-2-responsive neuronal progenitors reside in proliferative and quiescent regions of the adult rodent brain. Mol Cell Neurosci 6:474–486.

Palmer TD, Takahashi J, Gage FH (1997) The adult rat hippocampus contains premordial neural stem cells. Mol Cell Neurosci 8:389–404.

Palmer TD, Willhoite AR, Gage FH (2000) Vascular niche for adult hippocampal neurogenesis. J Comp Neurol 425:479–494.

Peirce JL, Chesler EJ, Williams RW, Lu L (2003) Genetic architecture of the mouse hippocampus: identification of gene loci with selective regional effects. Genes Brain Behav 2:238–252.

Priller J, Flugel A, Wehner T, Boentert M, Haas CA, Prinz M, Fernandez-Klett F, Prass K, Bechmann I, de Boer BA, Frotscher M, Kreutzberg GW, Persons DA, Dirnagl U (2001) Targeting gene-modified hematopoietic cells to the central nervous system: use of green fluorescent protein uncovers microglial engraftment. Nat Med 7:1356–1361.

Rao MS, Shetty AK (2004) Efficacy of doublecortin as a marker to analyse the absolute number and dendritic growth of newly generated neurons in the adult dentate gyrus. Eur J Neurosci 19:234–246.

Ray J, Peterson DA, Schinstine M, Gage FH (1993) Proliferation, differentiation, and long-term culture of primary hippocampal neurons. Proc Natl Acad Sci USA 90:3602–3606.

Ribak CE, Korn MJ, Shan Z, Obenaus A (2004) Dendritic growth cones and recurrent basal dendrites are typical features of newly generated dentate granule cells in the adult hippocampus. Brain Res 1000:195–199.

Rickmann M, Amaral DG, Cowan WM (1987) Organization of radial glial cells during the development of the rat dentate gyrus. J Comp Neurol 264:449–479.

Rietze R, Poulin P, Weiss S (2000) Mitotically active cells that generate neurons and astrocytes are present in multiple regions of the adult mouse hippocampus. J Comp Neurol 424:397–408.

Rochefort C, Gheusi G, Vincent JD, Lledo PM (2002) Enriched odor exposure increases the number of newborn neurons in the adult olfactory bulb and improves odor memory. J Neurosci 22:2679–2689.

Schanzer A, Wachs FP, Wilhelm D, Acker T, Cooper-Kuhn C, Beck H, Winkler J, Aigner L, Plate KH, Kuhn HG (2004) Direct stimulation of adult neural stem cells in vitro and neurogenesis in vivo by vascular endothelial growth factor. Brain Pathol 14:237–248.

Schmidt-Hieber C, Jonas P, Bischofberger J (2004) Enhanced synaptic plasticity in newly generated granule cells of the adult hippocampus. Nature 429:184–187.

Schwarzer C, Sperk G (1995) Hippocampal granule cells express glutamic acid decarboxylase-67 after limbic seizures in the rat. Neuroscience 69:705–709.

Seaberg RM, van der Kooy D (2002) Adult rodent neurogenic regions: the ventricular subependyma contains neural stem cells, but the dentate gyrus contains restricted progenitors. J Neurosci 22:1784–1793.

Seaberg RM, van der Kooy D (2003) Stem and progenitor cells: the premature desertion of rigorous definitions. Trends Neurosci 26:125–131.

Seki T (2002) Expression patterns of immature neuronal markers PSA-NCAM, CRMP-4 and NeuroD in the hippocampus of young adult and aged rodents. J Neurosci Res 70:327–334.

Seki T, Arai Y (1993) Highly polysialylated neural cell adhesion molecule (NCAM-H) is expressed by newly generated granule cells in the dentate gyrus of the adult rat. J Neurosci 13:2351–2358.

Seri B, Garcia-Verdugo JM, Collado-Morente L, McEwen BS, Alvarez-Buylla A (2004) Cell types, lineage, and architecture of the germinal zone in the adult dentate gyrus. J Comp Neurol 478:359.

Seri B, Garcia-Verdugo JM, McEwen BS, Alvarez-Buylla A (2001) Astrocytes give rise to new neurons in the adult mammalian hippocampus. J Neurosci 21:7153–7160.

Sloviter RS, Dichter MA, Rachinsky TL, Dean E, Goodman JH, Sollas AL, Martin DL (1996) Basal expression and induction of glutamate decarboxylase and GABA in excitatory granule cells of the rat and monkey hippocampal dentate gyrus. J Comp Neurol 373:593–618.

Stanfield BB, Cowan WM (1979) The development of the hippocampus and dentate gyrus in normal and reeler mice. J Comp Neurol 185:423–459.

Stanfield BB, Trice JE (1988) Evidence that granule cells generated in the dentate gyrus of adult rats extend axonal projections. Exp Brain Res 72:399–406.

Steiner B, Kronenberg G, Jessberger S, Brandt MD, Reuter K, Kempermann G (2004) Differential regulation of gliogenesis in the context of adult hippocampal neurogenesis in mice. Glia 46:41–52.

van Praag H, Schinder AF, Christie BR, Toni N, Palmer TD, Gage FH (2002) Functional neurogenesis in the adult hippocampus. Nature 415:1030–1034.

Vicario-Abejon C, Collin C, Tsoulfas P, McKay RD (2000) Hippocampal stem cells differentiate into excitatory and inhibitory neurons. Eur J Neurosci 12:677–688.

Wang S, Scott BW, Wojtowicz JM (2000) Heterogenous properties of dentate granule neurons in the adult rat. J Neurobiol 42:248–257.

West MJ, Gundersen HJG (1990) Unbiased stereological estimation of the number of neurons in the human hippocampus. Comp Neurol 296:1–22.

Yamashima T, Tonchev AB, Vachkov IH, Popivanova BK, Seki T, Sawamoto K, Okano H (2004) Vascular adventitia generates neuronal progenitors in the monkey hippocampus after ischemia. Hippocampus 14:861–875.

7

Technical Notes

A great deal of the present knowledge about adult neurogenesis in vivo relies on a rather limited repertoire of methods. This makes the body of information particularly sensitive to confounding technical problems. Consequently, critical evaluation of the methods used has been an important part of interpreting the data on adult neurogenesis. We discussed the problematic identity of precursor cells in Chapter 3. Here we ask the following questions: How can we reliably identify precursor cells in vivo and pay respect to their heterogeneity? How can we prove that a new cell has indeed become a functional neuron?

The first three decades after Altman's initial description of adult neurogenesis in the 1960s were dominated by fundamental skepticism of this phenomenon. Evidence of adult neurogenesis was not yet good enough. Since the mid-1990s, the mere existence of neurogenesis in the adult mammalian brain is no longer questioned. One reason for this acceptance is the rise of neural stem cell biology, another is technical progress. New techniques such as confocal microscopy and stereology are not without problems, however. The methodological issues fall into three categories.

- *Problems related to the identification of newly generated cells.* These issues circle around the use of tritiated thymidine and bromodeoxyuridine (BrdU) as persistent markers of proliferating cells. Do these methods reliably mark only dividing cells or is a contamination by DNA repair or cell death possible? How can these markers be used to identify precursor cells?
- *Problems related to identifying the phenotype of a cell already identified as new.* Here difficulties arise from the challenges of multichannel immunofluorescence and the potential ambiguities of the markers used in these experiments. The core problem is how to demonstrate the neuronal identity of a cell that has been generated in the adult brain. What are the minimal criteria for a neuron? Can they be addressed in vivo? What is a reasonable compromise between feasibility and validity?
- *Problems related to quantification.* This issue has to do with the not-so-trivial task of obtaining valid estimates of total cell numbers from counts of marked cells in the available sample. The solution to this problem is stereology, a solution that some researchers fear will pose greater problems than the pitfall it supposedly prevents. What are the consequences of sloppy quantification?

Some additional difficulties in interpreting data about adult neurogenesis, not covered here in detail, have to do with conclusions about a dynamic process being derived from essentially static data. How are our data influenced by the dynamics of the system? And even more difficult in this context, what do we define as our "system"? The brain? The hippocampus? The subgranular zone? In other words, our interpretations might depend on what we relate our data to.

TRITIATED THYMIDINE AND BROMODEOXYURININE

In most publications, demonstration of adult neurogenesis is based on the "birth-marking" of cells with bromodeoxyuridine (BrdU). The underlying principle is straightforward: a permanent marker is brought into a cell of interest at the time point of division and the later fate of this cell is studied. Because the marker is persistent, it is possible to retrospectively conclude with confidence that a marked cell must have undergone division at the time when the marker was injected (Fig. 7–1). Because neurons do not divide, the finding of a marked neuron signals that it must derive from a cell that could divide. It is thus inferred that these proliferative cells are precursor cells. Initially, *precursor* was more or less a descriptive term without the connotations of today's stem cell biology. In his first complete description of adult hippocampal neurogenesis, Joseph Altman already assumed that "some precursor" cell might have been responsible for the "birth-dating" marker found in the granule cells (Altman and Das, 1965).

The first widely used substance that allowed permanent labeling of cell divisions was tritiated thymidine. In the 1950s it was discovered that

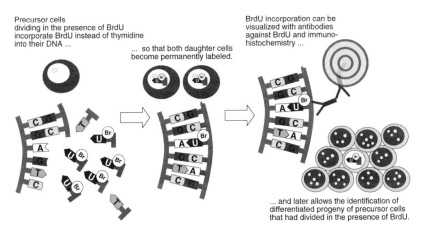

Precursor cells dividing in the presence of BrdU incorporate BrdU instead of thymidine into their DNA ...

... so that both daughter cells become permanently labeled.

BrdU incorporation can be visualized with antibodies against BrdU and immunohistochemistry ...

... and later allows the identification of differentiated progeny of precursor cells that had divided in the presence of BrdU.

Figure 7–1. The bromodeoxyuridine (BrdU) method to permanently label dividing cells. BrdU is an exogenously applied false base that competes with endogenous thymidine for incorporation into the DNA.

radioactively labeled nucleotides such as C14 marked thymidine were incorporated into the DNA of dividing cells during the S phase of the cell cycle and could be detected autoradiographically (see, e.g., Friedkin and Wood, 1956). But C14 thymidine was cumbersome to use and did not yield a resolution as high as that with tritiated thymidine, which was first applied to studies of brain by Messier and Leblond in 1958 (Messier et al., 1958). Thymidine, radioactively labeled with tritium, can be injected systemically. Once in the bloodstream, tritiated thymidine competes with endogenous thymidine in all cells in the S phase of cell division and is permanently incorporated into the DNA. Labeled thymidine has a short half-life in vivo (although the exact value for the rodent brain is not known and presumably varies). Thus tritiated thymidine labels all cells in the process of cell division when the label is injected. At a later time point, tissue sections can be prepared and coated with a photo emulsion. The radiation from the labeled thymidine molecules blackens the photo emulsion, thus making visible the typical grains of thymidine autoradiography.

All studies about adult neurogenesis from 1962 to 1993 were based on thymidine autoradiography (e.g., Fig. 2–3). From today's perspective the main disadvantage is that thymidine autoradiography cannot be easily combined with the increasing arsenal of cell type–specific markers that would allow a deeper and three-dimensional analysis of the labeled cells. In particular, a combination of radiography with immunofluorescence is not possible.

Nevertheless, in 1993 Gould and Cameron used thymidine autoradiography together with immunohistochemistry against neuron-specific enolase (NSE) to prove the existence of "new neurons" through double-labeling (Cameron et al., 1993). This technical advance enabled a description of adult neurogenesis that finally paved the way to wide acceptance of the phenomenon. That same year (1993) the next methodologic step was taken by Frank Corotto and coworkers, who first applied a nonradiographic technique, the BrdU-method, of birth-marking cells to the field of research on adult neurogenesis (Corotto et al., 1993). The first larger study that made full use of the potential of the new method came from H. Georg Kuhn, then with Fred H. Gage at the Salk Institute in La Jolla (Kuhn et al., 1996).

Because BrdU is detected with antibodies, its fluorescent visualization can be combined with two or more other markers. Analysis via the confocal microscope became possible (Kuhn et al., 1996). Today, most in vivo studies on adult neurogenesis rely on the BrdU method, thus we will cover it here in greater detail.

Like tritiated thymidine, 5-bromo-2-deoxyuridine (BrdU, or in older reports, BrdUrd or BUrd) is an analog to thymidine that can be administered systemically. BrdU is a false base that competes with endogenous thymidine during the synthesis phase of the cell cycle. BrdU was initially developed as a antitumorigenic agent used to sensitize tumor cells to radiotherapy (Sano et al., 1965, 1968). With the availability of more effective therapies, including other halogenated nucleotides such as fluorouracil with stronger antitumorigenic effects, this strategy was abandoned. That halogenated nucleotides can be incorporated into the DNA without interfering with transcription and the health of the cell was first described in the early 1950s (Dunn et al., 1954; Zamenhof and Gribiff, 1954). Nevertheless, very high doses of BrdU can kill dividing cells. With the development of specific antibodies, BrdU became detectable immunohistochemically (Gratzner, 1982). BrdU became a widely used marker for cell proliferation in vivo and in vitro (Dolbeare, 1995).

The estimated bioavailability that is most widely accepted suggests that in rodents BrdU labels cells for a maximum of 2 hours after injection, but this estimation is rough and no study can be cited to support it. Also, the sensitivity of the BrdU method depends on the dose of BrdU injected and on the immunohistochemical technique used to visualize it (Cameron and McKay, 2001). Others consider the bioavailability to be much shorter, around 30 minutes. In contrast to endogenous markers of cell division, such as Ki-67 or proliferating cell nuclear antigen (PCNA), BrdU and tritiated thymidine identify cells dividing at the time of marker injection, not when the tissue specimen was obtained. It is this fundamental difference that is the basis for the identification of new neurons with the BrdU method. Between the time point of birth-marking by BrdU injection and BrdU incorporation, and the collection of tissue and its analysis there can be days, weeks, or months, even years. This interval gives the labeled cell sufficient time to differentiate and mature into a neuron. Endogenous cell cycle–related antigens do not represent such a memory of a past cell division. Because neurons are strictly postmitotic, a BrdU-positive neuron that is detected weeks after BrdU injection must have originated from a cell that divided at exactly the time when BrdU was systemically available. The strength of the method lies in the fact that the experimenter can control the injection time point and the length of interval to analysis. Despite these advantages, the BrdU method has a number of pitfalls and problems that can severely confound results.

BrdU or Tritiated Thymidine?

For most researchers, BrdU has replaced tritiated thymidine as the method of choice. Tritiated thymidine cannot be detected immunohistochemically but requires autoradiography to identify labeled cells. The technical details of autoradiography require that the section be coated with a photo emulsion which then is blackened spotwise by the alpha radiation from the radioactivity in the underlying tissue section. Thus the spatial resolution of the method is low; to relate the black grains that represent the positive signal to a particular cell requires a projection of information between two different focal planes. Therefore the method can only be used in rather thin sections, making three-dimensional reconstructions difficult. At the same time, double-labelings are very challenging and triple-labelings are virtually impossible. Because the autoradiographic signal and the immunohisto-chemical for the marker of interest are not in the same focal plane, confocal microscopy cannot be used, thus making the decision whether a given cell is truly double-labeled problematic. On the other hand, autoradiography is very sensitive and, if done right, specific (Rakic, 2002). It even allows a certain quantification because the number of black grains per cell directly correlate with the amount of tritiated thymidine incorporated. The lack of high spatial resolution and compatibility with confocal microscopy largely outweigh these advantages and the use of tritiated thymidine is now re-served for some special applications.

Dosage of BrdU

In vivo, BrdU is normally used at a concentration of between 50 and 250 μg per gram body weight. Its solubility in normal saline is pH-dependent and prefers a basic milieu. Addition of NaOH to the injection solution, however, makes it aggressive to the animal's skin and other tissues. It is thus preferred that a pH as neutral as possible be used and that BrdU be slowly dissolved by warming the solution to about 40°C. Afterwards, the solution should be cooled to room temperature, sterile filtered, and used immediately. The solution should not be placed in the refrigerator because the white crystals that fall out are very difficult to bring back into solution (except by adding NaOH). No good data exist on how long the BrdU solution is stable, so to be on the safe side it should be prepared fresh before the injection. Expo-sure to light and ultraviolet sources should be avoided.

Cameron and McKay (2001) have reported that the yield of labeled cells is dependent on the individual dose of BrdU administered. However, more BrdU is not necessarily better because the total dose of BrdU and the pe-riod over which it is administered have to be taken into account. To increase the number of detectable BrdU-labeled cells for further analysis, the dose of the individual injection can be increased, or, at the price of a reduced temporal resolution, several injections can be spread out over consecutive days (cumulative labeling). There has been no systematic investigation of this trade-off, but it seems that single injections at higher doses can be tole-rated, as can multiple injections at lower doses.

For mice we recommend a single dose of 50 μg per gram body weight, given once per day over a period of 1 to 7 days. Longer injection periods do not give additional benefit. For rats single doses of up to 250 μg per gram body weight appear to be feasible, but in cumulative labeling paradigms one might want to reduce the dose to avoid overloading the cells and in-creasing toxicity.

BrdU incorporation into the DNA does not seem to interfere with tran-scription, perhaps because only a low number of thymidine nucleotides are replaced and endogenous DNA repair mechanisms can easily deal with the resulting mismatches. Even 1 year after BrdU injection (in mice), 2 years (in rats), or a maximum of over 2 years in humans, BrdU-labeled neurons have been detectable. If one assumes that a neuron with severely disturbed transcription machinery would not be viable and be eliminated, this can be taken as an indication of relative cellular health. But no data exist to prove this assumption.

Cells can, however, be overloaded with BrdU and die. Massive cumulative labeling thus reduces the number of BrdU-marked cells that can be detected at longer periods after BrdU administration.

Pretreating Tissue for BrdU Immunohistochemistry

To detect incorporated BrdU, denaturation of the DNA is necessary. Usually this is achieved by exposing the sections to 2N hydrochloric acid for 15 minutes at 37°C. Earlier protocols asked for an additional treatment with formamide at 65°C to precede the acid step, but it appears that the availability of new anti-BrdU antibodies has made this step dispensable.

Exposure to hydrochloric acid is helpful to unmask the BrdU antigen. However, it is potentially detrimental to other antigens of interest, particularly cell surface antigens and receptors. The result that certain immunoreactions might appear weaker or are absent has to be taken into consideration when interpreting double- and triple-labelings. The use of proper controls (omission of pretreatment steps) helps to assess the magnitude of this problem.

As an alternative to pretreatment with hydrochloric acid, treatment of the sections with DNAse can be tried (approximately 10 U/ml; see Gonchoroff et al., 1986). The method has to be carefully adjusted to individual requirements and yields a lower number of unambiguously labeled cells than the HCl treatment. It thus cannot be recommended for quantitative analysis, and because the signal-to-background ratio is not as good, the usefulness for qualitative questions is limited, too.

Pretreatment for BrdU incorporation must be carefully adjusted to the antibodies used. Some antibody clones recognize methylated thymidine as well, so that under harsh pretreatment essentially all nuclei can become positive.

Cell Cycle–Related Issues

The main advantage of the BrdU method is that the "false base" is permanently incorporated into the DNA of the dividing cell and thus allows posthoc analysis at late time points after division (and after injection of BrdU). At short time periods after injection, however, BrdU can also be used to estimate the proliferative activity itself, although the method is problematic because BrdU labels the S phase of the cell cycle only. The efficiency of detecting all dividing cells thus depends not only on the availability of BrdU but also on cell cycle parameters. The S phase comprises only half or less of the entire cell cycle. Hayes and Nowakowski (2002) have pointed out that estimates of proliferation are strongly distorted by a mismatch between the duration of the S phase and the availability of BrdU. Generally, the BrdU method will underestimate the number of cells that are in cell cycle.

If one can assume that the influence of a given experimental manipulation on the length of the cell cycle is negligible, relative statements can be made, for example, when comparing groups within the same experiment. In a straightforward comparison of proliferation in different experimental groups, the impact of cell cycle issues will be of much less importance. In most cases such incomplete comparisons will be sufficient (and the only feasible way to do this), but it must be remembered that this estimate of proliferation is not identical to the absolute size of the proliferating cell population.

Issues of cell cycle kinetics thus become potentially confounding if estimates of the total number of dividing cells need to be made or if a strong influence of experimental manipulation on cell cycle parameters is suspected. At the same time, the issue raised by Hayes and Nowakowski is complicated by the fact that dividing cells in the adult neurogenic zones are not homogeneous populations. In the dentate gyrus, at least seven morphologically and functionally distinct types of dividing cells can be distinguished (four types, or stages, of precursor cells plus microglia, endothelia, and NG2 cells). Nevertheless, the vast majority of proliferation is accounted for by the transiently amplifying progenitor cells (type 2). But all existing estimates of cell cycle durations in the adult hippocampus (no such data exist for the subventricular zone) relate to an average of all cell types that have incorporated BrdU (Nowakowski et al., 1989; Hayes and Nowakowski, 2002).

Does BrdU Detect DNA Repair and Cell Death?

The major argument brought forth against the BrdU method has been the suspicion that BrdU would not only label dividing cells but also pick up cell death or DNA repair (Cooper-Kuhn and Kuhn, 2002; Rakic, 2002). The cell death argument has two facets. One is that BrdU would be taken up during late stages of apoptotic cell death, when fragmented DNA can be found in the cell. Because DNA polymerase is not active under these conditions and this cellular condition is related to a distinct cellular and nuclear morphology of supposedly very brief existence, this argument can be dismissed rather easily. The concern, however, is that less obvious stages of apoptotic cell death might lead to false BrdU incorporation as well. This is particularly relevant for the reported cases of regenerative neurogenesis after ischemic or hypoxic cell damage, which are associated with apoptotic cell death (Magavi et al., 2000; Nakatomi et al., 2002).

The second variant of this argument has to do with the fact that induction of apoptosis can be preceded by an abortive attempt of the cell to enter into cell cycle. Damaged neurons initiate abortive DNA synthesis (Copani et al., 2001; Katchanov et al., 2001; Kuan et al., 2004). This event appears to take place, for example, in Alzheimer disease: mature neurons attempt to divide and activate the machinery for cell division (Neve et al., 2000). Because completion of the cell cycle is not possible in the postmitotic cells, the neuron dies instead. In this scenario it is difficult to exclude the possibility that the doomed neurons incorporate BrdU during the abortive S phase preceding their attempted division (Kuan et al., 2004); this issue can severely confound supposed evidence of regenerative neurogenesis. Little is known about the reasons for the initiation of division and the amount of BrdU taken up during this process. There is no indication that this process can be found in the normal brain. Also, the cells in the germinative matrices of the neurogenic zones that are identified by the BrdU method as proliferating are not mature neurons but fulfill immunohistochemical criteria of precursor cells. A BrdU signal in mature neurons at very early time points after the injection of BrdU would indeed raise the suspicion of a pathological event or a detection error. Some studies have reported BrdU incorporation in neurons very briefly after BrdU application—too soon to allow differentiation from a precursor cell (Gu et al., 2000). In contrast, the temporal pattern in many BrdU experiments with progression through the expression of different markers compatible with increasing neuronal maturation (e.g., in the hippocampus from nestin to doublecortin to calretinin to calbindin) resolves this suspicion (Arvidsson et al., 2002).

The argument that the BrdU method would actually detect DNA repair carries more weight. During DNA repair, the DNA polymerase is active and false nucleotides such as BrdU could be incorporated. However, brain irradiation as well as irradiation of isolated precursor cells, which induces DNA repair mechanisms, led to reduced immunohistochemical detection of BrdU, not an increased number of marked cells (Palmer et al., 2000; Mizumatsu et al., 2003). The second argument against BrdU labeling of DNA repair is again the marker progression indicative of cellular differentiation. Related to this is the observation that the number of BrdU-positive cells approximately doubles in the first 24 hours after the injection of BrdU. This is compatible with continuation of the cell cycle through the M and T phases and the appearance of two labeled daughter cells, but not with DNA repair.

Independent Confirmation of BrdU-Based Results: Cell Cycle–Related Antigens, Infection with a Retrovirus, and Absolute Cell Counts

BrdU-based results have also been confirmed by independent methods. In addition to the halogenated or tritiated thymidine analogs, retroviruses can be used to persistently label proliferating cells. Retroviruses can infect dividing cells only. They require a complete cell cycle and thus go beyond S-phase detection. Gene products from the incorporated viruses or viral genome can be detected at a later time in differentiated cells. In addition, however, transduction of proliferating cells with a retrovirus expressing the green fluorescent protein (GFP, or EGFP for enhanced GFP) allows visualization of living cells. This retrovirus-based approach could therefore successfully be used in electrophysiological studies of newly generated neurons (Carlen et al., 2002; van Praag et al., 2002; Schmidt-Hieber et al., 2004).

For many years, the BrdU-based method has been used to assess pathologic cell proliferation and has been the method of choice for determining the mitotic activity of tumors. Peter Eriksson's demonstration of adult neurogenesis in humans was done on postmortem tissue from patients who had received BrdU injections during their lifetime to determine the proliferative index of surgically treated laryngeal carcinoma (Eriksson et al., 1998). Today this invasive method of tumor staging has been replaced by use of other markers that do not require the injection of substances into the patient before surgery. Assessment of cell proliferation in tissue is now based on the expression of cell cycle–related antigens detected immunohistochemically. Some of the possible markers are found in Table 7–1. In situations where only proliferation needs to be assessed, cell cycle markers can be used instead of BrdU. However, the signal-to-background ratio of these markers can be lower than that of BrdU, which might justify the additional effort of administering BrdU. The strongest confirmation of neurogenesis is the demonstration of an increase in total cell number in the neuronal population, to which adult neurogenesis adds. Such demonstration can be achieved by use of stereological techniques, as described below.

Proliferating Cell Nuclear Antigen

Proliferating cell nuclear antigen, also called "cyclin," is a 36 kDa protein. It is an auxiliary protein to the delta-DNA-polymerase and is expressed in early G1 and S phase (Hall et al., 1990). In late S phase, PCNA is prominently found in the nucleoli. However, in formaldehyde-fixed tissue this does not become apparent and the staining tends to be diffuse. PCNA staining requires an antigen retrieval procedure consisting of brief boiling in citrate buffer. Although PCNA has been used in a few studies in the context of adult neurogenesis, its application is rather cumbersome and tends to yield a wide range of staining intensities that can be difficult to interpret. It is thus not recommended for routine use in rodents.

Ki67

Ki67 is the name of the original antibody clone that identifies a cell cycle–associated protein (mKi67) encoded on mouse chromosome 7. Although few functional data exist for mki67, it appears to be essential for cell cycle progression (Starborg et al., 1996; Endl and Gerdes, 2000). Ki stands for the Pathological Institute at the University of Kiel; the first antibody that could be used in paraffin-embedded sections was "made in Bostel," a place nearby, hence the mysterious synonymous name MIB. Ki67 antibodies identify cells in late G1, S, G2, and M phase (Scholzen and Gerdes, 2000). Thus only G0- and early G1-phase cells are not recognized. Mki67 is the broadest known cell cycle–associated antigen. Despite this wide specificity and presumably high sensitivity for identifying proliferating cells, in direct comparisons with analyses done shortly after BrdU injection, Ki67 immunohistochemistry yielded higher (Kee et al., 2002) or lower (McKeever et al., 1997) numbers. Except for one clone (available from Novocastra), most Ki67 antibodies require epitope retrieval procedures such as brief boiling in citrate buffer or microwaving.

IDENTIFYING NEW NEURONS: WHEN IS A CELL DOUBLE OR TRIPLE LABELED?

The immunohistochemical identification of new neurons is usually based on detection of BrdU in a cell that expresses neuronal markers. This straightforward approach poses two types of problems: (1) neuronal markers often cannot be unambiguously defined, (2) determination of an intracellular marker overlap that constitutes a double- or triple-labeling is technically challenging.

Dependencies on Markers

For the neurogenic regions of the adult brain, the immunohistochemical detection of neuronal markers in BrdU-positive cells has been validated by numerous studies. Particular problems arise, however, in non-neurogenic zones, when markers from the neurogenic regions are applied and their identical meaning is tacitly assumed. Here the rule that extraordinary claims require extraordinary evidence should be obeyed and independent, additional means of proving the neuronal identity of a cell need to be used.

In such cases, marker expression might not be stable. Pathological situations, most notably ischemia, pose particular challenges and the possibility that damaged cells might show a fluctuation in antigen expression has to be taken into account. As a worst-case scenario, a cell might be damaged and be at the brink of dying when cell death–related mechanisms trigger BrdU incorporation (Kuan et al., 2004) while at the same time proteins associated with neuronal maturity are down-regulated. If the cell recovers, its nucleus will contain BrdU and again the mature neuronal markers. This scenario has some plausibility and from a devil's advocat's point of view should be considered when difficult examples of evidence for neurogenesis are evaluated. As discussed above, hypothetical BrdU uptake during DNA repair and cell death cannot be used as a general argument against new neurons but remain potentially confounding aspects of the BrdU method that have to be taken into account. The best rule is to seek confirmation with an independent method, use more than one marker, and make every attempt

Table 7-1. Detection of Cell Proliferation

Marker	Description	Detects	Advantages	Disadvantages
Thymidine Analogs				
BrdU	Halogenated false nucleotide that competes with thymidine for incorporation into DNA	S phase	Simple use Allows birth-marking and analysis for long periods after division Can be combined with immuno-fluorescence for other markers and analyzed by confocal microscopy	For practical purposes, not quantitative on single-cell level theoretically, additional Br molecule might affect transcription
Tritiated thymidine	Radioactively labeled natural nucleotide that competes with regular thymidine for incorporation into DNA	S phase	Can be used semiquantiatively Very sensitive	Requires autoradiography Co-localization with other markers is difficult or impossible (no confocal analysis)
Cell Cycle Antigens				
Ki67	Protein expressed during cell cycle	Late G1, S, G2, M phases	Broadest sensitivity across cell cycle duration of all antibody-based methods	

PCNA	Protein expressed during cell cycle	Late G1, S phases	Cumbersome immunohistological detection with wide range of staining intensities
pH3	Phosphorylated form of histone H3	M phase	Detects very short period within cell cycle
			Visualizes M-phase chromatin and gives direct evidence of mitoses
Other			
Retrovirus		Completed cell cycle	Large differences in transduction rates
			Requires completed cell cycle for functional integration; abortive cell cycles (e.g., at initiation of cell death) or DNA repair will not be detected	No systemic application possible
			Reporter gene product visualizes entire cell morphology	Challenging and expensive handling
			Can be visualized in living tissue (electrophysiology)	

to demonstrate development. Cells that only re-express a mature marker are unlikely to go through a developmentally plausible sequence of transcription factors or other developmental molecules. A key example of this strategy was used in a study by Andreas Arvidsson and colleagues (2002), who showed regenerative neurogenesis in the ischemic striatum. These authors were able to show that the emerging new neurons went through a stage of transient Pbx and Meis2 expression, two transcripts associated with the development of striatal interneurons.

There are few antigens that are truly neuron-specific. Not all proteins known to have a high specificity for neurons, such as tau protein, are suitable for double- or triple-labeling studies with BrdU and other proliferation markers because they are not localized in or close to the nucleus. In the next chapter we will discuss the so-called NG2 cells (named after a key antigen they express) that in their antigen profile seem to stand somewhere between glia and immature neurons. It is not clear whether this duality also reflects a function between that of neurons and glia, but in any case the issue puts a simplified view of marker specificity into question. All markers have to be validated exactly for the population of cells they are intended for.

Neuron-Specific Enolase

Cameron and Gould's first double-labeling experiments to demonstrate adult hippocampal neurogenesis and Corotto's work in the olfactory bulb were based on the use of NSE (Cameron et al., 1993; Corotto et al., 1993). However, despite its name and original belief (Vinores et al., 1984; Schmechel, 1985), NSE is not entirely specific for neurons, especially if used in light microscopy. NSE immunoreaction is often diffuse and shows great variance in intensity even in neighboring cells. Immunoreaction in mice is lower than that in rats (Vinores et al., 1984). Currently better and more practical neuronal markers are available and NSE should no longer be used for this purpose.

NeuN

NeuN has become the most widely used marker to identify neurons. NeuN was first described by Richard J. Mullen in 1992 (Mullen et al., 1992). NeuN expression is restricted to postmitotic neurons, but a few neuronal populations, including photoreceptors of the retina, cerebellar Purkinje cells, mitral cells of the olfactory bulb, and a population of neurons in the cochlear nucleus, are negative for NeuN. The list of exceptions may not be complete, an important factor to remember if NeuN is used to demonstrate extraordinary cases of adult neurogenesis outside the neurogenic regions. The three populations of neurons known to be generated in adult neurogenesis—hippocampal granule cells and glomerular and periglomerular interneurons of the olfactory bulb—are NeuN positive. In no case has NeuN expression been noted in glial cells. *NeuN* stands for *Neu*ronal *N*uclei, and although NeuN is predominantly located in the nucleus, it can also be detected in purified cytoplasmic fractions from brain. Immunohistochemically, most neurons show a strong and reliable reaction in the nucleus and cytoplasm near the nucleus, occasionally reaching into some neurites.

NeuN is also expressed in neurons of the peripheral and autonomous nervous system. Neuroendocrine cells such as in the intestines, adrenal medulla, pituitary, and pineal gland are often negative for NeuN (Wolf et al., 1996). Also, sympathetic chain neurons do not show NeuN expression.

Remarkably, despite the wide acceptance of NeuN as a neuronal marker, only very few studies have addressed the properties of NeuN itself. The detailed biochemical and molecular properties of NeuN and its function are still not known. NeuN can bind to DNA, which suggests that it acts as a transcription factor that is switched on with the initiation of terminal differentiation (Mullen et al., 1992; Sarnat et al., 1998). Its peptide sequence and structure are not known.

Pathological conditions such as ischemia can down-regulate NeuN expression. The loss of immunoreactivity though does not necessarily relate to a loss of neurons (Unal-Cevik et al., 2004). Consequently, a reemergence of NeuN after recovery from a metabolical perturbation alone would not be indicative of newly generated neurons. Given the controversy about a potential BrdU incorporation during the initiation of cell death, this issue deserves close attention if regenerative neurogenesis is to be proven.

The main advantage of NeuN as a neuronal marker lies in its relatively high and under normal conditions stable expression in the nucleus, making it a good choice for confocal microscopic analyses in combination with BrdU. The presence of the two markers in the same compartment can be determined with high accuracy. See Chapter 6 for a discussion of whether NeuN necessarily identifies *mature* neurons.

β-III-tubulin

β-III-tubulin is an isotype of tubulin, one of the major constituents of the cytoskeleton. Class β-III has historically been labeled the "minor neuronal" isotype associated with neurons in the central and peripheral nervous systems, in contrast to "major neuronal" isotype β-II, expressed in both neurons and glia. β-III-tubulin is often also referred to as "TuJ1," which is not a true synonym but the clonal designation for a widely used antibody against this antigen. β-III-tubulin has found the most widespread application as a neuronal marker in cell culture work. Some groups have also used β-III-tubulin as an indicator of neurogenesis in vivo. However, in vivo, staining against β-III-tubulin is often unsatisfactory. Immature neurons in the neurogenic zones indeed seem to express β-III-tubulin, but nothing is known about re-expression in mature neurons, for example under stress. β-III-tubulin expression is switched on early in neuronal development and parallels NeuroD expression in vitro (Uittenbogaard and Chiaramello, 2002).

β-III-tubulin is not strictly brain-specific and is also found in testis. More worrying is the open question of β-III-tubulin for specific neuronal lineages. In the neurogenic zones in vivo, no overlap between β-III-tubulin and glial markers has been found, but elsewhere some NG2 cells have been found to be β-III-tubulin positive. The glial features of putatitive precursor cells that can generate neurons make it difficult to determine whether β-III-tubulin can be used as an indicator of neuronal lineage determination. As discussed previously, it has not yet been proven that glia-like stem cells are multipotent in vivo and putative lineage-determined progenitor cells are neuronal only. Consequently, the very early neuronal markers including β-III-tubulin remain somewhat problematic with respect to their sensitivity to detect fate choice and lineage determination. In cell culture these ambiguities become a potentially severely confounding issue. β-III-tubulin has, for example, been found in retinal pigment epithelial cells after prolonged periods of time in culture, but not constitutively (Vinores et al., 1993). In neurosphere cultures, β-III-tubulin expression can be found even under proliferation conditions. The specificity of β-III-tubulin as a neuronal marker is further reduced by the finding that during development, some types of non-neuronal cells can express β-III-tubulin, and its expression can be found in brain tumors of presumably glial origin (Ignatova et al., 2002). Although the latter point could also be taken as an argument that gliomas are in fact derived not from differentiated glial cells but from precursor cells, the point clearly requires further investigation. In any case, far-reaching conclusions about the neuronal nature of cells based solely on β-III-tubulin should be avoided.

TUC4 (Synonyms: TOAD-64, Ulip-1, DRP-3, CRMP4)

TUC4 is expressed by postmitotic neurons at the stage of initial differentiation and is associated with axonal outgrowth. Whereas β-III-tubulin is expressed along the entire axon, TUC4, or TOAD-64 (for Turned On After Division, 64 kDa) is found in the distal parts of the growth cones (Minturn et al., 1995). The TUC proteins are homolog to a *C. elegans* gene, *unc-33*, and like it presumably function as a collapsin-response mediator protein (CRMP) (Quinn et al., 1999). Collapsin belongs to the family of semaphorins, which are repulsive molecules active in axon pathfinding. TUC proteins mediate their effect by still unknown mechanisms.

In theory, because of its association with early postmitotic neuronal development, TUC4 should be an ideal marker for adult neurogenesis research. There are, however, a few caveats. The first is that the highest TUC4 expression is not necessarily found in the cell soma but in the growth cone. This makes double-labeling with nuclear markers (such as BrdU) difficult. Also, the intensity of positive cells thus tends to be highly variable. For qualitative statements, TUC4 can be useful, although background staining is often strong. Quantification, especially in tissue treated for BrdU immunohistochemistry, is tricky. There is also evidence that TUC4 might be weakly expressed in oligodendrocyte precursor cells, as they are found through-out the brain parenchyma (Ricard et al., 2001).

TUC4 is expressed very soon after the cells have become postmitotic, but it is not known how long it is expressed during maturation of the new cells. Because much of the quantitative regulation in hippocampal neurogenesis occurs during the postmitotic stage, quantification of TUC4 immunohis-tochemistry does not represent net neurogenesis but an intermediate stage of as-yet undefined length. TUC4, however, shares this limitation with other markers, such as DCX, PSA-NCAM, which can be used as markers for neu-ronal development but not necessarily the quantity of net neurogenesis.

Like β-III-tubulin, TUC4 should not be used as the sole marker to prove adult hippocampal neurogenesis. TUC4 is not expressed in the SVZ, but only in the olfactory bulb (where the new neurons begin to extend their axons).

PSA-NCAM

PSA-NCAM is the polysialyliated form of the neural cell adhesion molecule (NCAM). Polysialic acid (PSA) is only found on NCAM, making it rather specific to the neuronal lineage (Tomasiewicz et al., 1993). At least in some brain regions, such as the hypothalamohypophysial system, PSA is also found on glial cells (Kiss et al., 1993), reducing its sensitivity to detect po-tential neurogenesis outside the well-characterized neurogenic regions. The relationship between adult neurogenesis and PSA-NCAM expression was recognized and characterized early, most notably in the pioneering work by Tatsunori Seki (Seki and Arai, 1991, 1993a, 1993b; Seki, 2002).

In both the olfactory system and the hippocampus, PSA-NCAM is found on migratory neuronal cells. In these areas PSA-NCAM identifies type-2b and type-3 cells in the dentate gyrus and C cells in the SVZ and olfactory bulb. NeuroD expression precedes PSA-NCAM expression (Seki, 2002). The PSA residues reduce cell adhesion mediated by NCAM (Sadoul et al., 1983), thus PSA-NCAM is associated primarily with migratory stages. There is ex vivo evidence that glial progenitors after injury might require PSA-NCAM as well (Wang et al., 1996; Barral-Moran et al., 2003).

In addition, PSA-NCAM is still found on early postmitotic stages of neu-ronal development and those cells that extend dendrites and axon. In the hippocampus, developing neurons are often found in clusters, and the more immature cells are associated with the processes of the more mature cells, suggestive of a direct interaction (Seki, 2002). The details of this interac-tion are not known, however. PSA-NCAM expression on the cell surface is activity-dependently regulated and this process seems to be NMDA receptor-dependent (Wang et al., 1996). This finding, too, argues in favor of the hypothesis that PSA-NCAM is expressed after the neuronal fate choice has been made.

PSA-NCAM is also associated with non-neurogenic regions. In the piri-form cortex a region of particular strong expression is found, without any signs of neurogenesis. PSA-NCAM has functions independent of the adhesion mediated by NCAM, and these functions are beginning to be revealed. PSA plays a permissive role for axon pathfinding (Landmesser et al., 1990; Rutishauser and Landmesser, 1991) and in synaptogenesis (Seki and Rutishauser, 1998). PSA-NCAM is found on both the pre- and postsynaptic membrane (Muller et al., 1996) and is necessary for the structural plasticity following induction of long-term potentiation (LTP) in the hippocampus (Eckhardt et al., 2000).

PSA-NCAM might have a direct signaling function as well. For its function at synapses, activation of Trk B receptors, the receptors for brain-derived neurotrophic factor (BDNF), has been discussed (Muller et al., 2000).

In summary, PSA-NCAM is a very interesting molecule associated with embryonic and adult neurogenesis and other examples of plasticity (Bruses and Rutishauser, 2001; Kiss et al., 2001). Its value as a marker is context-dependent. Within the neurogenic regions, PSA-NCAM immunohistochemistry allows identification of cells at a transient stage of neuronal development. Outside the neurogenic regions, the specificity of PSA-NCAM is less clear, and its association with forms of gliogenesis is likely.

In the neurogenic zones, the time course of PSA-NCAM expression almost completely overlaps with doublecortin expression. Because PSA-NCAM is a surface molecule, immunohistochemical analysis can be difficult. Preservation of the glycoproteins and PSA residues depends on perfusion and fixation protocols. If the goal is only to identify the neuronal progenitor cells and their early postmitotic progeny, doublecortin immunohistochemistry is preferable. Even more than doublecortin, however, PSA-NCAM staining enables visualization of cells in their almost full dendritic morphology.

Doublecortin

Doublecortin (DCX) is a microtubule-associated protein enriched in migratory neuronal cells (Meyer et al., 2002), particularly in their leading processes (Schaar et al., 2004) and in the growth cones of neurites (Friocourt et al., 2003). Doublecortin was discovered because its mutation causes disturbed cortical lamination in humans. One of the resulting disorders is X-linked lissencephaly, associated with mental retardation and epilepsy (Gleeson et al., 1998, 1999). Here a four-layered cortex is found instead of the normal six layers and normal gyri and sulci are lacking. In other cases some neurons do not reach their appropriate position in the cortex and accumulate in the white matter below a layered cortex. This particular structural abnormality is called "subcortical band heterotopia" or "double cortex," hence the name of the protein. Silencing of DCX in developing mice by the RNAi technique has produced a similar phenotype in mice (Bai et al., 2003) but, oddly, not the classical gene knock-out (Corbo et al., 2002). During development, DCX extensively overlaps with reelin expression (Meyer et al., 2002).

Function of DCX is tightly regulated by a balance of kinase and phosphatase activities (Schaar et al., 2004). It has thus been suggested that several signaling pathways might converge at DCX, thereby modulating the stability of microtubules and consequently migratory behavior (LoTurco, 2004). In vitro data indicate that DCX stabilizes microtubules (Moores et al., 2004), but there might be other DCX-dependent mechanisms involved in migration as well (Tanaka et al., 2004).

In the neurogenic zones of the adult brain, DCX expression allows identification of type-2b and type-3 cells (or D cells) of the SGZ and C cells of the SVZ and olfactory bulb. Like PSA-NCAM, it is transiently expressed during adult neurogenesis, identifying the phases of migration and neurite extension (Brandt et al., 2003; Brown et al., 2003; Kronenberg et al., 2003; Ambrogini et al., 2004). DCX expression is found in proliferative cells but persists into the postmitotic stage of neuronal development in the adult hippocampus when it overlaps with calretinin expression (Brandt et al., 2003). An overlap between DCX and calretinin is also found in the developing brain (Meyer et al., 2002).

DCX is a very convenient and robust marker for defined stages of neuronal development in the neurogenic zones. Its cytoplasmic and nuclear expression make it ideally suited for double-labeling with nuclear antigens, such as proliferation marker BrdU. DCX is also detectable in the neurites and enables appreciation of dendritic morphology.

Both inside and outside the neurogenic regions, DCX expression overlaps almost completely with PSA-NCAM (Nacher et al., 2001). Expression by mature astrocytes or oligodendrocytes has not been reported, but NG2 cells throughout the brain might express DCX. As in the case of PSA-NCAM, sensitivity and specificity of DCX as a neurogenic marker in the non-neurogenic regions is reduced and largely undetermined. Both markers therefore cannot be used as sole indicators of neurogenesis.

Map2, Tau Protein, and Neurofilament 200

Microtubule-associated protein 2 (Map2), tau protein, and neurofilament 200 have good neuronal specificity and are widely used in vitro. In vivo, their applicability is limited because immunoreactions against these antigens visualize only neurites. This result makes it difficult to relate a BrdU-labeled nucleus to Map2- or neurofilament-positive processes or tau-positive axons. All three markers are expressed by mature neurons, which gives a very dense staining pattern. In vivo, dendrites of newly generated cells can be visualized more easily with DCX immunohistochemistry.

Pitfalls of Immunofluorescence and Confocal Microscopy

Analysis of double- and triple-stained fluorescent sections poses several challenges. Confocal microscopy has become the gold standard and some problems of classical fluorescent microscopy can be avoided with this technique. On the other hand, confocal microscopy can also add sources of errors. The three most important issues are

- Problems due to a lack of three-dimensional information
- Problems due to crosstalk between excitation and detection channels
- Problems due to incorrect detection sensitivity

In confocal microscopy, laser beams replace the light bulb as the source of light (Fig. 7–2). This allows one to focus the energy of the light very precisely. Filters (or in the most modern technology, acoustic-optical beam splitters) let only light of the desired wavelength pass through. Those excitation wavelengths are chosen at which the fluorophores used can be excited. If hit by light of this particular wavelength, the fluorophores coupled to the secondary antibodies used in the immunohistochemical reaction send out light with a wavelength that is longer than the excitation wavelength. A detector blind to the excitation wavelength thus allows one to distinguish emission from excitation light. This emission spectrum is not a sharp line but rather a distribution with a peak and more or less steep sides. Consequently, emission spectra corresponding to different excitation wavelengths can overlap. If more than one emission channel is analyzed at the same time, it is not possible to conclude from the recorded signal at which wavelength the excitation occurred and, consequently, which of the fluorophores was meant to be excited. This is the most common source of false-positive double-labelings. Confocal microscopy per se does not prevent this problem any more than good fluorescent microscope. The solution to this problem, com-

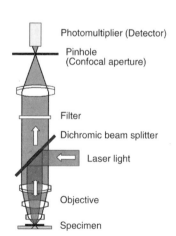

Confocal principle:

- Illuminate and detect from only a very small tissue volume and move the focal spot across the sample ("pixel by pixel")

- What is in the illumination focus is in the detection focus

- Pinhole blocks defracted light and allows optical sectioning

- Everything in focus appears bright, everything not in focus remains black

Photomultiplier (Detector)

Pinhole (Confocal aperture)

Filter

Dichromic beam splitter

Laser light

Objective

Specimen

Figure 7–2. The confocal principle. Confocal microscopy uses laser light to excite fluorescent dyes and generate digital microscopic images of high spatial resolution and strict separation of detection channels. The confocal principle allows placement of thin optical sections within a physical tissue section.

monly dubbed "bleeding," is to sequentially detect the different channels. For example, if the fluorophore FITC is excited at 488 nm, only the detection channel for FITC will be active; if TRTC is excited at 543 nm, only the detection channel for TRTC will be active. One advantage of confocal microscopy is that this sequential scanning is possible in a very straightforward way and a computerized system can immediately superimpose the independently generated images to allow evaluation of double-stainings. However, automated imaging systems can now accomplish this principle for conventional fluorescent light microscopy as well, offering a cheaper alternative to a confocal microscope.

The true (and name-giving) advantage of confocal microscopy lies in its sophisticated optical construction, which differs from that of a normal microscope. Because the laser light produces a sharp focus yielding high energy exactly at the right wavelength and in a tiny area, the image projected to the detection system is very sharp, albeit very small. Whatever is in focus in the specimen is in focus in the detector, thus the name *confocal*. By positioning an aperture in front of a detector that can be adjusted to variable width, it is possible to exclude diffracted, out-of-focus light from the image, producing a sharp image of the optical plane of focus. The full image is collected by moving the focal point over the specimen pixel by pixel and line by line. The confocal image is thus always digital.

In a normal microscope, in contrast, the full image has to be taken at one single time point and the light is distributed over a much larger area. Consequently, defracted light from one spot can interfere with emission of a neighboring spot. The spatial resolution of conventional light or fluorescent microscopy is thus much lower than that in confocal microscopy.

Because the confocal system works in all three dimensions, through confocal microscopy it is possible to place optical sections in the physical section. The laser beam can scan the specimen in x-, y-, and z-dimension, producing a stack of images. This application is called a "z-series." Special imaging software can reconstruct three-dimensional renderings from such z-series. Confocal microscopy thus allows three-dimensional analysis of cells. For proving double-labelings, this approach is often the only feasible way.

Conventional microscopes in contrast produce essentially two-dimensional information. The true optical depth is compressed along the view axis. The three-dimensional specimen is projected and the information in the z-axis is largely lost. To some degree, this can be overcome by manual focus through the section. Because of the limited spatial resolution, however, it can become difficult to distinguish closely neighboring structures (Peterson, 2004).

Satellite cells are glial cells that, especially in cortical regions, are tightly attached to the soma of neurons (Fig. 7–3). They often engulf one side of the neuron like a cap. Depending on the direction of the observer, the satellite cells can completely cover the neuron. Because of the close proximity and low spatial resolution, the BrdU-labeled nucleus of the satellite cell can

Adult Neurogenesis

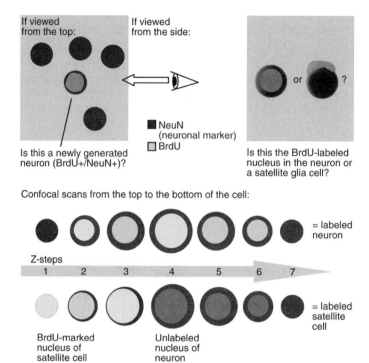

Figure 7–3. Satellite cells. Satellite glia are astrocytes that are tightly attached to neuronal cell bodies and often engulf the neuron like a cap. Depending on the viewing axis, satellite cells can be mistaken as the underlying neuron. BrdU incorporation in satellite glia might lead to the erroneous detection of neurogenesis (Kuhn et al., 1997). Z-series through the supposed new neuron can reveal that it actually consists of two cells with BrdU incorporation in the nucleus of the satellite cell.

be mistaken as the nucleus of the neuron. The neuron would be falsely identified as BrdU labeled and thus as new (Kuhn et al., 1997). The satellite phenomenon can even fool investigators who use a confocal microscope. An eccentric, kidney-shaped nucleus with dense chromatin found in a putative neuron should always raise suspicion.

Because in confocal microscopy the investigator can adjust both the energy of the excitation and the sensitivity of the detection, another problem is overamplification of spurious signals. In the path of light of the microscope, the pinhole corresponds to the iris of a camera. Opening the iris increases the amount of light that falls through it but reduces spatial resolution. The wider the pinhole, the brighter the image, but more of the confocal effect is given away. Also, the detection sensitivity (gain) needs to be adjusted carefully. If the gain is cranked up too far, more signal might seem present, but information is actually lost. Fine structures disappear and the image becomes patchy. If the sensitivity is adjusted to a signal of too low intensity, even though other stronger signals at the same wavelength are found in the same image, all one is doing is amplifying the background. It will become increasingly difficult to distinguish signal from noise. No simple rules exist for the correct adjustment of excitation intensity and detection sensitivity, although modern microscopes do offer software tools that help determine the optimal settings.

HOW TO QUANTIFY CELL NUMBERS: THE ISSUE OF STEREOLOGY

Reports on adult neurogenesis often contain quantitative statements reporting how much a given manipulation increased or decreased the production of new neurons. The parameter used to substantiate such claims is number of cells. Quantification becomes particularly relevant if far-reaching conclusions about regulation, function, and medical implications are made. Thus at one point or another in most studies on adult neurogenesis cells are counted. Although nothing seems to be as straightforward as counting something, this procedure is not without pitfalls because one simply cannot count all the cells that are there. Rather, cell counts are estimates based on an extrapolation from cell counts in samples such as tissue sections.

The following forms of reporting cell numbers are found in the literature:

- Cells per area or section
- Cells per volume
- Cells per anatomically defined structure

Only the last one represents meaningful absolute numbers; the first two will always raise questions about their validity and are difficult to interpret.

The Problem of Treating Tissue Sections as Two-Dimensional

A tissue section under the microscope is essentially two-dimensional. One can add some a third dimension by focusing through the section, but the spatial impression is limited because histological sections are thin, and in thicker sections the vision becomes blurred. Thus in many practical situations histological sections are used as flat images or prints. Their three-dimensional information is reduced to two dimensions, like a map. On a map it is simple to measure distances and areas as long as the scale is known. But for the third dimension, the heights of mountains, for example, one would have to turn to constructs such as altitude lines. Histological sections obviously do not come equipped with altitude lines.

When we count the number of cells in a histological section we are counting colored dots ("profiles") in an area (although it is actually a small volume of tissue). But in biological contexts we are rarely interested in the number per area because all organisms and their organs and cells are three-dimensional. The problem is that we usually do not know how the two-dimensional section represents the three-dimensional structure we are really interested in. After all, sections are not maps drawn with the idea of best possible representation. Sections are to a large degree random samples.

To display cell counts as cells per section is heavily confounded, even if we are seeking to "exactly match" sections between experimental groups. The slightest changes in orientation of a section according to the mean axes can have large effects on resulting cell counts. More fundamentally, because animals are three-dimensional creatures, expression of cell counts as number per area is biologically almost meaningless and extremely difficult to visualize for the reader.

The Problem of Giving Quantities as Densities

Most frequently, cell counts are incorrectly expressed as cells per volume. This is not an optimal way to present quantitative data either, and not just because it usually would be rather easy to obtain absolute cell counts with the same tissue and equipment. When the measurement cells per volume is mentioned, this volume is generally based on the volume of the samples in which the cells were counted. It therefore depends entirely on the relation between the sample volume and the volume of the complete structure of interest (reference volume) to determine whether this cell density is relevant and valid. The same cell density can refer to smaller or greater absolute numbers, depending on the size of the reference volume. If the size of the reference volume is not known, the reader cannot evaluate what a cell density tells about the entire structure. In the hippocampus of adult mice, for example, cell densities differ dramatically across even a structure as homogenous as the dentate gyrus. This problem is called the "reference trap" (Braendgaard and Gundersen, 1986): it can completely destroy the sense to be made out of quantitative statements in morphological studies. One of the key rules of stereology, the method for circumventing these problems, is "never, ever do not measure the reference volume" (H.J. Gundersen). A particularly interesting albeit controversial example is the neuroanatomical characterization of the p75 receptor null-mutant mouse. Depending on how the quantification was achieved, essentially opposite results were obtained by different groups (Van der Zee et al., 1996; Peterson et al., 1997).

Stereology as a Means of Obtaining Absolute Numbers

The only feasible way to give relatively valid quantitative data such as cell counts is to obtain absolute numbers, which are independent of the shape and size of the sample and relate to a meaningful anatomically defined structure. "Cells per dentate gyrus" tells us more about adult hippocampal neurogenesis than "cells per mm^3." The art of obtaining such data is called "stereology" (Haug, 1986) and is falsely accused of being complicated and time consuming. Because of its sometimes mysterious rules that at first sight can only be followed by the initiated, the entire construct has sometimes been mocked as "the holy church of stereology," a world that is rather detached from the realities of everyday science. The contrary is true. If a stereological analysis is carefully designed and carried out, it will actually save time. As much as one does not have to know how a four-stroke engine works in order to drive a car, one does not have to understand the mathematics underlying stereology in order to use the method effectively. The actual principle is fairly simple. Because research on adult neurogenesis in vivo is often heavily dependent on proper quantification, we will provide a more detailed discussion on stereology. The following few paragraphs cannot provide more than a coarse introduction explaining some key principles. For the exact protocols, original literature needs to be consulted.

Stereology is often called an "unbiased" counting technique. The term is thus used to describe improved, design-based tissue sampling that is assumption-free in terms of size, shape, or distribution of the cell within the tissue, and free from methodological biases that could result from incorrect assumptions. However, no scientific method is free of assumptions and thus bias is possible.

The pitfalls of estimating cell counts from samples can be visualized with the following example (Figs. 7–4 and 7–5). Imagine a cylindrical hippocampus of 100 μm length, for the sake of simplicity, with only one neuron every 10 μm (Fig. 7–4A). Stereology would be a way to estimate the total number of neurons in the cylinder from counting the cells in a sample slice of this cylinder.

One 10-μm slice is taken from the middle of the hippocampus; in the example it contains one neuron (Fig. 7–4B). As stated previously, depending on the angle of the cut, a 10-μm slice can comprise different volumes and if looked at from the cutting surface, cover different areas. All of these different volumes or areas still would contain one neuron. If expressed as neuron per volume (or even worse, per area), the resulting densities will differ, although the true total hippocampal volume and the true total number of neurons within it remain the same. To extrapolate from the slice to the hippocampus would yield greatly varying results.

On the other hand, if one knew which part of the hippocampus the sample slice came from, one could easily calculate the total number of neurons. If the slice were exactly one-tenth of the hippocampus, and the assumption could be reasonably made that the neurons are as evenly distributed as they are in the example, one could calculate the total number of neurons by dividing the number of neurons in the sample slice by the ratio of the volume, 1/10 (Fig. 7–4C, D). If the percentage of the volume occupied by the sample is known, the number of neurons in the entire brain can be calculated. In stereology, this principle is called the "fractionator."

In neurobiology, the reference objects are complex spatial anatomical structures, such as the dentate gyrus or the olfactory bulb. Although they can be defined anatomically, neither their boundaries nor their three-

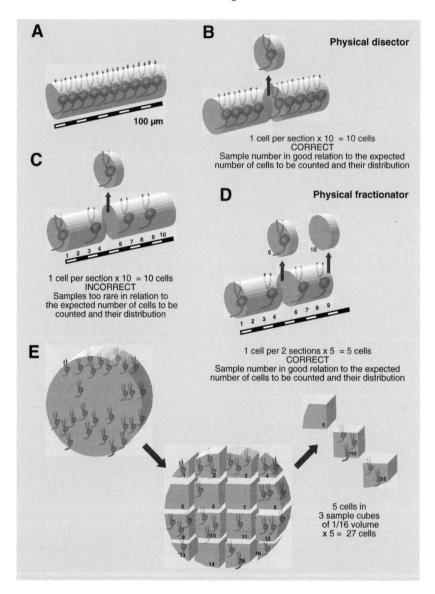

Figure 7–4. Stereology 1. See text for explanation.

dimensional extension are easily intelligible. This might be the reason why expressing cell counts as densities is so popular: a cube is a well-defined structure and easy to imagine. But biologically this cube needs to be related to the much more complicated three-dimensional representation of the anatomical structure of interest to convey the intended information. Densities are only a means of obtaining this absolute number, not an end in itself.

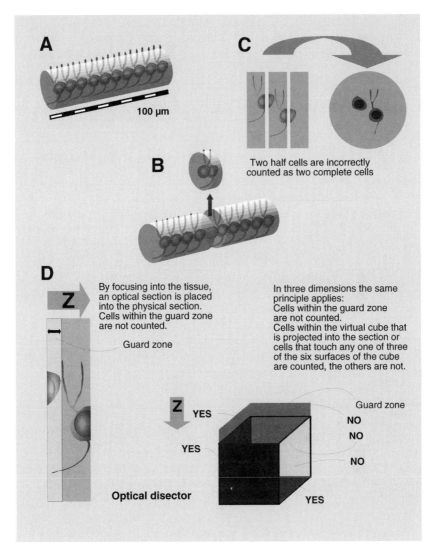

A

100 μm

C

Two half cells are incorrectly counted as two complete cells

B

D

Z

By focusing into the tissue, an optical section is placed into the physical section. Cells within the guard zone are not counted.

Guard zone

In three dimensions the same principle applies:
Cells within the guard zone are not counted.
Cells within the virtual cube that is projected into the section or cells that touch any one of three of the six surfaces of the cube are counted, the others are not.

Z YES

YES

Optical disector

YES

Guard zone

NO

NO

NO

YES

Figure 7–5. Stereology 2. See text for explanation.

With evenly distributed objects to count and knowledge of both the volume of the sample and of the total structure in which the objects are found, a very good estimate can be made with just one single sample. In reality this will never occur. The less evenly the objects are distributed, the more samples that need to be considered to lower the variance of the counted objects within each sample and to approximate the true mean.

For practical purposes, one should take series of slices (sections) and detect the number of neurons in every fifth or tenth section (or any other useful regular interval). The estimate of total counts based on counts made in this series of physical sections is called the "physical fractionator." The more irregular the shape of the entire structure, the more sections will be needed to produce a good estimate of the total volume. For this estimate the areas of the sections are measured and added. The result is then multiplied by the distance between the sections. This method thus transforms every object of complex three-dimensional structure into the equivalent approximation of a cube or cylinder of the same volume: ground area times height yields volume.

In the example of the cylindrical hippocampus, the entire slice is examined for the presence of neurons. If the neurons were very small in relation to the slice to be examined, this would not be practical. One could, however, cut the slice into many cubes of identical size and reapply the fractionator principle (Fig. 7–4E). For example, only every fifth or tenth tissue cube (or any other useful regular interval) would be examined. If the number of cubes per slice is known as well as the number of slices per hippocampus, the total number of neurons in the entire anatomical structure could be estimated. Again, the less evenly the objects to be counted are distributed in the slice, the more samples that need to be taken.

If we return to the simple version of one slice through the cylindrical brain with one neuron per every 10 μm, we can visualize another pitfall. (Fig. 7–5A). Imagine that the two cuts made for removing the slice are accidentally made in such a way that not one neuron is caught but two are cut in half. Each of these incomplete neurons could easily be miscounted as complete, yielding an estimate of two instead of one neuron per sample slice (Fig. 7–5B). The total number of neurons per brain would be overestimated by 100%. The obvious solution is to count only one-half of the incomplete cells. When looking from one side onto the slice the most superficial cells are disregarded. In histology this is accomplished by focusing into the section and disregarding the objects to be counted in the uppermost focal plane (Fig. 7–5D). This focusing into the section effectively transforms the as-if two-dimensional section (x- and y-axes) into a three-dimensional sample volume (x, y, and z), only part of which is used for counting. This method is called the *optical disector* (with only one *s*, as the term refers to two, hence *di*, sectors). The neglected uppermost part is called the "guard volume." If we have counts of the sample volume analyzed by the optical disector, as well as the total volume of the structure being examined, the total number of neurons in the hippocampus can be estimated. Combining the optical disector principle with the fractionator principle gives the *optical fractionator*. If the volume of the sample volume placed into the physical section with the optical disector method represents a known fraction of the total structure volume, the total number of counts can be estimated by multiplying the counts per sample volume with the reverse of the fraction that the sample volume represents. Again, the less evenly the objects to be counted are distributed, the more sample volumes are needed (although this issue is controversial in the field of stereology). These sample volumes are spaced evenly throughout the entire volume—first by using series of physical sections, then by dissecting the section into (virtual) cubes.

Disregarding the uppermost focal plane solves only part (to be precise, one-third) of the problem. If objects are counted in a virtual cube placed into the physical section, the same effect of cutting objects in two can occur on any two opposing surfaces of the cube, not just the uppermost and lowermost surfaces. Accordingly, only objects that are found within the cube or touch any one out of three of the six surfaces of the cube may be counted. Objects that touch the other surfaces have to be disregarded.

To be exact, the bottom of the disector should have a guard zone as well to ensure that a questionable profile observed in the bottom focal plane that could be counted can be brought into focus to validate that it really was the top of a cell. This strategy actually becomes rather important when using confocal stereology because the high resolution of the confocal microscope may make the investigator see signal in the bottom counting frame but not be sure that it is a real cell without focusing through further (Peterson, 1999).

Currently, stereology is normally done with a semiautomated system consisting of a motorized-stage microscope controlled by a computer. A video image is transferred to the monitor and counting frames can be superimposed so that the actual counting can be done on the screen. The software keeps track of the section series and enables measurement of area and volume. The program allows projection of a grid onto the sections, and when focusing through the section depicts the forbidden surfaces of the virtual counting cube as red, and those at which objects should be counted as green. A simplified version that can be done without computerized setup is based on determining cell densities at many randomly determined spots (with a randomly placed grid, for example) and relating them to the total volume of the olfactory bulb, which can be measured efficiently with a technique called the "Cavalieri estimator."

In the case of heterogeneous distributions, it is important to assess the amount of variance. There are a number of statistical estimators that can be employed to provide a critical evaluation of the amount of variance within the sample. Unfortunately, there is no absolute rule about how much variance is acceptable. A good rule of thumb is to look at the raw numbers produced by sampling at each optical disector and see how consistent the number of counted cells are at each site. For example, if the number of cells consistently ranges between zero and five at all counting sites, then the distribution is relatively homogeneous and the variance is likely acceptably low. However, if the sites produce mostly no cells counted and there are a couple of sites where 20–30 cells are counted, then the cells are heterogeneous in their distribution and the variance may be unacceptably high. In this case, many more sites should be sampled to reduce the sampling variance.

Stereology solves some but not all problems related to estimating cell counts. Although stereology is much less laborious than often assumed, it is complicated to apply to some specific questions and can lead to technical overkill. If small differences (10% to 20%) are detected and proven, however, stereology is the only feasible way to go. If differences are huge, they are unlikely to be greatly distorted by volume effects, as long as the anatomical structures of interest do not show gross differences. However, the general rule is never to not consider the reference volume.

For counting BrdU-labeled cells in the SGZ, one can use a full series of sections covering the entire dentate gyrus in its rostrocaudal extension and exhaustively count all labeled cells in the SGZ except those in the uppermost focal plane. The resulting number is multiplied by the number of sections in each interval (i.e., 6, if every sixth section is analyzed). This is not real stereology but is an often feasible compromise that still obeys some key stereological principles and avoids the reference trap.

REFERENCES

Altman J, Das GD (1965) Autoradiographic and histologic evidence of postnatal neurogenesis in rats. J Comp Neurol 124:319–335.

Ambrogini P, Lattanzi D, Ciuffoli S, Agostini D, Bertini L, Stocchi V, Santi S, Cuppini R (2004) Morpho-functional characterization of neuronal cells at different stages of maturation in granule cell layer of adult rat dentate gyrus. Brain Res 1017:21–31.

Arvidsson A, Collin T, Kirik D, Kokaia Z, Lindvall O (2002) Neuronal replacement from endogenous precursors in the adult brain after stroke. Nat Med 8:963–970.

Bai J, Ramos RL, Ackman JB, Thomas AM, Lee RV, LoTurco JJ (2003) RNAi reveals doublecortin is required for radial migration in rat neocortex. Nat Neurosci 6:1277–1283.

Barral-Moran MJ, Calaora V, Vutskits L, Wang C, Zhang H, Durbec P, Rougon G, Kiss JZ (2003) Oligodendrocyte progenitor migration in response to injury of glial monolayers requires the polysialic neural cell-adhesion molecule. J Neurosci Res 72:679–690.

Braendgaard H, Gundersen HJ (1986) The impact of recent stereological advances on quantitative studies of the nervous system. J Neurosci Methods 18:39–78.

Brandt MD, Jessberger S, Steiner B, Kronenberg G, Reuter K, Bick-Sander A, Von der Behrens W, Kempermann G (2003) Transient calretinin-expression defines early postmitotic step of neuronal differentiation in adult hippocampal neurogenesis of mice. Mol Cell Neurosci 24:603–613.

Brown JP, Couillard-Despres S, Cooper-Kuhn CM, Winkler J, Aigner L, Kuhn HG (2003) Transient expression of doublecortin during adult neurogenesis. J Comp Neurol 467:1–10.

Bruses JL, Rutishauser U (2001) Roles, regulation, and mechanism of polysialic acid function during neural development. Biochimie 83:635–643.

Cameron HA, McKay RD (2001) Adult neurogenesis produces a large pool of new granule cells in the dentate gyrus. J Comp Neurol 435:406–417.

Cameron HA, Woolley CS, McEwen BS, Gould E (1993) Differentiation of newly born neurons and glia in the dentate gyrus of the adult rat. Neuroscience 56:337–344.

Carlen M, Cassidy RM, Brismar H, Smith GA, Enquist LW, Frisen J (2002) Functional integration of adult-born neurons. Curr Biol 12:606–608.

Cooper-Kuhn CM, Kuhn HG (2002) Is it all DNA repair? Methodological considerations for detecting neurogenesis in the adult brain. Brain Res Dev Brain Res 134:13–21.

Copani A, Uberti D, Sortino MA, Bruno V, Nicoletti F, Memo M (2001) Activation of cell cycle–associated proteins in neuronal death: a mandatory or dispensable path? Trends Neurosci 24:25–31.

Corbo JC, Deuel TA, Long JM, LaPorte P, Tsai E, Wynshaw-Boris A, Walsh CA (2002) Doublecortin is required in mice for lamination of the hippocampus but not the neocortex. J Neurosci 22:7548–7557.

Corotto FS, Henegar JA, Maruniak JA (1993) Neurogenesis persists in the subependymal layer of the adult mouse brain. Neurosci Lett 149:111–114.

Dolbeare F (1995) Bromodeoxyuridine: a diagnostic tool in biology and medicine, Part I: historical perspectives, histochemical methods and cell kinetics. Histochem J 27:339–369.

Dunn DB, Smith JD, Zamenhof S, Griboff G (1954) Incorporation of halogenated pyrimidines into the deoxyribonucleic acids of *Bacterium coli* and its bacteriophages. Nature 174:305–307.

Eckhardt M, Bukalo O, Chazal G, Wang L, Goridis C, Schachner M, Gerardy-Schahn R, Cremer H, Dityatev A (2000) Mice deficient in the polysialyltransferase ST8SiaIV/PST-1 allow discrimination of the roles of neural cell adhesion molecule protein and polysialic acid in neural development and synaptic plasticity. J Neurosci 20:5234–5244.

Endl E, Gerdes J (2000) The Ki-67 protein: fascinating forms and an unknown function. Exp Cell Res 257:231–237.

Eriksson PS, Perfilieva E, Björk-Eriksson T, Alborn AM, Nordborg C, Peterson DA, Gage FH (1998) Neurogenesis in the adult human hippocampus. Nat Med 4:1313–1317.

Friedkin M, Wood HI (1956) Utilization of thymidine-C14 by bone marrow cells and isolated thymus nuclei. J Biol Chem 220:639–651.

Friocourt G, Koulakoff A, Chafey P, Boucher D, Fauchereau F, Chelly J, Francis F (2003) Doublecortin functions at the extremities of growing neuronal processes. Cereb Cortex 13:620–626.

Gleeson JG, Allen KM, Fox JW, Lamperti ED, Berkovic S, Scheffer I, Cooper EC, Dobyns WB, Minnerath SR, Ross ME, Walsh CA (1998) Doublecortin, a brain-specific gene mutated in human X-linked lissencephaly and double cortex syndrome, encodes a putative signaling protein. Cell 92:63–72.

Gleeson JG, Lin PT, Flanagan LA, Walsh CA (1999) Doublecortin is a microtubule-associated protein and is expressed widely by migrating neurons. Neuron 23:257–271.

Gonchoroff NJ, Katzmann JA, Currie RM, Evans EL, Houck DW, Kline BC, Greipp PR, Loken MR (1986) S-phase detection with an antibody to bromodeoxyuridine. Role of DNase pretreatment. J Immunol Methods 93:97–101.

Gratzner HG (1982) Monoclonal antibody to 5-bromo- and 5-iododeoxyuridine: a new reagent for detection of DNA replication. Science 218:474–475.

Gu W, Brannstrom T, Wester P (2000) Cortical neurogenesis in adult rats after reversible photothrombotic stroke. J Cereb Blood Flow Metab 20:1166–1173.

Hall PA, Levison DA, Woods AL, Yu CC, Kellock DB, Watkins JA, Barnes DM, Gillett CE, Camplejohn R, Dover R, et al. (1990) Proliferating cell nuclear antigen (PCNA) immunolocalization in paraffin sections: an index of cell proliferation with evidence of deregulated expression in some neoplasms. J Pathol 162:285–294.

Haug H (1986) History of neuromorphometry. J Neurosci Methods 18:1–17.

Hayes NL, Nowakowski RS (2002) Dynamics of cell proliferation in the adult dentate gyrus of two inbred strains of mice. Brain Res Dev Brain Res 134:77–85.

Ignatova TN, Kukekov VG, Laywell ED, Suslov ON, Vrionis FD, Steindler DA (2002) Human cortical glial tumors contain neural stem–like cells expressing astroglial and neuronal markers in vitro. Glia 39:193–206.

Katchanov J, Harms C, Gertz K, Hauck L, Waeber C, Hirt L, Priller J, von Harsdorf R, Bruck W, Hortnagl H, Dirnagl U, Bhide PG, Endres M (2001) Mild cerebral ischemia induces loss of cyclin-dependent kinase inhibitors and activation of cell cycle machinery before delayed neuronal cell death. J Neurosci 21:5045–5053.

Kee N, Sivalingam S, Boonstra R, Wojtowicz JM (2002) The utility of Ki-67 and BrdU as proliferative markers of adult neurogenesis. J Neurosci Methods 115:97–105.

Kiss JZ, Troncoso E, Djebbara Z, Vutskits L, Muller D (2001) The role of neural cell adhesion molecules in plasticity and repair. Brain Res Brain Res Rev 36:175–184.

Kiss JZ, Wang C, Rougon G (1993) Nerve-dependent expression of high polysialic acid neural cell adhesion molecule in neurohypophysial astrocytes of adult rats. Neuroscience 53:213–221.

Kronenberg G, Reuter K, Steiner B, Brandt MD, Jessberger S, Yamaguchi M, Kempermann G (2003) Subpopulations of proliferating cells of the adult hippocampus respond differently to physiologic neurogenic stimuli. J Comp Neurol 467:455–463.

Kuan CY, Schloemer AJ, Lu A, Burns KA, Weng WL, Williams MT, Strauss KI, Vorhees CV, Flavell RA, Davis RJ, Sharp FR, Rakic P (2004) Hypoxia-ischemia induces DNA synthesis without cell proliferation in dying neurons in adult rodent brain. J Neurosci 24:10763–10772.

Kuhn HG, Dickinson-Anson H, Gage FH (1996) Neurogenesis in the dentate gyrus of the adult rat: age-related decrease of neuronal progenitor proliferation. J Neurosci 16:2027–2033.

Kuhn HG, Winkler J, Kempermann G, Thal LJ, Gage FH (1997) Epidermal growth factor and fibroblast growth factor-2 have different effects on neural progenitors in the adult rat brain. J Neurosci 17:5820–5829.

Landmesser L, Dahm L, Tang JC, Rutishauser U (1990) Polysialic acid as a regulator of intramuscular nerve branching during embryonic development. Neuron 4:655–667.

LoTurco J (2004) Doublecortin and a tale of two serines. Neuron 41:175–177.

Magavi S, Leavitt B, Macklis J (2000) Induction of neurogenesis in the neocortex of adult mice. Nature 405:951–955.

McKeever PE, Ross DA, Strawderman MS, Brunberg JA, Greenberg HS, Junck L (1997) A comparison of the predictive power for survival in gliomas provided by MIB-1, bromodeoxyuridine and proliferating cell nuclear antigen with histopathologic and clinical parameters. J Neuropathol Exp Neurol 56:798–805.

Messier B, Leblond CP, Smart I (1958) Presence of DNA synthesis and mitosis in the brain of young adult mice. Exp Cell Res 14:224–226.

Meyer G, Perez-Garcia CG, Gleeson JG (2002) Selective expression of doublecortin and LIS1 in developing human cortex suggests unique modes of neuronal movement. Cereb Cortex 12:1225–1236.

Minturn JE, Geschwind DH, Fryer HJ, Hockfield S (1995) Early postmitotic neurons transiently express TOAD-64, a neural specific protein. J Comp Neurol 355:369–379.

Mizumatsu S, Monje ML, Morhardt DR, Rola R, Palmer TD, Fike JR (2003) Extreme sensitivity of adult neurogenesis to low doses of X-irradiation. Cancer Res 63:4021–4027.

Moores CA, Perderiset M, Francis F, Chelly J, Houdusse A, Milligan RA (2004) Mechanism of microtubule stabilization by doublecortin. Mol Cell 14:833–839.

Mullen RJ, Buck CR, Smith AM (1992) NeuN, a neuronal specific nuclear protein in vertebrates. Development 116:201–211.

Muller D, Djebbara-Hannas Z, Jourdain P, Vutskits L, Durbec P, Rougon G, Kiss JZ (2000) Brain-derived neurotrophic factor restores long-term potentiation in polysialic acid–neural cell adhesion molecule-deficient hippocampus. Proc Natl Acad Sci USA 97:4315–4320.

Muller D, Wang C, Skibo G, Toni N, Cremer H, Calaora V, Rougon G, Kiss JZ (1996) PSA-NCAM is required for activity-induced synaptic plasticity. Neuron 17:413–422.

Nacher J, Crespo C, McEwen BS (2001) Doublecortin expression in the adult rat telencephalon. Eur J Neurosci 14:629–644.

Nakatomi H, Kuriu T, Okabe S, Yamamoto S, Hatano O, Kawahara N, Tamura A, Kirino T, Nakafuku M (2002) Regeneration of hippocampal pyramidal neurons after ischemic brain injury by recruitment of endogenous neural progenitors. Cell 110:429–441.

Neve RL, McPhie DL, Chen Y (2000) Alzheimer's disease: a dysfunction of the amyloid precursor protein(1). Brain Res 886:54–66.

Nowakowski RS, Lewin SB, Miller MW (1989) Bromodeoxyuridine immunohistochemical determination of the lengths of the cell cycle and the DNA-synthetic phase for an anatomically defined population. J Neurocytol 18:311–318.

Palmer TD, Willhoite AR, Gage FH (2000) Vascular niche for adult hippocampal neurogenesis. J Comp Neurol 425:479–494.

Peterson DA (1999) Quantitative histology using confocal microscopy: implementation of unbiased stereology procedures. Methods 18:493–507.

Peterson DA (2004) The use of fluorescent probes in cell-counting procedures. In: Quantitative Methods in Neuroscience—A Neuroanatomical Approach (Evans ME, Janson AM, Nyengaard JR, eds), pp 85–115. Oxford: Oxford University Press.

Peterson DA, Leppert JT, Lee KF, Gage FH (1997) Basal forebrain neuronal loss in mice lacking neurotrophin receptor p75. Science 277:837–839.

Quinn CC, Gray GE, Hockfield S (1999) A family of proteins implicated in axon guidance and outgrowth. J Neurobiol 41:158–164.

Rakic P (2002) Adult neurogenesis in mammals: an identity crisis. J Neurosci 22:614–618.

Ricard D, Rogemond V, Charrier E, Aguera M, Bagnard D, Belin MF, Thomasset N, Honnorat J (2001) Isolation and expression pattern of human Unc-33-like phosphoprotein 6/collapsin response mediator protein 5 (Ulip6/CRMP5): coexistence with Ulip2/CRMP2 in Sema3a-sensitive oligodendrocytes. J Neurosci 21:7203–7214.

Rutishauser U, Landmesser L (1991) Polysialic acid on the surface of axons regulates patterns of normal and activity-dependent innervation. Trends Neurosci 14:528–532.

Sadoul R, Hirn M, Deagostini-Bazin H, Rougon G, Goridis C (1983) Adult and embryonic mouse neural cell adhesion molecules have different binding properties. Nature 304:347–349.

Sano K, Hoshino T, Nagai M (1968) Radiosensitization of brain tumor cells with a thymidine analogue (bromouridine). J Neurosurg 28:530–538.

Sano K, Sato F, Hoshino T, Nagai M (1965) Experimental and clinical studies of radiosensitizers in brain tumors, with special reference to BUdR-antimetabolite continuous regional infusion-radiation therapy (BAR therapy). Neurol Med Chir (Tokyo) 7:51–72.

Sarnat HB, Nochlin D, Born DE (1998) Neuronal nuclear antigen (NeuN): a marker of neuronal maturation in early human fetal nervous system. Brain Dev 20:88–94.

Schaar BT, Kinoshita K, McConnell SK (2004) Doublecortin microtubule affinity is regulated by a balance of kinase and phosphatase activity at the leading edge of migrating neurons. Neuron 41:203–213.

Schmechel DE (1985) Gamma-subunit of the glycolytic enzyme enolase: nonspecific or neuron specific? Lab Invest 52:239–242.

Schmidt-Hieber C, Jonas P, Bischofberger J (2004) Enhanced synaptic plasticity in newly generated granule cells of the adult hippocampus. Nature 429:184–187.

Scholzen T, Gerdes J (2000) The Ki-67 protein: from the known and the unknown. J Cell Physiol 182:311–322.

Seki T (2002) Expression patterns of immature neuronal markers PSA-NCAM, CRMP-4 and NeuroD in the hippocampus of young adult and aged rodents. J Neurosci Res 70:327–334.

Seki T, Arai Y (1991) The persistent expression of a highly polysialylated NCAM in the dentate gyrus of the adult rat. Neurosci Res 12:503–513.

Seki T, Arai Y (1993a) Distribution and possible roles of the highly polysialylated neural cell adhesion molecule (NCAM-H) in the developing and adult central nervous system. Neurosci Res 17:265–290.

Seki T, Arai Y (1993b) Highly polysialylated neural cell adhesion molecule (NCAM-H) is expressed by newly generated granule cells in the dentate gyrus of the adult rat. J Neurosci 13:2351–2358.

Seki T, Rutishauser U (1998) Removal of polysialic acid–neural cell adhesion molecule induces aberrant mossy fiber innervation and ectopic synaptogenesis in the hippocampus. J Neurosci 18:3757–3766.

Starborg M, Gell K, Brundell E, Hoog C (1996) The murine Ki-67 cell proliferation antigen accumulates in the nucleolar and heterochromatic regions of interphase cells and at the periphery of the mitotic chromosomes in a process essential for cell cycle progression. J Cell Sci 109 (Pt 1):143–153.

Tanaka T, Serneo FF, Higgins C, Gambello MJ, Wynshaw-Boris A, Gleeson JG (2004) Lis1 and doublecortin function with dynein to mediate coupling of the nucleus to the centrosome in neuronal migration. J Cell Biol 165:709–721.

Tomasiewicz H, Ono K, Yee D, Thompson C, Goridis C, Rutishauser U, Magnuson T (1993) Genetic deletion of a neural cell adhesion molecule variant (N-CAM-180) produces distinct defects in the central nervous system. Neuron 11:1163–1174.

Uittenbogaard M, Chiaramello A (2002) Constitutive overexpression of the basic helix-loop-helix Nex1/MATH-2 transcription factor promotes neuronal differentiation of PC12 cells and neurite regeneration. J Neurosci Res 67:235–245.

Unal-Cevik I, Kilinc M, Gursoy-Ozdemir Y, Gurer G, Dalkara T (2004) Loss of NeuN immunoreactivity after cerebral ischemia does not indicate neuronal cell loss: a cautionary note. Brain Res 1015:169–174.

Van der Zee CE, Ross GM, Riopelle RJ, Hagg T (1996) Survival of cholinergic forebrain neurons in developing p75NGFR-deficient mice. Science 274:1729–1732.

van Praag H, Schinder AF, Christie BR, Toni N, Palmer TD, Gage FH (2002) Functional neurogenesis in the adult hippocampus. Nature 415:1030–1034.

Vinores SA, Herman MM, Hackett SF, Campochiaro PA (1993) A morphological and immunohistochemical study of human retinal pigment epithelial cells, retinal glia, and fibroblasts grown on Gelfoam matrix in an organ culture system. A comparison of structural and nonstructural proteins and their application to cell type identification. Graefes Arch Clin Exp Ophthalmol 231:279–288.

Vinores SA, Herman MM, Rubinstein LJ, Marangos PJ (1984) Electron microscopic localization of neuron-specific enolase in rat and mouse brain. J Histochem Cytochem 32:1295–1302.

Wang C, Pralong WF, Schulz MF, Rougon G, Aubry JM, Pagliusi S, Robert A, Kiss JZ (1996) Functional N-methyl-D-aspartate receptors in O-2A glial precursor cells: a critical role in regulating polysialic acid–neural cell adhesion molecule expression and cell migration. J Cell Biol 135:1565–1581.

Wolf HK, Buslei R, Schmidt-Kastner R, Schmidt-Kastner PK, Pietsch T, Wiestler OD, Bluhmke I (1996) NeuN: a useful neuronal marker for diagnostic histopathology. J Histochem Cytochem 44:1167–1171.

Zamenhof S, Gribiff G (1954) E. coli containing 5-bromouracil in its deoxyribonucleic acid. Nature 174:307–308.

8

Neurogenic and
Non-neurogenic Regions

The neurogenic regions of the adult brain are characterized by the presence of a germinative matrix with a significant production of new neurons throughout life. As far as we know, in the adult mammalian brain only the subventricular zone (SVZ)/olfactory bulb and hippocampus qualify as neurogenic regions according to this definition. Consequently, the remainder of the brain would be the non-neurogenic regions. There are, however, reports on neurogenesis outside the classical neurogenic regions. Although many of these reports have raised methodological doubts (the reason for this chapter following the one on methods), today the widely held opinion is that in non-neurogenic regions, neurogenesis can occur even if it does not do so under physiological conditions (Magavi et al., 2000). This statement seems to be a contradiction in terms, consequently, some researchers refute the distinction between neurogenic and non-neurogenic regions altogether.

NEUROGENIC PERMISSIVENESS

There is one litmus test for a neurogenic region: a neural precursor cell implanted in a neurogenic region should develop into a neuron and when grafted onto a non-neurogenic region it should become a glial cell or die. Thus the definition of "neurogenicity" is based on a general and physiological neurogenic permissiveness. It is not based on the presence or absence of neural precursor cells alone, and it is not influenced by the possibility that such a promotion could be induced under certain unusual conditions. The key question becomes, then, what makes a neurogenic region neurogenic? How is neurogenic permissiveness defined on a molecular and cellular level?

Taken together, *neurogenic zones*, or *neurogenic regions*, are defined by (1) the presence of neural precursor cells *plus* (2) the presence of a microenvironment, consisting of cell–cell contacts and diffusible factors, that promotes neuronal development from intrinsic precursor cells and whose neurogenic potential can be tested by the implantation of neural precursor cells into this region. Consequently, non-neurogenic regions may contain precursor cells but lack distinctive germinative cell clusters as well as the permissive microenvironment that under physiologic conditions would promote neurogenesis from local or implanted precursor cells.

GERMINAL NICHES IN THE ADULT BRAIN

At the core of this concept is the idea that precursor cells in the neurogenic zones are embedded into a microenvironment with which they form a functional unit, the so-called stem cell niche, or germinative niche (Fig. 8–1). These niches consist of the precursor cell proper, astrocytes, endothelial cells, microglia or macrophages, extracellular matrix, and close contact with the basal membrane. This particular structure does not seem to be found outside the classical neurogenic zones in the hippocampus and olfactory bulb. Therefore, the germinative niche, rather than the presence of precursor cells alone, might provide the basis for adult neurogenesis. Precursor cells with a neurogenic potential can be isolated from many, if not all, brain areas (Palmer et al., 1999; Kondo and Raff, 2000). Germinative niches serve two functions: the maintenance of the stem and progenitor cell activity, and the promotion of neuronal differentiation. In non-neurogenic regions, precursor cells appear to be maintained in a different, niche-independent manner and no neuronal development occurs.

Astrocytes play a central role in germinative niches. First, radial glia–like, astrocyte-like cells are the precursor cells of these regions. Second, certain populations of astrocytes seem to have a region-specific potential to establish neurogenic permissiveness (Song et al., 2002). Astrocytes from the dentate gyrus promote precursor cell activity in hippocampal precursor cells, whereas cortical astrocytes do not. The close interaction between the developing neurons and S100β-negative astrocytes, which are presumably identical to the precursor cells of this region, indicates a dual function of astrocytes in this context: they function as precursor cells and form part of the niche.

Hippocampal astrocytes are also able to elicit a neurogenic potential in precursor cells from the spinal cord, a non-neurogenic region. Here spinal cord astrocytes have no effect. The same pattern applies to astrocytic effects on precursor cells isolated from the substantia nigra (Lie et al., 2002). Astrocytes from the neurogenic region elicited a potential for neuronal development, whereas astrocytes from non-neurogenic regions did not. Wnt-3 signaling has been suggested as one of the key mediators of this glial effect on precursor cells.

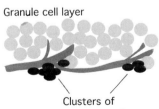

Granule cell layer

Clusters of proliferating cells associated with blood vessels

Figure 8–1. The vascular niche. Precursor cell activity in the subgranular zone occurs in close proximity to blood vessels. Vasculature is an integrative part of the germinative niche (Palmer et al., 2000). Clusters of BrdU-positive cells are found in close proximity to blood vessels.

The second cellular component of the germinative zones, other than pre-cursor cells and astrocytes, is blood vessels (Palmer et al., 2000; Fabel et al., 2003b). The definition of a vascular niche for neural stem cells raises the question of whether proximity to the blood vessels is required to allow neurogenesis. Endothelia or vascular smooth muscle cells might be impor-tant cell types involved in building the germinative niche. Precursor cell proliferation in the adult subgranular zone (SGZ) is paralleled by a prolif-eration of endothelial cells (Palmer et al., 2000). Induction of precursor cell proliferation can be accompanied by an induction of endothelial prolifera-tion (Hellsten et al., 2004). A link between angiogenesis and neurogenesis is further supported by the finding that vascular endothelial growth factor (VEGF) has strong effects on adult neurogenesis (Jin et al., 2002; Cao et al., 2004; Schanzer et al., 2004). Interestingly, however, the effect in vivo was survival promoting, whereas in vitro a pro-proliferative effect was seen (Schanzer et al., 2004). It seems that in vivo, doublecortin (DCX)-positive (type-2 and 3) progenitor cells of the SGZ express VEGF receptor 2, flk1.

The link between neurogenesis and angiogenesis might be even closer than just interdependency: in the presence of endothelial cells, neural pre-cursor cells were shown to transdifferentiate into endothelial cells (Wurmser et al., 2004). The possibility of reverse transdifferentiation, from endothelia to neurons, however, that has been hypothesized by some investigators, has not been found so far, although one report has suggested precursor cell properties in adventitia cells (Yamashima et al., 2004). Many questions re-main open in this context, but the evidence for a link between the local vasculature and neurogenesis in the dentate gyrus is strong.

Anatomical work by Mercier and colleagues (2002) suggests that in ad-dition to endothelia and astrocytes, microglia and macrophages are part of the germinative niche in both the SVZ and SGZ. Under pathological condi-tions, the activity of microglia and macrophages appears to dampen adult neurogenesis (Ekdahl et al., 2003; Monje et al., 2003). Whether these cells have a regulatory role under physiological conditions is not known.

Intimate contact of precursor cells and blood vessels with the basal lamina appears to be another characteristic of the germinative zones. Mercier and colleagues (2002) reported that the basal membrane surrounding the blood vessels could ensheathe the cell cluster that forms the germinative niche. Arturo Alvarez-Buylla has prosposed that the neurogenic niches in the adult brain are displaced neuroepithelium (Alvarez-Buylla and Lim, 2004). Dur-ing early embryonic brain development, neural precursor cells span the entire thickness of the future brain, coming into contact with both the ven-tricular lumen and the basal membrane at the pial surface. These radial glia–like stem cells produce neurons, very likely through expanding progenitor cell populations, and function as a guidance structure for migrating neu-rons that build up the layered cortex. Postnatally, the radial glia–like pre-cursor cells in the SGZ (type-1) are shortened, spanning only the distance between the SGZ and the inner molecular layer. In the SVZ they lose their radial glia–like appearance and become specialized astrocytes (B cells) that maintain contact with the ventricular surface and the basal membrane around the blood vessels. When the cortex thickens during development, the basal lamina around these blood vessels maintains contact between the astrocyte-like precursor cells in the SVZ and the pial surface. In the hippocampus this continuity is less obvious, because the germinative matrix of the SGZ is even further displaced from the original primary and secondary germinative zones in the ventricular wall. The basal membrane around blood vessels of the SGZ provides the basal contact for the radial elements, but in the inner molecular layer no counterpart is obvious. There, the cells branch and terminate between the fiber tracts.

Extracellular matrix (ECM) molecules are likely to play an important role in defining neurogenic conduciveness, but relatively little is known about the actual contributions. In precursor cell cultures, substrates such as laminin and fibronectin influence precursor cell survival and behavior, and integrins, which are receptors to laminin, influence the migration of neurosphere cells in vitro (Jacques et al., 1998). The adult neurogenic regions contain several ECM molecules such as tenascin-C, laminin, integrins, and different types of proteoglycans (Gates et al., 1995; Mercier et al., 2002). Heparan sulfate proteoglycans might bind to extracellular signaling molecules and thereby modify their action. When adult neurogenesis was stimulated by electroconvulsive seizures, gene expression profiling indicated a parallel increase in growth factors, angiogenic factors, and ECM constituents such as metalloproteinases (Newton et al., 2003). In the pancreas, for example, metalloproteinase-9 increased VEGF action and transformed normal tissue into angiogenic foci (Bergers et al., 2000). In bone marrow, metalloproteinase-9 increased the expression of soluble ligand to the kit-receptor and thereby promoted the recruitment of ckit-positive precursor cells from the stem cell niche (Heissig et al., 2002).

Taken together, our knowledge about the cellular composition and precise anatomy of neurogenic zones and about the contributions and relevance of identifiable components within them is still relatively scarce, although much progress has been made in this area.

TRANSPLANTATION STUDIES

The distinction between neurogenic and non-neurogenic region is based on a small number of fundamental transplantation studies. Implantation of cultured precursor cells from the adult hippocampus back into the hippocampus of adult rats demonstrated that the grafted cells incorporated adequately only into the granule cell layer and nowhere else (Gage et al., 1995). When the same hippocampal precursor cells were implanted in the rostral migratory stream (RMS), they generated olfactory interneurons (Suhonen et al., 1996). Implantation into the cerebellum did not result in neuronal differentiation, confirming that the implanted cells developed according to the local cues present in the neurogenic zones.

SVZ precursor cells implanted in the striatum, cortex, and olfactory bulb showed integration and neuronal differentiation only in the olfactory bulb but not in the other regions (Herrera et al., 1999). Another study, however, described neuronal differentiation in the striatum (Zhang et al., 2003). Also, neonatally isolated precursor cells differentiated into neurons when transplanted into the same region (Zigova et al., 1998).

Precursor cells from the non-neurogenic spinal cord and substantia nigra also developed into granule cell neurons when placed in the hippocampus (Shihabuddin et al., 2000; Lie et al., 2002). However, when spinal cord precursor cells were placed in the neocortex they failed to differentiate into neurons. Moreover, when substantia nigra precursor cells were grafted back into the substantia nigra they did not result in neurogenesis (Lie et al., 2002). In contrast to these findings, early postnatal cerebellar precursor cells implanted in the SVZ and RMS failed to differentiate into olfactory neurons and migrated only a brief distance into the RMS (Jankovski and Sotelo, 1996).

When hippocampal precursor cells were implanted in the retina, many stages of photoreceptor development were seen, including the highly characteristic morphology of photoreceptors. However, no terminal differentiation occurred (Takahashi et al., 1998). This finding indicates that neurogenic permissiveness might be graded and that the composition of neurogenic factors in different brain regions might vary. It is thus very likely that many factors have to act together to make a brain region fully neurogenic.

Taken together, these results argue that extrinsic factors are more important than cell-intrinsic parameters in neurogenesis but more transplantation studies would be necessary to fill the gaps. For example, neural precursor cells from the SVZ have not yet been implanted in the hippocampus.

NEURAL PRECURSOR CELLS IN NON-NEUROGENIC REGIONS

Neural precursor cells can be isolated from many brain regions, including by definition the neurogenic regions, but also from many other regions that apparently lack neurogenic permissiveness. It is not the presence of neural precursor cells alone that makes a neurogenic region neurogenic. Neural precursor cells may be found in very many brain areas, and lineage-determined progenitor cells for the glial lineage possibly in all. But the question of how cells with precursor cell properties and a neurogenic potential are distributed in the brain is extremely difficult to address. The only feasible available method to determine stemness is to isolate the cells and demonstrate self-renewal and multipotency in vitro. Nestin expression, for example, is not sufficient to identify precursor cells in vivo, nor is the detection of immunoreactivity for DCX or other markers. Even if these markers are sensitive, their specificity is not known. One must not extrapolate data from neurogenic regions to fit non-neurogenic regions. Precursor cell populations might be more heterogeneous in their properties than we are inclined to assume.

The first systematic study on this topic came from Theo D. Palmer, then with Fred H. Gage at the Salk Institute in La Jolla. Palmer found that fibroblast growth factor-2 (FGF-2) can elicit a neurogenic potential in cells isolated from the neocortex, septum, striatum, corpus callosum, and optic nerve (Palmer et al., 1999). He applied a culture method that had proven effective on hippocampal precursor cells (Palmer et al., 1997). The yield from the non-neurogenic regions was generally much lower (about three orders of magnitude) than that from neurogenic regions.

The most plausible location for persistent precursor cells in adulthood is along the ventricular system, and indeed it seems that cells with precursor cell properties can be derived from entire ventricular walls (not only from the lateral ventricles), including the central canal of the spinal cord (Shihabuddin et al., 1997; Martens et al., 2002).

Because of the important role in the dopaminergic system and thus its relevance for Parkinson disease, the adult substantia nigra has attracted particular interest from stem cell researchers. Whereas neural precursor cells could indeed be found in the substantia nigra (Lie et al., 2002), the question of whether physiologic adult neurogenesis occurs in the substantia nigra is still debated (Zhao et al., 2003); several studies have argued against it (Lie et al., 2002; Cooper and Isacson, 2004; Frielingsdorf et al., 2004).

The hypothalamus is another physiologically non-neurogenic region that contains neural precursor cells that can be isolated and propagated in vitro (Markakis et al., 2004). These precursor cells produce neuroendocrine phenotypes after initiation of differentiation. Surprisingly, they behaved almost indistinguishably from hippocampal cultures maintained in parallel. Instead of finding that hypothalamic precursor cells are special in that they are able to produce neuroendocrine phenotypes, it turns out that hippocampal precursor cells can do the same. Consequently, precursor cells in the adult brain, no matter which region they are from, share a wide spectrum of developmental potential. Obviously, this is not identical to the realization of this potential as it occurs under physiological conditions. In addition, only the initial stages of neuronal differentiation could be reproduced in vitro; beyond this stage the cells displayed signs of multiple phenotypes in parallel.

The most counterintuitive source of neural precursor cells in the adult brain might be the white-matter tracts, such as the corpus callosum and optic nerve (Palmer et al., 1999). Both contain neural precursor cells that can be propagated and clonally analyzed in vitro. Historically, the so-called O2A progenitor cell was first found in the rat optic nerve. The O2A cell is a glial precursor cell whose discovery by Raff, Miller, and Noble in 1983 initiated the research field of glial stem cell biology. O2A progenitor cells express the proteoglycan NG2, whose expression appears to be a common characteristic of precursor cells outside the neurogenic zones. However, it is not clear whether all of these parenchymal precursor cells express NG2 and whether all NG2 cells have precursor cell properties. It has also not been determined how the neural precursor cells that can be isolated from the white-matter tracts relate to the NG2 cells in the same region. But if one dares a quantitative evaluation (such as in the sphere-forming capacity), the neurogenic potential of cells from the fiber tracts is particularly high. In vivo, the corpus callosum and, even more, the region immediately below it, are rich with both nestin- and DCX-positive cells. It is not clear, however, whether these are indeed the cells that exert the neurogenic potential in vitro.

In the adult spinal cord, neural precursor cells have been found not only around the central canal (Martens et al., 2002) but also within the parenchyma, most notably the substantia gelatinosa, the dorsal tip of the dorsal horns (Horner et al., 2000). These appear to relate to the NG2-positive cells in this region (Horner et al., 2002) and give rise primarily to oligodendrocytes. Although regional differences exist, precursor cells from the spinal cord behaved very similarly to forebrain precursor cells in vitro and after implantation into the neurogenic zone. They were multipotent in vitro and generated astrocytes and neurons after transplantation (Shihabuddin et al., 2000). Although specific analysis is still lacking, it seems that the brain and spinal cord contain at least two types of precursor cells. This conjecture is reminiscent of very old concepts, depicted in the Penfield schema in Figure 2–1, which distinguishes between the neuroblasts and parenchymal "spongioblasts" as proposed by Wilhelm His and Alfred Schaper. Taken together, there is evidence of considerable precursor cell heterogeneity within and between different brain regions, despite the fact that some markers reliably identify precursor cells.

For both neurogenic regions, astrocyte-like cells function as precursor cells. Glial fibrillary acidic protein (GFAP) expression can be used as key criterion to isolate precursor cells from neurogenic regions (Laywell et al., 2000). Ablation of GFAP-positive cells efficiently eliminated stem cells from the SVZ but not from the non-neurogenic retina (Morshead et al., 2003), although another type of neural precursor cell with neurogenic potential could still be isolated from the retina (see below). GFAP-positive cells are not the only type of cell with neural precursor properties in neurogenic regions. They nonetheless might rank highest in the stem cell hierarchy of these regions (Alvarez-Buylla et al., 2001). This finding may not be used to extrapolate potential precursor-cell properties of astrocytes in non-neurogenic regions, however. Precursor cell astrocytes of neurogenic regions show coexpression of other precursor cell markers such as Sox2, brain lipid binding protein (BLBP), and nestin, but are negative for S100β, an astrocytic marker present in most astrocytes. Such distinguishing characteristics would have to be found in hypothetical astrocyte-like precursor cells as well. Not all astrocytes are stem cells.

What is the function of precursor cells in non-neurogenic regions? Adult neurogenesis resulting from precursor cell activity in the adult brain is only the tip of the iceberg of precursor cell–based cell genesis. The true wealth of precursor cell–based plasticity lies in gliogenesis. In the long run, adult neurogenesis will have to be seen increasingly in the context of cell genesis in the adult brain in general. The term *non-neurogenic* is thus somewhat unfortunate because it defines regions of presumably high cellular plasticity by the lack of potential, not by their positive characteristics.

Independent of the location and nature of neural precursor cells in different brain regions, a number of reports have contradicted the prevailing assumption that no new neurons can be generated outside the hippocampus and olfactory system in the absence of pathology. However, all of these claims have remained controversial, mainly for methodological reasons (see Chapter 7 and below). It has to be noted that in a peer-review situation, methodological concerns are more likely to be raised in cases of novel and unexpected claims, so these technical refutations need to be scrutinized as well. In addition, there is conflicting evidence. The most problematic conflict for the proponents of endogenous neurogenesis in non-neurogenic regions (an oxymoron that already reflects the dominant opinion) concerns the nature of neurogenic regions. Neurogenesis in non-neurogenic regions violates the concept of the precursor cell niche with its different factors contributing to neurogenic permissiveness. Consequently, in cases of putative neurogenesis in non-neurogenic regions, it becomes difficult to explain why precursor cells implanted in these regions fail to differentiate into neurons when the endogenous precursor cells supposedly did. In non-neurogenic regions there is a mismatch between precursor cells and the germinative niche. This conflict, however, is not a categorical argument, because neither our present knowledge about precursor cell heterogeneity nor the molecular bases of neurogenic permissiveness are sufficiently complete to rule out additional models of neurogenic permissiveness in the adult brain than realized in the neurogenic regions. A reasonable requirement for this extraordinary claim, however, is that the divergence from the predominant and otherwise well-supported concept be characterized in detail and with independent methods.

IDENTIFYING PRECURSOR CELLS IN NON-NEUROGENIC ZONES IN VIVO

Intermediate filament nestin is widely considered a simple and reliable precursor cell marker, and in fact it appears to recognize precursor cells in both the SVZ and SGZ (Palmer et al., 2000; Filippov et al., 2003). Endogenous nestin expression is relatively low in the neurogenic regions of adult mice and nestin immunohistochemistry shows a cross-reaction with blood vessels. The development of transgenic reporter gene mice, which express green fluorescent protein (GFP) under neurally specific elements of the nestin promoter, made the study of nestin-expressing cells feasible (Yamaguchi et al., 2000; Sawamoto et al., 2001). Nestin-GFP-positive cells can be found in essentially the entire brain. Nestin–GFP expression can also be used to prospectively isolate precursor cells from the adult mouse brain (Sawamoto et al., 2001). But although many precursor cells express nestin, the reverse does not appear to be necessarily true.

Even more surprising than the widespread nestin expression is the abundance of DCX-positive cells throughout the brain, sometimes overlapping with nestin expression. DCX is associated with the initiation of neuronal differentiation and migration during development and in the adult neurogenic zones. Its function in non-neurogenic regions is not clear. The presence of proliferative DCX-positive cells in non-neurogenic regions is often taken to indicate that very early stages of neurogenesis are possible in these regions. It is not clear, however, if this interpretation is justified and if DCX is truly specific to the neuronal lineage. In the neurogenic zones, this appears to be the case.

If taken at face value, however, the detection of DCX in non-neurogenic regions might suggest that neuronal development up to this immature stage is either autonomous or induced by the microenvironment of non-neurogenic regions. This interpretation is supported by the finding that in response to trauma, ischemia, or tumors, nestin- and DCX-positive cells can be found around the lesion site, but there is no (or only very limited) neurogenesis. The early stages of neuronal development might thus be possible even in non-neurogenic regions, but neuronal development is physiologically aborted in later stages. The question is whether non-neurogenic regions actively suppress neuronal development or just lack the factors necessary to promote it. There is evidence that the answer is a combination of both. Alternatively, it is possible that, analogous to cell classification in the neurogenic zones, identification of nestin-DCX-positive cells as neural precursor cells or even immature neurons might not be justified.

In addition, the presence or absence of precursor cells in many brain regions might underlie fluctuations. The concept of local precursor cells might in fact be misleading and these cells might be in constant exchange, migration, and turnover. There is little direct evidence for this idea, but the assumption of a static precursor cell distribution in the non-neurogenic regions of the adult brain might not be justified either.

A general problem is that many conclusions about the nature and identity of precursor cells have to be derived from ex vivo data. The multipotent adult precursor cells (MAPC) from adult bone marrow that were first described by Catherine Verfaillie can serve as an example of cell properties that appear only after prolonged exposure to specified cell culture conditions (Jiang et al., 2002). The detection of precursor cell properties thus depends on the conditions applied. Therefore, the identification of neurogenic potential in cells derived from a given brain region is to some degree relative to the methods used. The challenge lies in the fact that stem cell properties can hardly be directly assessed in vivo, but ex vivo methods influence or possibly even determine the properties that should be studied.

In both neurogenic regions of the adult brain, precursor cell activity has been linked to radial glia–like cells: B cells in the SVZ and type-1 cells in the SGZ. Although all precursor cells of the adult brain are supposedly derived from radial glia in the embryonic ventricular zone (Fishell and Kriegstein, 2003; Anthony et al., 2004), the immediate relationship between the putative precursor cells in non-neurogenic regions and radial glia is not clear at present.

NG2 AS PRECURSOR CELL MARKER

Given the expression of nestin–GFP (and with the discussed caveats about nestin as a precursor cell marker), many putative nestin-positive precursor cells in many non-neurogenic regions differ from those in neurogenic zones by their co-expression of chondroitin-sulfate proteoglycan NG2. This co-localization is absent in neurogenic zones.

Neuron-glia 2 (NG2) is a transmembrane protein containing extracellular laminin-like domains, which is suggestive of a function in cell adhesion, recognition, and migration. In vitro, a blocking antibody against NG2 inhibits migration of NG2-expressing cells (Niehaus et al., 1999). The mouse homologue was originally called AN2 (Schneider et al., 2001) but the name NG2 is now generally used for all species. Antibodies against NG2 label about 3% – 5% of glial cells in the adult rodent central nervous system (CNS). NG2 cells are distributed throughout gray- and white-matter areas. A small percentage of NG2 cells is proliferative, but the degree of proliferative activity is highly region-dependent.

A current working hypothesis holds that there are two types of NG2-positive cells in the developing and adult CNS (Mallon et al., 2002; Nishiyama et al., 2002). First, NG2 is thought to identify precursor cells in the oligodendrocytic lineage (Keirstead et al., 1998; Chari and Blakemore, 2002; Watanabe et al., 2002). Second, NG2-positive glia might be a highly specific type of astrocyte, closely related to synapses and nodes of Ranvier (Butt et al., 1999; Ong and Levine, 1999). Morphologically, there are also two types of NG2 cells. One type is bipolar and has a small nucleus, whereas the other has a ramified appearance. It is not clear how these anatomical phenotypes relate to the functional distinction. Consequently, neither the sensitivity nor the specificity of NG2 as a precursor cell marker are known. If the precursor-like cells and the astrocyte-like cells were in fact identical, the situation would resemble radial glia, which also has dual functions, one of them being a precursor cell. On the other hand, not all NG2-positive cells are nestin–GFP expressing, and other obvious differences exist as well. Consequently, NG2 remains an interesting but still problematic marker.

Ex vivo, NG2-expressing cells were initially described as giving rise to oligodendrocytes and one type of astrocyte (Stallcup and Beasley, 1987). They have thus been considered more or less identical to the classical O2A precursor cell as described by Raff, Miller, and Noble (1983). During development, NG2 cells characteristically express platelet-derived growth factor (PDGF) receptor alpha (Nishiyama et al., 1996, 1999). PDGF is secreted by neurons and astrocytes and maintains oligodendrocyte progenitor cells in a proliferative stage (Hart et al., 1989).

Despite the fact that NG2-positive cells are negative for oligodendrocyte marker CNP, the CNP promoter could be used to isolate multipotent cells (Belachew et al., 2003; Aguirre et al., 2004). The evidence that NG2 is expressed by some sort of precursor cell is therefore quite strong. It is not clear, however, whether all NG2 cells have precursor cell properties, and if so, to what degree. It is also not known whether NG2 protein itself plays a role in inducing or maintaining this state.

Interestingly, in vivo, even over longer time periods, most dividing NG2 cells seem to generate primarily other NG2 cells not differentiating oligodendroglia (Horner et al., 2000). Some NG2-expressing cells can also show immunoreactivity for DCX and PSA-NCAM as two markers associated with neuronal immaturity, but there is no indication that new neurons would arise from NG2-expressing cells in the adult brain in vivo. However, when precursor cells were isolated on the basis of activity of the CNPase promoter and implanted in the developing hippocampus, they gave rise to local interneurons (Aguirre et al., 2004).

In astrocytic differentiation, NG2 cells are consistently negative for GFAP, but they might express low levels of S100β. Reporter gene mice with the S100β promoter showed enhanced GFP expression in both astrocytes and NG2-positive cells of the hippocampus (Lin and Bergles, 2002). On the basis of electrophysiological examinations, two types of astrocytes can be distinguished: one with classical passive properties, the other called "complex," with a very high input resistance, lower resting conductance to potassium, and lower expression of glutamate transporters (Steinhauser et al., 1992, 1994). This pattern was originally described for O2A precursor cells in vitro (Steinhauser et al., 1992), later for one type of astrocyte (Akopian et al., 1997), NG2-expressing hippocampal cells (Bergles et al., 2000), and finally for type-2 precursor cells in the adult hippocampus (Filippov et al., 2003). This characteristic functional measure further supports the idea of some identity between these cells. They share an involvement in cellular or synaptic plasticity.

NG2 expression and the proliferation of NG2-expressing cells are upregulated after many different types of injury (Levine et al., 2001). NG2 cells are part of the glial scar. The response is not limited to mechanical damage. Demyelination induces a very focal response of NG2-positive cells, which initiate differentiation into new oligodendrocytes (Keirstead et al., 1998; Redwine and Armstrong, 1998). However, remyelination from these cells is not always successful, especially not in locations of chronic damage (Reynolds et al., 2002).

NG2 protein itself might have several functions. The cytoplasmic domain contains a PDZ-binding site that can bind to glutamate receptor interacting protein (GRIP), which in turn interacts with AMPA receptors (Stegmuller et al., 2003). NG2 cells have AMPA receptors and sense neuronal glutamate release (Bergles et al., 2000). This might be one pathway through which NG2-expressing cells are involved in synaptic or other forms of plasticity. NG2 cells might therefore play a particular role in neuron–glia communication underlying forms of plasticity. This function could be very subtle because NG2 null-mutant mice do not have an obvious phenotype (Grako et al., 1999).

NG2 increases cell migration in vitro (Fang et al., 1999), but in the adult brain, it does not appear to be expressed in migratory cells (Gensert and Goldman, 1996, 1997; Horner et al., 2002). NG2-expressing cells thus predominantly divide in loco.

NG2 inhibits axonal growth (Dou and Levine, 1994) by inducing a growth cone collapse (Ughrin et al., 2003). During development, NG2 is expressed in regions that should be avoided by growing axons—for example, the mesenchyma (Chen et al., 2002). If one interprets this finding from a precursor cell perspective, as the other face of NG2 cells, it seems that NG2 cells are geared toward maintaining an immature stage and act against a maturing plasticity. If NG2 cells are indeed only one type of cell, they might normally modulate and stabilize neuronal function at synapses or nodes of Ranvier and prevent axonal sprouting. They are usually in a relatively repressed state, presumably by contact inhibition or factors secreted from neighboring cells (Miller, 1999). In cases of pathology, NG2 cells become disinhibited and generate new oligodendrocytes that remyelinate damage but at the same time are part of the glial scar, further preventing axonal regeneration.

In sum, despite some intriguing relations to neuronal development and plasticity, at present NG2 cannot be viewed as an unambiguous marker of precursor cells with neurogenic potential in the adult brain. Although NG2 cells are involved in multiple types of plasticity, including cellular plasticity, the few available markers that allow this conclusion indicate that only immature stages of neuronal development are reached. These stages coincide with a complex electrophysiological phenotype whose exact meaning is not yet clear but which is again associated with states of synaptic or cellular plasticity. It is not known whether NG2 cells are involved in the proposed exceptional cases of neurogenesis in non-neurogenic regions, which we will discuss below.

NEUROGENESIS IN THE ADULT NEOCORTEX?

Non-neurogenic regions withhold cues necessary for neurogenic development of not only endogenous precursor cells but also implanted cells, which would turn into neurons when placed in the hippocampus or olfactory system. This definition of neurogenicity is thus independent of issues related to precursor cell heterogeneity. Unfortunately, only a few transplantation studies have been carried out and thus not all presumably non-neurogenic brain regions have been tested by this vigorous standard. Consequently, the debate about the stringency of the dichotomy of neurogenic versus non-neurogenic regions has repeatedly been questioned and considered biased.

This is particularly true for the cerebral cortex. Altman's initial descriptions of adult neurogenesis as well as several studies by Kaplan in the 1980s reported neurogenesis in the neocortex (Altman, 1963; Kaplan, 1981). Unlike their reports on neurogenesis in the hippocampus and olfactory system, these claims were not confirmed by others. However, in 1999, Elisabeth Gould and colleagues published a report claiming that large numbers of new neurons could be found in the neocortex of adult macaque monkeys (Gould et al., 1999). Presumably, these cells originated from the SVZ, branched away from the RMS, and migrated into prefrontal, parietal, and temporal areas. The study contained only a few examples and neither three-dimensional reconstructions nor retrograde labeling. There was also no description of neuronal development in the sense that different stages of neuronal maturation in new neurons could be demonstrated. The study received much attention but also raised substantial critique (Nowakowski and Hayes, 2000; Rakic, 2002).

In previous series of experiments involving a total of 127 macaque monkeys up to 17 years of age, Pasko Rakic and his coworkers at Harvard University and Yale University had not found any new neurons in the adult neocortex (see Rakic, 2002, and Chapter 7 for details).

What struck many investigators as problematic regarding the reports on cortical neurogenesis in adult primates was the fact that the many groups working in rodents had never found evidence of adult cortical neurogenesis in the cortex of rats or mice. Although the possibility could not be categorically denied that primates had the ability of adult cortical neurogenesis and rodents did not, this seemed very unlikely given the overall reduction in neurogenesis with increasing brain complexity during evolution. Somewhat in line with these thoughts, Gould and colleagues (2001) later reported that new neurons in the cortex of adult monkeys had only a transient existence and now showed examples of cortical neurogenesis in rodents.

An alternate interpretation is that the new cells never reached a stage of complete neuronal maturation. The detection of immature neurons in the cortex might be equivalent to other reports indicating that the earliest but not more mature stages of neuronal development might in fact be found in non-neurogenic regions of the adult brain. If this is true, the lack of neurogenic permissiveness in non-neurogenic regions would affect primarily the stages of neuronal maturation, not the (short-term) maintenance of neuronal progenitor cells. Many NG2-expressing cells show (an often weak) coexpression of DCX. DCX was not studied in the experiments by Gould and coworkers, but TUC4 was. TUC4 expression, however, is not sufficient evidence of neuronal maturation, because it can also be found in the putative oligodendrocyte precursor cells of the adult brain (Ricard et al., 2001). It thus seems possible that presumed signs of adult cortical neurogenesis actually reflect activity on the level of NG2 cells that did not lead to completed neurogenesis. It is questionable whether such aborted neuronal development should be termed *neurogenesis*. This interpretation of aborted neurogenesis is entirely based on marker analogies to neuronal development in the neurogenic zones. These analogies might not be justified because the specificity of the markers is not known. A more parsimonious interpretation is that in the adult brain, renewing cells can be found that show marker expression from both the glial and neuronal lineage, whose functional significance is not known at present.

Several studies have searched further for completed neurogenesis in the adult primate and rodent brain and found not evidence of it (Magavi et al., 2000; Kornack and Rakic, 2001; Ehninger and Kempermann, 2003; Koketsu et al., 2003). The methodological issues that have been brought forth against the reports claiming neurogenesis in the adult cortex are essentially those reviewed in Chapter 7: the pitfalls of BrdU immunohistochemistry, the lack of demonstration of development, and the problems of unambiguous neuronal markers.

THE SPECIAL CASE OF THE RETINA

In fish, amphibians, and birds, a ring of retinal precursor cells lies along the junction between the retina and iris. These precursor cells generate new retinal neurons throughout life, and adult retinal neurogenesis is stimulated after retinal cell loss (Hollyfield, 1968; Johns, 1977; Johns and Easter, 1977; Reh and Constantine-Paton, 1983; Marcus et al., 1999; Fischer and Reh, 2000, for a review see Hitchcock et al., 2004). In frogs, these precursor cells are multipotent and can generate all cell types in the retina (Wetts and Fraser, 1988).

In mammals, retinal neurogenesis ceases early postnatally (Young, 1985), and to date no reports on spontaneous adult neurogenesis in the retina have been published. However, the ciliary body, the structural equivalent to the germinative annulus in the amphibian eye, contains multipotent precursor cells (Ahmad et al., 2000; Tropepe et al., 2000) (Fig. 8–2). In the retina, outside the ciliary body a second population of precursor cells with neurogenic potential is found, and these cells share a number of markers with precursor cells from the SVZ. They express BLPB, nestin, Pax6, and flk1 (Yang and Cepko, 1996; Engelhardt et al., 2004). Müller cells, which are the radial glial elements of the eye, might also act as precursor cells in the adult mammalian retina (Fischer and Reh, 2001). Retinal precursor cells, like their ontogenetic predecessors in the wall of the developing optic vesicle, are bipotent and generate neurons and astrocytes, but no oligodendrocytes (Alexiades and Cepko, 1997; Ahmad et al., 1999; Engelhardt et al., 2004). The two types of precursor cells share many characteristics but differ in their potential of self-renewal (Ahmad et al., 2004).

After implantation of precursor cells from other brain regions, the retina seems to allow an astonishing degree of neuronal development, but no full

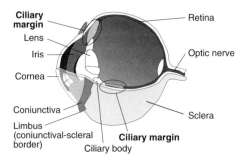

Figure 8–2. Anatomy of the eye. The adult mammalian eye appears to contain three different populations of precursor cells: one in the limbic margin and one in the retina itself. There is still controversy about the relationship between these cell types and their potential. In addition, there is a non-neural precursor cell population in the limbus that replaces corneal epithelium.

maturation (Takahashi et al., 1998; Young et al., 2000; Warfvinge et al., 2001; Akita et al., 2002; Chacko et al., 2003; Mellough et al., 2004). This support of multilineage integration sets the retina apart from the other non-neurogenic regions and makes the retinal precursor cell niche particularly interesting. A change in its classification as non-neurogenic is not yet justified however. Little is known about the role of retinal and ciliary body precursor cells for normal and diseased physiology of the eye, but as in other brain regions, many efforts are directed at finding ways to tap the regenerative potential of the precursor cells of the eye (Boulton and Albon, 2004).

To avoid any misunderstanding it should be mentioned that the eye contains yet another important population of precursor cells that are not part of the central nervous system: limbal stem cells continuously maintain the corneal epithelium (Fig. 8–2).

ADULT NEUROGENESIS IN OTHER BRAIN REGIONS

In the case of the substantia nigra the discrepancy between one study that claimed to have found new neurons in the adult mouse substantia nigra and others that did not is particularly confusing. Ming Zhao, Jonas Frisén, and coworkers from Karolinska Insitute in Stockholm used several methods to support their claim (Zhao et al., 2003). Newly generated cells were labeled with BrdU as usual, but their migration from the ventricular wall was also tracked by injecting dye DiI or fluorescence-labeled latex beads into the ventricle. Only cells having contact with the ventricular surface can pick up and store these markers. A cell labeled with the marker later found in the substantia nigra (or theoretically elsewhere) must have migrated in from a spot where it had contact with the ventricular lumen. The study also included retrograde labeling of the axonal projections of newly generated cells to the striatum. Besides physiological neurogenesis, an induction of neurogenesis in response to models of Parkinson disease was found. This finding was not replicated by others (Lie et al., 2002; Cooper and Isacson, 2004; Frielingsdorf et al., 2004), although neural precursor cells were found in the substantia nigra (Lie et al., 2002). Methodological differences might explain part of any discrepancy, but because the Zhao method did not rely on just one method, the situation remains difficult to understand.

Whereas one study reported new neurons in region CA1 of adult rat hippocampus (Rietze et al., 2000), others did not find evidence for adult neurogenesis in CA1 of mice (Kempermann et al., 1997; Nakatomi et al., 2002). However, neurogenesis in CA1 might be inducible by ischemia and growth factor infusion (Nakatomi et al., 2002).

The question of neurogenesis in the adult amygdala has not been conclusively answered either. Like for the neocortex, one report found evidence of new neurons in the adult amygdala in primates (Bernier et al., 2002), whereas others could not detect it in rodents. Species and technical differences could be partially responsible for this discrepancy without solving the problem. As in the cortex and substantia nigra, the pro-side has the burden of proof beyond reasonable doubt, whereas the contra-side has the fundamental problem of proving the complete absence of a trait.

REGENERATIVE AND TARGETED ADULT NEUROGENESIS

A few studies have demonstrated that the lack of neurogenic permissiveness in some brain regions can be overcome by a pathological stimulus. It is not clear whether pathology (and if so, which cellular aspects of it) disinhibits an endogenous program or actively induces neurogenesis. Neural precursor cells are not only present in many brain regions, they are also attracted to migrate to the damage site from the SVZ. In any case, two conditions have to be fulfilled to make regenerative neurogenesis possible: neural precursor cells must be present at the site of regeneration, and the local microenvironment must be switched to neurogenic permissiveness.

Jeffrey Macklis, Constance Scharff, and colleagues pioneered this work with a study on targeted neurogenesis in the bird brain (Scharff et al., 2000). The method consists of the stereotaxic application of a phototoxic drug into the area to which the cells of interest project. The cells take up the compound and become vulnerable to light. To induce cell death, laser light is shone onto the brain region of interest. Only the loaded neurons die. Because they die by apoptosis, the tissue reaction is minimal or absent. This is the great advantage of this experimental model: the lesion is precisely on the level of single cells from a targeted population.

In 2000, Sanjay S. Magavi and Jeffrey D. Macklis at Harvard University applied the same method to the rodent brain (Figures 8–3, and 8–4, Color Plate 11). With the described method of targeted photolysis, they selectively killed corticothalamic neurons in layer VI of the anterior cortex. They then observed that presumably precursor cells, some of them DCX positive,

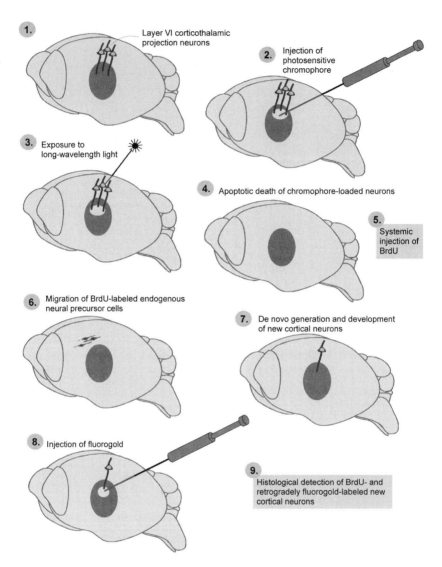

Figure 8–3. Targeted neurogenesis in the adult murine neocortex. Magavi et al. (2000) reported cortical neurogenesis after the selective phototoxic ablation of corticothalamic neurons in the anterior cortex of adult mice. Integration of new BrdU-labeled neurons was confirmed by retrograde fluorogold tracing from the thalamus (see Fig. 8–4, Color Plate 11).

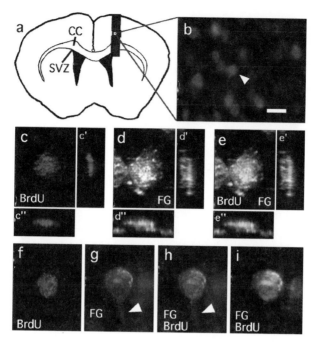

Figure 8–4 (Color Plate 11). Targeted neurogenesis in the adult murine neo-cortex. In the experiment by Magavi et al. (2000) explained in Figure 8–2, new cortical neurons made appropriate target connections in the thalamus, here visualized with retrograde fluorogold tracing (FG) in BrdU-positive cells. *a* and *b*: Camera lucida drawing and photo of a BrdU-positive (red)/FG (white) retro-gradely labeled neuron. CC, corpus callosum; SVZ, subventricular zone. Ar-rowhead indicates labeled neuron. Scale bar: 20μm. *c–e*: Confocal three-dimensional reconstruction of the neuron. *f*: BrdU-positive (red) nucleus of a new FG-positive corticothalamic neuron. *g–i*: FG-positive (blue) cell body with labeled axon (arrowheads). Reprinted with kind permission by Jeffrey D. Macklis, Cambridge, Massachusetts, and *Nature* Publishing Group.

migrated toward the lesion site. For at least 28 weeks after the lesion, they detected new neurons with the BrdU method. By retrograde tracing they were able to confirm that the new cells adequately projected to the thala-mus. This study was a milestone in that it showed that adult neurogenesis could be induced in adult mammalian non-neurogenic regions and that cell death is sufficient to trigger it. The key requirement might be that the lesion has to be small enough to prevent a general reaction of the surrounding tissue. In the absence of an inflammatory response, for example, neuro-genesis might become possible. The damage, however, would have to fun-damentally change the level of neurogenic permissiveness. This was also shown by implanting neural progenitor cells in the cortex of rats in which targeted apoptosis had been induced; the transplanted cells developed into neurons (Sheen and Macklis, 1995; Snyder et al., 1997; Shin et al., 2000). The model was extended in a study in which corticospinal projection neurons were regenerated after targeted photolysis (Chen et al., 2004).

In a middle cerebral artery occlusion model in which transient block-age of the blood flow to the brain mimics the situation of focal cerebral ischemia in patients, the size of the infarct can be titrated by varying the ischemic interval. Andreas Arvidsson from Olle Lindvall's group in Lund, Sweden, showed that when the ischemia damaged only the striatum, a very small number of degenerating medium spiny interneurons in the striatum were replaced, presumably by progenitor cells migrating in from the neighboring SVZ (Arvidsson et al., 2002). Because other studies have shown that the overexpression of BDNF in the ventricular wall can lead to striatal neurogenesis as well (Benraiss et al., 2001; Chmielnicki et al., 2004), striatal damage might result in a shift in the neurotrophic balance toward neurogenic permissiveness in the adult striatum. Also, striatal damage might lead to a down-regulation of slit, the factor that has been made responsible for keeping SVZ precursor cells out of the striatum and directing them toward the RMS and olfactory bulb. Both mechanistic interpretations remain speculative, though. The number of new neurons in the ischemic striatum was extremely low and thus unlikely to lead to a substantial functional recovery. In the controls no new neurons were detected. In this sense, the Arvidsson study could serve as further proof of principle that regenerative neurogenesis is possible in non-neurogenic regions. The Swedish group was able to show that, over weeks after the damage, the new cells progressed through developmental stages typical for medium spiny interneurons and identifiable by the expression of transcription factors Pbx and Meis2 (Arvidsson et al., 2002).

Hirofumi Nakatomi, Masato Nakafuko, and colleagues from Tokyo used a similar ischemia model in which ischemia caused damage of hippocampal region CA1 (Nakatomi et al., 2002). After the ischemic stimulus, and boosted by massive intraventricular infusions of growth factors EGF and FGF-2, they found that migratory precursor cells from the SVZ contributed to an impressive structural reconstitution of CA1. This finding suggests that in addition to interneurons in the olfactory bulb, SVZ precursor cells might be able to generate not only other interneurons in the striatum but also excitatory principal neurons in CA1. Whether this range of developmental potential reflects precursor cell heterogeneity in the SVZ (for example, in the sense of a dorsal vs. ventral positional identity of the precursor cells) or, alternatively, by which instructive cues this specification is achieved, is not known. In the Nakatomi study, the unprecedented extent of the presumably precursor cell based regeneration surprised many researchers. One skeptical question is whether BrdU-incorporation might have labeled dying neurons (Kuan et al., 2004), which survived as "zombies" without normal function and antigenic properties but could be rescued by the massive growth factor application.

THE CELLULAR AND MOLECULAR BASIS
OF NEUROGENIC PERMISSIVENESS

At present it is not clear to what degree the factors that define the stem cell niche are identical to those that determine neurogenic permissiveness. Both sets of parameters do not completely overlap, as suggested by the distribution of different stages of neuronal development in adult olfactory bulb neurogenesis over the distance between the SVZ, RMS, and the olfactory bulb. This distinction would mirror the situation in the developing brain, where factors that determine positional identity need not be identical to those controlling neuronal differentiation.

Some of the regulatory molecules involved in the early stages of brain development might also influence adult neurogenesis. Bone morphogenic proteins (BMPs), for example, actively antagonize neurogenesis in non-neurogenic regions. When Daniel Lim and Arturo Alvarez-Buylla used noggin to inhibit BMP activity in the adult SVZ, they found neurogenesis in the otherwise non-neurogenic striatum (Lim et al., 2000).

Astrocytes might provide the cell-cell interaction necessary for precursor cell function. However, astrocytes in neurogenic regions appear to be specialized and even encompass the stem cells themselves, so that the argument becomes somewhat circular. Not all astrocytes are stem cells though, and not all astrocytes are neurogenic. At present it remains also unclear by which means astrocytes induce neurogenic permissiveness. To some degree, cell–cell contact is required (Lim and Alvarez-Buylla, 1999), but astrocytes also exert contact-independent effects (Song et al., 2002).

Astrocytes form functional networks through gap junctions and calcium waves can travel through this network. It is plausible to assume that astrocytes as precursor cells take part in such networks, but this remains to be shown. During development, calcium waves in radial glia modulate the proliferative activity of the precursor cells (Weissman et al., 2004). Similarly, precursor cell activity in the adult brain is calcium-dependent (Deisseroth et al., 2004). The link to a gap junction–mediated process has yet to be made.

Very little is known about extracellular matrix components as promoters of adult neurogenesis. The success of precursor cell culture experiments is heavily influenced by the choice of the coating for the culture dish. Of these, laminin, for example, is also found in vivo. The basal membrane forms complex invaginations in the stem cell niches; Mercier and colleagues (2002) have speculated that contact of precursor cells to the basal membrane might be required for their activity.

Between cell–cell contacts and extra-cellular matrix-mediated effects lies the conspicuous connection between the stem cell niche and the vasculature (Palmer et al., 2000). Type-1 cells in the SGZ have vascular endfeet characteristic of astrocytes, and these endfeet rest on the basal membrane of the endothelial cells (Filippov et al., 2003). In the SVZ, B cells come into contact with both the ventricular wall and basal membrane invaginations associated with blood vessels. The vascular basal membrane from the vessels in the subependymal tissue engulfs the cells of the stem cell niche. Vascular endothelial growth factor is one of the key molecules suspected to modulate precursor cell activity. In fact, the VEGF receptor 2, flk-1, is expressed on type-2b and type-3 cells because it co-localizes with DCX (Jin et al., 2002) and inhibition of VEGF action prevents the exercise-induced up-regulation of adult hippocampal neurogenesis (Fabel et al., 2003a). Despite its name and the suggestive spatial situation, however, VEGF action in neurogenic zones might be entirely independent of the vasculature. The cellular and molecular key mechanisms of the vascular niche remain to be identified (Palmer, 2002).

Fabienne Agasse, Michel Roger, and Valérie Coronas from the University of Poitiers in France have discovered that proteins secreted in an autocrine or paracrine fashion by SVZ cells promote neurogenesis in vitro, whereas protein factors from cortex actively inhibit neurogenesis (Agasse et al., 2004). Intriguingly, if apoptosis was induced in the cortical explants used in the co-culture systems of these studies, the inhibitory effect was reversed and cell proliferation in the SVZ samples increased. These data indicate that beyond cell–cell interaction and extracellular matrix effects, neurogenic permissiveness is determined by both permissive and inhibitory diffusible cues. Non-neurogenic regions actively block neurogenesis, whereas neurogenic regions actively promote it. The interesting question is whether the removal of the blocking effects in non-neurogenic regions is sufficient to allow an intrinsic neurogenic program to unfold, or whether below the normal inhibitory effect of non-neurogenic regions a pro-neurogenic effect awaits and is up-regulated when the inhibition ceases. This question is of central importance for cases of targeted or induced regenerative neurogenesis. Does the tissue damage do more than remove the negative influence blocking neurogenic permissiveness? Does apoptosis actively induce pro-neurogenic factors in non-neurogenic regions?

The degree to which more extensive cell death can trigger adult neurogenesis has been debated for many years (Gould and Cameron, 1996). The data are ambiguous. On the one hand, the induction of highly selective cell death in individual cells could trigger neurogenesis (Magavi and Macklis, 2002). On the other hand, however, cell death under pathological conditions can be associated with an antineurogenic inflammatory response (Monje et al., 2003). It might thus be that apoptotic cell death is compatible with neurogenesis and even conducive, whereas the necrotic forms are not. There are no indications, however, that neurogenesis is necessarily linked to cell death, because adult neurogenesis in the neurogenic zones is not primarily a regenerative event. In non-neurogenic regions, this is fundamentally different and neurogenesis in non-neurogenic regions might thus be affected more by death signals.

REFERENCES

Agasse F, Roger M, Coronas V (2004) Neurogenic and intact or apoptotic non-neurogenic areas of adult brain release diffusible molecules that differentially modulate the development of subventricular zone cell cultures. Eur J Neurosci 19:1459–1468.

Aguirre AA, Chittajallu R, Belachew S, Gallo V (2004) NG2-expressing cells in the subventricular zone are type C–like cells and contribute to interneuron generation in the postnatal hippocampus. J Cell Biol 165:575–589.

Ahmad I, Das AV, James J, Bhattacharya S, Zhao X (2004) Neural stem cells in the mammalian eye: types and regulation. Semin Cell Dev Biol 15:53–62.

Ahmad I, Dooley CM, Thoreson WB, Rogers JA, Afiat S (1999) In vitro analysis of a mammalian retinal progenitor that gives rise to neurons and glia. Brain Res 831:1–10.

Ahmad I, Tang L, Pham H (2000) Identification of neural progenitors in the adult mammalian eye. Biochem Biophys Res Commun 270:517–521.

Akita J, Takahashi M, Hojo M, Nishida A, Haruta M, Honda Y (2002) Neuronal differentiation of adult rat hippocampus-derived neural stem cells transplanted into embryonic rat explanted retinas with retinoic acid pretreatment. Brain Res 954:286–293.

Akopian G, Kuprijanova E, Kressin K, Steinhuser C (1997) Analysis of ion channel expression by astrocytes in red nucleus brain stem slices of the rat. Glia 19:234–246.

Alexiades MR, Cepko CL (1997) Subsets of retinal progenitors display temporally regulated and distinct biases in the fates of their progeny. Development 124:1119–1131.

Altman J (1963) Autoradiographic investigation of cell proliferation in the brains of rats and cats. Anat Rec 145:573–591.

Alvarez-Buylla A, Garcia-Verdugo JM, Tramontin AD (2001) A unified hypothesis on the lineage of neural stem cells. Nat Rev Neurosci 2:287–293.

Alvarez-Buylla A, Lim DA (2004) For the long run: maintaining germinal niches in the adult brain. Neuron 41:683–686.

Anthony TE, Klein C, Fishell G, Heintz N (2004) Radial glia serve as neuronal progenitors in all regions of the central nervous system. Neuron 41:881–890.

Arvidsson A, Collin T, Kirik D, Kokaia Z, Lindvall O (2002) Neuronal replacement from endogenous precursors in the adult brain after stroke. Nat Med 8:963–970.

Belachew S, Chittajallu R, Aguirre AA, Yuan X, Kirby M, Anderson S, Gallo V (2003) Postnatal NG2 proteoglycan-expressing progenitor cells are intrinsically multipotent and generate functional neurons. J Cell Biol 161:169–186.

Benraiss A, Chmielnicki E, Lerner K, Roh D, Goldman SA (2001) Adenoviral brain-derived neurotrophic factor induces both neostriatal and olfactory neuronal recruitment from endogenous progenitor cells in the adult forebrain. J Neurosci 21:6718–6731.

Bergers G, Brekken R, McMahon G, Vu TH, Itoh T, Tamaki K, Tanzawa K, Thorpe P, Itohara S, Werb Z, Hanahan D (2000) Matrix metalloproteinase-9 triggers the angiogenic switch during carcinogenesis. Nat Cell Biol 2:737–744.

Bergles DE, Roberts JD, Somogyi P, Jahr CE (2000) Glutamatergic synapses on oligodendrocyte precursor cells in the hippocampus. Nature 405:187–191.

Bernier PJ, Bedard A, Vinet J, Levesque M, Parent A (2002) Newly generated neurons in the amygdala and adjoining cortex of adult primates. Proc Natl Acad Sci USA 99:11464–11469.

Boulton M, Albon J (2004) Stem cells in the eye. Int J Biochem Cell Biol 36:643–657.

Butt AM, Duncan A, Hornby MF, Kirvell SL, Hunter A, Levine JM, Berry M (1999) Cells expressing the NG2 antigen contact nodes of Ranvier in adult CNS white matter. Glia 26:84–91.

Cao L, Jiao X, Zuzga DS, Liu Y, Fong DM, Young D, During MJ (2004) VEGF links hippocampal activity with neurogenesis, learning and memory. Nat Genet 36:827–835.

Chacko DM, Das AV, Zhao X, James J, Bhattacharya S, Ahmad I (2003) Transplantation of ocular stem cells: the role of injury in incorporation and differentiation of grafted cells in the retina. Vision Res 43:937–946.

Chari DM, Blakemore WF (2002) Efficient recolonisation of progenitor-depleted areas of the CNS by adult oligodendrocyte progenitor cells. Glia 37:307–313.

Chen J, Magavi SS, Macklis JD (2004) Neurogenesis of corticospinal motor neurons extending spinal projections in adult mice. Proc Natl Acad Sci USA 101:16357–16362.

Chen ZJ, Negra M, Levine A, Ughrin Y, Levine JM (2002) Oligodendrocyte precursor cells: reactive cells that inhibit axon growth and regeneration. J Neurocytol 31:481–495.

Chmielnicki E, Benraiss A, Economides AN, Goldman SA (2004) Adenovirally expressed noggin and brain-derived neurotrophic factor cooperate to induce new medium spiny neurons from resident progenitor cells in the adult striatal ventricular zone. J Neurosci 24:2133–2142.

Cooper O, Isacson O (2004) Intrastriatal transforming growth factor alpha delivery to a model of Parkinson's disease induces proliferation and migration of endogenous adult neural progenitor cells without differentiation into dopaminergic neurons. J Neurosci 24:8924–8931.

Deisseroth K, Singla S, Toda H, Monje M, Palmer TD, Malenka RC (2004) Excitation–neurogenesis coupling in adult neural stem/progenitor cells. Neuron 42:535–552.

Dou CL, Levine JM (1994) Inhibition of neurite growth by the NG2 chondroitin sulfate proteoglycan. J Neurosci 14:7616–7628.

Ehninger D, Kempermann G (2003) Regional effects of wheel running and environmental enrichment on cell genesis and microglia proliferation in the adult murine neocortex. Cereb Cortex 13:845–851.

Ekdahl CT, Claasen JH, Bonde S, Kokaia Z, Lindvall O (2003) Inflammation is detrimental for neurogenesis in adult brain. Proc Natl Acad Sci USA 100:13632–13637.

Engelhardt M, Wachs FP, Couillard-Despres S, Aigner L (2004) The neurogenic competence of progenitors from the postnatal rat retina in vitro. Exp Eye Res 78:1025–1036.

Fabel K, Tam B, Kaufer D, Baiker A, Simmons N, Kuo CJ, Palmer TD (2003a) VEGF is necessary for exercise-induced adult hippocampal neurogenesis. Eur J Neurosci 18:2803–2812.

Fabel K, Toda H, Palmer T (2003b) Copernican stem cells: regulatory constellations in adult hippocampal neurogenesis. J Cell Biochem 88:41–50.

Fang X, Burg MA, Barritt D, Dahlin-Huppe K, Nishiyama A, Stallcup WB (1999) Cytoskeletal reorganization induced by engagement of the NG2 proteoglycan leads to cell spreading and migration. Mol Biol Cell 10:3373–3387.

Filippov V, Kronenberg G, Pivneva T, Reuter K, Steiner B, Wang LP, Yamaguchi M, Kettenmann H, Kempermann G (2003) Subpopulation of nestin-expressing progenitor cells in the adult murine hippocampus shows electrophysiological and morphological characteristics of astrocytes. Mol Cell Neurosci 23:373–382.

Fischer AJ, Reh TA (2000) Identification of a proliferating marginal zone of retinal progenitors in postnatal chickens. Dev Biol 220:197–210.

Fischer AJ, Reh TA (2001) Müller glia are a potential source of neural regeneration in the postnatal chicken retina. Nat Neurosci 4:247–252.

Fishell G, Kriegstein AR (2003) Neurons from radial glia: the consequences of asymmetric inheritance. Curr Opin Neurobiol 13:34–41.

Frielingsdorf H, Schwarz K, Brundin P, Mohapel P (2004) No evidence for new dopaminergic neurons in the adult mammalian substantia nigra. Proc Natl Acad Sci USA 101:10177–10182.

Gage FH, Coates PW, Palmer TD, Kuhn HG, Fisher LJ, Suhonen JO, Peterson DA, Suhr ST, Ray J (1995) Survival and differentiation of adult neuronal progenitor cells transplanted to the adult brain. Proc Natl Acad Sci USA 92:11879–11883.

Gates MA, Thomas LB, Howard EM, Laywell ED, Sajin B, Faissner A, Gotz B, Silver J, Steindler DA (1995) Cell and molecular analysis of the developing and adult mouse subventricular zone of the cerebral hemispheres. J Comp Neurol 361:249–266.

Gensert JM, Goldman JE (1996) In vivo characterization of endogenous proliferating cells in adult rat subcortical white matter. Glia 17:39–51.

Gensert JM, Goldman JE (1997) Endogenous progenitors remyelinate demyelinated axons in the adult CNS. Neuron 19:197–203.

Gould E, Cameron HA (1996) Regulation of neuronal birth, migration and death in the rat dentate gyrus. Dev Neurosci 18:22–35.

Gould E, Reeves AJ, Graziano MS, Gross CG (1999) Neurogenesis in the neocortex of adult primates. Science 286:548–552.

Gould E, Vail N, Wagers M, Gross CG (2001) Adult-generated hippocampal and neocortical neurons in macaques have a transient existence. Proc Natl Acad Sci USA 98:10910–10917.

Grako KA, Ochiya T, Barritt D, Nishiyama A, Stallcup WB (1999) PDGF (alpha)-receptor is unresponsive to PDGF-AA in aortic smooth muscle cells from the NG2 knockout mouse. J Cell Sci 112(Pt 6):905–915.

Hart IK, Richardson WD, Heldin CH, Westermark B, Raff MC (1989) PDGF receptors on cells of the oligodendrocyte-type-2 astrocyte (O-2A) cell lineage. Development 105:595–603.

Heissig B, Hattori K, Dias S, Friedrich M, Ferris B, Hackett NR, Crystal RG, Besmer P, Lyden D, Moore MA, Werb Z, Rafii S (2002) Recruitment of stem and progenitor cells from the bone marrow niche requires MMP-9 mediated release of kit-ligand. Cell 109:625–637.

Hellsten J, Wennstrom M, Bengzon J, Mohapel P, Tingstrom A (2004) Electroconvulsive seizures induce endothelial cell proliferation in adult rat hippocampus. Biol Psychiatry 55:420–427.

Herrera DG, Garcia-Verdugo JM, Alvarez-Buylla A (1999) Adult-derived neural precursors transplanted into multiple regions in the adult brain. Ann Neurol 46:867–877.

Hitchcock P, Ochocinska M, Sieh A, Otteson D (2004) Persistent and injury-induced neurogenesis in the vertebrate retina. Prog Retin Eye Res 23:183–194.

Hollyfield JG (1968) Differential addition of cells to the retina in Rana pipiens tadpoles. Dev Biol 18:163–179.

Horner PJ, Power AE, Kempermann G, Kuhn HG, Palmer TD, Winkler J, Thal LJ, Gage FH (2000) Proliferation and differentiation of progenitor cells throughout the intact adult rat spinal cord. J Neurosci 20:2218–2228.

Horner PJ, Thallmair M, Gage FH (2002) Defining the NG2-expressing cell of the adult CNS. J Neurocytol 31:469–480.

Jacques TS, Relvas JB, Nishimura S, Pytela R, Edwards GM, Streuli CH, ffrench-Constant C (1998) Neural precursor cell chain migration and division are regulated through different beta1 integrins. Development 125:3167–3177.

Jankovski A, Sotelo C (1996) Subventricular zone-olfactory bulb migratory pathway in the adult mouse: cellular composition and specificity as determined by heterochronic and heterotopic transplantation. J Comp Neurol 371:376–396.

Jiang Y, Jahagirdar BN, Reinhardt RL, Schwartz RE, Keene CD, Ortiz-Gonzalez XR, Reyes M, Lenvik T, Lund T, Blackstad M, Du J, Aldrich S, Lisberg A, Low WC, Largaespada DA, Verfaillie CM (2002) Pluripotency of mesenchymal stem cells derived from adult marrow. Nature 418:41–49.

Jin K, Zhu Y, Sun Y, Mao XO, Xie L, Greenberg DA (2002) Vascular endothelial growth factor (VEGF) stimulates neurogenesis in vitro and in vivo. Proc Natl Acad Sci USA 99:11946–11950.

Johns PR (1977) Growth of the adult goldfish eye. III. Source of the new retinal cells. J Comp Neurol 176:343–357.

Johns PR, Easter SS Jr. (1977) Growth of the adult goldfish eye. II. Increase in retinal cell number. J Comp Neurol 176:331–341.

Kaplan MS (1981) Neurogenesis in the 3-month-old rat visual cortex. J Comp Neurol 195:323–338.

Keirstead HS, Levine JM, Blakemore WF (1998) Response of the oligodendrocyte progenitor cell population (defined by NG2 labelling) to demyelination of the adult spinal cord. Glia 22:161–170.

Kempermann G, Kuhn HG, Gage FH (1997) More hippocampal neurons in adult mice living in an enriched environment. Nature 386:493–495.

Koketsu D, Mikami A, Miyamoto Y, Hisatsune T (2003) Nonrenewal of neurons in the cerebral neocortex of adult macaque monkeys. J Neurosci 23:937–942.

Kondo T, Raff M (2000) Oligodendrocyte precursor cells reprogrammed to become multipotential CNS stem cells. Science 289:1754–1757.

Kornack DR, Rakic P (2001) Cell proliferation without neurogenesis in adult primate neocortex. Science 294:2127–2130.

Kuan CY, Schloemer AJ, Lu A, Burns KA, Weng WL, Williams MT, Strauss KI, Vorhees CV, Flavell RA, Davis RJ, Sharp FR, Rakic P (2004) Hypoxia-ischemia induces DNA synthesis without cell proliferation in dying neurons in adult rodent brain. J Neurosci 24:10763–10772.

Laywell ED, Rakic P, Kukekov VG, Holland EC, Steindler DA (2000) Identification of a multipotent astrocytic stem cell in the immature and adult mouse brain. Proc Natl Acad Sci USA 97:13883–13888.

Levine JM, Reynolds R, Fawcett JW (2001) The oligodendrocyte precursor cell in health and disease. Trends Neurosci 24:39–47.

Lie DC, Dziewczapolski G, Willhoite AR, Kaspar BK, Shults CW, Gage FH (2002) The adult substantia nigra contains progenitor cells with neurogenic potential. J Neurosci 22:6639–6649.

Lim DA, Alvarez-Buylla A (1999) Interaction between astrocytes and adult subventricular zone precursors stimulates neurogenesis. Proc Natl Acad Sci USA 96:7526–7531.

Lim DA, Tramontin AD, Trevejo JM, Herrera DG, Garcia-Verdugo JM, Alvarez-Buylla A (2000) Noggin antagonizes BMP signaling to create a niche for adult neurogenesis. Neuron 28:713–726.

Lin SC, Bergles DE (2002) Physiological characteristics of NG2–expressing glial cells. J Neurocytol 31:537–549.

Magavi S, Leavitt B, Macklis J (2000) Induction of neurogenesis in the neocortex of adult mice. Nature 405:951–955.

Magavi SS, Macklis JD (2002) Induction of neuronal type-specific neurogenesis in the cerebral cortex of adult mice: manipulation of neural precursors in situ. Brain Res Dev Brain Res 134:57–76.

Mallon BS, Shick HE, Kidd GJ, Macklin WB (2002) Proteolipid promoter activity distinguishes two populations of NG2-positive cells throughout neonatal cortical development. J Neurosci 22:876–885.

Marcus RC, Delaney CL, Easter SS Jr. (1999) Neurogenesis in the visual system of embryonic and adult zebrafish (*Danio rerio*). Vis Neurosci 16:417–424.

Markakis EA, Palmer TD, Randolph-Moore L, Rakic P, Gage FH (2004) Novel neuronal phenotypes from neural progenitor cells. J Neurosci 24:2886–2897.

Martens DJ, Seaberg RM, van der Kooy D (2002) In vivo infusions of exogenous growth factors into the fourth ventricle of the adult mouse brain increase the proliferation of neural progenitors around the fourth ventricle and the central canal of the spinal cord. Eur J Neurosci 16:1045–1057.

Mellough CB, Cui Q, Spalding KL, Symons NA, Pollett MA, Snyder EY, Macklis JD, Harvey AR (2004) Fate of multipotent neural precursor cells transplanted into mouse retina selectively depleted of retinal ganglion cells. Exp Neurol 186:6–19.

Mercier F, Kitasako JT, Hatton GI (2002) Anatomy of the brain neurogenic zones revisited: fractones and the fibroblast/macrophage network. J Comp Neurol 451:170–188.

Miller RH (1999) Contact with central nervous system myelin inhibits oligodendrocyte progenitor maturation. Dev Biol 216:359–368.

Monje ML, Toda H, Palmer TD (2003) Inflammatory blockade restores adult hippocampal neurogenesis. Science 302:1760–1765.

Morshead CM, Garcia AD, Sofroniew MV, van Der Kooy D (2003) The ablation of glial fibrillary acidic protein–positive cells from the adult central nervous system results in the loss of forebrain neural stem cells but not retinal stem cells. Eur J Neurosci 18:76–84.

Nakatomi H, Kuriu T, Okabe S, Yamamoto S, Hatano O, Kawahara N, Tamura A, Kirino T, Nakafuku M (2002) Regeneration of hippocampal pyramidal neurons after ischemic brain injury by recruitment of endogenous neural progenitors. Cell 110:429–441.

Newton SS, Collier EF, Hunsberger J, Adams D, Terwilliger R, Selvanayagam E, Duman RS (2003) Gene profile of electroconvulsive seizures: induction of neurotrophic and angiogenic factors. J Neurosci 23:10841–10851.

Niehaus A, Stegmuller J, Diers-Fenger M, Trotter J (1999) Cell-surface glycoprotein of oligodendrocyte progenitors involved in migration. J Neurosci 19:4948–4961.

Nishiyama A, Chang A, Trapp BD (1999) NG2+ glial cells: a novel glial cell population in the adult brain. J Neuropathol Exp Neurol 58:1113–1124.

Nishiyama A, Lin XH, Giese N, Heldin CH, Stallcup WB (1996) Co-localization of NG2 proteoglycan and PDGF alpha-receptor on O2A progenitor cells in the developing rat brain. J Neurosci Res 43:299–314.

Nishiyama A, Watanabe M, Yang Z, Bu J (2002) Identity, distribution, and development of polydendrocytes: NG2–expressing glial cells. J Neurocytol 31:437–455.

Nowakowski RS, Hayes NL (2000) New neurons: extraordinary evidence or extraordinary conclusion? Science 288:771.

Ong WY, Levine JM (1999) A light and electron microscopic study of NG2 chondroitin sulfate proteoglycan–positive oligodendrocyte precursor cells in the normal and kainate-lesioned rat hippocampus. Neuroscience 92:83–95.

Palmer TD (2002) Adult neurogenesis and the vascular Nietzsche. Neuron 34:856–858.

Palmer TD, Markakis EA, Willhoite AR, Safar F, Gage FH (1999) Fibroblast growth factor-2 activates a latent neurogenic program in neural stem cells from divers regions of the adult CNS. J Neurosci 19:8487–8497.

Palmer TD, Takahashi J, Gage FH (1997) The adult rat hippocampus contains premordial neural stem cells. Mol Cell Neurosci 8:389–404.

Palmer TD, Willhoite AR, Gage FH (2000) Vascular niche for adult hippocampal neurogenesis. J Comp Neurol 425:479–494.

Raff MC, Miller RH, Noble M (1983) A glial progenitor cell that develops in vitro into an astrocyte or an oligodendrocyte depending on culture medium. Nature 303:390–396.

Rakic P (2002) Neurogenesis in adult primate neocortex: an evaluation of the evidence. Nat Rev Neurosci 3:65–71.

Redwine JM, Armstrong RC (1998) In vivo proliferation of oligodendrocyte progenitors expressing PDGF-αR during early remyelination. J Neurobiol 37:413–428.

Reh TA, Constantine-Paton M (1983) Qualitative and quantitative measures of plasticity during the normal development of the *Rana pipiens* retinotectal projection. Brain Res 312:187–200.

Reynolds R, Dawson M, Papadopoulos D, Polito A, Di Bello IC, Pham-Dinh D, Levine J (2002) The response of NG2–expressing oligodendrocyte progenitors to demyelination in MOG-EAE and MS. J Neurocytol 31:523–536.

Ricard D, Rogemond V, Charrier E, Aguera M, Bagnard D, Belin MF, Thomasset N, Honnorat J (2001) Isolation and expression pattern of human Unc-33-like phosphoprotein 6/collapsin response mediator protein 5 (Ulip6/CRMP5): coexistence with Ulip2/CRMP2 in Sema3a-sensitive oligodendrocytes. J Neurosci 21:7203–7214.

Rietze R, Poulin P, Weiss S (2000) Mitotically active cells that generate neurons and astrocytes are present in multiple regions of the adult mouse hippocampus. J Comp Neurol 424:397–408.

Sawamoto K, Yamamoto A, Kawaguchi A, Yamaguchi M, Mori K, Goldman SA, Okano H (2001) Direct isolation of committed neuronal progenitor cells from transgenic mice coexpressing spectrally distinct fluorescent proteins regulated by stage-specific neural promoters. J Neurosci Res 65:220–227.

Schanzer A, Wachs FP, Wilhelm D, Acker T, Cooper-Kuhn C, Beck H, Winkler J, Aigner L, Plate KH, Kuhn HG (2004) Direct stimulation of adult neural stem cells in vitro and neurogenesis in vivo by vascular endothelial growth factor. Brain Pathol 14:237–248.

Scharff C, Kirn JR, Grossman M, Macklis JD, Nottebohm F (2000) Targeted neuronal death affects neuronal replacement and vocal behavior in adult songbirds. Neuron 25:481–492.

Schneider S, Bosse F, D'Urso D, Muller H, Sereda MW, Nave K, Niehaus A, Kempf T, Schnolzer M, Trotter J (2001) The AN2 protein is a novel marker for the Schwann cell lineage expressed by immature and nonmyelinating Schwann cells. J Neurosci 21:920–933.

Sheen VL, Macklis JD (1995) Targeted neocortical cell death in adult mice guides migration and differentiation of transplanted embryonic neurons. J Neurosci 15:8378–8392.

Shihabuddin LS, Horner PJ, Ray J, Gage FH (2000) Adult spinal cord stem cells generate neurons after transplantation in the adult dentate gyrus. J Neurosci 20:8727–8735.

Shihabuddin LS, Ray J, Gage FH (1997) FGF-2 is sufficient to isolate progenitors found in the adult mammalian spinal cord. Exp Neurol 148:577–586.

Shin JJ, Fricker-Gates RA, Perez FA, Leavitt BR, Zurakowski D, Macklis JD (2000) Transplanted neuroblasts differentiate appropriately into projection neurons with correct neurotransmitter and receptor phenotype in neocortex undergoing targeted projection neuron degeneration. J Neurosci 20:7404–7416.

Snyder EY, Yoon C, Flax JD, Macklis JD (1997) Multipotent neural precursors can differentiate toward replacement of neurons undergoing targeted apoptotic degeneration in adult mouse neocortex. Proc Natl Acad Sci USA 94:11663–11668.

Song H, Stevens CF, Gage FH (2002) Astroglia induce neurogenesis from adult neural stem cells. Nature 417:39–44.

Stallcup WB, Beasley L (1987) Bipotential glial precursor cells of the optic nerve express the NG2 proteoglycan. J Neurosci 7:2737–2744.

Stegmuller J, Werner H, Nave KA, Trotter J (2003) The proteoglycan NG2 is complexed with alpha-amino-3-hydroxy-5-methyl-4-isoxazolepropionic acid (AMPA) receptors by the PDZ glutamate receptor interaction protein (GRIP) in glial progenitor cells. Implications for glial–neuronal signaling. J Biol Chem 278:3590–3598.

Steinhauser C, Berger T, Frotscher M, Kettenmann H (1992) Heterogeneity in the membrane current pattern of identified glial cells in the hippocampal slice. Eur J Neurosci 4:472–484.

Steinhauser C, Kressin K, Kuprijanova E, Weber M, Seifert G (1994) Properties of voltage-activated Na+ and K+ currents in mouse hippocampal glial cells in situ and after acute isolation from tissue slices. Pflugers Arch 428:610–620.

Suhonen JO, Peterson DA, Ray J, Gage FH (1996) Differentiation of adult hippocampus-derived progenitors into olfactory neurons in vivo. Nature 383:624–627.

Takahashi M, Palmer TD, Takahashi J, Gage FH (1998) Widespread integration and survival of adult-derived neural progenitor cells in the developing optic retina. Mol Cell Neurosci 12:340–348.

Tropepe V, Coles BL, Chiasson BJ, Horsford DJ, Elia AJ, McInnes RR, van der Kooy D (2000) Retinal stem cells in the adult mammalian eye. Science 287:2032–2036.

Ughrin YM, Chen ZJ, Levine JM (2003) Multiple regions of the NG2 proteoglycan inhibit neurite growth and induce growth cone collapse. J Neurosci 23:175–186.

Warfvinge K, Kamme C, Englund U, Wictorin K (2001) Retinal integration of grafts of brain-derived precursor cell lines implanted subretinally into adult, normal rats. Exp Neurol 169:1–12.

Watanabe M, Toyama Y, Nishiyama A (2002) Differentiation of proliferated NG2-positive glial progenitor cells in a remyelinating lesion. J Neurosci Res 69:826–836.

Weissman TA, Riquelme PA, Ivic L, Flint AC, Kriegstein AR (2004) Calcium waves propagate through radial glial cells and modulate proliferation in the developing neocortex. Neuron 43:647–661.

Wetts R, Fraser SE (1988) Multipotent precursors can give rise to all major cell types of the frog retina. Science 239:1142–1145.

Wurmser AE, Nakashima K, Summers RG, Toni N, D'Amour KA, Lie DC, Gage FH (2004) Cell fusion–independent differentiation of neural stem cells to the endothelial lineage. Nature 430:350–356.

Yamaguchi M, Saito H, Suzuki M, Mori K (2000) Visualization of neurogenesis in the central nervous system using nestin promoter–GFP transgenic mice. Neuroreport 11:1991–1996.

Yamashima T, Tonchev AB, Vachkov IH, Popivanova BK, Seki T, Sawamoto K, Okano H (2004) Vascular adventitia generates neuronal progenitors in the monkey hippocampus after ischemia. Hippocampus 14:861–875.

Yang K, Cepko CL (1996) Flk-1, a receptor for vascular endothelial growth factor (VEGF), is expressed by retinal progenitor cells. J Neurosci 16:6089–6099.

Young MJ, Ray J, Whiteley SJ, Klassen H, Gage FH (2000) Neuronal differentiation and morphological integration of hippocampal progenitor cells transplanted to the retina of immature and mature dystrophic rats. Mol Cell Neurosci 16:197–205.

Young RW (1985) Cell proliferation during postnatal development of the retina in the mouse. Brain Res 353:229–239.

Zhang RL, Zhang L, Zhang ZG, Morris D, Jiang Q, Wang L, Zhang LJ, Chopp M (2003) Migration and differentiation of adult rat subventricular zone progenitor cells transplanted into the adult rat striatum. Neuroscience 116:373–382.

Zhao M, Momma S, Delfani K, Carlen M, Cassidy RM, Johansson CB, Brismar H, Shupliakov O, Frisen J, Janson AM (2003) Evidence for neurogenesis in the adult mammalian substantia nigra. Proc Natl Acad Sci USA 100:7925–7930.

Zigova T, Pencea V, Betarbet R, Wiegand SJ, Alexander C, Bakay RA, Luskin MB (1998) Neuronal progenitor cells of the neonatal subventricular zone differentiate and disperse following transplantation into the adult rat striatum. Cell Transplant 7:137–156.

9

Regulation

Most original publications on adult neurogenesis are in one form or another concerned with its regulation. Factors as diverse as neurotrophins, stress, opioids, seizures, odors, diabetes, gingko biloba, physical activity, acupuncture, ischemia, learning, nitric oxide, alcohol, electromagnetic waves, and many others have been reported to regulate neurogenesis. Often it remains undecided whether influence actually reflects regulation. Many regulators might share a common mechanism or be entirely nonspecific. This flood of reports is likely to continue and a book is not the place to review this literature in its entirety; the overview would be neither timely nor complete. In this chapter we will thus focus on the emerging principles behind the regulation of adult neurogenesis and examine a number of important key regulators. One general observation from the large variety of studies on this topic is that the regulation of adult neurogenesis seems to be almost seismographically sensitive to almost any stimulus. This observation is certainly misleading.

In the reality of experimental situations, *regulation* usually means a change in quantity and only rarely changes in quality. Therefore, important aspects of regulation might be missed because only selected parameters were measured. In most studies, regulation of adult neurogenesis is equivalent to an increase or decrease in the number of newly generated cells. The readout of these studies is the number of cells labeled with bromodeoxyuridine (BrdU) before or during the experimental manipulation. As we have seen, the number of BrdU-positive cells is only a good indicator of the number of new neurons if long enough survival times are allowed after the injection of BrdU. Thus many studies that report changes in adult neurogenesis but base their claim only on an acute measurement of BrdU incorporation (or some other measure of proliferation; see Chapter 7) do not necessarily deliver a meaningful quantitative assessment of regulation as far as the resulting number of new neurons is concerned.

The growing awareness of this pitfall and increasing knowledge about the details of adult neuronal development are changing this situation. The use of electrophysiological methods and the characterization of complex regulatory situations by gene or protein expression profiling will enable us to define regulation on more levels than are possible today. Our concepts of how adult neurogenesis is controlled are thus bound to improve in the near future. Qualitatively, the end-point of adult neurogenesis—that is, the existence of new neurons—will not be as homogenous as it has appeared for some time. Regulation of adult neurogenesis might also cause the new neurons to not so much change in number but in aspects of their neuronal functionality.

REGULATION MEANS INTEGRATION OF MANY COFACTORS

Regulation is a multidimensional event. There are regulatory cascades and sequences of cause–effect relationships that can create a scenario in which, for example, the experience of a new odor causes phosphorylated cAMP response binding protein (CREB) to activate the gene for brain-derived neurotrophic factor (BDNF) and thereby promote neuronal survival. Another scenario is voluntary wheel-running, in mice, which by itself requires preceding brain activity, via a multitude of systemic responses in the central nervous system (CNS) and bodily systems, reaches the germinative niches and through a variety of cell-to-cell interactions that find continuation in intracellular signaling pathways, finally effects transcriptional control of the relevant genes (Fig. 9–1). We can get first impressions of how regulation proceeds from the behavioral level down to the action of a single transcription factor. In reality, however, this identified path is only part of an immense network of interactions. The net effect is often not indicative of the regulation that let to it. Both kainic acid (KA) receptor activation and epidermal growth factor (EGF) receptor activation cause an increase in hippocampal precursor cell proliferation but involve different cascades: many regulatory pathways are redundant. Finally, the effectiveness of a regula-

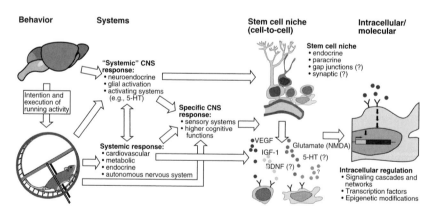

Figure 9–1. Regulation occurs on many conceptual levels. The example of physical activity inducing adult hippocampal neurogenesis is used here as an example to demonstrate that *regulation* is a multifaceted term that encompasses effects on levels from behavior to single transcription factors. Note that the behavior that causes the regulation within the brain is itself dependent on brain activity. BDNF, brain-derived neurotrophic factor; IGF-1, insulin-like growth factor-1; VEGF, vascular endothelial growth factor; 5-HT, serotonin.

tor in a reductionistic experimental situation does not necessarily elucidate the relevance of the individual stimuli to physiologic situations, so that mechanistically, regulation remains a rather ephemeral construct.

On a transcriptional level and on the level of controlling transcriptional control, many pathways in the net regulation of neurogenesis may share identical components. Although we have to study the small pieces of regulatory networks one by one, in reality they compete and interact with each other and are interdependent. The complex challenge is thus to understand not only the mechanisms of regulation but also their hierarchy and interdependencies. Net regulation is the result of integration of all these influences and is high-dimensional. From a phenomenological point of view, the net result of regulation ("seizures lead to more new neurons") might be predictable, but describing, understanding, and manipulating the state of the precursor cell or the immature neuron during this process remains a tremendous challenge. This situation underscores the importance of reductionism and the underestimated value of phenomenology in biological research. But the relevance of individually identified factors should not be overemphasized.

NATURAL VARIATION IN ADULT HIPPOCAMPAL NEUROGENESIS

Comparison of adult hippocampal neurogenesis in different strains of inbred (Kempermann et al., 1997b; Kempermann and Gage, 2002a, 2002b) and wild (Amrein et al., 2004) strains of mice has revealed large, natural variation in this trait. In rats a comparison of two strains also showed differences in adult hippocampal neurogenesis (Perfilieva et al., 2001). Many other parameters such as total granule cell number and hippocampal weight show a similar variability (Wimer and Wimer, 1989; Peirce et al., 2003). Especially in inbred mice, this variation mainly reflects the influence of genetic background. The data are not devoid of all environmental influence because animals might react differently to an identical environment, but the environment can be held constant. Under these conditions, the variation in net hippocampal neurogenesis can be larger than with any other experimental manipulation examined so far: the largest difference between two strains of mice was 25-fold in one study (Kempermann and Gage, 2002b).

These comparisons have further revealed that regulation of adult neurogenesis does not follow a simple on–off pattern but is differentially regulated at different stages of development, such as cell proliferation, rate of survival and the relative contributions to neurogenesis and gliogenesis (Kempermann et al., 1997b; Kempermann and Gage, 2002a). This observation can be interpreted as a differential contribution of different sets of genes to the regulation of adult neurogenesis. Adult neurogenesis is a polygenic trait and numerous genes will interact in determining the rate of neurogenesis and its regulation in response to external or internal neurogenic stimuli. Consequently, results from studies manipulating single genes erroneously treat adult neurogenesis as a monogenic Mendelian trait, which limits the conclusions that can be drawn from such experiments for understanding neurogenic regulation as a whole.

The genetic contribution to the variation in total granule cell number is 86% (Abusaad et al., 1999). RI strains of mice are essentially inbred progeny of F2 generations from a cross of two genetically defined parental strains such as C57BL/6 and DBA/2. The breeding paradigm leads to different strains within one set of strains (called "BXD" in the case of C57BL/6 and DBA/2) that contain roughly 50% genome from each parental strain in various compositions. Because they are inbred, RI strains are homologous at every locus and can be used for linkage studies (Abiola et al., 2003). Figure 9–2 displays how the different mix of parental genomes in such strains results in large variation in the genetically determined baseline level of adult neurogenesis (data from Kempermann and Gage, 2002b).

REGULATION OF THE BALANCE BETWEEN CELL PRODUCTION AND CELL DEATH

There is little evidence that adult neurogenesis contributes to neuronal turnover in the hippocampus. Rather, new neurons are added to the existing

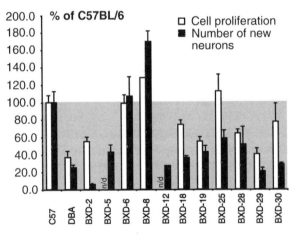

Figure 9–2. Natural variation in adult hippocampal neurogenesis. Adult hippocampal neurogenesis in mice is to a large degree genetically controlled and shows large strain differences. Strains C57BL/6 and DBA/2 show a fourfold difference in the baseline rate of neurogenesis (number of new neurons, open bars). The other strains are recombinant inbred strains of mice derived from these two parental strains and are essentially inbred F2 generation animals. The strains thus differ only in the genetic mix but all have approximately half C57BL/6 and half DBA/2 genome. C57BL/6 has been set as 100%. The data show how extensive the influence of genetic background is on adult neurogenesis. Data are taken from Kempermann and Gage (2002b).

networks and the dentate gyrus grows throughout life, although in a rodent this absolute growth becomes minute and not measurable after the first
months of life. In the olfactory bulb the situation is more complex; both
turnover and long-term addition of new neurons seem to occur. Of all regions in the adult brain, the neurogenic zones show the highest incidence
of apoptotic cell death, being about a hundred times higher than in the rest
of the brain (Blaschke et al., 1996; Biebl et al., 2000). In the dentate gyrus,
the highest number of apoptotic cells is found in the subgranular zone (SGZ);
in the olfactory system, approximately 80% are detected in the olfactory
bulb, the remainder in the rostral migratory stream (RMS) and the subventricular zone (SVZ). In both the SVZ and SGZ the counts of BrdU-labeled
cells at different times after BrdU reflect a strong initial expansion followed
by a dramatic decrease in the number of newly generated cells (Winner et al.,
2002; Kempermann et al., 2003). This elimination of cells is achieved by
programmed cell death of immature neurons. Consequently, measures of
cell proliferation and cell death are related; in a model of chronic stress that
resulted in a large decrease in cell proliferation in the dentate gyrus (see
below), the number of apoptotic cells was reduced accordingly (Heine et al.,
2004b).

Analogous to the prevailing mechanism during embryonic brain development there is a surplus of new neurons generated in adult neurogenesis.
From these cells only those survive that make useful functional connections.
Over a period of several weeks the new cells mature in responsiveness to
synaptic activation (Jessberger and Kempermann, 2003) and become electrophysiologically indistinguishable from older granule cells (van Praag
et al., 2002). This sensitive period coincides with the phase of elimination
during neuronal development in the adult (Kempermann et al., 2004). The
primary principle underlying the regulation of adult neurogenesis thus
seems to be a Hebbian mechanism. The cells that are functionally beneficial survive, while the others die.

A large number of factors have been identified that influence the expansion phase ("proliferation"). This does not mean that such factors would
necessarily be mitogens; their pro-proliferative action might be indirect.
Regulation of precursor cell proliferation is largely considered to be rather
nonspecific. Nevertheless, loss-of-function experiments with E2F, a transcription factor involved in the control of cell cycle progression, led to a
reduction in adult neurogenesis without grossly affecting prenatal neurogenesis (Cooper-Kuhn et al., 2002). Similarly, loss of cyclin D2 (but not D1)
reduced adult neurogenesis (Kowalczyk et al., 2004).

Specificity is brought into the net regulation not primarily on the expansion side but also by means of a selection process accompanied by the specific elimination of cells. At the highest conceptual level, benefit from adult
neurogenesis would be measured as an improvement in cognitive function
as a consequence of the addition of new neurons. Consistent with this concept, cognitive stimuli such as environmental enrichment and learning

stimuli affect primarily the survival period during adult neurogenesis, although this distinction is not clear-cut (Kempermann et al., 1997a, 1998a; Gould et al., 1999; Dobrossy et al., 2003; Leuner et al., 2004). For many factors that can influence adult neurogenesis it is not clear how their net effect on adult neurogenesis is achieved. Many paths might lead to the same net result. Cell proliferation during the expansion phase and survival of newly generated cells during the selection phase might be independently affected. However, some factors might act indirectly and influence both aspects through different pathways.

The strongest candidates for extracellular signaling molecules that promote survival of newly generated cells are neurotrophic factors (see below). These factors exert a balanced action; on the one hand they promote survival through activation of trk receptors, on the other they can stimulate apoptotic cell death via the low-affinity p75 receptor. TrkA activation counteracts the proapoptotic signal at the p75 receptor. For details on the intracellular mechanisms following receptor activation leading to cell survival or death the reader is referred to specialized reviews (Miller and Kaplan, 2001).

Related to the idea of a balance between cell birth and death is the concept of *quiescence*: precursor cells can withdraw from the cell cycle and remain in a dormant, nonproliferative stage from which they can be recruited. Protein p27 kip1 is associated with a transitional stage of cell cycle arrest in precursor cells albeit not classical "quiescence": both neurogenic zones of the adult brain show p27kip1 expression (Doetsch et al., 2002; Heine et al., 2004b). When p27kip1 function was abolished, proliferation in the SVZ increased (Doetsch et al., 2002). A chronic stress model resulting in reduced adult neurogenesis caused a relative increase in p27kip1-positive cells. This finding indicates that the experimental manipulation caused an arrest of further neuronal development (Heine et al., 2004b).

MAINTAINING THE PRECURSOR POOL

Adult neurogenesis is dependent on the existence of precursor cells. The precursor cell pool is maintained by self-renewal and the possible quiescence of some of the cells. This maintenance requires the specific conditions of the stem cell niche (see Chapter 8 and below) as well as cell-intrinsic properties. Long-term self-renewal in stem cells requires the activity of the enzyme telomerase, which counteracts the shortening of chromosome ends, the telomeres, that occurs during every cell division because the DNA polymerase misses the first nucleotides when synthesizing the new strand. Without telomerase activity this increasing loss of telomeres would limit the number of possible divisions without chromosomal damage. Telomerase activity is thus a characteristic of stem cells. Telomerases add repetitive noncoding DNA sequence to the ends of chromosomes. Telomerase activity has been detected in the SVZ and remained present at low levels even after cytostatic treatment, a finding consistent with the idea that relatively quiescent stem cells can survive such treatment. Telomerase activity has also been found to be regulated in association with the regulation of neurogenesis (Caporaso et al., 2003). Whereas telomerase activity is widespread during development, it is restricted to the regions of high proliferative activity in the adult brain. Adult neural stem cells, however, seem to rely on telomerase activity even more than stem cells from the embryonic brain, possibly because redundant protection mechanisms exist in the embryo (Ferron et al., 2004). In vitro, telomerase activity was down-regulated when differentiation of primary neuronal precursor cells was initiated (Haik et al., 2000; Ostenfeld et al., 2000). In regenerative tissues of telomerase null-mutants, cell proliferation was not abolished but reduced and cell death increased. This result further suggests that telomerase activity is necessary to maintain precursor cell proliferation over long periods of time and across generations (Lee et al., 1998; Herrera et al., 1999a, 1999b).

REGULATION OCCURS ON DIFFERENT CONCEPTUAL LEVELS

The use of only quantitative readouts for measuring the regulation of neurogenesis tends to blur the fact that regulation can occur during many different aspects of neuronal development and thus mechanistically can mean very different things. We can distinguish the following three levels:

- *Regulation on the level of function and behavior.* How does adult neurogenesis respond to the animal's behavior? Specifically, how do changes in the functional states of the olfactory system or the hippocampus that are related to certain behaviors affect adult neurogenesis?
- *Regulation on the level of cell–cell interactions.* Independent of the way in which the functional system detects the need for new neurons, how is the message conveyed to a precursor cell or a differentiating young neuron that it should divide, live or die, migrate, extend an axon and dendrites, or form synapses? What kind of extracellular signaling is involved in the regulation of adult neurogenesis?
- *Regulation on the level of the individual cell.* What is the nature of the intracellular signaling involved in the regulation of precursor cell activity and adult neurogenesis? Which genes are involved and how are they controlled? What are the transcriptional regulators? How do the many different signal transduction cascades interact in determining the next step in adult neurogenesis for the given cell?

For the full picture, one level cannot be understood without the others. Systematic distinctions might be necessary but they are artificial. Exposure to a complex environment, for example, stimulates adult hippocampal neurogenesis, but the ephemeral cognitive stimuli induced by the environment do not directly interfere with precursor cells. There is a network of regulatory pathways whose activation over many intermediate steps, supposedly in many different brain regions, ultimately leads to a particular change in the cellular niche engulfing the precursor cell. Such influences can come from neurotransmitters, hormones, growth factors, cell–cell contacts, extracellular matrix components, and others. Through intracellular second-messenger machinery, cells integrate across a large number of concurrent stimuli. These regulatory intracellular networks link activity at the many different receptors a cell carries as well as other intracellular events with the effects of transcription factors that interact with the DNA. Induction of proliferation is thus the consequence of a cell sensing a condition that is promitogenic and reacting to it accordingly. The same principle applies to the regulation of all consecutive stages of adult neurogenesis.

Reductionistic experimental settings tend to suggest that single, identifiable stimuli are necessary and sufficient to elicit certain responses in biological systems, although this is usually nothing more than a direct consequence of the experimental design. Epidermal growth factor, for example, is a strong mitogen in vitro and in vivo, but that does not mean that EGF is the one and only factor responsible for control of proliferation. Excess of EGF can override other stimuli and lack of EGF can block proliferation. Control, however, is more than all-or-nothing decisions. Control means integrating all available relevant stimuli. Nonspecific stimuli might override the complex pathways of specific regulation.

Although regulation of adult neurogenesis that deserves this name in the stricter sense should have an effect on net neurogenesis—that is, on the quantity (and possibly the quality) of new neurons—the target of regulation in the course of adult neuronal development can vary. Theoretically, any identifiable step during neuronal development can be subject to regulatory influences resulting in the net effect. Consequently, the degree to which the results of an experiment are meaningful depends on the specificity to which the readout is adjusted to the needs of the regulatory mechanism of interest. The impression that adult neurogenesis boldly and nonspecifically reacts to many different stimuli in an apparently identical way might be a problem of gross methodology.

In many studies, three key parameters of adult neurogenesis have been addressed: the proliferation of presumed precursor cells, the survival of their progeny, and the neuronal (vs. glial) differentiation of the new cells. By comparing neurogenesis in different strains of mice, i.e., mice who differ only in their genetic background but not in their experience and parameters such as age, it was found that these three stages are influenced differently by inheritable traits (Kempermann et al., 1997b; Kempermann and Gage, 2002a, 2002b). This finding also implies that these stages can be regulated with some degree of independence from each other.

An identical net effect on adult neurogenesis can thus result from many different combinations of effects on individual stages of development. Increased proliferation with decreased survival, for example, could lead to no net change at all. Decreased proliferation with much increased survival of the reduced progeny could still result in more new neurons at the end of the day. One thus cannot extrapolate information from effects on individual stages of neuronal development and apply this to net effects. Nevertheless, discrete and specific effects on neuronal development are relevant and conceptually might provide more useful information than the report of a generic net effect. Precise language needs to be used in such discussions. For the uninitiated reader, an effect on adult neurogenesis implies a measurable net effect on the number (or function) of new neurons. Subeffects during development without known consequences for this net neurogenesis need to be clearly identified as such. Effects on cell proliferation are interesting but not the same as an effect on adult neurogenesis.

REGULATION OF SYSTEMS AND BEHAVIOR

Stress

Stress might be the most notorious negative regulator of adult hippocampal neurogenesis. Historically, the first research on adult neurogenesis that captured the imagination of a wider circle of scientists had to do with the effects of stress on the brain. As reviewed in Chapter 2, Elizabeth Gould and Bruce McEwen's work on adult neurogenesis originated from the question of why stress did not lead to smaller hippocampal dentate gyri even though many dying cells could be detected (Gould et al., 1992; Gould and McEwen, 1993). Gould reasoned that the new neurons generated in adult hippocampal neurogenesis could be involved in maintaining this cellular balance. On the basis of the idea that stress hormone cortisol or corticosterone mediates stress effects, Gould published a first study in 1994 on the up-regulating effects of adrenalectomy and down-regulating effects of exogenous glucocorticoids on adult hippocampal neurogenesis (Cameron et al., 1993; Cameron and Gould, 1994). Two influential studies on the effects of psychosocial stress on adult neurogenesis in primates followed (Gould et al., 1997, 1998).

Since the publication of the first studies in 1992 and 1994, a number of other studies have confirmed the initial central finding: stress downregulates cell proliferation in the dentate gyrus and the consecutive stages of neuronal development, although much less is known about this latter stage. Prenatal stress has been found to have long-lasting effects on adult neurogenesis and appears to lower the baseline level of adult hippocampal neurogenesis (Lemaire et al., 2000; Coe et al., 2003). It is not known how persistent the effects of stress in adulthood are, but negative effects of even prolonged stress on adult hippocampal neurogenesis are reversible (Heine et al., 2004b).

From the available data it can be concluded that severe, acute stress dramatically decreases cell proliferation in the adult dentate gyrus. The experimental models that have been used to demonstrate this link have included psychosocial stress—for example, the resident-intruder model in territorial tree shrews (Gould et al., 1997; Czeh et al., 2002) (Fig. 9–3), predator odor

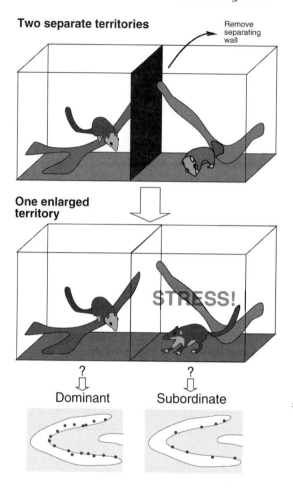

Two separate territories

Remove separating wall

One enlarged territory

STRESS!

? Dominant

? Subordinate

Figure 9–3. Resident intruder model of stress. In the resident intruder model of psychosocial stress, territorial tree shrews are confronted with another male in an enlarged territory. A dominant–subordinate relationship rapidly evolves that results in greater stress in the subordinate tree shrew, with elevated cortisol levels and reduced adult hippocampal neurogenesis (Gould et al., 1997).

(Tanapat et al., 2001), restraint (Pham et al., 2003), social isolation (Lu et al., 2003b), or electrical foot shocks in rodents (Malberg and Duman, 2003; Vollmayr et al., 2003). Importantly, these experimental paradigms usually consist of unusual, nonphysiological stress situations. Consequently, from the negative effects of severe stress on adult neurogenesis some researches have implicitly concluded that down-regulating effects on adult neuro-genesis are induced by any measure that is remotely stressful. However, many situations associated with mild to moderate and more chronic stress actually seem to increase adult neurogenesis. Voluntary physical activity and environmental enrichment are two prime examples of such conditions. In contrast, chronic mild stress has down-regulating effects on cell prolif-eration (Alonso et al., 2004). Although detailed experimental analysis is still lacking, it seems that the dose-response relationship between stress and adult neurogenesis follows an inverted-*U* curve. At low stress levels, experienced more as challenge, there is a positive effect; at high levels, a negative effect is seen. The details of this regulation are highly relevant because stress-related effects on the brain play an important role in current concepts on the cellular bases of psychiatric disorders and age-related cognitive decline. In Chapter 12 we will see how adult neurogenesis might fit into these concepts.

The biological key parameter for measuring stress in an organism is the serum level of the glucocorticoid hormones cortisol (in humans and nonhuman primates) or corticosterone (in rodents). High levels of stress lead to chronically high levels of glucocorticoids and over time to a failure of feedback mechanisms that control glucocorticoid secretion on the one hand and glucocorticoid receptor expression on the other. Depression, for example, is associated with disturbed regulation of cortisol levels, resulting in an abnormal circadian pattern of hormone secretion and chronically elevated glucocorticoid levels. Glucocorticoids as regulators of adult neurogenesis are discussed further below.

Stress also affects the number of sphere-forming cells that can be derived from the brain, which serves as an estimate of the number of neural precursor cells in the SVZ (Kippin et al., 2004). In one study, whereas prenatal stress decreased the number of spheres that could be generated at both postnatal day 1 and the age of 14 months, postnatal handling (as a paradigm with well-known positive effects on reducing stress responses [Meaney et al., 1991]) reversed this decline. Postnatal handling alone increased the yield of sphere-forming cells (Kippin et al., 2004). In contrast to this finding, the similarly stress-protective paradigm of preweaning enrichment did not have lasting effects on neurogenesis in the adult hippocampus in vivo (Kohl et al., 2002).

Odors

Odors are important carriers of information for many animals. For dogs, smelling is the primary way of extracting information from the outside world. Rodents, too, rely very much on their olfactory sense, although they complement it with tactile input from their whiskers. In experimental contexts, manipulation of the experience of odors is a paradigm that is relatively close to the animal's physiologic range of experience.

Odors can evoke stress in rodents. When rodents were exposed to fox odor and thus the smell of a natural enemy that preys upon them, severe stress reactions resulted that consequently led to a down-regulation of cell proliferation in the hippocampus (Tanapat et al., 2001).

But odors have other effects that relate to situations more within the physiological range of experiences. Neurogenesis in the olfactory bulb has sometimes been conceptualized as a consequence of high cellular turnover in the olfactory epithelium. Accordingly, the continuous exchange of primary olfactory neurons would call for a consecutive turnover in downstream neurons within the neuronal network of the olfactory system. Interestingly, however, adult neurogenesis in the olfactory bulb does not generate new second (projection) neurons but interneurons. Also, the olfactory bulb is not a topographical representation of the receptor neurons but a map of the many different receptor subtypes.

Nevertheless, damage to the olfactory epithelium has negative consequences for olfactory bulb neurogenesis (Chapter 5). Acutely, there is an increase in cell proliferation in the SVZ, the RMS, and especially the olfactory bulb that later gives way to a long-lasting decrease if the damage in the epithelium persists. It is tempting to believe that this negative regulation is due to sensory deprivation, a hypothesis supported by a number of arguments, but the lesion itself with its axonal damage might also have a lasting effect.

The net effect of decreased olfactory bulb neurogenesis is due to an interesting combination of effects on different stages of development. The axotomy of olfactory receptor neurons increased not only cell division in the SVZ but also cell death of the migrating neuroblasts. The two effects canceled each other out. Structural input to the olfactory bulb in the form of axons of the olfactory receptor neurons appears to be necessary to control the balance of cell birth and death in the regulation of adult olfactory bulb neurogenesis (Mandairon et al., 2003).

Similar effects can be observed in less invasive paradigms. Closure of one naris, which deprives the receptor neurons of olfactory stimuli, downregulated adult neurogenesis in the olfactory epithelium on the same side and secondarily decreases olfactory bulb neurogenesis (Corotto et al., 1994). This finding supports the hypothesis that beyond axonal integrity, the sensory activity itself is important for regulating adult olfactory bulb neurogenesis. However, sensory deprivation has been found to induce apoptosis in the olfactory glomeruli. Reopening of the closed naris caused a rebound in adult olfactory bulb neurogenesis (Cummings et al., 1997) and decreased cell death in the olfactory bulb (Fiske and Brunjes, 2001).

Even more compelling than these negative and compensatory effects are direct positive effects of odors on adult olfactory bulb neurogenesis. When Christelle Rochefort, Pierre-Marie Lledo, and colleagues from the Institut Pasteur in Paris exposed mice to a large number of odors over several days, they found that this enriched odor experience resulted in an increased number of BrdU-labeled neurons in the olfactory bulb at 3 weeks after BrdU injections (Rochefort et al., 2002). This result was interpreted as a survival-promoting effect, similar to the effects of environmental enrichment on adult hippocampal neurogenesis (see below). There was no effect of odor enrichment on cell proliferation in the SVZ and there was also no effect on adult neurogenesis in the hippocampus. Whereas olfactory enrichment was associated with improved olfactory learning, there was no effect on hippocampus-dependent learning.

Although the integrity of the olfactory bulb appears to be important in maintaining adult olfactory bulb neurogenesis, it is not clear how this regulation is mediated. It could be direct and local by increasing the attraction of migrating neuroblasts. This presumably chemical attractant could be sensitive to apoptotic cell death in the bulb, reducing migration and survival of incoming cells. The precursor cells in the SVZ would not be reached by these gradients. Alternatively, the effect could be mediated systemically by a similarly unknown humoral factor and a differential expression of the relevant receptors. Finally, regulation might occur through activity in the neuronal networks.

Enriched Environment and Learning

In 1997, the first report on a positive regulator of adult hippocampal neurogenesis was published and intriguingly, this up-regulation could be linked to hippocampal function. Mice living in an enriched environment had more new hippocampal granule cells than those of controls (Kempermann et al., 1997a) (Fig. 9–4). The same effect was later reported for rats as well (Nilsson et al., 1999). If the complexity of the enriched environment was experienced

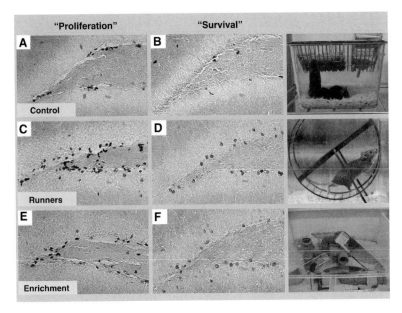

Figure 9–4. Environmental enrichment increases adult hippocampal neurogenesis. Exposure to an enriched environment has a survival-promoting effect on newly generated cells in the adult dentate gyrus; physical activity also induces precursor cell proliferation. The survival-promoting effect of environmental enrichment affects primarily young postmitotic neurons, whereas the pro-proliferative effect of wheel running has a strong effect on type-2 progenitor cells in the dentate gyrus. Both manipulations do not affect neurogenesis in the adult olfactory bulb.

in early adulthood, when adult hippocampal neurogenesis still generated a very high number of neurons, this increase in adult hippocampal neurogenesis led to a measurable increase in the absolute number of granule cells (Kempermann et al., 1997a). In C57Bl/6 mice this effect was due to a survival-promoting effect on the progeny of the dividing precursor cells in the SGZ (calretinin stage) but not to increased divisions of the precursor cells (Brandt et al., 2003; Kronenberg et al., 2003). However, this specificity was influenced by the genetic background. In contrast to C57BL/6, mouse strain 129/SvJ showed a strong induction of cell proliferation after environmental enrichment (Kempermann et al., 1998a). Because 129/SvJ mice have very low endogenous levels of adult neurogenesis, this resulted in a net induction that was similar in the two strains. In 129/SvJ mice, in contrast, environmental enrichment also affected cell proliferation. Inheritable traits thus influence the mechanism by which adult neurogenesis is regulated. It seems that when faced with a challenging situation, the hippocampus can activate its neurogenic resources to increase adult neurogenesis and can achieve this by different means. The survival-promoting effect of environmental enrichment was found to be diminished in presenilin-1 null-mutants (Feng et al., 2001).

Even in the absence of a pro-proliferative effect, environmental enrichment affected precursor cells in the SGZ identified by nestin–GFP expression. In the enriched living animals, the number of nestin-GFP-positive cells that also expressed transcription factor Prox1, which is expressed early during granule cell development and stays expressed in all mature granule cells, was significantly increased (Kronenberg et al., 2003). This suggests that the neurogenic effect of environmental enrichment reaches rather early stages of neuronal development, even if most of the survival-promoting factors will affect the later stages.

Environmental enrichment is a very straightforward experimental concept that historically has taught much about activity-dependent brain plasticity (Chapter 2). An enriched environment typically consists of a larger cage, larger groups of animals, toys, and, for example, a tunnel system that is rearranged frequently. In some of the early experiments, changes in diet were also part of the experimental program (because it was assumed that cheese would be most appropriate for enriching mice). This led some readers to believe that dietary factors were the main mediators of the effect of an enriched environment. However, when identical food was given to enriched animals and controls, the results of enrichment on adult neurogenesis were maintained (Kempermann et al., 1998a, 1998b). Ironically, diet can influence adult hippocampal neurogenesis. Caloric restriction is a classic experimental paradigm in which rodents receive about one-third less food than what they would eat on their own and is the only manipulation known to prolong life. In addition, caloric restriction induced cell proliferation in the dentate gyrus (Lee et al., 2000a, 2002). Caloric restriction might be one of the mild stressors alluded to above that have a positive effect on adult neurogenesis, but the mechanism might be more complicated. Given the effects on life span, it might also be that caloric restriction slows the age-dependent decrease in adult neurogenesis.

The effects of environmental enrichment on adult neurogenesis were maintained in old age: here, the relative increase was even larger than in younger age, although the absolute numbers of new neurons were very low (Kempermann et al., 1998b). More details about the effects of environmental enrichment on age-dependent decrease in adult neurogenesis are discussed below.

Independent of nutrition it is not known which of the many potential components of an enriched environment are responsible for the neurogenic effects. We hypothesize, however, that the key stimuli are complexity and novelty (Kempermann, 2002; Kempermann and Wiskott, 2004). In this sense, experiencing an enriched environment could be a form of continued learning. In fact, more or less isolated learning stimuli have been reported to have a similar survival-promoting effect on adult hippocampal neurogenesis to that of environmental enrichment (Gould et al., 1999; Leuner et al., 2004). One study found a complex effect on late stages of the downward-sloping survival curve of new hippocampal neurons in rats and a small but specific increase in cell proliferation (Dobrossy et al., 2003). In other modifications of the experimental settings, however, other groups could not detect such effects (van Praag et al., 1999b; Ambrogini et al., 2004b), so the question of whether learning per se can directly recruit new neurons into function remains open. The central problem is that learning as a stimulus cannot be presented in a pure form and always is embedded in situations that by themselves might influence neurogenesis by additional means. Whether learning is a form of environmental enrichment or whether experience of enrichment is a form of learning remains undecided. The idea that learning could have a survival-promoting effect on newly generated cells, however, is in line with current concepts about the functional relevance of adult hippocampal neurogenesis (Chapter 10).

Environmental enrichment has a strong neurogenic effect on the hippocampus, but no effect on adult olfactory bulb neurogenesis (Brown et al., 2003). These results are the opposite of effects of olfactory enrichment (Rochefort et al., 2002).

Physical Activity

Rodents provided with a running wheel in their cage make extensive use of this opportunity to exercise during their active period of the day. As nocturnal animals, mice run as much as 3 to 8 kilometers a night, an amount that has been estimated to reflect natural physical activity. Voluntary physical activity is a very robust inducer of adult neurogenesis (Van Praag et al., 1999a, 1999b). Running has an acute and strong effect on cell proliferation that wears off over a number of days and weeks (Fig. 9–4). This mitogenic effect affects primarily type-2 progenitor cells in the hippocampus (Kronenberg et al., 2003). There is an independent effect on subsequent stages of neuronal development, most importantly a survival-promoting effect. The increase in adult hippocampal neurogenesis is accompanied by increased long-term potentiation (LTP) in the dentate gyrus and improved performance in the hippocampus-dependent learning task of the Morris water maze (Van Praag et al., 1999a). Like environmental enrichment (Kempermann et al., 2002), prolonged physical activity maintains adult hippocampal neurogenesis on a higher level and thus slows the age-dependent decline. There are two different, activity-dependent effects: one acute that affects cell proliferation and is transient, and one that affects the stem cell niche as a whole and is long-lasting. If voluntary wheel-running is interpreted less as exercise and more as a way to measure the level of intrinsic activity (as the paradigm is widely used in research on circadian rhythms) an additional aspect becomes apparent. There is an activity-dependent component in the regulation of adult hippocampal neurogenesis that is not related to physical exercise itself, because circadian phase, and thus activity in a more general sense, also correlates with levels of adult hippocampal neurogenesis (Holmes et al., 2004). At least under acute conditions, forced physical activity on a treadmill seems to have similar effects on cell proliferation (Trejo et al., 2001; Ra et al., 2002; Kim et al., 2004).

Details of the mechanisms underlying the effects of physical activity on adult neurogenesis have not yet been unraveled. Growth factors, most notably insulin-like growth factor-1 (IGF-1), have been discussed as key mediators because IGF-1, like other growth factors (Gomez-Pinilla et al., 1997), is increased in running animals, and the running-induced increase in cell proliferation can be blocked by scavenging circulating IGF-1 and is missing in IGF-1 null-mutants (Carro et al., 2000; Trejo et al., 2001). Similarly, but also contradicting the solitary role of IGF-1, blockade of vascular endothelial growth factor (VEGF) prevents the induction of cell proliferation and adult neurogenesis (Fabel et al., 2003).

One conceptual problem is to define activity. Like function, which will be considered in the next chapter, activity has different (although often related) meanings on different conceptual levels. Equating the reductionistic physical activity in rodents with exercise in humans might be a misleading simplification. Arguably, most aspects of cognition in a rodent are inseparable from physical activity. Exploration, spatial navigation, and most types of learning accessible in a rodent are based on physical activity. Only language would allow a separation of motor and cognitive activity and something like pure thought (and even executed language is arguably a motor activity). This consideration might seem far-fetched, but the finding of running-induced neurogenesis appears less counterintuitive if one regards physical activity as a basis for cognition. In line with this speculation, it is very likely that serotonin and N-methyl-D-asparatate (NMDA) receptor–dependent mechanisms contribute to the proneurogenic effect of physical activity. In vitro,

NMDA receptor–mediated pathways are involved in determining the state of activation of neural precursor cells and consequently influence the cell's behavior and potential (Deisseroth et al., 2004). Walking has a noted effect on LTP, the electrophysiological correlate of learning (Leung et al., 2003), and it is thought that the induction of theta rhythms in the brain, which is promoted by repetitive regular movements, might underlie this finding. The direct link between theta waves (or other endogenous oscillations) and the regulation of adult neurogenesis has not yet been made.

Surprisingly, voluntary physical activity does not influence neurogenesis in the olfactory system (Brown et al., 2003). Cell proliferation in other brain regions without evidence of adult neurogenesis is regulated by exercise, but the patterns are complex and not yet fully understood (Ehninger and Kempermann, 2003).

Age

The strongest known negative regulator of adult hippocampal neurogenesis is age. This decrease over time is not linear but almost hyperbolic. Joseph Altman's first complete description of adult hippocampal neurogenesis in 1965 already contained an account of this decrease over months in the life of rodents (Altman and Das, 1965). Several studies have confirmed this initial report for both rats (Seki and Arai, 1995; Kuhn et al., 1996; Cameron and McKay, 1999; Bizon and Gallagher, 2003) and mice (Kempermann et al., 1998b).

A stereological longitudinal study linking this decline to other morphological, biochemical, and molecular parameters and the total number of granule cells is still lacking. In any case, adult neurogenesis has the highest level in early adulthood, during and after puberty, and quickly decreases thereafter. Figure 6–8 displays a rough estimate of the quantitative relations. Importantly, however, even in very old age, adult neurogenesis can be detected, although the levels are very low. The nonlinearity of the decline precludes simple calculations of lifetime gains in neuron numbers based one snapshot measurement of adult neurogenesis. The estimates from studies based on quantification in young rodents consequently tend to be too high.

The finding that adult neurogenesis declines but does not completely disappear with age apparently also applies to humans, in whom adult hippocampal neurogenesis was detected in postmortem samples from 72-year-old individuals (Eriksson et al., 1998).

Environmental enrichment is also effective in regulating adult hippocampal neurogenesis in old age. In relative terms, the effect was even stronger than in young animals (Kempermann et al., 1998b). It seems that the functional stimulus provided by environmental complexity previously unknown to an animal challenged adult neurogenesis to deliver the maximum number of new neurons possible.

Even in the absence of significant inductions of cell proliferation, in most experiments with enriched environments cell counts in the enriched animals have tended to be somewhat higher than those in controls. In mice exposed to an enriched environment for 3 months and returned afterwards to standard housing for an additional 3 months this difference became significant (Kempermann and Gage, 1999). It appears that early stimulation of adult neurogenesis as a result of experiencing an enriched environment maintained neurogenesis at levels corresponding roughly to those of this much earlier age and the stimulation thus counteracted the age effect. Even withdrawal for 3 months after environmental enrichment did not allow these animals to catch up with the age-related decline in precursor cell proliferation witnessed in the control mice.

This finding was confirmed when adult hippocampal neurogenesis was studied in mice that lived the second half of their life, from age 10 to 20 months, in an enriched environment (Kempermann et al., 2002). Although the environment might have been more complex than that for controls, the aspect of novelty disappeared during this chronic paradigm. These long-term-enriched mice not only had less age pigment in their dentate granule cells (and thus presumably a biologically younger hippocampus), their rate of adult hippocampal neurogenesis also corresponded to that of a much younger age. The baseline level was five times as high as that in controls. Both sustained physical and cognitive activity might underlie this effect.

Insulin-like growth factor-1 is one of the possible key mediators in the effects of physical activity on adult hippocampal neurogenesis (Carro et al., 2000; Trejo et al., 2001). Similarly, exogenous application of IGF-1 to restore endogenous levels of IGF-1 associated with younger age acutely counteracted the age-dependent decrease in adult hippocampal neurogenesis (Lichtenwalner et al., 2001). Although a long-term experiment has not yet been done, the correlative result nonetheless suggests that a reduction in neurogenic signals should contribute to the age-dependent decrease in adult neurogenesis.

Conversely, and as in the case of stress, chronically increased levels of corticosteroids have been proposed to be the main negative mediators of age-dependent loss of adult hippocampal neurogenesis. Indeed, Cameron and coworkers showed that adrenalectomy was able to restore adult neurogenesis to a level similar to that of a much younger age (Cameron and McKay, 1999). On the other hand, age-dependent decline is not necessarily associated with increased corticosterone levels (Heine et al., 2004a). With increasing age, the expression of corticosteroids receptors in the course of neuronal development shifts to more immature stages, which suggests that in older age, adult neurogenesis might become more sensitive to corticocorticoid action (Garcia et al., 2004).

Chronological age, and thus time by itself, is unlikely to be a regulator of neurogenesis, but many changes associated with age might influence neuronal development in the adult. For example, the stem cell niche and its vascular component are substantially affected by age. Also, the number of precursor cells that can be isolated from the adult brain decreases with increasing age (Maslov et al., 2004), although a contradicting report does not support this idea (Goldman et al., 1997).

Seizures

Seizures are synchronized hyperexcitation in neuronal networks. Clinically, several classes of seizures can be distinguished, depending on the site of origin and the symptoms. In the context of adult hippocampal neurogenesis, generalized seizures as models of temporal lobe epilepsy are of particular relevance. The more medical aspects are discussed in Chapter 12. The induction of seizures can be achieved by systemic or local application of, for example, kainic acid (KA), which causes hyperexcitation via glutamate receptors of the KA type, or by inhibiting GABAergic inhibition with pentylenetetrazole. The common principle is a massive overactivity of excitatory synapses. Other models are variations of this principle. Independent of the chosen experimental paradigm, seizures invariably cause a strong induction of cell proliferation in the adult hippocampus (Bengzon et al., 1997; Parent et al., 1997; Scott et al., 1998, 2000; Madsen et al., 2000; Nakagawa et al., 2000; Jiang et al., 2003) (Fig. 9–5). This increase is followed by a similar rise in net neurogenesis, leading to long-lasting presence of new neurons. Using a glial fibrillary acidic protein–green fluorescent protein (GFAP-GFP) reporter mouse, it was found that seizures induce proliferation of GFAP-positive cells (Huttmann et al., 2003). At 4 weeks after BrdU and KA injections, a significantly increased number of calretinin-expressing cells was found (Brandt et al., 2003). It is not yet known, which stage of neuronal development is primarily affected by seizure-activity. It seems likely that type-2 and -3 cells, which receive synaptic input, are responsible for the massive expansion of dividing cells. In addition, seizures seem to interfere with other aspects of adult neurogenesis. Migration is disturbed, leading to ectopic granule cells near CA3 (Scharfman et al., 2000). This effect might be relevant to explaining the so-called granule cell dispersion found in many patients with temporal lobe epilepsy.

The degree to which disturbed adult hippocampal neurogenesis is responsible for propagating seizures is not clear. When precursor cell proliferation was blocked by irradiation (see below), the sprouting of mossy fibers that is characteristic for temporal lobe epilepsy still occurred (Parent et al., 1999). This finding suggests that overinduced neurogenesis is not solely responsible for structural and subsequent functional abnormalities.

In a model of electroconvulsive seizures (with externally applied electrodes), the induction of precursor cell proliferation was paralleled by an induction of endothelial proliferation in the SGZ (Hellsten et al., 2004). Other components of the precursor cell niche have not yet been studied in detail, but it is likely that after seizures profound structural alterations in the stem

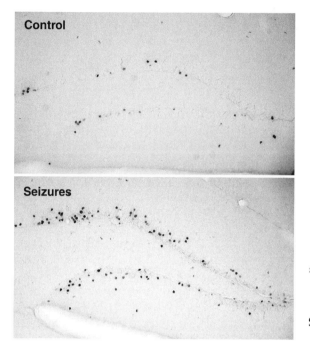

Figure 9–5. Epileptic seizures induce cell proliferation in the adult dentate gyrus. Systemic application of glutamate receptor agonist kainic acid strongly up-regulates cell proliferation in the subgranular zone. Image by Sebastian Jessberger, La Jolla CA.

cell niche are found. Experimental seizures also affected neurogenesis in the olfactory bulb (Parent et al., 2002a).

Ischemia and Hypoxia

The effects of ischemia and hypoxia have been studied primarily in the context of animal models for stroke. They will be discussed in greater detail in Chapter 12. Ischemia causes a complex response of local precursor cells in the neurogenic and non-neurogenic zones of the adult brain (Fig. 9–6). Cell proliferation in the SGZ has been found to be induced in many models of ischemic brain injury (Takagi et al., 1999; Liu et al., 2000; Arvidsson et al., 2001; Iwai et al., 2001; Jin et al., 2001; Kee et al., 2001; Yagita et al., 2001; Komitova et al., 2002; Takasawa et al., 2002). This effect is seen even in the absence of direct visible damage to the hippocampus, supporting the idea that not just gross local regulatory mechanisms apply (Arvidsson et al., 2001). This increase in cell proliferation is NMDA receptor activation–dependent (Arvidsson et al., 2001).

A number of studies have reported regenerative neurogenesis in non-neurogenic regions after ischemia (Arvidsson et al., 2002; Nakatomi et al., 2002; Parent et al., 2002b, see Chapter 8). The important problem of falsely identifying BrdU incorporation in dying neurons as evidence of neurogenesis applies to both non-neurogenic and neurogenic regions (Kuan et al.,

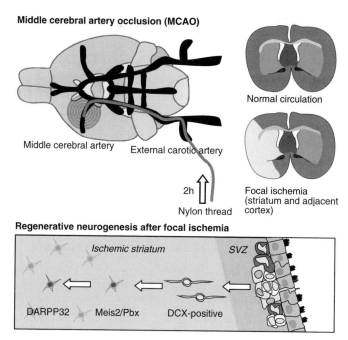

Figure 9–6. Regenerative neurogenesis after ischemia. Middle cerebral artery occlusion induced regenerative neurogenesis in the striatum (Arvidsson et al., 2002). Precursor cells migration in from the subventricular zone (SVZ) resulted in a low level of neuronal replacement. The new cells went through an identifiable intermediate stage of development depicted in Figure 9–7 (Color Plate 12), a result arguing against the concern that neurons dying in response to ischemia had taken up BrdU and were falsely identified as new. DCX, doublecortin.

2004; see also Chapter 7) but in non-neurogenic regions, proof of these regenerative neurogenesis is much harder to find, because no undisputed baseline exist. There is little doubt, however, that ischemia and hypoxia can influence precursor cells and adult neurogenesis in neurogenic regions. Blockade of CREB, for example, inhibited ischemia-induced neurogenesis in the dentate gyrus of rats (Zhu et al., 2004), an effect that would not be observable in a case of falsely detected cell death. Otherwise, evidence of neuronal development, e.g., in the sense of a marker progression, can circumvent this problem because dying cells would not show signs of gradual maturation.

A study by Andreas Arvidsson, Olle Lindvall and colleagues from Lund University is particularly noteworthy in this context, because the ischemia-induced generation of new striatal neurons was followed over different stages of development. About 2 weeks after the insult, the attracted migrating cells expressed transcription factors Pbx and Meis2 (Fig. 9–7, Color Plate 12), which are characteristic for the development of medium spiny

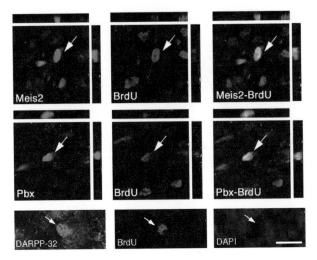

Figure 9–7 (Color Plate 12). Regenerative neurogenesis after ischemia. During ischemia-induced regenerative neurogenesis in the adult striatum, the new neurons went through an intermediate transient stage, at which they expressed transcription factors Pbx and Meis2. Mature neurons expressed DARP-32. See text and Figure 9–6 for details. Figure from Arvidsson et al. (2002), reprinted with kind permission of Olle Lindvall, Lund, and *Nature Medicine*.

interneurons in the striatum (Toresson et al., 2000). About 2 or 3 weeks later, the new cells expressed DARPP-32, a marker of mature striatal neurons (Arvidsson et al., 2002; Parent et al., 2002b). This result is perplexing because the neuronal phenotypes into which SVZ cells normally differentiate are interneurons in the olfactory bulb. These express neither Pbx and Meis2 during development nor DARPP-32 in their mature condition. This point is similarly surprising in the study by Nakatomi et al. (2002), in which SVZ cells obviously differentiated into yet another neuronal phenotype, pyramidal neurons in CA1, which are glutamatergic principal neurons, not interneurons. The key question is thus how this phenotypic specification is achieved.

Additional studies have reported specifically cortical neurogenesis after stroke (Gu et al., 2000; Jiang et al., 2001), but they are contradicted by other studies that did not find new neurons in or around the ischemic cortex (Arvidsson et al., 2002; Parent et al., 2002b).

As in other cases of pathology-induced plasticity, NMDA receptor activation seems to play a prominent role in mediating the neurogenic response to stroke. Blockade of NMDA receptors prevented the induction of hippocampal neurogenesis in both global and focal ischemia models (Bernabeu and Sharp, 2000; Arvidsson et al., 2001).

Hypoxia induces a number of factors that might underlie the neurogenic response to ischemia, including erythropoetin (Shingo et al., 2001), VEGF

(Jin et al., 2002c; Schanzer et al., 2004), stem cell factor (Jin et al., 2002a), and heparin-binding EGF (Jin et al., 2002b). The receptors for all of these are expressed in the SVZ, making their involvement plausible. Their relative contributions and the necessity of their involvement in the regulation remain unclear, however. Nitric oxide (NO) might also take part in ischemia-induced induction of adult hippocampal neurogenesis, because inhibition of inducible nitric oxide synthase (iNOS) or an iNOS null mutation blocked the increase in neurogenesis (Zhu et al., 2003).

Brain-derived neurotrophic factor is another likely candidate mediator of the neurogenic response to stroke. In the healthy rat, infusion of BDNF into the ventricle and overexpression of BDNF through use of an adenovirus were reported to not only increase neurogenesis in the olfactory bulb but also induce neurogenesis in the striatum (Zigova et al., 1998; Benraiss et al., 2001; Pencea et al., 2001). Under ischemic conditions, however, no proneurogenic effect of BDNF overexpression in the striatum was found (Larsson et al., 2002). It therefore remains to be discovered whether ischemia-induced tissue conditions counteract BDNF action. Blockage of BDNF action in vivo by means of a TrkB fusion protein (TrkB being the receptor for BDNF) increased neuronal differentiation after ischemia without affecting cell proliferation (Gustafsson et al., 2003).

Ischemia can also damage precursor cells. When neonatal rats were exposed to ischemia persistent damage to the SVZ resulted. Interestingly, oligodendrocyte precursor cells, which are very numerous at this stage of brain development, were particularly vulnerable to ischemia. This resulted in white matter defects and a reduced SVZ (Levison et al., 2001; Back et al., 2002). That precursor cells show such a marked sensitivity dependent on the developmental stage might underlie the neurological consequences of hypoxia in utero or during birth.

Irradiation

In cell culture, irradiation blocks proliferation of neural precursor cells (Palmer et al., 2000). Gamma- and X-rays damage DNA so extensively during mitosis that endogenous repair mechanisms are overwhelmed and apoptotic elimination is induced. In vivo, exposure to X-rays efficiently wiped out cell proliferation from the SGZ (Parent et al., 1999; Monje et al., 2002; Santarelli et al., 2003; Raber et al., 2004). The sensitivity of the precursor cells in vivo was dose-dependent and caused long-lasting damage (Mizumatsu et al., 2003; Rola et al., 2004a). Irradiation not only ablated cell proliferation but also caused gliosis in the stem cell niche of the adult hippocampus (Monje et al., 2002). In addition, angiogenesis in the SGZ, normally associated with adult neurogenesis, was diminished, whereas the number of microglia increased. A large part of the damage to the stem cell niche after irradiation is due to inflammation and microglia activation (Monje et al., 2003). Irradiation-induced disturbance of adult neurogenesis might have profound medical implications because it might contribute to long-term cognitive impairment after brain irradiation (Raber et al., 2004; Rola et al., 2004b; see Chapter 12).

Irradiation has been used to block adult hippocampal neurogenesis for experimental purposes (Parent et al., 1999). The effects of antidepressants on both anxiety-related behavior and adult hippocampal neurogenesis were eliminated in mice in which the hippocampus had been irradiated (Santarelli et al., 2003) (see also Fig. 10–4). Fractionated irradiation also reduced performance in a hippocampus-dependent learning task (Madsen et al., 2003a). In both cases, effects of X-rays beyond the direct damage to precursor cells are difficult to rule out (and actually very likely), but the findings are nevertheless compelling. The link between irradiation-induced effects and inflammation, for example, should lead to the discovery of other indirect but related pathogenic mechanisms related to a disturbance of the stem cell niche.

Because highly proliferative cells are more sensitive to radiation damage than postmitotic and quiescent cells, irradiation should primarily affect the transiently amplifying progenitor cells and only to a lesser degree, the stem cells (Mizumatsu et al., 2003; Limoli et al., 2004). The proposed mechanism of irradiation-induced precursor cell dysfunction, besides inflammation, is an increased sensitivity to oxidative stress as well as an increase in the phosphorylation of cell cycle–associated protein transformation-related protein 53 (Trp53), which leads to higher rates of apoptosis (Limoli et al., 2004). Consequently, precursor cells in Trp53 null-mutant mice were less sensitive to irradiation than wild types.

CELL–CELL COMMUNICATION

The Stem Cell Niche

One of the most influential ideas in neural stem cell biology in vivo has been the concept of the stem cell niche (see also Chapters 3 and 8). This niche can be thought of as the functional unit of stem cell biology, consisting of the precursor cells and those cells that form the permissive microenvironment. The niche itself is a structure, not a regulatory mechanism. It is the place where cell-to-cell communication occurs and where the precursor cells receive local regulatory cues. The stem cell niche is the smallest and foremost unit of interaction between precursor cells and the environment.

Dividing cells in the neurogenic regions, particularly in older animals, are not evenly distributed (Kuhn et al., 1996). Through labeling of proliferating cells with BrdU over a number of consecutive days, one finds that the dividing cells form clusters. In these clusters, cells at different stages of neuronal development are found. Theo D. Palmer described the close relationship of these clusters to blood vessels in the adult dentate gyrus and formulated the theory of a vascular niche for precursor cells in the adult brain (Palmer et al., 2000). The type-1 cells, the putative stem cells of this region, have vascular endfeet and are thus particularly suited to react to blood-borne factors (Filippov et al., 2003). The degree to which they do so is not known. The vascular endfeet of normal astrocytes induce the blood–brain barrier. There normal function does not seem to be primarily the uptake of circulating factors.

In the SVZ, the formation of clusters is less prominent and here the relationship to blood vessels is not as obvious as in the SGZ. However, the ventricle plays a comparable role: B cells of the SVZ have a cilia-bearing process that reaches the ventricular surface. Here again, it is not known if and how putative circulating regulators enter the niche through these cells.

During development, cell–cell contact between progenitor or immature cells plays an important role in the communication between cells. For example, in *Drosophila*, cell communication through adherens junctions controls the proliferation of stem cells in the germline (Spradling et al., 2001). Because adherens junctions contain β-catenin, which is an important downstream part of Wnt signaling (see below), a similar role in maintenance of the precursor cell niche in the adult brain is conceivable.

Gap junctions allow communication between neural cells before the appearance of chemical synapses. Small molecules and electrical currents can cross the cell membrane between coupled cells. In the developing neocortex, immature cells form a functional syncytium—a nonsynaptic system for neuronal communication. There are many examples from embryology in which precursor cells can be coupled (Bittman et al., 1997), including hippocampal progenitor cells in vitro (Rozental et al., 1995, 1998). In the postnatal SVZ of rats, cell coupling has been visualized by dye effusion from one cell to the other (Menezes et al., 2000), although the range of coupled cell types and the reasons for the varying degree of coupling have not yet been determined. Connexins are molecules involved in the formation of gap junctions. As one example, in the SGZ, NG2-positive oligodendrocyte precursor cells but not GFAP-positive cells expressed connexin-32. In the connexin-32 null-mutant mouse, the turnover of NG2-positive cells in the SGZ was increased (Melanson-Drapeau et al., 2003).

The concept of the stem cell niche is covered in greater detail in Chapter 8. Surface molecules that appear to play key roles in mediating regulation based on cell-to-cell contacts, such as PSA-NCAM, are discussed in Chapters 5, 6, and 8.

Immune Cells and Inflammatory Cytokines

Microglia, one of the cell types that constitute the stem cell niche, are the immune-competent cells of the brain. They are activated by many pathological stimuli and can secrete factors associated with inflammation. Very little is known about their function in the absence of pathology. Michelle Monje, Theo Palmer, and colleagues found that reduction in adult neurogenesis inflicted by irradiation or injection of bacterial lipopolysaccharide (LPS) can be reversed and normal levels restored by treating the irradiated animals with a common anti-inflammatory drug, indomethacin (Monje et al., 2003) (Fig. 9–8). The number of activated microglia correlated with the amount of damage. Christine Ekdahl, Olle Lindvall, and colleagues from Lund University in Sweden showed that microglia activation after LPS injections is detrimental to adult hippocampal neurogenesis (Ekdahl et al., 2003). Inhibition of microglia prevented the damage. In cell culture, activated (but not resting) microglia inhibited neuronal development from neural precursor cells. One of the humoral mediators that is a likely candidate for being prominently involved in eliciting such effects is interleukin-6 (Il-6). Overexpression of Il-6 in astrocytes strongly decreased adult hippocampal neurogenesis, but left gliogenesis and glial cell counts unaffected (Vallieres et al., 2002). In vitro, cytokines influence neuronal development of hippocampal precursor cells (Mehler et al., 1993) and Il-6 can steer development of cortical precursor cells to an astrocytic fate (Bonni et al., 1997). This fate shift, as well as direct effects on precursor cell proliferation or survival mechanisms, might help to explain the negative effects of inflammatory processes on adult hippocampal neurogenesis. On the other hand, microglia might also have positive, trophic effects. For example, BDNF can be secreted by microglia. And at least in some cortical regions, microglia was induced to proliferate through physical activity in the absence of pathological stimuli (Ehninger and Kempermann, 2003). Although there is little doubt that inflammation acts negatively on adult neurogenesis, the potentially double-edged role of microglia in the control of adult neurogenesis remains to be elucidated.

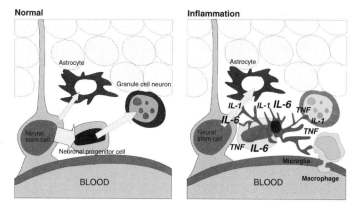

Figure 9–8. Effects of inflammation on adult neurogenesis. Inflammation inhibits adult neurogenesis through microglial activation and secreted inflammatory molecules. Gliogenesis is increased. Anti-inflammatory treatment and depletion of microglia prevented this effect. (Monje et al., 2003; Ekdahl et al., 2003). IL, interleukin; TNF, tumor necrosis factor.

Another class of inflammatory molecules potentially involved in the regulation of adult neurogenesis are prostaglandins (Uchida et al., 2002). Inhibition of prostaglandin synthesis with acetyl salicilic acid led to a reduction in ischemia-induced cell proliferation (Kumihashi et al., 2001). The rate-limiting enzyme in prostaglandin synthesis in the brain is cyclooxygenase-2 (COX2). COX2 knockout mice and the pharmacological inhibition of COX2 caused a reduction in ischemia-induced up-regulation of cell proliferation in the SGZ, but did not have a significant effect under physiological conditions (Sasaki et al., 2003).

In cell cultures of neural progenitor cell lines from humans and rodents, various types of cytokines are expressed (Klassen et al., 2003). It is not clear, however, to what degree this expression pattern is directly dependent on culture conditions.

Corticosteroid Hormones

Corticosteroids play a complex modulatory role in adult hippocampal neurogenesis (Table 9–1). It was first hypothesized that both the stress-induced and the age-dependent decline in hippocampal neurogenesis might be due to the accumulated negative effects of endogenous corticosteroids. Adrenalectomy, a radical experimental way of abolishing glucocorticoid effects, has been shown to prevent some of the age-related losses in adult neurogenesis (Cameron and McKay, 1999). Similarly, stress-induced responses in adult neurogenesis were reduced (Tanapat et al., 2001). At first glance, this finding might seem confusing because adrenalectomy also induces cell death in the hippocampus (Gould et al., 1991). However, it is primarily the older cells and cells outside the dentate gyrus whose death rate is increased, not necessarily the new neurons in the dentate gyrus (Cameron and Gould, 1996). The mature and developing cells differ in their glucocorticoid receptor expression and thus presumably in their sensitivity to corticosterone (Cameron et al., 1993; Garcia et al., 2004). Cell generation and cell death have to be balanced during adult neuronal development, because elimination of surplus cells is one of the key mechanisms in controlling adult neurogenesis quantitatively and, presumably, qualitatively. Corticosteroids are good candidates for being centrally involved in regulating this balance by adjusting the baseline level of cell proliferation, survival, and differentiation. Many details, however, are still lacking in how this differential regulation is achieved and how corticosterone interacts with other regulatory factors. Adrenalectomy after cell division increased the survival of BrdU-labeled cells, whereas exogenous corticosterone decreased it. Adrenalectomy before cell division, in contrast, decreased cell survival (Wong and Herbert, 2004).

There are also many open questions regarding the dose–response relationship between corticosterone and adult neurogenesis. There is no strict correlation between serum corticosterone levels and adult hippocampal neurogenesis. But acute and strong stress (and therefore acute and strong

Table 9–1. Effects of Corticosterone on Adult Hippocampal Neurogenesis

Reference	Aged?	Species	Model	Receptor Block	Exogenous Application of	Effect on Cell Proliferation	Other Effects
Cameron and Gould, 1994	No	Rat			Corticosterone	(−)	
			Adrenalectomy			(+)	
					Corticosterone	No effect	
Gould et al., 1997	No	Tree shrew	Psychosocial stress			(−)	
				NMDA		(+)	
Cameron et al., 1998	No	Rat	Adrenalectomy	NMDA		Prevents decrease	
					NMDA agonist	Blocks increase	
Cameron and McKay, 1999	Yes	Rat	Adrenalectomy			(+)	Net neurogenesis (+)
Montaron et al., 1999)	Yes	Rat	Adrenalectomy			(+)	PSA (+)
					Corticosterone	Blocks increase	No effect on PSA
Montaron et al., 2003	No	Rat	Adrenalectomy		Low-dose aldosterone	No effect.	Reduced death of mature cells
					High dose aldosterone	Blocks increase	No effect on PSA
					GR agonist		Normalizes PSA

(+), increase; (−), decrease; GR, gluticocorticoid receptor; NMDA, *N*-methyl-ᴅ-aspartate; PSA, PSA-NCAM.

increases in blood corticosterone) lead to the described down-regulation of adult neurogenesis. Chronic and more moderate increases in corticosteroids, in contrast, seem to have no or even the opposite effect. In aged rats that were not adrenalectomized, a dissociation between the number of new cells and corticosterone levels was found (Heine et al., 2004a). Many physiological situations associated with increased adult neurogenesis are accompanied by high, not low, serum corticosterone levels. This apparent paradox can only be explained by a differential sensitivity of different cells to corticosteroids. This in turn implies that corticosterone effects on adult neurogenesis are at least to some degree controlled or modulated by other regulatory instances.

Corticosterone acts through two receptors with different binding affinity. These are the glucocorticoid receptor (GR, or glucorticoid receptor I) and the mineralocorticoid receptor (MR, or glucocorticoid receptor II). The GR is abundantly expressed throughout the brain but enriched in the hippocampus; the MR is found primarily in the hippocampus. Both receptors are expressed on the nuclear membrane. In hippocampal granule cells (and some other neuronal populations), GR and MR co-localize. Functionally, both receptors can heterodimerize and alone or together they act as hormone-activated transcription factors. To put it simply, the GR mediates relatively acute and suppressive responses, and the MR mediates more tonic and lasting, conducive corticoid effects (Sapolsky et al., 2000). This difference in function might help to explain why acute and chronic corticosteroid effects on adult hippocampal neurogenesis differ: acute increases in corticosterone decrease cell proliferation, whereas lasting increases are actually compatible with elevated proliferation rates. These respective proliferation rates may result from the fact that the MR is not expressed on proliferating hippocampal precursor cells but only on mature cells, whereas the GR is also found at the earliest progenitor stages, including type-2a, cells, which is the population responsible for quantitative expansion (Garcia et al., 2004). Along with this observation, treatment with MR agonist aldosterone has been found to be associated with increased cell survival, albeit in a model of adrenalectomy-induced cell death (Montaron et al., 1999). Conditional MR knockout mice in which the receptor was eliminated only in the brain had a reduced level of adult neurogenesis and lower total number of granule cells (Gass et al., 2000), consistent with the idea that MR activation might have a survival-promoting effect on new neurons.

The GR, in contrast, is expressed on precursor cells, except for type-2b cells, but to a variable degree. Aged animals tend to have relatively more cells that express the GR at different stages, which might explain the strong effects of manipulating the corticoid level on neurogenesis in aging. In aged rats, for example, adrenalectomy caused an increase in neurogenesis that could be counteracted by treating the animals with corticosterone (Montaron et al., 1999). The number of polysialylated acid–neural cell adhesion molecule (PSA-NCAM)-expressing cells, which was also elevated after adrenalectomy, in contrast, was not affected by exogenously applied corticosterone. Blockage of the GR in younger rats, however, restored the number of PSA-NCAM-positive cells in the adrenalectomy model (Montaron et al., 1999). Conditional brain-specific GR knockout mice did not have altered levels of adult neurogenesis or total granule cell numbers (Gass et al., 2000).

In vitro, GR activation was sufficient to suppress divisions of fetal hippocampal progenitor cells (Yu et al., 2004). However, at present it is not clear whether glucocorticoid-dependent regulation of adult neurogenesis is due to direct effects on precursor cells. Indirect pathways within the hippocampal stem cell niche might be involved as well and even predominate. On the basis of receptor immunohistochemistry one can even hypothesize that neuronal differentiation occurs physiologically in the absence of GR expression on the developing cells and thus is presumably insensitive to direct corticosterone action (Garcia et al., 2004).

The effects of glucocorticoids on cell proliferation are dependent on NMDA receptor activity. If the NMDA receptor is blocked, no decrease in response to glucocorticoid treatment is found (Cameron et al., 1998). This result suggests that the regulation through corticosteroids is upstream of the transmitter-dependent regulation and is probably less specific. This observation also indicates that several signaling pathways act together in eliciting the net response on adult neurogenesis. NMDA-dependent mechanisms are the best candidates for modulating global corticosterone effects on adult neurogenesis.

Other hormonal systems might play a role in modifying corticosterone effects as well. Dehydroepiandrosterone (DHEA) is a steroid hormone from the adrenal gland that can modulate and even counteract glucocorticoid activity. For example, DHEA levels in serum and cerebrospinal fluid (CSF) decrease not only with age (Orentreich et al., 1992; Guazzo et al., 1996) but also in major depression, a condition associated with cortisol dysregulation (Michael et al., 2000). In the adult rodent hippocampus, DHEA on its own had a significantly inductive effect on cell proliferation and adult neurogenesis, which could dose-dependently counteract the down-regulating effect of corticosterone (Karishma and Herbert, 2002).

Sex Hormones

There is no evidence of strong gender differences in adult neurogenesis. However, sex hormones can influence adult neurogenesis and both female and male hormones seem to do so. The data to support this remain far from conclusive however.

In song birds, testosterone is a positive regulator of neurogenesis in the adult higher vocal center (HVC), the brain region responsible for song learning (Rasika et al., 1994; Alvarez-Borda and Nottebohm, 2002; Louissaint et al., 2002). Female hormones have also been studied in canaries (Nordeen and Nordeen, 1989; Hidalgo et al., 1995) because the HVC is close to a subventriular layer of cells that express estrogen receptors. In these birds, estrogen induced cell proliferation, supported survival of the new neurons, and resulted in a higher number of neurons in the HVC.

In the female rodent hippocampus, cell proliferation has been found to peak in proestrous, when estrogen levels are high, and to be reduced in the phases when estrogen is low (Tanapat et al., 1999). Exogenously applied estradiol acutely increased cell proliferation in vivo but then led to a consecutive decrease within 48 hours, probably reflecting a feedback loop activating other adrenal hormone pathways (Ormerod et al., 2003). In male meadow voles, estradiol had survival-promoting effects when administered 6 to 10 days after BrdU, a finding suggesting a sensitive period in neuronal development that is possibly associated with axon elongation (Ormerod et al., 2004). Many studies on the effects of hormone levels in the ovary cycle have been conducted in female prairie voles, because in this species the entry into estrus can be provoked by exposure to the odor of a male. The number of proliferating cells in the SVZ and RMS almost doubled in female voles exposed to a male compared to those exposed to another female (Smith et al., 2001). The effect disappeared in ovariectomized animals but could be rescued when estrogen was injected. Increased estrogen levels during pregnancy did not induce cell proliferation in the dentate gyrus, but the total number of PSA-NCAM-positive cells increased (Smith et al., 2001). Pregnancy was indeed shown to induce net adult hippocampal neurogenesis, but this effect was mediated by prolactin, not estrogen (Shingo et al., 2003). Conversely, in meadow voles a seasonal influence (which is tightly correlated with hormonal status) on cell proliferation in the dentate gyrus was found. In winter, high cell proliferation and survival coincided with reproductive inactivity (Galea and McEwen, 1999).

The effects of estrogen on olfactory bulb neurogenesis have so far received less attention. Prolactin has been found to induce cell proliferation in the SVZ and neurogenesis in the adult olfactory bulb (Shingo et al., 2003). This finding has been connected with the increased sense of smell experienced by many pregnant women, but at present this link is speculation.

Rat neural precursor cells in vitro express receptors for estrogen, and treatment with estrogen results in reduced mitogenic effectiveness of EGF. Embryonic precursor cells, by contrast, were induced to proliferate by estradiol (Brannvall et al., 2002).

Just as corticosteroids might require NMDA receptor activity to exert their effect on adult neurogenesis, estrogen might depend on activation of the serotonergic system (Banasr et al., 2001). However, blockade of the estrogen receptor inhibited the effect of IGF-1 on adult hippocampal neurogenesis (Perez-Martin et al., 2003), which further illustrates the complex interdependence of the many regulatory systems.

Growth Factors

Growth factors are extracellular signaling molecules that increase cell growth and maintenance. They have diverse effects on neurogenesis. Historically, growth factors such as EGF and fibroblast growth factor (FGF) have been distinguished from the neurotrophic factors. Neurotrophic factors such as nerve growth factor (NGF) were considered primarily survival factors giving trophic support to neurons and thus maintaining the integrity of nervous tissue. However, in many contexts this distinction seems arbitrary and often the distinction between the biological net effects of growth factors and neurotrophic factors is not clear-cut. Neurotrophins are a class of factors that share signaling through trk and p75 receptors.

Epidermal Growth Factor

Neurospheres from the mouse forebrain grow in the presence of EGF (Reynolds et al., 1992). In vitro, EGF has a strong mitogenic effect. Upon withdrawal of EGF the neural precursor cells can be induced to differentiate.

Putative stem cells, however, differ with respect to their expression of EGF receptor. Some cells express EGF receptors only, some express only FGF receptors, and some express both. This distribution is species-, region-, and time-dependent (Represa et al., 2001). When neural stem cells were first discovered, this varying dependence on EGF caused misunderstandings, because the growth factor requirements of stem cells seemed to differ among different studies. In fact, however, across these studies there were species differences and different populations of cells. Hippocampal progenitor cells from rats, for example, rely on FGF-2 in vitro but do not require EGF (Palmer et al., 1995). Neural precursor cells from the adult human brain are responsive to both FGF-2 and EGF (Kirschenbaum et al., 1994; Arsenijevic et al., 2001).

When EGF was infused into the ventricles, proliferation in the SVZ increased dramatically (Fig. 9–9) and could lead to hyperplasias that protruded into the ventricle but resolved after discontinuation of the infusion (Kuhn et al., 1997). A similar effect was achieved when a form of EGF was administered intranasally (Jin et al., 2003b). Intracerebroventricular infusion of EGF did not induce proliferation in the SGZ, possibly because the growth factor did not diffuse the longer distance from the ventricle to the SGZ (Kuhn et al., 1997). In contrast, there was an increased number of BrdU-labeled cells in the striatum, reflecting cell migration from the SVZ or the induction of local responsive cells. Under normal conditions, no neuronal differentiation of these EGF-induced striatal cells was found. In both the olfactory bulb and hippocampus, EGF reduced the number of new neurons but increased the number of new astrocytes.

Nevertheless, EGF has been used successfully to boost regenerative neurogenesis in the ischemic striatum (Teramoto et al., 2003) and the is-

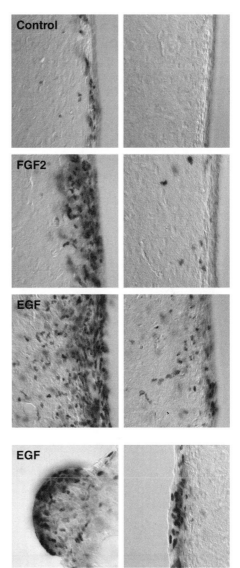

Figure 9–9. Effects of growth factors on adult neurogenesis. Cell proliferation in the sub-ventricular zone (SVZ) was differentially affected by the infusion of growth factors epidermal growth factor (EGF) and fibroblast growth factor-2 (FGF-2) into the ventricles of adult rats. EGF had a stronger effect and resulted in increased numbers of BrdU-labeled cells not only in the SVZ but also in the adjacent striatum. EGF-induced cell proliferation resulted in protrusions into the ventricle that resolved after discontinuation of the treatment (Kuhn et al., 1997). Image reproduced with kind permission of H. Georg Kuhn, Gothenburg. Copyright 1997 by The Society for Neuroscience.

chemic CA1 region of the hippocampus (Nakatomi et al., 2002). As discussed in Chapters 7 and 8, there remains considerable controversy over regenerative neurogenesis in non-neurogenic regions, but it might well be that the ischemic environment provides additional stimuli that facilitate the growth factor effects. Alternatively, growth factors might rescue dying neurons that incorporated BrdU (Kuan et al., 2004).

A molecule related to EGF and having similar properties, heparin-binding epidermal growth factor–like growth factor (HB-EGF) is induced by hypoxia and might be involved in mediating an endogenous response to ischemia (Jin et al., 2002b).

Fibroblast Growth Factor-2

When precursor cells were first isolated from the adult rat hippocampus, they were described as being FGF-2-dependent, not EGF-dependent stem cells (Palmer et al., 1995, 1997). It was later found that their murine counterpart also required EGF. To some degree, EGF and FGF-2 thus appear to have redundant functions in precursor cells—they are both mitogenic. However, the mitogenic effect of FGF-2 appears to be lower than that of EGF. FGF-2 is also sufficient to successfully elicit a neurogenic potential in precursor cells isolated from non-neurogenic regions in rats (Palmer et al., 1999).

When infused into the ventricle, FGF-2, unlike EGF, not only expanded the dividing cells of the SVZ but also induced net neurogenesis in the olfactory bulb (Kuhn et al., 1997). Thus FGF-2 function might have a proneurogenic component. This finding shares an unexplained link with data from embryogenesis, where microinjected FGF-2 induced neurogenesis at embryonic day 15.5 (E15.5) but induced gliogenesis at E20.5 (Vaccarino et al., 1999). Like EGF, FGF-2 can be applied systemically and crosses the blood–brain barrier (Wagner et al., 1999), which suggests that it can act like a hormone. In FGF knockout mice, no increase in hippocampal cell proliferation was found in response to KA-induced seizures or ischemia, normally two strong inducers of precursor cell division (Yoshimura et al., 2001). This effect could be rescued when FGF-2 expression was reintroduced with a viral vector. This finding does not prove a solitary role for FGF-2 in regulating adult neurogenesis (because not all mechanisms possibly capable of rescuing the phenotype could be examined), but it does underscore the fact that FGF-2 can profoundly modulate adult neurogenesis. Growth factors like FGF-2 might, for example, require autocrine and paracrine cofactors for their action on neural stem cells in vivo and in vitro; cystatin C is the first identified example (Taupin et al., 2000).

The finding that FGF-2 induces telomerase activity in neural precursor cells might indicate that FGF-2 also plays a role in maintaining precursor cell function (Haik et al., 2000) (see Maintaining the Precuror Pool, above, for the role of telomerase activity in neural stem cells).

Insulin-Like Growth Factor-1

Whereas most of the trophic support for neurons originates from the local microenvironment, glia, and other neurons, IGF-1 is an example of a systemically acting factor. IGF-1 is part of a major signaling pathway affecting many body systems. Growth hormone induces IGF-1 levels, which in turn increase the action of BDNF. Thus in addition to other potential direct mechanisms, IGF-1 essentially mediates BDNF action.

When infused peripherally or intracerebroventricularly, IGF-1 induced both cell proliferation and net neurogenesis (Aberg et al., 2000, 2003; Lichtenwalner et al., 2001). Not surprisingly, IGF-1 has been with the increase in adult neurogenesis in response to physical activity. With physical activity, IGF-1 accumulates in neurons and at least some of the exercise-induced effects on neurons can be inhibited by blocking the uptake of IGF-1 into the brain (Carro et al., 2000; Trejo et al., 2001). Administration of an antibody that blocks IGF-1 activity prevailed many positive effects of physical activity on the brain (Carro et al., 2001). This shows that IGF1 is necessary but not that it is sufficient to elicit activity-dependent effects. Nevertheless, the finding supports the idea that lack of activity (a sedentary life) causes a decrease in systemic trophic support that neurons receive. This tonic effect (to which not only IGF-1, but also FGF-2 and the neurotrophins contribute) has been called "neuroprotective surveillance" (Torres-Aleman, 2000). Like adrenalectomy (Cameron and McKay, 1999), FGF-2, and HB-EGF (Jin et al., 2003a), IGF-1 administration can prevent some of the age-related decline in adult hippocampal neurogenesis (Lichtenwalner et al., 2001).

The exact function of IGF-1 is not clear: It has a comparatively mild mitogenic effect that is physiologically modulated by specific IGF-binding proteins (Clemmons, 1991; Hill and Han, 1991). Interaction with estrogen signaling is evident in that IGF-1-mediated increase in cell proliferation can be prevented by blocking the estrogen receptor (Perez-Martin et al., 2003). Both IGF-1 and its binding proteins are found in the CSF (Ferry et al., 1999) and the blood. The main source of endogenous IGF-1 is the liver, although there is restricted production in the brain as well (Werther et al., 1990).

Besides the effect on neuronal development, IGF-1 preferentially induces oligodendrocyte differentiation from hippocampal precursor cells both in vitro and in vivo (Hsieh et al., 2004).

Vascular Endothelial Growth Factor

Vascular endothelial growth factor was first identified as a hypoxia-induced growth factor primarily thought to be involved in angiogenesis. However, in the songbird brain, angiogenesis and adult neurogenesis are coordinated (Louissaint et al., 2002). Testosterone increased neurogenesis in the HVC of songbirds and induced BDNF expression in endothelial cells in the adult HVC. This BDNF expression was preceded by an induced expression of both VEGF proteins and the endothelial VEGF receptor. When the receptor was blocked, both the angiogenic and the neurogenic response was abolished. Parallel to this finding by Steven Goldman's group at Cornell University, David Greenberg and colleagues at the Buck Institute for Age Research in Novato reported that VEGF induced neural precursor cell proliferation in vivo and in vitro. VEGF receptor 2 (Flk1) was found to be expressed on cells expressing DCX (Jin et al., 2002c). This finding suggests that VEGF acts on late progenitor cells in vivo. However, flk-1 was also expressed on clonal precursor cells from the rat brain (Schanzer et al., 2004). Blockage of Flk1 inhibited the VEGF effect on cultured precursor cells.

After infusion into the lateral ventricle, VEGF did not increase precursor cell proliferation but acted as a survival-promoting factor (Schanzer et al., 2004). In conflict with this result, another study that used viral gene transfer found an induction of cell proliferation in vivo as well (Cao et al., 2004). In contrast, stimulation of VEGF receptor 1 (Flt1) with its specific agonist, placental growth factor, reduced hippocampal neurogenesis. In that study, the positive and negative effects of signaling through the VEGF receptors were paralleled by a suggestive change in hippocampal learning parameters (Cao et al., 2004).

Blocking of peripheral action of VEGF in vivo inhibited the induction of adult neurogenesis in response to physical activity (Fabel et al., 2003), just as was shown for IGF-1 earlier (Trejo et al., 2001). Inhibition of VEGF had no effect on baseline neurogenesis, however.

Neurotrophic Factors

Neurotrophic factors are extracellular signaling molecules that exert a wide range of functions in brain development and maintenance (Lewin and Barde, 1996). Several classes of neurotrophic factors can be distinguished: (1) neurotrophins—that is, NGF, BDNF, and the other factors that act through the trk receptors and p75; (2) the Glial cell–derived neurotrophic factor (GDNF); (3) the hepatocyte growth factor (HGF) families of neurotrophic factors; and (4) the neurotrophic cytokines such as ciliary neurotrophic factor (CNTF), Il-6, and others. The neurotrophin hypothesis proposes that a lack of this trophic support causes neurodegeneration. This trophic support can be mediated through retrograde transport from the innervated target, through anterograde transport from afferent regions (Altar et al., 1997), or in autocrine loops as has been found for developing retinal ganglion cells (Wright et al., 1992). The neurotrophins and CNTF are discussed below. No data exist on the regulation of adult neurogenesis through GDNF and HGF, although HGF promotes survival of sympathetic neuroblasts in an autocrine fashion (Maina and Klein, 1999).

Brain-Derived Neurotrophic Factors, Nerve Growth Factor, and Neurotrophins 3, 4, and 5

Brain-derived neurotrophic factor, NGF and the NTs, that is NT-3, NT-4, and NT-5, act through the same class of receptors, the trk receptors, and show some cross-reaction on the different receptors. On the basis of this shared receptor binding and certain functional characteristics, neurotrophic factors have been distinguished from growth factors, but biologically this distinction is not always strong. BDNF is by far the best-studied factor of this family, and even if one concedes a certain bias in research, BDNF seems in fact to be the most relevant representative. BDNF is often considered *the* secreted factor modulating brain plasticity. For example, BDNF plays a major role in synaptic plasticity during learning; LTP is BDNF-dependent (Korte et al., 1996; Minichiello et al., 2002). Physical activity induces hippocampal BDNF mRNA expression, and BDNF might thus be responsible for the inductive effects of physical activity on LTP (Farmer et al., 2004). At the same time, BDNF also influences adult neurogenesis. Infusion of BDNF into the ventricles induced neurogenesis originating from the SVZ (Pencea et al., 2001). Because BDNF sticks to cellular surfaces, the effectiveness of infusion studies has been limited. BDNF also does not cross the blood–brain barrier. But infection of ependymal cells with an adenovirus constituitively overexpressing BDNF caused long-lasting induction of olfactory bulb neurogenesis (Benraiss et al., 2001). In contrast, heterozygous BDNF knockout mice have reduced levels of adult hippocampal neurogenesis (homozygotes do not survive into adulthood) (Lee et al., 2002). Unexpectedly, virus-mediated overexpression of BDNF in the ischemic hippocampus dampened the normal endogenous neurogenic response to ischemia (Larsson et al., 2002). When endogenous BDNF was inhibited by intraventricular infusion of a BDNF blocker, induction of hippocampal neurogenesis by ischemia was stimulated (Gustafsson et al., 2003). Under pathological conditions, BDNF thus appears to have an effect opposite its normal action and blocks neuronal differentiation. Interpretation of this finding is difficult but it might indicate that ischemia-induced neurogenesis is in fact distinguishable from normal neurogenesis and that one of BDNF's functions is to keep adult neurogenesis within a physiologic range.

BDNF has gained further interest because of the hypothesis that the action of antidepressants might include effects on adult neurogenesis, and that BDNF is a key regulator of this mechanism (D'Sa and Duman, 2002). Many antidepressants induce the phosphorylation of CREB, after which CREB binds to the BDNF promoter and induces BDNF transcription. BDNF is involved in inducing neuronal differentiation; the details of the underlying mechanism are still unknown.

In vitro, BDNF is a differentiation factor that can down-regulate precursor cell proliferation (Cheng et al., 2003a). Purified precursor cells that have been expanded with FGF-2 can be primed to become responsive to BDNF by the application of retinoic acid (RA) (Takahashi et al., 1999). Upon contact with RA, hippocampal progenitor cells in vitro up-regulated trk receptors and p75 (the low-affinity neurotrophin receptor), expressed p21 as a molecule associated with exit from the cell cycle, and expressed NeuroD, indicating neuronal determination. Although the role of RA signaling (or that of other nuclear steroid receptors) in adult neurogenesis is not known, these data also suggest that part of the initiation of neuronal differentiation is independent of BDNF.

Nerve growth factor binds to tyrosine kinase receptors trk-A and trk-B. Consequently, its effects should overlap somewhat with those of BDNF. Like

BDNF and NT3, NGF is highly expressed in the adult hippocampus (Maison-pierre et al., 1990). Despite its suggestive name, the role of NGF in regulating adult neurogenesis appears to be limited. Intracerebroventricular infusion of NGF did not have any effect on SVZ or SGZ precursor cells or on net neurogenesis (Kuhn et al., 1997).

Similarly, little is known about the effects of the NTs on adult neurogenesis. Both BDNF and NT3 are induced by dietary restriction (Lee et al., 2002), an experimental paradigm that not only has robust positive effects on life expectancy in rodents but also induces cell proliferation in the SGZ. In vitro, RA induced expression of not only primary BDNF receptor trkB, but also of trkC, to which NT-3 preferentially binds. Retinoic acid also sensitized cultured precursor cells to differentiation-inducing effects of NT-3 (Takahashi et al., 1999). During embryonic neural development, NT-3 is the most highly expressed neurotrophic factor; this does not seem to be the case in adult neurogenesis.

Ciliary Neurotrophic Factor

Injection of CNTF into the adult mouse brain caused an induction of precursor cell proliferation and net neurogenesis. The CNTF receptor alpha was expressed solely by GFAP-positive cells of the SVZ (Emsley and Hagg, 2003). Thus CNTF might be one of the factors that reaches specifically the initial stages of adult neurogenesis.

Nitric Oxide

Nitric oxide (NO) is the smallest known signaling molecule. Among other mechanisms of action, it induces the synthesis of cGMP and this step is a key restriction point in the regulation of neurogenesis in many invertebrates. In general, NO is antiproliferative and induces differentiation but does so in concert with other factors. For example, NO inhibits the EGF receptor and thus reduces the mitogenic effects of EGF (Peranovich et al., 1995; Estrada et al., 1997). Among its numerous other functions, NO might be involved in the control of adult mammalian neurogenesis (Moreno-Lopez et al., 2000). External application of NO leads to an enhancement of regenerative neurogenesis after ischemia or trauma (Cheng et al., 2003b; Lu et al., 2003a). Nitric oxide has a very short range of action and acts primarily at its site of production. The key enzyme is nitric oxide synthase (NOS). The major constitutive producers are neurons (nNOS) and endothelial cells (eNOS). These forms are involved in physiological pathways of regulation. In cases of pathology, an inducible isoform (iNOS) is up-regulated. Consequently, after damage the first response involves primarily nNOS activity, which is followed by a later stage of iNOS effects. Null-mutants for iNOS do not show an induction of neurogenesis after ischemia (Zhu et al., 2003).

In vitro, NO scavengers such as hemoglobin increase cell proliferation and reduce differentiation. NO donors do the reverse (Cheng et al., 2003a). Thus, NO inhibits precursor cell proliferation and initiates differentiation. Many growth factors induce NOS in precursor cells; rising levels of NO will then lead to exit from the cell cycle. Thus NO might serve as an in-built brake that prevents continued divisions. In vivo, administration of an NO donor induced cell proliferation in the SVZ and SGZ as well as consecutive neuronal differentiation. (Zhang et al., 2001; Cheng et al., 2003a). BDNF causes an induction of NOS, which in turn is associated with the cessation of proliferation and the beginning of differentiation (Cheng et al., 2003a). This does not necessarily prove that NO is an obligatory downstream factor of BDNF. Consistent with a role at the transition stage between proliferation phase and differentiation, NOS has been found in PSA-NCAM-positive cells of the dentate gyrus (Islam et al., 2003).

Neurotransmitters

The dentate gyrus receives input from a variety of brain regions and axonal terminals of several neurotransmitter classes project to the dentate gyrus.

- *Glutamate.* The main afferent to the dentate gyrus is the perforant path from the entorhinal cortex. The synapses of perforant path projections on the dendrites of the granule cells are glutamatergic and thus excitatory. They occupy primarily the outer molecular layer. In the inner molecular layer, excitatory commissural fibers terminate from the contralateral hippocampus.
- *Acetylcholine.* In the inner molecular layer commissural projections from the contralateral hippocampus end. These axons use acetylcholine as a neurotransmitter. A second acetylcholinergic input comes from the septum and the nucleus basalis Meynert (NBM).
- *Serotonin (5-HT).* Serotonergic afferents project from the raphe nuclei in the brain stem to the SGZ.
- *Dopamine.* From the ventral tegmental area, dopaminergic fibers reach the SGZ and presumably the SVZ. Direct dopaminergic innervation of the SGZ is very sparse. Fibers from the substantia nigra reach the striatum, immediately adjoining the SVZ and possibly the SVZ itself.
- *Catecholamines.* These include adrenaline and noradrenaline. Noradrenergic projections reach the SGZ from the locus coeruleus.
- *GABA.* GABAergic inhibitory systems are a local network of interneurons. The architecture of this system is not completely understood. In the dentate gyrus at least seven classes of interneurons can be found (Freund and Buzsaki, 1996). Their distinguishing characteristics are their morphology and exact location, their

pattern of connectivity, and their expression of different calcium-binding proteins (calretinin, calbindin, parvalbumin) and other markers (VIP, NPY, STR). Their general function is to modulate the activity of the granule cells, for example, through negative feedback mechanisms.

Glutamate

Glutamatergic fibers from the entorhinal cortex reach the dentate gyrus through the perforant path. Lesioning of this main excitatory input up-regulated cell proliferation in the dentate gyrus of adult rats (Gould, 1994; Cameron et al., 1995). From this finding the hypothesis was developed that under physiological conditions, excitatory input would put a lid on adult neurogenesis. However, a later study found no such effect in mice; lesioning of the perforant path left cell proliferation unaffected but led to a transient increase in cell survival (Gama Sosa et al., 2004).

In addition, blockade of the NMDA receptors with antagonist MK-801 increased adult neurogenesis under physiological and pathological conditions (Gould et al., 1994; Cameron et al., 1995, 1998; Bernabeu and Sharp, 2000; Arvidsson et al., 2001; Nacher et al., 2001; Okuyama et al., 2004). Excitation would thus limit neurogenesis by inhibiting cell proliferation in the dentate gyrus.

Activation of KA receptors as another class of glutamate receptors, how-ever, caused a strong induction of cell proliferation and net neurogenesis (Parent et al., 1997). The discrepancy between the action mediated by NMDA- and KA-receptor activation suggests that excitatory input to the dentate gyrus has a balanced effect on adult neurogenesis, which is then modulated by other systems. KA-receptor activation would stimulate neurogenesis according to the incoming excitation, being equivalent to the data flow into the dentate gyrus. NMDA-receptor activation would limit this proneuro-genic response and allow other systems to take part in fine-tuning it. This interpretation, however, is not undisputed: in vitro, NMDA receptor–mediated activity induced neurogenesis from hippocampal precursor cells via L-type calcium channels and directly changed transcription factor pat-terns to a neuronal program (Deisseroth et al., 2004). Similarly, synaptic plas-ticity as in models of LTP is NMDA receptor dependent and can be blocked by application of MK-801.

The finding that excessive stimulation of KA receptors induces adult neurogenesis, whereas stimulation of NMDA receptors might limit it (al-though these data are not yet conclusive, see below), suggests the existence of a balanced regulatory mechanism based on excitatory glutamatergic input.

AMPA receptors are ionotropic glutamate receptors and are responsible for the fast transmission of an excitation across the synaptic cleft. The ef-fects of NMDA-receptor activation, in contrast, are slower and mediate the plastic structural alterations that might follow the excitation. Interestingly, when AMPA receptor–dependent transmission is enhanced by special pharmacological potentiators, the result is an effect on plasticity as well. BDNF mRNA, for example, is up-regulated in the adult rat hippocampus (Macko-wiak et al., 2002) and these compounds are considered a new class of antide-pressants (Li et al., 2001). Upon chronic administration, an AMPA potentiator increased cell proliferation in the adult hippocampus and did so at a lower dose than had been necessary for a detectable induction of BDNF mRNA (Bai et al., 2003). The pharmacology and effects of AMPA potentiators clearly go beyond the physiological activation of AMPA receptors. Nothing is known about their direct role in controlling adult neurogenesis.

Acetylcholine

Most data on the acetylcholinergic regulation of adult neurogenesis have been gathered by manipulating the nicotinergic acetylcholine receptor in the brain with nicotine. This aspect is discussed below. Both the hippocam-pus and the SVZ receive acetylcholinergic input from the septal region and the nucleus basalis Meynert. This input plays an important role in hippo-campal function. In Alzheimer disease, cholinergic neurons in the basal fore-brain are the primary target of degeneration. The reduced cholinergic input to the hippocampus is made responsible for some parts of the loss of hip-pocampal function during the course of the disease (Leanza et al., 1996; Pizzo et al., 2002). Lesioning of the fimbria fornix, which contains the major cho-linergic projections between the septum and the hippocampus, resulted in increased cell proliferation in the SGZ (Weinstein et al., 1996), but this may have been a nonspecific effect. In a more specific approach, lesioning of acetylcholinergic neurons in the basal forebrain, reliably achieved with an immunotoxin, caused a reduction in adult neurogenesis in both the hippo-campus and the olfactory bulb (Cooper-Kuhn et al., 2004). The cholinergic system appears to exert a survival-promoting effect, because in the dener-vated rats, the numbers of apoptotic cells in the germinative regions in-creased. An interesting detail is that the small number of new neurons in the periglomerular layer of the olfactory bulb seemed to increase (although not significantly), despite the significant overall decrease in neurogenesis in the entire bulb. The meaning of this finding is not clear, but it might be one of the first examples of differential regulation of neurogenesis of the different types of new interneurons in the adult olfactory bulb (Cooper-Kuhn et al., 2004).

Serotonin

Serotonergic innervation from the median and dorsal raphe nuclei in the brain stem reaches the entire brain and provides signals of general activity and alertness. Serotonergic activity correlates well with general activity. The widespread distribution notwithstanding, serotonin effects can be very specific in different neuronal populations. This specificity is primarily achieved by the differential expression of the 15 known serotonin receptors.

Serotonergic input to the hippocampus and SVZ up-regulates adult neurogenesis (Brezun and Daszuta, 1999). This has been shown by lesioning the input fibers from the median raphe, causing a sharp decline in adult neurogenesis that could be rescued by transplanting serotonergic tissue into the lesion area (Brezun and Daszuta, 2000). Substances that increase the activity of serotonin, such as serotonin reuptake inhibitors (SSRI), which are effective antidepressants, increase adult hippocampal neurogenesis, but they seem to do so only after a latency period of several weeks (Malberg et al., 2000).

The 5-HT antagonist tianeptin, a so-called atypical antidepressant because it inhibits serotonergic effects rather than stimulating them, also increased adult neurogenesis (Czeh et al., 2002). The explanation for this might lie in the activation of different 5-HT-receptor subtypes, leading to different net effects. As in the case of glutamate, serotonin-mediated regulation of adult neurogenesis consists of several balanced partial effects mediated by the various receptors. Distribution of 5-HT receptors in the SGZ is heterogeneous and appears to change in the course of neuronal development. This phenomenon has not been studied in enough detail to determine the specific individual contributions of the different precursor cell types (Banasr et al., 2004). Thus, in the case of tianeptin, the effect on adult neurogenesis could be indirect. In a knockout mouse for the 5-HT 1A receptor, in contrast, the effects on adult neurogenesis by fluoxetine (the most widely used SSRI, sold as Prozac or Fluctine) were abolished (Santarelli et al., 2003).

Dopamine

Together with acetylcholine and serotonin, the dopamine system belongs to the ubiquitous regulatory systems that reach out from a few control centers and allow fine-tuning and orchestrating of complex functions. Dopaminergic fibers from the ventral tegmental area reach almost the entire brain and are involved in mood functions. Dopaminergic input from the substantia nigra to the basal ganglia plays an important role in the extrapyramidal motor system. When rodents were treated with dopamine antagonist haloperidol, the results on neurogenesis were ambiguous. One study using an unorthodox way of quantification reported a small stimulating effect on cell proliferation in the adult SGZ (Dawirs et al., 1998), a result that was not seen by others (Malberg et al., 2000). Olanzapine, in contrast, enhanced adult neurogenesis (Wang et al., 2004). Low doses of clozapine induced cell proliferation but did not increase net neurogenesis (Halim et al., 2004).

Similarly, in the SVZ, one study reported an increase in cell proliferation, although in early postnatal rodents (Backhouse et al., 1982), while another report did not find an effect (Wakade et al., 2002). The diversity of results might simply reflect the fact that haloperidol is not a specifically antidopaminergic agent but has numerous other effects at glutamatergic, adrenergic, and serotonergic synapses, all of which might affect adult neurogenesis. The different effects of the various antipsychotic drugs are likely due to their different binding properties at the dopamine receptors.

Gunter Höglinger, Etienne Hirsch, and colleagues at the Hôpital de la Salpetrière in Paris demonstrated that C cells of the SVZ expressed dopamine receptors, dopaminergic denervation caused reduced olfactory bulb neurogenesis in vivo, and, conversely activation of the dopaminergic receptor D2 resulted in an increase in proliferation in vitro (Höglinger et al., 2004). For the SGZ, the group also reported a negative effect on cell proliferation after dopaminergic denervation.

In contrast to this report, another study claimed that damage to the dopamergic system by application of MPTP (1-methyl-4-phenyl-1,2,3,6-tetrahydropyridine) caused a reactive increase in the production of dopaminergic periglomerular interneurons in the olfactory bulb (Yamada et al., 2004).

Adrenaline (Epinephrine) and Noradrenaline (Norepinephrine)

Few data exist on the role of the other catecholamines besides dopamine, adrenaline (epinephrine) and noradrenaline (norepinephrine), in the control of adult neurogenesis. There are extensive noradrenergic fiber connections into the dentate gyrus (Loy et al., 1980). In the dentate gyrus depletion of norepinephrine by a selective neurotoxin decreased cell proliferation without affecting consecutive stages of neuronal development (Kulkarni et al., 2002). Given the overall abundance of adrenergic and noradrenergic effects throughout the body, it is likely that catecholamines can indeed affect precursor cell activity and adult neurogenesis, but this mechanism is tightly controlled by other systems. Especially in the context of activity-dependent regulation of adult neurogenesis and the many stress effects on adult neurogenesis, the role of catecholamines will be important to study.

GABA

Of the transmitter systems with plausible relevance to the context of adult hippocampal neurogenesis, the least is known about GABA. Because of the complexity of the interneuron network in the dentate gyrus, mechanical lesion studies are impossible. Inhibiting inhibition systemically by applying pentylenetetrazole (PTZ) has been shown to induce hippocampal seizures and consequently adult neurogenesis (Jiang et al., 2003). This result fits with the role of glutamatergic innervation in modulating adult neurogenesis. Inhibitory circuits tend to counteract the proneurogenic effects of KA-receptor activation and enforce the NMDA receptor–mediated balancing effects.

The benzodiazepine receptor is a co-receptor to the GABA receptor. Chronic treatment with diazepam caused a reduction in the fraction of newly generated cells turning into neurons in the adult hippocampus (Deisseroth et al., 2004).

Activity-Dependent Regulation of Precursor Cell Proliferation

In a pioneering study, Karl Deisseroth, Robert Malenka, and colleagues at Stanford University showed that hippocampal precursor cells in vitro can directly sense excitation (Deisseroth et al., 2004) (Fig. 9–10). The underlying fundamental question is whether the precursor cells are able to directly respond to local excitatory activity or whether such reaction is always a function of the local network and the precursor cell niche. There is a discrepancy between the effects of activity in a more general sense and those in the sense of direct excitation on adult hippocampal neurogenesis. Whereas voluntary wheel-running activity increased neurogenesis (Van Praag et al., 1999b), blocking NMDA receptors (and thus reducing excitatory activity) decreased the production of new neurons (Cameron et al., 1995). However, in models of seizures, overexcitation drastically increased neurogenesis (Bengzon et al., 1997; Parent et al., 1997). Deisseroth and colleagues cultured hippocampal precursor cells on either living or fixed hippocampal astrocyte cultures, an experimental paradigm that favors neuronal differentiation (Song et al., 2002). Under these conditions, even short-lasting and mild depolarization caused long-lasting increases in the number of newly generated neurons. This effect was specific in that cell proliferation was not broadly enhanced. Rather, in the proliferating cells, a fast up-regulation of NeuroD was found, accompanied by a down-regulation of transcription factors favoring glial phenotypes, such as Hes1 and Id2. Depolarization of postmitotic cells had no effect.

The NMDA receptor–dependent effect was mediated by calcium signaling. Accordingly, in vivo, calcium-antagonist nifidipine decreased adult hippocampal neurogenesis, whereas treatment with a calcium channel agonist induced adult neurogenesis (Deisseroth et al., 2004).

Endogenous Psychotropic Systems

Cannabinoids

Cannabinoids have a short-term enhancing effect on learning capabilities, but in the long run can lead to dementive symptoms and depression. Consistent with such gross effects, the picture that can be drawn from available data on cannabinoid effects on adult neurogenesis is incoherent and contradictory. In vitro, endocannabinoids inhibited NGF-induced neuronal differentiation of PC12 cells (a commonly used yet somewhat artificial neuronal progenitor cell line) and other cell lines by blocking trkA effects (Rueda et al., 2002). However, evidence for physiological action of endogenous trkA-

Excitation increases neurogenesis

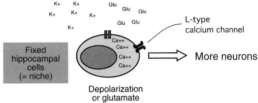

Excitation acts directly on neural precursor cells via L-type calcium channels

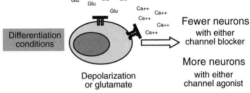

Bidirectional effects of NMDA- or L-type calcium channel blockade or agonism on excitation-induced neurogenesis

Figure 9–10. Direct effects of activity on precursor cells. Precursor cells in culture can react to excitatory stimuli via NMDA receptors on their surface. The drawing summarizes work by Deisseroth et al. (1994).

Excitation or calcium channel activation causes rapid down-regulation of antineurogenic transcription factors

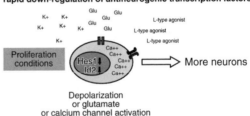

ligand NGF on adult neurogenesis in situ is limited, so the finding remains difficult to interpret and generalize. In vivo, Rueda and colleagues (2002) reported a slight phenotypic shift in adult hippocampal neurogenesis of rats treated with a CB1 antagonist to relatively more glial cells. In cannabinoid receptor 1 (CB1) knockout mice, adult neurogenesis was impaired: cell proliferation was only half that of the wild-type animals (Jin et al., 2004). However, in that study, a CB1 antagonist did not change hippocampal cell proliferation in wild types but paradoxically quadrupled it in the knockouts. In the SVZ the pattern was similar but less strong, except that an effect on cell proliferation in wild-type mice was seen.

The endocannabinoid system's possible effects on adult neurogenesis are a good example of the difficulties that can arise from very straightforward pharmacologic and genetic models of complex regulatory systems. From all we know about the other physiological functions of the endocannabinoid system, its role in adult neurogenesis is likely modulatory. Such regulatory systems tend to be tightly bound into feedback loops and interact with many other systems. Acute and chronic effects might differ. Consequently, from the available data, no specific conclusions can be drawn on how the endocannabinoid system is involved in the regulation of adult neurogenesis.

Opioids

Expression of the μ-opioid receptor during development correlates with regions and times of neurogenesis, suggesting a functional role of the endorphins in the regulation of neurogenesis (Tong et al., 2000). Adult hippocampal precursor cells in culture release β-endorphin and express the μ- and α-opioid receptors. Exogenous activation of the receptors caused a decrease in cell proliferation. Under differentiation conditions, receptor activation lead to increased neuronal but decreased glial differentiation (Persson et al., 2003). In contrast, chronic application of morphine and heroin decreased adult hippocampal neurogenesis in vivo (Eisch et al., 2000). No in vivo data on acute effects of opioid receptor activation on adult neurogenesis exist yet. Because endorphins are up-regulated in many situations that induce adult neurogenesis (for example, wheel running), the available experimental data suggest that acute and chronic effects on adult neurogenesis differ. As for the endocannabinoids, however, the exact physiological role of the opioid receptor system in the control of adult neurogenesis is difficult to determine.

Nicotine

Nora Abrous and colleagues from Bordeaux allowed rats self-administration of nicotine and found that cell death in the dentate gyrus increased whereas adult neurogenesis decreased, both in a dose-dependent manner (Abrous et al., 2002). Assuming a positive role of adult neurogenesis in hippocampal function, the finding may conflict with the claims that nicotine might actually improve cognitive performance and that heavy smokers who quit showed impaired cognition (Changeux et al., 1998). Nicotinic receptors are down-regulated in many neurodegenerative disorders, including Alzheimer disease and Parkinson disease (James and Nordberg, 1995). This finding has led to the controversial recommendation that smoking is beneficial because it helps prevent neurodegeneration. The Abrous study clarified this statement, claiming that this generalized conclusion is not justified from a hippocampal perspective. In addition, a range of negative effects of nicotine on other aspects of brain morphology are known (Aramakis et al.,

2000). Generally, the abundance of nicotinic receptors in the brain, the multitude of effects of nicotine in different cell types and brain regions, the complexity of cognition, and the problem of different net effects of the same molecule on different time scales make it difficult to draw a clear picture. The interesting observation for our context is that precursor cells seem to directly respond to nicotine. This is supported by in vitro findings in neural cell lines (Newman et al., 2002).

PARACRINE SIGNALING MOLECULES

In the regulation of development, gradients of paracrine factors play an important role (see Chapter 4). Nevertheless, so far relatively little is known about their potential roles in adult neurogenesis.

Bone Morphogenic Proteins and Noggin

Bone morphogenic proteins (BMPs) are extracellular signaling molecules that play many different roles at various stages of neuronal development. The BMPs generally antagonize neurogenesis. One of the factors that disinhibits neurogenesis by attenuating BMP action is noggin (Wilson and Hemmati-Brivanlou, 1997). In the adult SVZ, ependymal cells secrete noggin and by counteracting the antineurogenic effects of local BMP4 contribute to creating a region of neurogenic permissiveness. Overexpression of noggin consequently further promoted neurogenesis (Lim et al., 2000). In the adult SGZ, both noggin and BMP4 are expressed (Fan et al., 2003) and inhibition of noggin activity by the application of anti-sense oligonucleotides in vivo resulted in a decrease in cell proliferation (Fan et al., 2004).

Wnt

Wnt (Wingless) plays an important role in maintaining self-renewal in hematopoetic stem cells (van de Wetering et al., 2002; Reya et al., 2003; Willert et al., 2003) and in the induction of neural specification (Munoz-Sanjuan and Brivanlou, 2002; Muroyama et al., 2002). Wnt signaling occurs through two complex signal transduction pathways that are tightly controlled by a large number of interacting factors. This multifaceted regulation converges to β-catenin as a downstream target. In the presence of Wnt, the concentration of β-catenin in the cell rises because its degradation is inhibited. In the cell nucleus, β-catenin associates with transcription factors TCF/Lef and induces the transcription of Wnt-dependent genes. The loss of appropriate β-catenin signaling is thought to play an important role in cancer development (Morin, 1999), possibly including brain tumors, including medulloblastomas (Itoh et al., 1993; Zurawel et al., 1998).

The effects of Wnt are cell type specific and dependent on the Wnt family members involved. Different *Wnt* genes show different distinct expression patterns in the course of brain development. In embryonic stem cells in vitro, Wnt3 is sufficient to induce neuronal lineage commitment (Otero et al., 2004). Wnt1 and Wnt5a increase the number of dopaminergic neurons through two different mechanisms (Castelo-Branco et al., 2003). In midbrain development Wnt3a stimulates the proliferation of ventral precursor cells. In neural precursor cells of the CNS, Wnt controls self-renewal, whereas in neural crest stem cells Wnt additionally induces the generation of sensory neurons at the expense of other cell types (Ikeya et al., 1997; Lee et al., 2004).

Wnt signaling seems to be particularly relevant for dorsal brain development (Dickinson et al., 1994; Liem et al., 1995; Muroyama et al., 2002), particularly in the spinal cord. But speculatively, dysfunctional Wnt signaling has been linked with the pathogenesis of mood disorders (Gould and Manji, 2002), Alzheimer disease (De Ferrari and Inestrosa, 2000), and schizophrenia (Kozlovsky et al., 2002). In fact, Wnt3a signaling is also necessary for normal hippocampal development by controlling the expansion of neural precursor cells in the cortical SVZ (Lee et al., 2000b). In the adult hippocampus, proliferative (BrdU-incorporating) cells are associated with β-catenin immunoreactivity. When experimental seizures were induced by electroconvulsive seizures, β-catenin in BrdU-labeled cells and expression of Wnt2 in the dentate gyrus were induced (Madsen et al., 2003b). Thus, although direct experimental evidence is still lacking, Wnt signaling is likely to play an important role in the control of neurogenesis in the adult dentate gyrus. As a dorsal factor, Wnt signaling might be one of the systems that distinguishes regulation of neurogenesis in the adult hippocampus from its counterpart in the olfactory bulb.

Sonic Hedgehog

Sonic hedgehog (Shh) serves a multitude of functions during development and is required in the brain for patterning of the ventral brain (McMahon et al., 2003). Ectopic expression of Shh causes ventralization (Kohtz et al., 1998); in Shh null-mutants the telencephalon is greatly reduced, dorsoventral patterning is disturbed, and precursor cell divisions throughout the brain are disturbed (Chiang et al., 1996). Using a conditional mutant based on the neural enhancer element of the nestin promoter, and restricting the loss of Shh function to nestin-expressing cells in the brain, Robert Machold, Gord Fishell, and colleagues studied the role of Shh signaling in neural precursor cells. In terms of the general patterning during development, the phenotype of these mice was minor. Those that reached adulthood had a much smaller brain and enlarged ventricles. In the postnatal neurogenic zones the number of precursor cells was strongly reduced. Both the olfactory bulb and dentate gyrus were reduced in size (Machold et al., 2003). Although this postnatal phenotype is not independent of a role of Shh signaling during prior development, an interesting hypothesis has been proposed: consistent with earlier findings of a pro-proliferative effect of Shh

(Wechsler-Reya and Scott, 1999), Shh might serve a dual function in the precursor cell niches by promoting proliferative activity and maintaining the precursor cell populations. If this hypothesis is right, Shh might act as a self-renewal factor. Shh receptors patched and smoothed are expressed in the hippocampus of adult rats, but the expression is not restricted to precursor cells in the SGZ (Traiffort et al., 1999; Lai et al., 2003). In addition, nestin-positive precursor cells from the adult rat hippocampus expressed Patched in vitro (Sakurada et al., 1999; Lai et al., 2003). Administration of Shh in vitro and in vivo resulted in an increase in the proliferation of multipotent precursor cells (Lai et al., 2003).

Notch

Notch1 is another factor with multiple functions during brain development. In general, activation of Notch1 appears to maintain cells in a precursor cell state and prevent neuronal differentiation (Chojnacki et al., 2003). In Notch1 null-mutants, neural stem cells were depleted although at early stages of development they could be generated independent of Notch signaling (Hitoshi et al., 2002). When key downstream regulators of Notch signaling, such as presenilin 1, which cleaves Notch after ligand binding, were mutated a similar situation occurred (Hitoshi et al., 2002). In other contexts, however, Notch1 has been reported to actively induce gliogenesis. In neural crest stem cells even a transient overexpression of Notch1 caused a switch from neurogenesis to gliogenesis (Morrison et al., 2000). The apparent conflict between maintenance of the precursor cell state and active promotion of gliogenesis might be resolved, if the astrocytic nature of neural precursor cells in the adult SVZ and SGZ turns out to be a sufficient explanation. This possibility is supported by the finding that when Notch1 and a marker gene were overexpressed retrovirally in the embryonic SVZ, radial glia became labeled in the fetal brain, and many of the transduced cells became SVZ astrocytes postnatally (Gaiano et al., 2000). This finding strongly not only supports the idea of a lineage relationship between radial glia and adult SVZ precursor cells, but also suggests how the apparently contradictory function of Notch1 might actually be resolved.

INTRACELLULAR AND TRANSCRIPTIONAL REGULATION

Methodical Challenges in Studying Transcriptional and Molecular Regulation of Neurogenesis in the Adult Brain

The list of extracellular signaling factors during neuronal development is still growing and gives a vivid impression of the complexity of neuronal development in the embryo. In comparison, our knowledge about the analogous events during adult neurogenesis is limited. The overall lack of genetic and molecular information on the regulation of adult neurogenesis might be surprising if adult neurogenesis were considered a continuation of embryonic development in the adult brain. But this perspective may be wrong. During embryonic brain development, the entire nervous system is jointly moving toward differentiation and does so in massively parallel actions. During this time, brain function essentially consists of building up its structure and laying the foundation for its mature cognitive functions. This situation is different from that of the adult, when neurogenesis occurs only in privileged niches of an environment that is otherwise non-permissive or even hostile to neuronal development. Even if the mechanisms underlying adult neurogenesis within the niches were similar (or identical) to embryonic neuronal development, the molecular activity and transcriptional control necessary to maintain the neurogenic niches would be special. One not immediately obvious consequence of this observation is that neurogenic niches in the adult rely on normal brain development to establish their specific permissive environment. In other words, to study the neurogenic privilege, the rest of the brain must be in a condition to grant that privilege. This is the limiting problem with knockout models and transgenic animals tailored to study the role of neurogenic genes and transcription factors in the context of adult neurogenesis. Mutation of a gene of high relevance to neurogenesis will severely disturb neuronal development and preclude the existence of a mature (if largely non-neurogenic) brain in which the special case of neurogenic permissiveness and adult neurogenesis could be studied. Many of the mutations are even lethal. The specific genetic and transcriptional control of adult neurogenesis can only be studied in brains with normal embryonic neurodevelopment.

The only solution to this problem is conditional mutants that would allow restriction of the targeted mutation both locally (to the brain or the neurogenic zones) and temporally (to adulthood). Because of the highly specific design of conditional mutants, they tend to be less universally exploitable than classical knockouts and transgenic models. With few exceptions, the lack of promoter systems specific enough to restrict the mutation to adult neurogenesis, the general technical demands of this method, and the complex study designs have thus far precluded the successful and efficient use of this strategy for study of adult neurogenesis. Consequently, present knowledge about the transcriptional regulation of adult neurogenesis is limited.

Pax6 is an example of a transcription factor whose eminent role in embryonic neurogenesis makes it a likely candidate as a key regulator in adult neurogenesis. However, the Pax6 null-mutant (smalleye) is embryonically lethal. Pax6 is expressed in the SVZ but not the SGZ, a pattern suggesting a differential role in the two neurogenic regions.

cAMP and cAMP Response Element Binding Protein

Two of the few intracellular mediators studied in the context of adult neurogenesis in any detail thus far are cAMP and CREB. As mentioned before, phosphorylation allows CREB to bind to the BDNF promoter and thus modulate BDNF action. Phosphorylated CREB highly co-localizes with PSA-NCAM in the dentate gyrus (Nakagawa et al., 2002a). Consequently, in a situation of induced neurogenesis, such as in response to focal ischemia, CREB expression is increased as well (Zhu et al., 2004). The link does not appear to be merely correlational, because blockade of CREB prevented the induction of adult neurogenesis, whereas overexpression of CREB further stimulated it (Zhu et al., 2004). The same pattern applied to physiological situations where hippocampus-specific expression of a dominant negative mutant of CREB led to reduced cell proliferation (Nakagawa et al., 2002b). Similarly, blocking the metabolism of cAMP by application of the drug rolipram increased both the number of dividing cells and the number of surviving newly generated cells (Nakagawa et al., 2002a, 2002b).

Sox

Sox1 is involved in fate choice decision and the initiation of neuronal differentiation. Sox1 is first expressed during formation of the neural plate (Collignon et al., 1996). It later becomes restricted to neural precursor cells. Null-mutants for Sox1 show a loss of ventral brain structures (Malas et al., 2003). In neural progenitor cell lines and neurosphere cultures from the embryonic brain, Sox1 induced neurogenesis by blocking Notch activity and by attenuating Wnt signaling (Kan et al., 2004).

Sox2 (Sry-related HMG box 2) is a transcription factor that controls the development of the nervous system from its earliest stages (Gubbay et al., 1990; Uwanogho et al., 1995). Sox2 is expressed in embryonic stem cells in the inner cell mass of the blastocyst and persists in many multipotent cell lineages. In the neurogenic zones of the adult brain, Sox2 is expressed by the radial glia–like stem cells (B cells/type-1 cells) and their progenitor progeny (C cells/type-2 cells), but not all cells within these populations express Sox2 (Ferri et al., 2004; Komitova and Eriksson, 2004). Adult neurogenesis was decreased in mice in which the neural enhancer element of the Sox2 promoter had been deleted, thus preventing embryonic lethality. Nestin-GFAP-positive cells were greatly decreased (Ferri et al., 2004). On the basis of Sox2 expression, both pluripotent embryonic stem cells and multipotent neural precursor cells could be isolated from the mouse brain (D'Amour and Gage, 2003). This isolation technique allowed comparison of the two precursor cell populations. Sox2-positive multipotent neural precursor cells differed from Sox2-positive embryonic stem cells in the expression of a total of about 270 identified genes, which were present in one and absent in the other population. This finding suggests that Sox2 exerts its function in precursor cells whose positional identity has already been determined. In this determination, the neural enhancer element of the Sox2 promoter is involved, which suggests that despite its early expression in embryonic stem cells, Sox2 in adult neural precursor cells is controlled by yet another factor.

Nevertheless, to date, Sox2 is the one transcription factor that is most closely associated with "stemness" in adult neurogenesis.

Tailless

In the case of tailless (TLX), researchers were in an unusually advantageous situation, because the role of TLX during development appears to shift and becomes more pronounced in late neurogenesis than during embryonic brain development. TLX is not necessary for intrauterine survival and general formation of the brain, although it is primarily expressed in the ventricular walls from which neurons and glia originate (Monaghan et al., 1997). In TLX null-mutants cortical development was disturbed and led to a premature specification of cortical layers (Roy et al., 2004). Adult TLX null-mutants showed hypotrophic limbic structures, notably including the postnatally developing brain regions such as the dentate gyrus and olfactory bulb, partially because the late progenitor cells have a prolonged cell cycle time (Roy et al., 2004). Although TLX function is thus not specific to adult neurogenesis and is not independent of a developmental phenotype, relevance of TLX to precursor cell function appears to increase in postnatal and adult neurogenesis. TLX-expressing cells derived from wild-type mice were self-renewing and multipotent, but TLX−/− mice lacked nestin-expressing precursor cells in adult neurogenic zones (Shi et al., 2004). TLX also down-regulates the expression of glial proteins such as GFAP, which suggests that TLX is expressed not in the radial glia–like cells but in the transiently amplifying progenitor cells of the neurogenic zones. This interpretation also suggests that TLX could serve a relatively specific function in adult neurogenesis and might be involved in determining precursor cells in neuronal lineage.

Epigenetic Modifications and dsRNA

Transcription factor binding is controlled by additional mechanisms. Epigenetic regulation controls gene activity by altering chromatin structure. DNA methylation and acetylation in promoter regions, for example, make them unavailable for transcription factor binding (see Fisher and Merkenschlager, 2002, for review). This type of control might bundle many different genes and help to coordinate regulation in complex developmental processes.

Null-mutants for methyl-CpG binding protein 1 (MBD1), a member of a family of proteins that bind to methylated promoters and facilitate transcriptional repression, showed decreased precursor cell activity in vitro and in vivo. Adult hippocampal neurogenesis was decreased and hippocampal function impaired (Zhao et al., 2003).

Numerous genes involved in neuronal development contain a highly conserved DNA responsive element, NRSE/RE1, to which a key transcription factor NRSF/REST (for neuronal-restricted silencing factor/RE-1 silencing transcription factor) can bind. NRSF/REST binding suppresses activation of the neuronal genes and is thus antineurogenic. The system plays an important role in preventing the expression of neuronal genes in non-neuronal cells (Schoenherr and Anderson, 1995).

Tomoko Kuwabara and colleagues from Fred H. Gage's group at the Salk Institute discovered that a small noncoding piece of double-stranded RNA (NRSE dsRNA) binds to NRSF/REST in hippocampal precursor cells in vitro and by suppressing the inhibitory action of NRSF/REST, induces a fate choice decision toward neuronal differentiation (Kuwabara et al., 2004). In the presence of NRSE, dsRNA NRSF/REST acted as an activator of neuronal genes. If the uptake of NRSE dsRNA into the nucleus was blocked, no neuronal differentiation of hippocampal precursor cells occurred.

This finding helps explain how neural precursor cells switch from the suppression of neuronal genes associated with the stemness state to their activation when differentiation is induced. Because the NRSE/RE1 sequence is part of so many neuronal genes, a great number of genes are efficiently controlled at the same time.

REFERENCES

Aberg MA, Aberg ND, Hedbacker H, Oscarsson J, Eriksson PS (2000) Peripheral infusion of IGF-I selectively induces neurogenesis in the adult rat hippocampus. J Neurosci 20:2896–2903.

Aberg MA, Aberg ND, Palmer TD, Alborn AM, Carlsson-Skwirut C, Bang P, Rosengren LE, Olsson T, Gage FH, Eriksson PS (2003) IGF-I has a direct proliferative effect in adult hippocampal progenitor cells. Mol Cell Neurosci 24:23–40.

Abiola O, Angel JM, Avner P, Bachmanov AA, Belknap JK, Bennett B, Blankenhorn EP, Blizard DA, Bolivar V, Brockmann GA, Buck KJ, Bureau JF, Casley WL, Chesler EJ, Cheverud JM, Churchill GA, Cook M, Crabbe JC, Crusio WE, Darvasi A, de Haan G, Dermant P, Doerge RW, Elliot RW, Farber CR, Flaherty L, Flint J, Gershenfeld H, Gibson JP, Gu J, Gu W, Himmelbauer H, Hitzemann R, Hsu HC, Hunter K, Iraqi FF, Jansen RC, Johnson TE, Jones BC, Kempermann G, Lammert F, Lu L, Manly KF, Matthews DB, Medrano JF, Mehrabian M, Mittlemann G, Mock BA, Mogil JS, Montagutelli X, Morahan G, Mountz JD, Nagase H, Nowakowski RS, O'Hara BF, Osadchuk AV, Paigen B, Palmer AA, Peirce JL, Pomp D, Rosemann M, Rosen GD, Schalkwyk LC, Seltzer Z, Settle S, Shimomura K, Shou S, Sikela JM, Siracusa LD, Spearow JL, Teuscher C, Threadgill DW, Toth LA, Toye AA, Vadasz C, Van Zant G, Wakeland E, Williams RW, Zhang HG, Zou F (2003) The nature and identification of quantitative trait loci: a community's view. Nat Rev Genet 4:911–916.

Abrous DN, Adriani W, Montaron MF, Aurousseau C, Rougon G, Le Moal M, Piazza PV (2002) Nicotine self-administration impairs hippocampal plasticity. J Neurosci 22:3656–3662.

Abusaad I, MacKay D, Zhao J, Stanford P, Collier DA, Everall IP (1999) Stereological estimation of the total number of neurons in the murine hippocampus using the optical disector. J Comp Neurol 408:560–566.

Alonso R, Griebel G, Pavone G, Stemmelin J, Le Fur G, Soubrie P (2004) Blockade of CRF(1) or V(1b) receptors reverses stress-induced suppression of neurogenesis in a mouse model of depression. Mol Psychiatry 9:278–286, 224.

Altar CA, Cai N, Bliven T, Juhasz M, Conner JM, Acheson AL, Lindsay RM, Wiegand SJ (1997) Anterograde transport of brain-derived neurotrophic factor and its role in the brain. Nature 389:856–860.

Altman J, Das GD (1965) Autoradiographic and histologic evidence of postnatal neurogenesis in rats. J Comp Neurol 124:319–335.

Alvarez-Borda B, Nottebohm F (2002) Gonads and singing play separate, additive roles in new neuron recruitment in adult canary brain. J Neurosci 22:8684–8690.

Ambrogini P, Lattanzi D, Ciuffoli S, Agostini D, Bertini L, Stocchi V, Santi S, Cuppini R (2004a) Morpho-functional characterization of neuronal cells at different stages of maturation in granule cell layer of adult rat dentate gyrus. Brain Res 1017:21–31.

Ambrogini P, Orsini L, Mancini C, Ferri P, Ciaroni S, Cuppini R (2004b) Learning may reduce neurogenesis in adult rat dentate gyrus. Neurosci Lett 359:13–16.

Amrein I, Slomianka L, Poletaeva, II, Bologova NV, Lipp HP (2004) Marked species and age-dependent differences in cell proliferation and neurogenesis in the hippocampus of wild-living rodents. Hippocampus 14:1000–1010.

Aramakis VB, Hsieh CY, Leslie FM, Metherate R (2000) A critical period for nicotine-induced disruption of synaptic development in rat auditory cortex. J Neurosci 20:6106–6116.

Arsenijevic Y, Villemure JG, Brunet JF, Bloch JJ, Deglon N, Kostic C, Zurn A, Aebischer P (2001) Isolation of multipotent neural precursors residing in the cortex of the adult human brain. Exp Neurol 170:48–62.

Arvidsson A, Collin T, Kirik D, Kokaia Z, Lindvall O (2002) Neuronal replacement from endogenous precursors in the adult brain after stroke. Nat Med 8:963–970.

Arvidsson A, Kokaia Z, Lindvall O (2001) N-methyl-D-aspartate receptor–mediated increase of neurogenesis in adult rat dentate gyrus following stroke. Eur J Neurosci 14:10–18.

Back SA, Han BH, Luo NL, Chricton CA, Xanthoudakis S, Tam J, Arvin KL, Holtzman DM (2002) Selective vulnerability of late oligodendrocyte progenitors to hypoxia-ischemia. J Neurosci 22:455–463.

Backhouse B, Barochovsky O, Malik C, Patel AJ, Lewis PD (1982) Effects of haloperidol on cell proliferation in the early postnatal rat brain. Neuropathol Appl Neurobiol 8:109–116.

Bai F, Bergeron M, Nelson DL (2003) Chronic AMPA receptor potentiator (LY451646) treatment increases cell proliferation in adult rat hippocampus. Neuropharmacology 44:1013–1021.

Banasr M, Hery M, Brezun JM, Daszuta A (2001) Serotonin mediates oestrogen stimulation of cell proliferation in the adult dentate gyrus. Eur J Neurosci 14:1417–1424.

Banasr M, Hery M, Printemps R, Daszuta A (2004) Serotonin-induced increases in adult cell proliferation and neurogenesis are mediated through different and common 5-HT receptor subtypes in the dentate gyrus and the subventricular zone. Neuropsychopharmacology 29:450–460.

Bengzon J, Kokaia Z, Elmér E, Nanobashvili A, Kokaia M, Lindvall O (1997) Apoptosis and proliferation of dentate gyrus neurons after single and intermittent limbic seizures. Proc Natl Acad Sci USA 94:10432–10437.

Benraiss A, Chmielnicki E, Lerner K, Roh D, Goldman SA (2001) Adenoviral brain-derived neurotrophic factor induces both neostriatal and olfactory neuronal recruitment from endogenous progenitor cells in the adult forebrain. J Neurosci 21:6718–6731.

Bernabeu R, Sharp FR (2000) NMDA and AMPA/kainate glutamate receptors modulate dentate neurogenesis and CA3 synapsin-I in normal and ischemic hippocampus. J Cereb Blood Flow Metab 20:1669–1680.

Biebl M, Cooper CM, Winkler J, Kuhn HG (2000) Analysis of neurogenesis and programmed cell death reveals a self-renewing capacity in the adult rat brain. Neurosci Lett 291:17–20.

Bittman K, Owens DF, Kriegstein AR, LoTurco JJ (1997) Cell coupling and uncoupling in the ventricular zone of developing neocortex. J Neurosci 17:7037–7044.

Bizon JL, Gallagher M (2003) Production of new cells in the rat dentate gyrus over the lifespan: relation to cognitive decline. Eur J Neurosci 18:215–219.

Blaschke AJ, Staley K, Chun J (1996) Widespread programmed cell death in proliferative and postmitotic regions of the fetal cerebral cortex. Development 122:1165–1174.

Bonni A, Sun Y, Nadal-Vicens M, Bhatt A, Frank DA, Rozovsky I, Stahl N, Yancopoulos GD, Greenberg ME (1997) Regulation of gliogenesis in the central nervous system by the JAK-STAT signaling pathway. Science 278:477–483.

Brandt MD, Jessberger S, Steiner B, Kronenberg G, Reuter K, Bick-Sander A, Von der Behrens W, Kempermann G (2003) Transient calretinin-expression defines early postmitotic step of neuronal differentiation in adult hippocampal neurogenesis of mice. Mol Cell Neurosci 24:603–613.

Brannvall K, Korhonen L, Lindholm D (2002) Estrogen-receptor-dependent regulation of neural stem cell proliferation and differentiation. Mol Cell Neurosci 21:512–520.

Brezun JM, Daszuta A (1999) Depletion in serotonin decreases neurogenesis in the dentate gyrus and the subventricular zone of adult rats. Neuroscience 89:999–1002.

Brezun JM, Daszuta A (2000) Serotonin may stimulate granule cell proliferation in the adult hippocampus, as observed in rats grafted with foetal raphe neurons. Eur J Neurosci 12:391–396.

Brown J, Cooper-Kuhn CM, Kempermann G, Van Praag H, Winkler J, Gage FH, Kuhn HG (2003) Enriched environment and physical activity stimulate hippocampal but not olfactory bulb neurogenesis. Eur J Neurosci 17:2042–2046.

Cameron HA, Gould E (1994) Adult neurogenesis is regulated by adrenal steroids in the dentate gyrus. Neuroscience 61:203–209.

Cameron HA, Gould E (1996) Distinct populations of cells in the adult dentate gyrus undergo mitosis or apoptosis in response to adrenalectomy. J Comp Neurol 369:56–63.

Cameron HA, McKay RD (1999) Restoring production of hippocampal neurons in old age. Nat Neurosci 2:894–897.

Cameron HA, McEwen BS, Gould E (1995) Regulation of adult neurogenesis by excitatory input and NMDA receptor activation in the dentate gyrus. J Neurosci 15:4687–4692.

Cameron HA, Tanapat P, Gould E (1998) Adrenal steroids and N-methyl-D-aspartate receptor activation regulate neurogenesis in the dentate gyrus of adult rats through a common pathway. Neuroscience 82:349–354.

Cameron HA, Woolley CS, Gould E (1993) Adrenal steroid receptor immunoreactivity in cells born in the adult rat dentate gyrus. Brain Res 611:342–346.

Cao L, Jiao X, Zuzga DS, Liu Y, Fong DM, Young D, During MJ (2004) VEGF links hippocampal activity with neurogenesis, learning and memory. Nat Genet 36:827–835.

Caporaso GL, Lim DA, Alvarez-Buylla A, Chao MV (2003) Telomerase activity in the subventricular zone of adult mice. Mol Cell Neurosci 23:693–702.

Carro E, Nunez A, Busiguina S, Torres-Aleman I (2000) Circulating insulin-like growth factor I mediates effects of exercise on the brain. J Neurosci 20:2926–2933.

Carro E, Trejo JL, Busiguina S, Torres-Aleman I (2001) Circulating insulin-like growth factor I mediates the protective effects of physical exercise against brain insults of different etiology and anatomy. J Neurosci 21:5678–5684.

Castelo-Branco G, Wagner J, Rodriguez FJ, Kele J, Sousa K, Rawal N, Pasolli HA, Fuchs E, Kitajewski J, Arenas E (2003) Differential regulation of midbrain dopaminergic neuron development by Wnt-1, Wnt-3a, and Wnt-5a. Proc Natl Acad Sci USA 100:12747–12752.

Changeux JP, Bertrand D, Corringer PJ, Dehaene S, Edelstein S, Lena C, Le Novere N, Marubio L, Picciotto M, Zoli M (1998) Brain nicotinic receptors: structure and regulation, role in learning and reinforcement. Brain Res Brain Res Rev 26:198–216.

Cheng A, Wang S, Cai J, Rao MS, Mattson MP (2003a) Nitric oxide acts in a positive feedback loop with BDNF to regulate neural progenitor cell proliferation and differentiation in the mammalian brain. Dev Biol 258:319–333.

Cheng YH, Wang WD, Sun LS, Cheng ZJ, Xu JP (2003b) [Effects of nitric oxide synthase inhibitor on dentate gyrus neurogenesis after diffuse brain injury in adult rats]. Di Yi Jun Yi Da Xue Xue Bao 23:1074–1077.

Chiang C, Litingtung Y, Lee E, Young KE, Corden JL, Westphal H, Beachy PA (1996) Cyclopia and defective axial patterning in mice lacking Sonic hedgehog gene function. Nature 383:407–413.

Chojnacki A, Shimazaki T, Gregg C, Weinmaster G, Weiss S (2003) Glycoprotein 130 signaling regulates Notch1 expression and activation in the self-renewal of mammalian forebrain neural stem cells. J Neurosci 23:1730–1741.

Clemmons DR (1991) Insulin-like growth factor binding proteins: roles in regulating IGF physiology. J Dev Physiol 15:105–110.

Coe CL, Kramer M, Czeh B, Gould E, Reeves AJ, Kirschbaum C, Fuchs E (2003) Prenatal stress diminishes neurogenesis in the dentate gyrus of juvenile rhesus monkeys. Biol Psychiatry 54:1025–1034.

Collignon J, Sockanathan S, Hacker A, Cohen-Tannoudji M, Norris D, Rastan S, Stevanovic M, Goodfellow PN, Lovell-Badge R (1996) A comparison of the properties of Sox-3 with Sry and two related genes, Sox-1 and Sox-2. Development 122:509–520.

Cooper-Kuhn CM, Vroemen M, Brown J, Ye H, Thompson MA, Winkler J, Kuhn HG (2002) Impaired adult neurogenesis in mice lacking the transcription factor E2F1. Mol Cell Neurosci 21:312–323.

Cooper-Kuhn CM, Winkler J, Kuhn HG (2004) Decreased neurogenesis after cholinergic forebrain lesion in the adult rat. J Neurosci Res 77:155–165.

Corotto FS, Henegar JR, Maruniak JA (1994) Odor deprivation leads to reduced neurogenesis and reduced neuronal survival in the olfactory bulb of the adult mouse. Neuroscience 61:739–744.

Cummings DM, Henning HE, Brunjes PC (1997) Olfactory bulb recovery after early sensory deprivation. J Neurosci 17:7433–7440.

Czeh B, Welt T, Fischer AK, Erhardt A, Schmitt W, Muller MB, Toschi N, Fuchs E, Keck ME (2002) Chronic psychosocial stress and concomitant repetitive transcranial magnetic stimulation: effects on stress hormone levels and adult hippocampal neurogenesis. Biol Psychiatry 52:1057–1065.

D'Amour KA, Gage FH (2003) Genetic and functional differences between multipotent neural and pluripotent embryonic stem cells. Proc Natl Acad Sci USA 100 (Suppl 1):11866–11872.

Dawirs RR, Hildebrandt K, Teuchert-Noodt G (1998) Adult treatment with haloperidol increases dentate granule cell proliferation in the gerbil hippocampus. J Neural Transm 105:317–127.

De Ferrari GV, Inestrosa NC (2000) Wnt signaling function in Alzheimer's disease. Brain Res Brain Res Rev 33:1–12.

Deisseroth K, Singla S, Toda H, Monje M, Palmer TD, Malenka RC (2004) Excitation–neurogenesis coupling in adult neural stem/progenitor cells. Neuron 42:535–552.

Dickinson ME, Krumlauf R, McMahon AP (1994) Evidence for a mitogenic effect of Wnt-1 in the developing mammalian central nervous system. Development 120:1453–1471.

Dobrossy MD, Drapeau E, Aurousseau C, Le Moal M, Piazza PV, Abrous DN (2003) Differential effects of learning on neurogenesis: learning increases or decreases the number of newly born cells depending on their birth date. Mol Psychiatry 8:974–982.

Doetsch F, Verdugo JM, Caille I, Alvarez-Buylla A, Chao MV, Casaccia-Bonnefil P (2002) Lack of the cell-cycle inhibitor p27Kip1 results in selective increase of transit-amplifying cells for adult neurogenesis. J Neurosci 22:2255–2264.

D'Sa C, Duman RS (2002) Antidepressants and neuroplasticity. Bipolar Disord 4:183–194.

Ehninger D, Kempermann G (2003) Regional effects of wheel running and environmental enrichment on cell genesis and microglia proliferation in the adult murine neocortex. Cereb Cortex 13:845–851.

Eisch AJ, Barrot M, Schad CA, Self DW, Nestler EJ (2000) Opiates inhibit neurogenesis in the adult rat hippocampus. Proc Natl Acad Sci USA 97:7579–7584.

Ekdahl CT, Claasen JH, Bonde S, Kokaia Z, Lindvall O (2003) Inflammation is detrimental for neurogenesis in adult brain. Proc Natl Acad Sci USA 100:13632–13637.

Emsley JG, Hagg T (2003) Endogenous and exogenous ciliary neurotrophic factor enhances forebrain neurogenesis in adult mice. Exp Neurol 183:298–310.

Eriksson PS, Perfilieva E, Björk-Eriksson T, Alborn AM, Nordborg C, Peterson DA, Gage FH (1998) Neurogenesis in the adult human hippocampus. Nat Med 4:1313–1317.

Estrada C, Gomez C, Martin-Nieto J, De Frutos T, Jimenez A, Villalobo A (1997) Nitric oxide reversibly inhibits the epidermal growth factor receptor tyrosine kinase. Biochem J 326(Pt 2):369–376.

Fabel K, Tam B, Kaufer D, Baiker A, Simmons N, Kuo CJ, Palmer TD (2003) VEGF is necessary for exercise-induced adult hippocampal neurogenesis. Eur J Neurosci 18:2803–2812.

Fan X, Xu H, Cai W, Yang Z, Zhang J (2003) Spatial and temporal patterns of expression of Noggin and BMP4 in embryonic and postnatal rat hippocampus. Brain Res Dev Brain Res 146:51–58.

Fan XT, Xu HW, Cai WQ, Yang H, Liu S (2004) Antisense Noggin oligodeoxynucleotide administration decreases cell proliferation in the dentate gyrus of adult rats. Neurosci Lett 366:107–111.

Farmer J, Zhao X, van Praag H, Wodtke K, Gage FH, Christie BR (2004) Effects of voluntary exercise on synaptic plasticity and gene expression in the dentate gyrus of adult male Sprague-Dawley rats in vivo. Neuroscience 124:71–79.

Feng R, Rampon C, Tang YP, Shrom D, Jin J, Kyin M, Sopher B, Martin GM, Kim SH, Langdon RB, Sisodia SS, Tsien JZ (2001) Deficient neurogenesis in forebrain-specific presenilin-1 knockout mice is associated with reduced clearance of hippocampal memory traces. Neuron 32:911–926.

Ferri AL, Cavallaro M, Braida D, Di Cristofano A, Canta A, Vezzani A, Ottolenghi S, Pandolfi PP, Sala M, DeBiasi S, Nicolis SK (2004) Sox2 deficiency causes neurodegeneration and impaired neurogenesis in the adult mouse brain. Development 131:3805–3819.

Ferron S, Mira H, Franco S, Cano-Jaimez M, Bellmunt E, Ramirez C, Farinas I, Blasco

MA (2004) Telomere shortening and chromosomal instability abrogates proliferation of adult but not embryonic neural stem cells. Development 131:4059–4070.

Ferry RJ Jr, Katz LE, Grimberg A, Cohen P, Weinzimer SA (1999) Cellular actions of insulin-like growth factor binding proteins. Horm Metab Res 31:192–202.

Filippov V, Kronenberg G, Pivneva T, Reuter K, Steiner B, Wang LP, Yamaguchi M, Kettenmann H, Kempermann G (2003) Subpopulation of nestin-expressing progenitor cells in the adult murine hippocampus shows electrophysiological and morphological characteristics of astrocytes. Mol Cell Neurosci 23:373–382.

Fisher AG, Merkenschlager M (2002) Gene silencing, cell fate and nuclear organisation. Curr Opin Genet Dev 12:193–197.

Fiske BK, Brunjes PC (2001) Cell death in the developing and sensory-deprived rat olfactory bulb. J Comp Neurol 431:311–319.

Freund TF, Buzsaki G (1996) Interneurons of the hippocampus. Hippocampus 6:347–470.

Gaiano N, Nye JS, Fishell G (2000) Radial glial identity is promoted by Notch1 signaling in the murine forebrain. Neuron 26:395–404.

Galea LA, McEwen BS (1999) Sex and seasonal differences in the rate of cell proliferation in the dentate gyrus of adult wild meadow voles. Neuroscience 89:955–964.

Gama Sosa MA, Wen PH, De Gasperi R, Perez GM, Senturk E, Friedrich VL Jr, Elder GA (2004) Entorhinal cortex lesioning promotes neurogenesis in the hippocampus of adult mice. Neuroscience 127:881–891.

Garcia A, Steiner B, Kronenberg G, Bick-Sander A, Kempermann G (2004) Age-dependent expression of glucocorticoid and mineralocorticoid receptors on neural precursor cell populations in the adult murine hippocampus. Aging Cell 3:363–371.

Gass P, Kretz O, Wolfer DP, Berger S, Tronche F, Reichardt HM, Kellendonk C, Lipp HP, Schmid W, Schutz G (2000) Genetic disruption of mineralocorticoid receptor leads to impaired neurogenesis and granule cell degeneration in the hippocampus of adult mice. EMBO Rep 1:447–451.

Goldman SA, Kirschenbaum B, Harrison-Restelli C, Thaler HT (1997) Neuronal precursors of the adult rat subependymal zone persist into senescence, with no decline in spatial extent or response to BDNF. J Neurobiol 32:554–566.

Gomez-Pinilla F, Dao L, So V (1997) Physical exercise induces FGF-2 and its mRNA in the hippocampus. Brain Res 764:1–8.

Gould E (1994) The effects of adrenal steroids and excitatory input on neuronal birth and survival. Ann NY Acad Sci 743:73–92; discussion 92–73.

Gould E, Beylin A, Tanapat P, Reeves A, Shors TJ (1999) Learning enhances adult neurogenesis in the hippoampal formation. Nat Neurosci 2:260–265.

Gould E, Cameron HA, Daniels DC, Woolley CS, McEwen BS (1992) Adrenal hormones suppress cell division in the adult rat dentate gyrus. J Neurosci 12:3642–3650.

Gould E, Cameron HA, McEwen BS (1994) Blockade of NMDA receptors increases cell death and birth in the developing rat dentate gyrus. J Comp Neurol 340:551–565.

Gould E, McEwen BS (1993) Neuronal birth and death. Curr Opin Neurobiol 3:676–682.

Gould E, McEwen BS, Tanapat P, Galea LAM, Fuchs E (1997) Neurogenesis in the dentate gyrus of the adult tree shrew is regulated by psychosocial stress and NMDA receptor activation. J Neurosci 17:2492–2498.

Gould E, Tanapat P, McEwen BS, Flügge G, Fuchs E (1998) Proliferation of granule cell precursors in the dentate gyrus of adult monkeys is diminished by stress. Proc Natl Acad Sci USA 95:3168–3171.

Gould E, Woolley CS, McEwen BS (1991) Adrenal steroids regulate postnatal development of the rat dentate gyrus: I. Effects of glucocorticoids on cell death. J Comp Neurol 313:479–485.

Gould TD, Manji HK (2002) The Wnt signaling pathway in bipolar disorder. Neuroscientist 8:497–511.

Gu W, Brannstrom T, Wester P (2000) Cortical neurogenesis in adult rats after reversible photothrombotic stroke. J Cereb Blood Flow Metab 20:1166–1173.

Guazzo EP, Kirkpatrick PJ, Goodyer IM, Shiers HM, Herbert J (1996) Cortisol, dehydroepiandrosterone (DHEA), and DHEA sulfate in the cerebrospinal fluid of man: relation to blood levels and the effects of age. J Clin Endocrinol Metab 81:3951–3960.

Gubbay J, Collignon J, Koopman P, Capel B, Economou A, Munsterberg A, Vivian N, Goodfellow P, Lovell-Badge R (1990) A gene mapping to the sex-determining region of the mouse Y chromosome is a member of a novel family of embryonically expressed genes. Nature 346:245–250.

Gustafsson E, Lindvall O, Kokaia Z (2003) Intraventricular infusion of TrkB-Fc fusion protein promotes ischemia-induced neurogenesis in adult rat dentate gyrus. Stroke 34:2710–2715.

Haik S, Gauthier LR, Granotier C, Peyrin JM, Lages CS, Dormont D, Boussin FD (2000) Fibroblast growth factor 2 up-regulates telomerase activity in neural precursor cells. Oncogene 19:2957–2966.

Halim ND, Weickert CS, McClintock BW, Weinberger DR, Lipska BK (2004) Effects of chronic haloperidol and clozapine treatment on neurogenesis in the adult rat hippocampus. Neuropsychopharmacology 29:1063–1069.

Heine VM, Maslam S, Joels M, Lucassen PJ (2004a) Prominent decline of newborn cell proliferation, differentiation, and apoptosis in the aging dentate gyrus, in absence of an age-related hypothalamus-pituitary-adrenal axis activation. Neurobiol Aging 25:361–375.

Heine VM, Maslam S, Zareno J, Joels M, Lucassen PJ (2004b) Suppressed proliferation and apoptotic changes in the rat dentate gyrus after acute and chronic stress are reversible. Eur J Neurosci 19:131–144.

Hellsten J, Wennstrom M, Bengzon J, Mohapel P, Tingstrom A (2004) Electroconvulsive seizures induce endothelial cell proliferation in adult rat hippocampus. Biol Psychiatry 55:420–427.

Herrera E, Samper E, Blasco MA (1999a) Telomere shortening in mTR−/− embryos is associated with failure to close the neural tube. EMBO J 18:1172–1181.

Herrera E, Samper E, Martin-Caballero J, Flores JM, Lee HW, Blasco MA (1999b) Disease states associated with telomerase deficiency appear earlier in mice with short telomeres. EMBO J 18:2950–2960.

Hidalgo A, Barami K, Iversen K, Goldman SA (1995) Estrogens and non-estrogenic ovarian influences combine to promote the recruitment and decrease the turnover of new neurons in the adult female canary brain. J Neurobiol 27:470–487.

Hill DJ, Han VK (1991) Paracrinology of growth regulation. J Dev Physiol 15:91–104.

Hitoshi S, Alexson T, Tropepe V, Donoviel D, Elia AJ, Nye JS, Conlon RA, Mak TW, Bernstein A, van der Kooy D (2002) Notch pathway molecules are essential for the maintenance, but not the generation, of mammalian neural stem cells. Genes Dev 16:846–858.

Höglinger GU, Rizk P, Muriel MP, Duyckaerts C, Oertel WH, Caille I, Hirsch EC (2004) Dopamine depletion impairs precursor cell proliferation in Parkinson disease. Nat Neurosci 7:726–735.

Holmes MM, Galea LA, Mistlberger RE, Kempermann G (2004) Adult hippocampal neurogenesis and voluntary running activity: circadian and dose-dependent effects. J Neurosci Res 76:216–222.

Hsieh J, Aimone JB, Kaspar BK, Kuwabara T, Nakashima K, Gage FH (2004) IGF-I instructs multipotent adult neural progenitor cells to become oligodendrocytes. J Cell Biol 164:111–122.

Huttmann K, Sadgrove M, Wallraff A, Hinterkeuser S, Kirchhoff F, Steinhauser C, Gray WP (2003) Seizures preferentially stimulate proliferation of radial glia–like astrocytes in the adult dentate gyrus: functional and immunocytochemical analysis. Eur J Neurosci 18:2769–2778.

Ikeya M, Lee SM, Johnson JE, McMahon AP, Takada S (1997) Wnt signalling required for expansion of neural crest and CNS progenitors. Nature 389:966–970.

Islam AT, Kuraoka A, Kawabuchi M (2003) Morphological basis of nitric oxide production and its correlation with the polysialylated precursor cells in the dentate gyrus of the adult guinea pig hippocampus. Anat Sci Int 78:98–103.

Itoh H, Hirata K, Ohsato K (1993) Turcot's syndrome and familial adenomatous polyposis associated with brain tumor: review of related literature. Int J Colorectal Dis 8:87–94.

Iwai M, Hayashi T, Zhang WR, Sato K, Manabe Y, Abe K (2001) Induction of highly polysialylated neural cell adhesion molecule (PSA-NCAM) in postischemic gerbil hippocampus mainly dissociated with neural stem cell proliferation. Brain Res 902:288–293.

James JR, Nordberg A (1995) Genetic and environmental aspects of the role of nicotinic receptors in neurodegenerative disorders: emphasis on Alzheimer's disease and Parkinson's disease. Behav Genet 25:149–159.

Jessberger S, Kempermann G (2003) Adult-born hippocampal neurons mature into activity-dependent responsiveness. Eur J Neurosci 18:2707–2712.

Jiang W, Gu W, Brannstrom T, Rosqvist R, Wester P (2001) Cortical neurogenesis in adult rats after transient middle cerebral artery occlusion. Stroke 32:1201–1207.

Jiang W, Wan Q, Zhang ZJ, Wang WD, Huang YG, Rao ZR, Zhang X (2003) Dentate granule cell neurogenesis after seizures induced by pentylenetrazol in rats. Brain Res 977:141–148.

Jin K, Mao XO, Sun Y, Xie L, Greenberg DA (2002a) Stem cell factor stimulates neurogenesis in vitro and in vivo. J Clin Invest 110:311–319.

Jin K, Minami M, Lan JQ, Mao XO, Batteur S, Simon RP, Greenberg DA (2001) Neurogenesis in dentate subgranular zone and rostral subventricular zone after focal cerebral ischemia in the rat. Proc Natl Acad Sci USA 98:4710–4715.

Jin K, Mao XO, Sun Y, Xie L, Jin L, Nishi E, Klagsbrun M, Greenberg DA (2002b) Heparin-binding epidermal growth factor-like growth factor: hypoxia-inducible expression in vitro and stimulation of neurogenesis in vitro and in vivo. J Neurosci 22:5365–5373.

Jin K, Sun Y, Xie L, Batteur S, Mao XO, Smelick C, Logvinova A, Greenberg DA (2003a) Neurogenesis and aging: FGF-2 and HB-EGF restore neurogenesis in hippocampus and subventricular zone of aged mice. Aging Cell 2:175–183.

Jin K, Xie L, Childs J, Sun Y, Mao XO, Logvinova A, Greenberg DA (2003b) Cerebral neurogenesis is induced by intranasal administration of growth factors. Ann Neurol 53:405–409.

Jin K, Xie L, Kim SH, Parmentier-Batteur S, Sun Y, Mao XO, Childs J, Greenberg DA (2004) Defective adult neurogenesis in CB1 cannabinoid receptor knockout mice. Mol Pharmacol 66:204–208.

Jin K, Zhu Y, Sun Y, Mao XO, Xie L, Greenberg DA (2002c) Vascular endothelial growth factor (VEGF) stimulates neurogenesis in vitro and in vivo. Proc Natl Acad Sci USA 99:11946–11950.

Kan L, Israsena N, Zhang Z, Hu M, Zhao LR, Jalali A, Sahni V, Kessler JA (2004)

Sox1 acts through multiple independent pathways to promote neurogenesis. Dev Biol 269:580–594.

Karishma KK, Herbert J (2002) Dehydroepiandrosterone (DHEA) stimulates neurogenesis in the hippocampus of the rat, promotes survival of newly formed neurons and prevents corticosterone-induced suppression. Eur J Neurosci 16:445–453.

Kee NJ, Preston E, Wojtowicz JM (2001) Enhanced neurogenesis after transient global ischemia in the dentate gyrus of the rat. Exp Brain Res 136:313–320.

Kempermann G (2002) Why new neurons? Possible functions for adult hippocampal neurogenesis. J Neurosci 22:635–638.

Kempermann G, Brandon EP, Gage FH (1998a) Environmental stimulation of 129/SvJ mice results in increased cell proliferation and neurogenesis in the adult dentate gyrus. Curr Biol 8:939–942.

Kempermann G, Gage FH (1999) Experience-dependent regulation of adult hippocampal neurogenesis: effects of long-term stimulation and stimulus withdrawal. Hippocampus 9:321–332.

Kempermann G, Gage FH (2002a) Genetic influence on phenotypic differentiation in adult hippocampal neurogenesis. Brain Res Dev Brain Res 134:1–12.

Kempermann G, Gage FH (2002b) Genetic determinants of adult hippocampal neurogenesis correlate with acquisition, but not probe trial performance in the water maze task. Eur J Neurosci 16:129–136.

Kempermann G, Gast D, Gage FH (2002) Neuroplasticity in old age: sustained five-fold induction of hippocampal neurogenesis by long-term environmental enrichment. Ann Neurol 52:135–143.

Kempermann G, Gast D, Kronenberg G, Yamaguchi M, Gage FH (2003) Early determination and long-term persistence of adult-generated new neurons in the hippocampus of mice. Development 130:391–399.

Kempermann G, Jessberger S, Steiner B, Kronenberg G (2004) Milestones of neuronal development in the adult hippocampus. Trends Neurosci 27:447–452.

Kempermann G, Kuhn HG, Gage FH (1997a) More hippocampal neurons in adult mice living in an enriched environment. Nature 386:493–495.

Kempermann G, Kuhn HG, Gage FH (1997b) Genetic influence on neurogenesis in the dentate gyrus of adult mice. Proc Natl Acad Sci USA 94:10409–10414.

Kempermann G, Kuhn HG, Gage FH (1998b) Experience-induced neurogenesis in the senescent dentate gyrus. J Neurosci 18:3206–3212.

Kempermann G, Wiskott L (2004) What is the functional role of new neurons in the adult dentate gyrus? In: Stem Cells in the Nervous System: Function and Clinical Implications (Gage F, Björklund A, Prochiatz A, Christen Y, eds), pp 57–65. Berlin and Heidelberg: Springer.

Kim YP, Kim H, Shin MS, Chang HK, Jang MH, Shin MC, Lee SJ, Lee HH, Yoon JH, Jeong IG, Kim CJ (2004) Age-dependence of the effect of treadmill exercise on cell proliferation in the dentate gyrus of rats. Neurosci Lett 355:152–154.

Kippin TE, Cain SW, Masum Z, Ralph MR (2004) Neural stem cells show bidirectional experience-dependent plasticity in the perinatal mammalian brain. J Neurosci 24:2832–2836.

Kirschenbaum B, Nedergaard M, Preuss A, Barami K, Fraser RA, Goldman SA (1994) In vitro neuronal production and differentiation by precursor cells derived from the adult human forebrain. Cereb Cortex 6:576–589.

Klassen HJ, Imfeld KL, Kirov, II, Tai L, Gage FH, Young MJ, Berman MA (2003) Expression of cytokines by multipotent neural progenitor cells. Cytokine 22:101–106.

Kohl Z, Kuhn HG, Cooper-Kuhn CM, Winkler J, Aigner L, Kempermann G (2002) Preweaning enrichment has no lasting effect on adult hippocampal neurogenesis in four-month old mice. Genes Brain Behav 1:46–54.

Kohtz JD, Baker DP, Corte G, Fishell G (1998) Regionalization within the mammalian telencephalon is mediated by changes in responsiveness to Sonic hedgehog. Development 125:5079–5089.

Komitova M, Eriksson PS (2004) Sox-2 is expressed by neural progenitors and astroglia in the adult rat brain. Neurosci Lett 369:24–27.

Komitova M, Perfilieva E, Mattsson B, Eriksson PS, Johansson BB (2002) Effects of cortical ischemia and postischemic environmental enrichment on hippocampal cell genesis and differentiation in the adult rat. J Cereb Blood Flow Metab 22:852–860.

Korte M, Griesbeck O, Gravel C, Carroll P, Staiger V, Thoenen H, Bonhoeffer T (1996) Virus-mediated gene transfer into hippocampal CA1 region restores long-term potentiation in brain-derived neurotrophic factor mutant mice. Proc Natl Acad Sci USA 93:12547–12552.

Kowalczyk A, Filipkowski RK, Rylski M, Wilczynski GM, Konopacki FA, Jaworski J, Ciemerych MA, Sicinski P, Kaczmarek L (2004) The critical role of cyclin D2 in adult neurogenesis. J Cell Biol 167:209–213.

Kozlovsky N, Belmaker RH, Agam G (2002) GSK-3 and the neurodevelopmental hypothesis of schizophrenia. Eur Neuropsychopharmacol 12:13–25.

Kronenberg G, Reuter K, Steiner B, Brandt MD, Jessberger S, Yamaguchi M, Kempermann G (2003) Subpopulations of proliferating cells of the adult hippocampus respond differently to physiologic neurogenic stimuli. J Comp Neurol 467:455–463.

Kuan CY, Schloemer AJ, Lu A, Burns KA, Weng WL, Williams MT, Strauss KI, Vorhees CV, Flavell RA, Davis RJ, Sharp FR, Rakic P (2004) Hypoxia-ischemia induces DNA synthesis without cell proliferation in dying neurons in adult rodent brain. J Neurosci 24:10763–10772.

Kuhn HG, Dickinson-Anson H, Gage FH (1996) Neurogenesis in the dentate gyrus of the adult rat: age-related decrease of neuronal progenitor proliferation. J Neurosci 16:2027–2033.

Kuhn HG, Winkler J, Kempermann G, Thal LJ, Gage FH (1997) Epidermal growth factor and fibroblast growth factor-2 have different effects on neural progenitors in the adult rat brain. J Neurosci 17:5820–5829.

Kulkarni VA, Jha S, Vaidya VA (2002) Depletion of norepinephrine decreases the proliferation, but does not influence the survival and differentiation, of granule cell progenitors in the adult rat hippocampus. Eur J Neurosci 16:2008–2012.

Kumihashi K, Uchida K, Miyazaki H, Kobayashi J, Tsushima T, Machida T (2001) Acetylsalicylic acid reduces ischemia-induced proliferation of dentate cells in gerbils. Neuroreport 12:915–917.

Kuwabara T, Hsieh J, Nakashima K, Taira K, Gage FH (2004) A small modulatory dsRNA specifies the fate of adult neural stem cells. Cell 116:779–793.

Lai K, Kaspar BK, Gage FH, Schaffer DV (2003) Sonic hedgehog regulates adult neural progenitor proliferation in vitro and in vivo. Nat Neurosci 6:21–27.

Larsson E, Mandel RJ, Klein RL, Muzyczka N, Lindvall O, Kokaia Z (2002) Suppression of insult-induced neurogenesis in adult rat brain by brain-derived neurotrophic factor. Exp Neurol 177:1–8.

Leanza G, Muir J, Nilsson OG, Wiley RG, Dunnett SB, Bjorklund A (1996) Selective immunolesioning of the basal forebrain cholinergic system disrupts short-term memory in rats. Eur J Neurosci 8:1535–1544.

Lee HW, Blasco MA, Gottlieb GJ, Horner JW 2nd, Greider CW, DePinho RA (1998) Essential role of mouse telomerase in highly proliferative organs. Nature 392:569–574.

Lee HY, Kleber M, Hari L, Brault V, Suter U, Taketo MM, Kemler R, Sommer L (2004) Instructive role of Wnt/beta-catenin in sensory fate specification in neural crest stem cells. Science 303:1020–1023.

Lee J, Duan W, Long JM, Ingram DK, Mattson MP (2000a) Dietary restriction increases the number of newly generated neural cells, and induces BDNF expression, in the dentate gyrus of rats. J Mol Neurosci 15:99–108.

Lee J, Duan W, Mattson MP (2002) Evidence that brain-derived neurotrophic factor is required for basal neurogenesis and mediates, in part, the enhancement of neurogenesis by dietary restriction in the hippocampus of adult mice. J Neurochem 82:1367–1375.

Lee SM, Tole S, Grove E, McMahon AP (2000b) A local Wnt-3a signal is required for development of the mammalian hippocampus. Development 127:457–467.

Lemaire V, Koehl M, Le Moal M, Abrous DN (2000) Prenatal stress produces learning deficits associated with an inhibition of neurogenesis in the hippocampus. Proc Natl Acad Sci USA 97:11032–11037.

Leuner B, Mendolia-Loffredo S, Kozorovitskiy Y, Samburg D, Gould E, Shors TJ (2004) Learning enhances the survival of new neurons beyond the time when the hippocampus is required for memory. J Neurosci 24:7477–7481.

Leung LS, Shen B, Rajakumar N, Ma J (2003) Cholinergic activity enhances hippocampal long-term potentiation in CA1 during walking in rats. J Neurosci 23:9297–9304.

Levison SW, Rothstein RP, Romanko MJ, Snyder MJ, Meyers RL, Vannucci SJ (2001) Hypoxia/ischemia depletes the rat perinatal subventricular zone of oligodendrocyte progenitors and neural stem cells. Dev Neurosci 23:234–247.

Lewin GR, Barde YA (1996) Physiology of the neurotrophins. Annu Rev Neurosci 19:289–317.

Li X, Tizzano JP, Griffey K, Clay M, Lindstrom T, Skolnick P (2001) Antidepressant-like actions of an AMPA receptor potentiator (LY392098). Neuropharmacology 40:1028–1033.

Lichtenwalner RJ, Forbes ME, Bennett SA, Lynch CD, Sonntag WE, Riddle DR (2001) Intracerebroventricular infusion of insulin-like growth factor-I ameliorates the age-related decline in hippocampal neurogenesis. Neuroscience 107:603–613.

Liem KF Jr, Tremml G, Roelink H, Jessell TM (1995) Dorsal differentiation of neural plate cells induced by BMP-mediated signals from epidermal ectoderm. Cell 82:969–979.

Lim DA, Tramontin AD, Trevejo JM, Herrera DG, Garcia-Verdugo JM, Alvarez-Buylla A (2000) Noggin antagonizes BMP signaling to create a niche for adult neurogenesis. Neuron 28:713–726.

Limoli CL, Giedzinski E, Rola R, Otsuka S, Palmer TD, Fike JR (2004) Radiation response of neural precursor cells: linking cellular sensitivity to cell cycle checkpoints, apoptosis and oxidative stress. Radiat Res 161:17–27.

Liu D, Caldji C, Sharma S, Plotsky PM, Meaney MJ (2000) Influence of neonatal rearing conditions on stress-induced adrenocorticotropin responses and norepinepherine release in the hypothalamic paraventricular nucleus. J Neuroendocrinol 12:5–12.

Louissaint A Jr, Rao S, Leventhal C, Goldman SA (2002) Coordinated interaction of neurogenesis and angiogenesis in the adult songbird brain. Neuron 34:945–960.

Loy R, Koziell DA, Lindsey JD, Moore RY (1980) Noradrenergic innervation of the adult rat hippocampal formation. J Comp Neurol 189:699–710.

Lu D, Mahmood A, Zhang R, Copp M (2003a) Upregulation of neurogenesis and reduction in functional deficits following administration of DEtA/NONOate, a nitric oxide donor, after traumatic brain injury in rats. J Neurosurg 99:351–361.

Lu L, Bao G, Chen H, Xia P, Fan X, Zhang J, Pei G, Ma L (2003b) Modification of hippocampal neurogenesis and neuroplasticity by social environments. Exp Neurol 183:600–609.

Machold R, Hayashi S, Rutlin M, Muzumdar MD, Nery S, Corbin JG, Gritli-Linde A, Dellovade T, Porter JA, Rubin LL, Dudek H, McMahon AP, Fishell G (2003) Sonic hedgehog is required for progenitor cell maintenance in telencephalic stem cell niches. Neuron 39:937–950.

Mackowiak M, O'Neill MJ, Hicks CA, Bleakman D, Skolnick P (2002) An AMPA receptor potentiator modulates hippocampal expression of BDNF: an in vivo study. Neuropharmacology 43:1–10.

Madsen TM, Kristjansen PE, Bolwig TG, Wortwein G (2003a) Arrested neuronal proliferation and impaired hippocampal function following fractionated brain irradiation in the adult rat. Neuroscience 119:635–642.

Madsen TM, Newton SS, Eaton ME, Russell DS, Duman RS (2003b) Chronic electroconvulsive seizure up-regulates beta-catenin expression in rat hippocampus: role in adult neurogenesis. Biol Psychiatry 54:1006–1014.

Madsen TM, Treschow A, Bengzon J, Bolwig TG, Lindvall O, Tingstrom A (2000) Increased neurogenesis in a model of electroconvulsive therapy. Biol Psychiatry 47:1043–1049.

Maina F, Klein R (1999) Hepatocyte growth factor, a versatile signal for developing neurons. Nat Neurosci 2:213–217.

Maisonpierre PC, Belluscio L, Friedman B, Alderson RF, Wiegand SJ, Furth ME, Lindsay RM, Yancopoulos GD (1990) NT-3, BDNF, and NGF in the developing rat nervous system: parallel as well as reciprocal patterns of expression. Neuron 5:501–509.

Malas S, Postlethwaite M, Ekonomou A, Whalley B, Nishiguchi S, Wood H, Meldrum B, Constanti A, Episkopou V (2003) Sox1-deficient mice suffer from epilepsy associated with abnormal ventral forebrain development and olfactory cortex hyperexcitability. Neuroscience 119:421–432.

Malberg JE, Duman RS (2003) Cell proliferation in adult hippocampus is decreased by inescapable stress: reversal by fluoxetine treatment. Neuropsychopharmacology 28:1562–1571.

Malberg JE, Eisch AJ, Nestler EJ, Duman RS (2000) Chronic antidepressant treatment increases neurogenesis in adult rat hippocampus. J Neurosci 20:9104–9110.

Mandairon N, Jourdan F, Didier A (2003) Deprivation of sensory inputs to the olfactory bulb up-regulates cell death and proliferation in the subventricular zone of adult mice. Neuroscience 119:507–516.

Maslov AY, Barone TA, Plunkett RJ, Pruitt SC (2004) Neural stem cell detection, characterization, and age-related changes in the subventricular zone of mice. J Neurosci 24:1726–1733.

McMahon AP, Ingham PW, Tabin CJ (2003) Developmental roles and clinical significance of hedgehog signaling. Curr Top Dev Biol 53:1–114.

Meaney MJ, Aitken DH, Bhatnagar S, Sapolsky RM (1991) Postnatal handling attenuates certain neuroendocrine, anatomical, and cognitive dysfunctions associated with aging in female rats. Neurobiol Aging 12:31–38.

Mehler MF, Rozental R, Dougherty M, Spray DC, Kessler JA (1993) Cytokine regulation of neuronal differentiation of hippocampal progenitor cells. Nature 362:62–65.

Melanson-Drapeau L, Beyko S, Dave S, Hebb AL, Franks DJ, Sellitto C, Paul DL, Bennett SA (2003) Oligodendrocyte progenitor enrichment in the connexin32 null-mutant mouse. J Neurosci 23:1759–1768.

Menezes JR, Froes MM, Moura Neto V, Lent R (2000) Gap junction-mediated coupling in the postnatal anterior subventricular zone. Dev Neurosci 22:34–43.

Michael A, Jenaway A, Paykel ES, Herbert J (2000) Altered salivary dehydroepiandrosterone levels in major depression in adults. Biol Psychiatry 48:989–995.

Miller FD, Kaplan DR (2001) Neurotrophin signalling pathways regulating neuronal apoptosis. Cell Mol Life Sci 58:1045–1053.

Minichiello L, Calella AM, Medina DL, Bonhoeffer T, Klein R, Korte M (2002) Mechanism of TrkB-mediated hippocampal long-term potentiation. Neuron 36:121–137.

Mizumatsu S, Monje ML, Morhardt DR, Rola R, Palmer TD, Fike JR (2003) Extreme sensitivity of adult neurogenesis to low doses of X-irradiation. Cancer Res 63:4021–4027.

Monaghan AP, Bock D, Gass P, Schwager A, Wolfer DP, Lipp HP, Schutz G (1997) Defective limbic system in mice lacking the *tailless* gene. Nature 390:515–517.

Monje ML, Mizumatsu S, Fike JR, Palmer TD (2002) Irradiation induces neural precursor-cell dysfunction. Nat Med 8:955–962.

Monje ML, Toda H, Palmer TD (2003) Inflammatory blockade restores adult hippocampal neurogenesis. Science 302:1760–1765.

Montaron MF, Petry KG, Rodriguez JJ, Marinelli M, Aurousseau C, Rougon G, Le Moal M, Abrous DN (1999) Adrenalectomy increases neurogenesis but not PSA-NCAM expression in aged dentate gyrus. Eur J Neurosci 11:1479–1485.

Montaron MF, Piazza PV, Aurousseau C, Urani A, Le Moal M, Abrous DN (2003) Implication of corticosteroid receptors in the regulation of hippocampal structural plasticity. Eur J Neurosci 18:3105–3111.

Moreno-Lopez B, Noval JA, Gonzalez-Bonet LG, Estrada C (2000) Morphological bases for a role of nitric oxide in adult neurogenesis. Brain Res 869:244–250.

Morin PJ (1999) Beta-catenin signaling and cancer. Bioessays 21:1021–1030.

Morrison SJ, Perez SE, Qiao Z, Verdi JM, Hicks C, Weinmaster G, Anderson DJ (2000) Transient Notch activation initiates an irreversible switch from neurogenesis to gliogenesis by neural crest stem cells. Cell 101:499–510.

Munoz-Sanjuan I, Brivanlou AH (2002) Neural induction, the default model and embryonic stem cells. Nat Rev Neurosci 3:271–280.

Muroyama Y, Fujihara M, Ikeya M, Kondoh H, Takada S (2002) Wnt signaling plays an essential role in neuronal specification of the dorsal spinal cord. Genes Dev 16:548–553.

Nacher J, Rosell DR, Alonso-Llosa G, McEwen BS (2001) NMDA receptor antagonist treatment induces a long-lasting increase in the number of proliferating cells, PSA-NCAM-immunoreactive granule neurons and radial glia in the adult rat dentate gyrus. Eur J Neurosci 13:512–520.

Nakagawa E, Aimi Y, Yasuhara O, Tooyama I, Shimada M, McGeer PL, Kimura H (2000) Enhancement of progenitor cell division in the dentate gyrus triggered by initial limbic seizures in rat models of epilepsy. Epilepsia 41:10–18.

Nakagawa S, Kim JE, Lee R, Chen J, Fujioka T, Malberg J, Tsuji S, Duman RS (2002a) Localization of phosphorylated cAMP response element–binding protein in immature neurons of adult hippocampus. J Neurosci 22:9868–9876.

Nakagawa S, Kim JE, Lee R, Malberg JE, Chen J, Steffen C, Zhang YJ, Nestler EJ, Duman RS (2002b) Regulation of neurogenesis in adult mouse hippocampus by cAMP and the cAMP response element–binding protein. J Neurosci 22:3673–3682.

Nakatomi H, Kuriu T, Okabe S, Yamamoto S, Hatano O, Kawahara N, Tamura A, Kirino T, Nakafuku M (2002) Regeneration of hippocampal pyramidal neurons after ischemic brain injury by recruitment of endogenous neural progenitors. Cell 110:429–441.

Newman MB, Kuo YP, Lukas RJ, Sanberg PR, Douglas Shytle R, McGrogan MP, Zigova T (2002) Nicotinic acetylcholine receptors on NT2 precursor cells and hNT (NT2-N) neurons. Brain Res Dev Brain Res 139:73–86.

Nilsson M, Perflilieva E, Johansson U, Orwar O, Eriksson P (1999) Enriched environment increases neurogenesis in the adult rat dentate gyrus and improves spatial memory. J Neurobiol 39:569–578.

Nordeen EJ, Nordeen KW (1989) Estrogen stimulates the incorporation of new neurons into avian song nuclei during adolescence. Brain Res Dev Brain Res 49:27–32.

Okuyama N, Takagi N, Kawai T, Miyake-Takagi K, Takeo S (2004) Phosphorylation of extracellular-regulating kinase in NMDA receptor antagonist-induced newly generated neurons in the adult rat dentate gyrus. J Neurochem 88:717–725.

Orentreich N, Brind JL, Vogelman JH, Andres R, Baldwin H (1992) Long-term longitudinal measurements of plasma dehydroepiandrosterone sulfate in normal men. J Clin Endocrinol Metab 75:1002–1004.

Ormerod BK, Lee TT, Galea LA (2003) Estradiol initially enhances but subsequently suppresses (via adrenal steroids) granule cell proliferation in the dentate gyrus of adult female rats. J Neurobiol 55:247–260.

Ormerod BK, Lee TT, Galea LA (2004) Estradiol enhances neurogenesis in the dentate gyri of adult male meadow voles by increasing the survival of young granule neurons. Neuroscience 128:645–654.

Ostenfeld T, Caldwell MA, Prowse KR, Linskens MH, Jauniaux E, Svendsen CN (2000) Human neural precursor cells express low levels of telomerase in vitro and show diminishing cell proliferation with extensive axonal outgrowth following transplantation. Exp Neurol 164:215–226.

Otero JJ, Fu W, Kan L, Cuadra AE, Kessler JA (2004) Beta-catenin signaling is required for neural differentiation of embryonic stem cells. Development 131:3545–3557.

Palmer TD, Markakis EA, Willhoite AR, Safar F, Gage FH (1999) Fibroblast growth factor-2 activates a latent neurogenic program in neural stem cells from divers regions of the adult CNS. J Neurosci 19:8487–8497.

Palmer TD, Ray J, Gage FH (1995) FGF-2-responsive neuronal progenitors reside in proliferative and quiescent regions of the adult rodent brain. Mol Cell Neurosci 6:474–486.

Palmer TD, Takahashi J, Gage FH (1997) The adult rat hippocampus contains premordial neural stem cells. Mol Cell Neurosci 8:389–404.

Palmer TD, Willhoite AR, Gage FH (2000) Vascular niche for adult hippocampal neurogenesis. J Comp Neurol 425:479–494.

Parent JM, Tada E, Fike JR, Lowenstein DH (1999) Inhibition of dentate granule cell neurogenesis with brain irradiation does not prevent seizure-induced mossy fiber synaptic reorganization in the rat. J Neurosci 19:4508–4519.

Parent JM, Valentin VV, Lowenstein DH (2002a) Prolonged seizures increase proliferating neuroblasts in the adult rat subventricular zone-olfactory bulb pathway. J Neurosci 22:3174–3188.

Parent JM, Vexler ZS, Gong C, Derugin N, Ferriero DM (2002b) Rat forebrain neurogenesis and striatal neuron replacement after focal stroke. Ann Neurol 52:802–813.

Parent JM, Yu TW, Leibowitz RT, Geschwind DH, Sloviter RS, Lowenstein DH (1997) Dentate granule cell neurogenesis is increased by seizures and contributes to aberrant network reorganization in the adult rat hippocampus. J Neurosci 17:3727–3738.

Peirce JL, Chesler EJ, Williams RW, Lu L (2003) Genetic architecture of the mouse hippocampus: identification of gene loci with selective regional effects. Genes Brain Behav 2:238–252.

Pencea V, Bingaman KD, Wiegand SJ, Luskin MB (2001) Infusion of brain-derived neurotrophic factor into the lateral ventricle of the adult rat leads to new neurons in the parenchyma of the striatum, septum, thalamus, and hypothalamus. J Neurosci 21:6706–6717.

Peranovich TM, da Silva AM, Fries DM, Stern A, Monteiro HP (1995) Nitric oxide stimulates tyrosine phosphorylation in murine fibroblasts in the absence and presence of epidermal growth factor. Biochem J 305(Pt 2):613–619.

Perez-Martin M, Azcoitia I, Trejo JL, Sierra A, Garcia-Segura LM (2003) An antagonist of estrogen receptors blocks the induction of adult neurogenesis by insulin-like growth factor-I in the dentate gyrus of adult female rat. Eur J
Neurosci 18:923–930.

Perfilieva E, Risedal A, Nyberg J, Johansson BB, Eriksson PS (2001) Gender and strain
influence on neurogenesis in dentate gyrus of young rats. J Cereb Blood Flow
Metab 21:211–217.

Persson AI, Thorlin T, Bull C, Zarnegar P, Ekman R, Terenius L, Eriksson PS (2003)
Mu- and delta-opioid receptor antagonists decrease proliferation and increase
neurogenesis in cultures of rat adult hippocampal progenitors. Eur J Neurosci
17:1159–1172.

Pham K, Nacher J, Hof PR, McEwen BS (2003) Repeated restraint stress suppresses
neurogenesis and induces biphasic PSA-NCAM expression in the adult rat
dentate gyrus. Eur J Neurosci 17:879–886.

Pizzo DP, Thal LJ, Winkler J (2002) Mnemonic deficits in animals depend upon the
degree of cholinergic deficit and task complexity. Exp Neurol 177:292–305.

Ra SM, Kim H, Jang MH, Shin MC, Lee TH, Lim BV, Kim CJ, Kim EH, Kim KM,
Kim SS (2002) Treadmill running and swimming increase cell proliferation
in the hippocampal dentate gyrus of rats. Neurosci Lett 333:123–126.

Raber J, Fan Y, Matsumori Y, Liu Z, Weinstein PR, Fike JR, Liu J (2004) Irradiation
attenuates neurogenesis and exacerbates ischemia-induced deficits. Ann
Neurol 55:381–389.

Rasika S, Nottebohm F, Alvarez-Buylla A (1994) Testosterone increases the recruitment and/or survival of new high vocal center neurons in adult female canaries. Proc Natl Acad Sci USA 91:7854–7858.

Represa A, Shimazaki T, Simmonds M, Weiss S (2001) EGF-responsive neural stem
cells are a transient population in the developing mouse spinal cord. Eur J
Neurosci 14:452–462.

Reya T, Duncan AW, Ailles L, Domen J, Scherer DC, Willert K, Hintz L, Nusse R,
Weissman IL (2003) A role for Wnt signalling in self-renewal of haemato-
poietic stem cells. Nature 423:409–414.

Reynolds BA, Tetzlaff W, Weiss S (1992) A multipotent EGF-responsive striatal
embryonic progenitor cell produces neurons and astrocytes. J Neurosci
12:4565–4574.

Rochefort C, Gheusi G, Vincent JD, Lledo PM (2002) Enriched odor exposure increases the number of newborn neurons in the adult olfactory bulb and improves odor memory. J Neurosci 22:2679–2689.

Rola R, Otsuka S, Obenaus A, Nelson GA, Limoli CL, VandenBerg SR, Fike JR (2004a)
Indicators of hippocampal neurogenesis are altered by 56Fe-particle irradiation in a dose-dependent manner. Radiat Res 162:442–446.

Rola R, Raber J, Rizk A, Otsuka S, VandenBerg SR, Morhardt DR, Fike JR (2004b)
Radiation-induced impairment of hippocampal neurogenesis is associated
with cognitive deficits in young mice. Exp Neurol 188:316–330.

Roy K, Kuznicki K, Wu Q, Sun Z, Bock D, Schutz G, Vranich N, Monaghan AP (2004)
The *Tlx* gene regulates the timing of neurogenesis in the cortex. J Neurosci
24:8333–8345.

Rozental R, Mehler MF, Morales M, Andrade-Rozental AF, Kessler JA, Spray DC
(1995) Differentiation of hippocampal progenitor cells in vitro: temporal
expression of intercellular coupling and voltage- and ligand-gated responses.
Dev Biol 167:350–362.

Rozental R, Morales M, Mehler MF, Urban M, Kremer M, Dermietzel R, Kessler JA,
Spray DC (1998) Changes in the properties of gap junctions during neuronal
differentiation of hippocampal progenitor cells. J Neurosci 18:1753–1762.

Rueda D, Navarro B, Martinez-Serrano A, Guzman M, Galve-Roperh I (2002) The endocannabinoid anandamide inhibits neuronal progenitor cell differentiation through attenuation of the Rap1/B-Raf/ERK pathway. J Biol Chem 277:46645–46650.

Sakurada K, Ohshima-Sakurada M, Palmer TD, Gage FH (1999) Nurr1, an orphan nuclear receptor, is a transcriptional activator of endogenous tyrosine hydroxylase in neural progenitor cells derived from the adult brain. Development 126:4017–4026.

Santarelli L, Saxe M, Gross C, Surget A, Battaglia F, Dulawa S, Weisstaub N, Lee J, Duman R, Arancio O, Belzung C, Hen R (2003) Requirement of hippocampal neurogenesis for the behavioral effects of antidepressants. Science 301:805–809.

Sapolsky RM, Romero LM, Munck AU (2000) How do glucocorticoids influence stress responses? Integrating permissive, suppressive, stimulatory, and preparative actions. Endocr Rev 21:55–89.

Sasaki T, Kitagawa K, Sugiura S, Omura-Matsuoka E, Tanaka S, Yagita Y, Okano H, Matsumoto M, Hori M (2003) Implication of cyclooxygenase-2 on enhanced proliferation of neural progenitor cells in the adult mouse hippocampus after ischemia. J Neurosci Res 72:461–471.

Schanzer A, Wachs FP, Wilhelm D, Acker T, Cooper-Kuhn C, Beck H, Winkler J, Aigner L, Plate KH, Kuhn HG (2004) Direct stimulation of adult neural stem cells in vitro and neurogenesis in vivo by vascular endothelial growth factor. Brain Pathol 14:237–248.

Scharfman HE, Goodman JH, Sollas AL (2000) Granule-like neurons at the hilar/CA3 border after status epilepticus and their synchrony with area CA3 pyramidal cells: functional implications of seizure-induced neurogenesis. J Neurosci 20:6144–6158.

Schoenherr CJ, Anderson DJ (1995) The neuron-restrictive silencer factor (NRSF): a coordinate repressor of multiple neuron-specific genes. Science 267:1360–1363.

Scott BW, Wang S, Burnham WM, De Boni U, Wojtowicz JM (1998) Kindling-induced neurogenesis in the dentate gyrus of the rat. Neurosci Lett 248:73–76.

Scott BW, Wojtowicz JM, Burnham WM (2000) Neurogenesis in the dentate gyrus of the rat following electroconvulsive shock seizures Exp Neurol 165:231–236.

Seki T, Arai Y (1995) Age-related production of new granule cells in the adult dentate gyrus. Neuroreport 6:2479–2482.

Shi Y, Chichung Lie D, Taupin P, Nakashima K, Ray J, Yu RT, Gage FH, Evans RM (2004) Expression and function of orphan nuclear receptor TLX in adult neural stem cells. Nature 427:78–83.

Shingo T, Gregg C, Enwere E, Fujikawa H, Hassam R, Geary C, Cross JC, Weiss S (2003) Pregnancy-stimulated neurogenesis in the adult female forebrain mediated by prolactin. Science 299:117–120.

Shingo T, Sorokan ST, Shimazaki T, Weiss S (2001) Erythropoietin regulates the in vitro and in vivo production of neuronal progenitors by mammalian forebrain neural stem cells. J Neurosci 21:9733–9743.

Smith MT, Pencea V, Wang Z, Luskin MB, Insel TR (2001) Increased number of BrdU-labeled neurons in the rostral migratory stream of the estrous prairie vole. Horm Behav 39:11–21.

Song H, Stevens CF, Gage FH (2002) Astroglia induce neurogenesis from adult neural stem cells. Nature 417:39–44.

Spradling A, Drummond-Barbosa D, Kai T (2001) Stem cells find their niche. Nature 414:98–104.

Takagi Y, Nozaki K, Takahashi J, Yodoi J, Ishikawa M, Hashimoto N (1999) Proliferation of neuronal precursor cells in the dentate gyrus is accelerated after transient forebrain ischemia in mice. Brain Res 831:283–287.

Takahashi J, Palmer TD, Gage FH (1999) Retinoic acid and neurotrophins collaborate to regulate neurogenesis in adult-derived neural stem cell cultures. J Neurobiol 38:65–81.

Takasawa K, Kitagawa K, Yagita Y, Sasaki T, Tanaka S, Matsushita K, Ohstuki T, Miyata T, Okano H, Hori M, Matsumoto M (2002) Increased proliferation of neural progenitor cells but reduced survival of newborn cells in the contralateral hippocampus after focal cerebral ischemia in rats. J Cereb Blood Flow Metab 22:299–307.

Tanapat P, Hastings NB, Reeves AJ, Gould E (1999) Estrogen stimulates a transient increase in the number of new neurons in the dentate gyrus of the adult female rat. J Neurosci 19:5792–5801.

Tanapat P, Hastings NB, Rydel TA, Galea LA, Gould E (2001) Exposure to fox odor inhibits cell proliferation in the hippocampus of adult rats via an adrenal hormone–dependent mechanism. J Comp Neurol 437:496–504.

Taupin P, Ray J, Fischer WH, Suhr ST, Hakansson K, Grubb A, Gage FH (2000) FGF-2-responsive neural stem cell proliferation requires CCg, a novel autocrine/paracrine cofactor. Neuron 28:385–397.

Teramoto T, Qiu J, Plumier JC, Moskowitz MA (2003) EGF amplifies the replacement of parvalbumin-expressing striatal interneurons after ischemia. J Clin Invest 111:1125–1132.

Tong Y, Chabot JG, Shen SH, O'Dowd BF, George SR, Quirion R (2000) Ontogenic profile of the expression of the mu opioid receptor gene in the rat telencephalon and diencephalon: an in situ hybridization study. J Chem Neuroanat 18:209–222.

Toresson H, Parmar M, Campbell K (2000) Expression of *Meis* and *Pbx* genes and their protein products in the developing telencephalon: implications for regional differentiation. Mech Dev 94:183–187.

Torres-Aleman I (2000) Serum growth factors and neuroprotective surveillance: focus on IGF-1. Mol Neurobiol 21:153–160.

Traiffort E, Charytoniuk D, Watroba L, Faure H, Sales N, Ruat M (1999) Discrete localizations of hedgehog signalling components in the developing and adult rat nervous system. Eur J Neurosci 11:3199–3214.

Trejo JL, Carro E, Torres-Aleman I (2001) Circulating insulin-like growth factor I mediates exercise-induced increases in the number of new neurons in the adult hippocampus. J Neurosci 21:1628–1634.

Uchida K, Kumihashi K, Kurosawa S, Kobayashi T, Itoi K, Machida T (2002) Stimulatory effects of prostaglandin E2 on neurogenesis in the dentate gyrus of the adult rat. Zoolog Sci 19:1211–1216.

Uwanogho D, Rex M, Cartwright EJ, Pearl G, Healy C, Scotting PJ, Sharpe PT (1995) Embryonic expression of the chicken *Sox2*, *Sox3* and *Sox11* genes suggests an interactive role in neuronal development. Mech Dev 49:23–36.

Vaccarino FM, Schwartz ML, Raballo R, Nilsen J, Rhee J, Zhou M, Doetschman T, Coffin JD, Wyland JJ, Hung YT (1999) Changes in cerebral cortex size are governed by fibroblast growth factor during embryogenesis. Nat Neurosci 2:246–253.

Vallieres L, Campbell IL, Gage FH, Sawchenko PE (2002) Reduced hippocampal neurogenesis in adult transgenic mice with chronic astrocytic production of interleukin-6. J Neurosci 22:486–492.

van de Wetering M, de Lau W, Clevers H (2002) WNT signaling and lymphocyte development. Cell 109 Suppl:S13–19.

Van Praag H, Christie BR, Sejnowski TJ, Gage FH (1999a) Running enhances neurogenesis, learning and long-term potentiation in mice. Proc Natl Acad Sci USA 96:13427–13431.

Van Praag H, Kempermann G, Gage FH (1999b) Running increases cell proliferation and neurogenesis in the adult mouse dentate gyrus. Nat Neurosci 2:266–270.

Van Praag H, Schinder AF, Christie BR, Toni N, Palmer TD, Gage FH (2002) Functional neurogenesis in the adult hippocampus. Nature 415:1030–1034.

Vollmayr B, Simonis C, Weber S, Gass P, Henn F (2003) Reduced cell proliferation in the dentate gyrus is not correlated with the development of learned helplessness. Biol Psychiatry 54:1035–1040.

Wagner JP, Black IB, DiCicco-Bloom E (1999) Stimulation of neonatal and adult brain neurogenesis by subcutaneous injection of basic fibroblast growth factor. J Neurosci 19:6006–6016.

Wakade CG, Mahadik SP, Waller JL, Chiu FC (2002) Atypical neuroleptics stimulate neurogenesis in adult rat brain. J Neurosci Res 69:72–79.

Wang HD, Dunnavant FD, Jarman T, Deutch AY (2004) Effects of antipsychotic drugs on neurogenesis in the forebrain of the adult rat. Neuropsychopharmacology 29:1230–1238.

Wechsler-Reya RJ, Scott MP (1999) Control of neuronal precursor proliferation in the cerebellum by Sonic hedgehog. Neuron 22:103–114.

Weinstein DE, Burrola P, Kilpatrick TJ (1996) Increased proliferation of precursor cells in the adult rat brain after targeted lesioning. Brain Res 743:11–16.

Werther GA, Abate M, Hogg A, Cheesman H, Oldfield B, Hards D, Hudson P, Power B, Freed K, Herington AC (1990) Localization of insulin-like growth factor-I mRNA in rat brain by in situ hybridization—relationship to IGF-I receptors. Mol Endocrinol 4:773–778.

Willert K, Brown JD, Danenberg E, Duncan AW, Weissman IL, Reya T, Yates JR 3rd, Nusse R (2003) Wnt proteins are lipid-modified and can act as stem cell growth factors. Nature 423:448–452.

Wilson PA, Hemmati-Brivanlou A (1997) Vertebrate neural induction: inducers, inhibitors, and a new synthesis. Neuron 18:699–710.

Wimer CC, Wimer RE (1989) On the sources of strain and sex differences in granule cell number in the dentate area of house mice. Brain Res Dev Brain Res 48:167–176.

Winner B, Cooper-Kuhn CM, Aigner R, Winkler J, Kuhn HG (2002) Long-term survival and cell death of newly generated neurons in the adult rat olfactory bulb. Eur J Neurosci 16:1681–1689.

Wong EY, Herbert J (2004) The corticoid environment: a determining factor for neural progenitors' survival in the adult hippocampus. Eur J Neurosci 20:2491–2498.

Wright EM, Vogel KS, Davies AM (1992) Neurotrophic factors promote the maturation of developing sensory neurons before they become dependent on these factors for survival. Neuron 9:139–150.

Yagita Y, Kitagawa K, Ohtsuki T, Takasawa K, Miyata T, Okano H, Hori M, Matsumoto M (2001) Neurogenesis by progenitor cells in the ischemic adult rat hippocampus. Stroke 32:1890–1896.

Yamada M, Onodera M, Mizuno Y, Mochizuki H (2004) Neurogenesis in olfactory bulb identified by retroviral labeling in normal and 1-methyl-4-phenyl-1,2,3,6-tetrahydropyridine-treated adult mice. Neuroscience 124:173–181.

Yoshimura S, Takagi Y, Harada J, Teramoto T, Thomas SS, Waeber C, Bakowska JC, Breakefield XO, Moskowitz MA (2001) FGF-2 regulation of neurogenesis in adult hippocampus after brain injury. Proc Natl Acad Sci USA 98:5874–5879.

Yu IT, Lee SH, Lee YS, Son H (2004) Differential effects of corticosterone and dexamethasone on hippocampal neurogenesis in vitro. Biochem Biophys Res Commun 317:484–490.

Zhang R, Zhang L, Zhang Z, Wang Y, Lu M, Lapointe M, Chopp M (2001) A nitric oxide donor induces neurogenesis and reduces functional deficits after stroke in rats. Ann Neurol 50:602–611.

Zhao X, Ueba T, Christie BR, Barkho B, McConnell MJ, Nakashima K, Lein ES, Eadie BD, Willhoite AR, Muotri AR, Summers RG, Chun J, Lee KF, Gage FH (2003) Mice lacking methyl-CpG binding protein 1 have deficits in adult neurogenesis and hippocampal function. Proc Natl Acad Sci USA 100:6777–6782.

Zhu DY, Lau L, Liu SH, Wei JS, Lu YM (2004) Activation of cAMP-response-element-binding protein (CREB) after focal cerebral ischemia stimulates neurogenesis in the adult dentate gyrus. Proc Natl Acad Sci USA 101:9453–9457.

Zhu DY, Liu SH, Sun HS, Lu YM (2003) Expression of inducible nitric oxide synthase after focal cerebral ischemia stimulates neurogenesis in the adult rodent dentate gyrus. J Neurosci 23:223–229.

Zigova T, Pencea V, Wiegand SJ, Luskin MB (1998) Intraventricular administration of BDNF increases the number of newly generated neurons in the adult olfactory bulb. Mol Cell Neurosci 11:234–245.

Zurawel RH, Chiappa SA, Allen C, Raffel C (1998) Sporadic medulloblastomas contain oncogenic beta-catenin mutations. Cancer Res 58:896–899.

10

Function

Adult neurogenesis elicits fascination because new neurons might contribute to brain function in health and disease. Most people intuitively assume that new neurons in the adult brain are beneficial and might provide a means to actively improve brain function and cognition. It seems almost trivial that a neuron is not a true neuron unless it functions as one. However, the findings that learning stimuli and experience might specifically recruit new neurons in the hippocampus and induce their long-term survival (Kempermann et al., 1997, 1998; Leuner et al., 2004) and that immature new granule cells show signs of increased synaptic plasticity (Wang et al., 2000; Schmidt-Hieber et al., 2004), as well as theoretical considerations (Feng et al., 2001; Deisseroth et al., 2004), have raised the possibility that adult neurogenesis might be beneficial to hippocampal activity through a functional contribution of precursor cells and immature neurons. Although there are good arguments against the idea that in adult neurogenesis "the path is the goal," rather than the long-term alteration to the hippocampal or olfactory network, the theory raises important issues. Most importantly, we need to investigate what exactly is meant by function.

During the course of evolution, the ability to undergo adult neurogenesis decreased with growing brain complexity. From this observation one might be tempted to conclude that the most complex brain functions as found in primates and humans are not compatible with the ability to produce new neurons and integrate them into the functional networks. However, it is difficult to evaluate whether function of the spinal cord in lizards, which show robust and extensive adult neurogenesis, is in a fundamental sense less complex than that in a human.

In 1985, Pasko Rakic hypothesized that during in the course of evolution, adult cortical neurogenesis might have been reduced and was not found in the primate brain (Rakic, 1985). One of his arguments was based on the stability–plasticity dilemma, a fundamental issue in network theory: new neurons can be thought of as being disruptive to existing networks. In the region with the highest cortical function the addition of new neurons might have more disadvantages than benefits. This plausible argument does not hold up, however, for all types of networks. Modeling studies show that neuronal networks exist that not only accommodate new neurons but actually call for them. The number of new neurons in these situations, however, appears to be relatively small. Thus, while the general observation of a decrease in adult neurogenesis with increasing brain complexity

is certainly correct and the stability–plasticity dilemma is an important issue in neuronal network architecture, it is not clear whether this alone could
rule out adult neurogenesis in the primate neocortex.

Independent of the degree to which different species rely on adult neurogenesis and why, there is likely a balance between the benefits that can be
gained from new neurons and the problems the integration of new cells
causes for the network structure. In the two neurogenic regions of the adult
mammalian brain, the benefits seem to outweigh the disadvantages. Given
the fact that we generally still know relatively little about the exact function of individual brain parts (and this even applies to the heavily studied
hippocampus), and much less is known about their precise contribution to
cognition, the role of new neurons within these functions is difficult to
determine.

The term *function* has theoretical and practical meanings on different
conceptual levels. To speak of *function* therefore often remains vague. Consequently, we are left with a considerable challenge to develop concepts of
what function should mean in the context of adult neurogenesis. To date,
adult neurogenesis has been examined on the levels of individual cells,
neuronal networks, and neuronal systems (Fig. 10–1). Function can be at-
tributed to all of these levels. In the olfactory bulb, the *cellular* level refers
to the physiology of the new granule cells, the *network* level to the integration of these cells into the circuitry of the olfactory bulb, and the *systems*
level to the question of how the new neurons might contribute to olfaction.
Analogously, in the hippocampus, study at the cellular level involves the
functional properties of individual new granule cells; at the network level,
analysis of the means by which how the new granule cells are integrated
into the neuronal circuits of the dentate gyrus and the mossy fiber tract; and
at the systems level, investigation of ways in which new granule cells might
contribute to hippocampus-dependent learning and memory. Tests of function are very different at the different conceptual levels. Thus *function* will
mean very different things, depending on the experimental situation.

In addition, the conceptual levels overlap. They are helpful constructs but
are not strictly separated in reality. Neurons form synapses to build networks.
Integration of different local networks leads to the establishment of the complex circuitry in functional systems, such as the hippocampus or the olfactory system. Neither synapses, neurons, local networks, nor systems are
functionally self-sustained islands. The higher the conceptual level the more
its functions rely on the integrity of function at the levels below. Action potentials can be detected in neurons in vitro, but olfaction, which clearly depends on action potential in many neurons, cannot be fully represented in
single cells. This is not a trivial point, because the mechanism of synaptic
strengthening, long-term potentiation (LTP), that can be studied in living
hippocampal slices (and thus on a network level) is thought to be the synaptic
mechanism underlying learning. When *learning* is implicitly used in a behavioral sense (which is not the same as the learning of the neuronal networks of

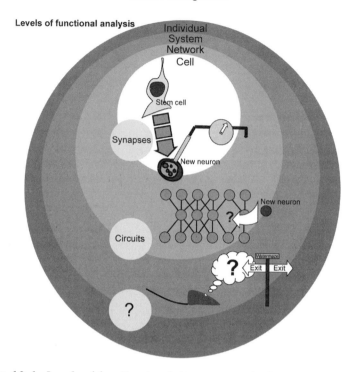

Figure 10–1. Levels of function in adult neurogenesis. Just as regulation occurs on several conceptual levels (Fig. 9–1), *function* is an elusive term that can be addressed with different meaning from single-cell level to complex behaviors. Figure from Kempermann et al. (2004); reprinted with kind permission of Elsevier.

computational neurosciences), this tacit transfer can become problematic. Consequently, whether LTP is learning has been debated for decades, despite very good evidence that a profound link between them exists. But the fundamental problem is that the similar language and concepts used at the different levels are not identical; implications vary with the concepts.

Matters become even more complicated when a functional significance of the new neurons is inferred from the three levels of cells, networks, and systems leading to a fourth level, the cognitive level. This is the level of the individual as it behaves and is integrated into its psychological, historical, and social contexts. Such extrapolations can provide insight into the broader picture of neuronal function, but they nevertheless usually remain problematic.

SIGNS OF NEURONAL FUNCTION IN INDIVIDUAL NEW NEURONS

The essence of neuronal function is communication. Consequently, only limited conclusions about function can be drawn from individual neurons. Nevertheless, in many experimental contexts single cells are the only available objects of functional investigations and it is thus useful to consider function of single new neurons.

With patch-clamp techniques the membrane properties and currents of individual identified cells can be studied in the course of neuronal development. For both the olfactory system and the hippocampus, signs of "electrophysiological maturation" have been described (Carlen et al., 2002; Filippov et al., 2003; Fukuda et al., 2003; Ambrogini et al., 2004) (Fig. 10–2). The radial glia–like precursor cells of the subgranular zone (SGZ) and the subventricular zone (SVZ) share not only morphological characteristics but also electrophysiological features with astrocytes: they have passive mem-

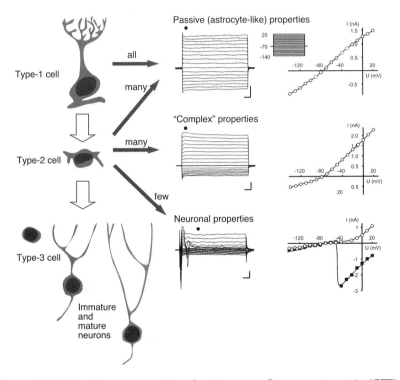

Figure 10–2. Membrane properties of nestin green fluorescent protein (GFP)-expressing precursor cells in the dentate gyrus. Radial glia–like type-1 cells show the electrophysiological characteristics of astrocytes: passive membrane properties and potassium currents Type-2 cells can have astrocytic or "complex" properties The complex pattern was originally described for oligodendrocyte precursor cells (Steinhauser et al., 1994) and appears to be a shared feature of many nestin- and NG2-expressing cells throughout the brain. A small percentage of the nestin-GFP-expressing cells show neuronal characteristics with sodium currents, indicative of the first stages of neuronal differentiation. The presented data are based on patch-clamp recordings by Li-Ping Wang and Helmut Kettenmann, Berlin.

brane properties and show potassium currents (Filippov et al., 2003; Fukuda et al., 2003). Many type-2 progenitor cells of the SGZ have electrophysiological properties that have been named "complex" and originally were described for glial precursor cells (Steinhauser et al., 1994). Nevertheless, the transiently amplifying type-2 progenitor cells, identified by their nestin-expression, contribute to the neuronal lineage because early neuronal markers and sodium currents can be found in a small portion of type-2 cells (Filippov et al., 2003). However, type-2 cells are electrophysiologically not homogeneous.

Patrizia Ambrogini, Ricardo Cuppini, and colleagues (2004) from Urbino described the pattern of electrophysiological differentiation based on an immunohistochemical post-hoc identification of the patch-clamped cells filled with biocytin during the course of the recordings. They used the expression of β-III-tubulin to identify the immature neurons. From their findings they concluded that in the course of the development, these cells became increasingly hyperpolarized, progressed from low to high capacitance and from receiving GABAergic input to glutamatergic input (see below). Shortly after the cell-cycle exit the new neurons show signs of high synaptic plasticity and immediately begin to show large differences from the progenitor cell stages (Wang et al., 2000; van Praag et al., 2002; Ambrogini et al., 2004; Schmidt-Hieber et al., 2004).

The diversity of implicit functional concepts becomes particularly obvious in another context. A large part of neural stem cell biology aims at producing neuronal progenitor cells or neurons in vitro as a source for cell transplants. In such in vitro contexts, functional evaluation is particularly problematic. Obviously, the ultimate proof that an implanted cell behaves like the desired neuronal cell type can only be assessed in vivo. Providing this proof is a major technical challenge, and no studies have fully succeeded in this regard. Because the proof in vivo is possible only post hoc and is technically challenging, functional predictions from in vitro studies are particularly important. The standards for demonstration of neuronal functionality have been raised considerably over the last few years, as exemplified in the generation of dopaminergic neurons from precursor cells in vitro. Dopaminergic neurons are a foremost target for tissue engineers, because in Parkinson disease a relatively circumscribed population of dopaminergic neurons is lost because of the disease. The transplantation of fetal dopaminergic neurons into patients has led to the conclusion that cell transplantation therapies of Parkinson disease are generally feasible. In many early studies the expression of tyrosine hydroxylase (TH), the key enzyme of dopamine synthesis, was taken as evidence of dopaminergic differentiation in vitro. But TH is not sufficient to indicate full maturation and thus additional key enzymes of the dopamine synthesis pathway as well as characteristic transcription factors such as Nurr1 have to be demonstrated. As a further step toward functional characterization, dopamine secretion into the culture medium has been shown. All of these criteria, even the most descriptive ones such as the detection of a key enzyme, allow conclusions about aspects of function. But for an appreciation of function in a sense that is meaningful beyond the immediate experimental context, multiple parameters have to be assessed. Function can usually not be assessed by measuring a single parameter.

Coculture systems and organotypic slice cultures add a moment of cellular interaction to in vitro studies and cross the border into studies on the network level. Hongjun Song and colleagues from the Salk Institute cocultured adult hippocampal precursor cells with astrocytes from the same region and showed that this induced the development of electrically active neurons that formed synaptic networks in the culture dish (Song et al., 2002). This was the first demonstration that, within the highly reductionistic system in vitro, a meaningful level of neuronal function can be achieved by specifically introducing a natural cellular environment. When neurons derived from embryonic stem cells in vitro were implanted in early postnatal hippocampal slice cultures, over time the new cells expressed voltage-gated ion channels and a mature profile of receptors and synaptically integrated into the host tissue (Benninger et al., 2003).

LOCAL NETWORK INTEGRATION OF NEW NEURONS IN VIVO

Functional integration on a network level in vivo requires the establishment of synapses. A small number of nestin-expressing cells and many β-III-tubulin- or doublecortin (DCX)-positive cells in the dentate gyrus receive synaptic input (Wang et al., 2000; Fillippov et al., 2003; Ambrogini et al., 2004; Schmidt-Hieber et al., 2004). These findings imply that the first signs of synaptic activity and thus network integration are found at a putative precursor cell stage. The first synapses should be found on the soma of newly generated cells and presumably primarily influence further neuronal differentiation. They have not yet been unambiguously visualized. Because it has been speculated that immature neurons serve a specific function independent of their full maturation, relevance of their first synaptic integration might go beyond the modulation of further development.

Henriette van Praag and colleagues were the first to succeed in a prospective electrophysiological characterization of newly generated granule cells (van Praag et al., 2002). Their study provided the first direct proof that adult-generated neurons become electrophysiologically functional in vivo and are integrated as granule cells. The new neurons were not identified post hoc but dividing cells were labeled with a retrovirus expressing green fluorescent protein (GFP) in vivo. Their living progeny could thus be identified under the fluorescent microscope. After a maturation period of about 7 weeks, the new granule cells showed electrophysiological properties very similar to those of the older granule cells. The finding of increased synaptic plasticity during the course of granule cell development (Wang et al., 2000; Schmidt-Hieber et al., 2004) suggests that the cautious statement of "similarity" opens opportunities for further research. Also, there is considerable heterogeneity among granule cells and it is tempting to link these even subtle differences to stages of further maturation or to specialized function of new cells.

During neuronal development in the adult olfactory bulb with its long migratory phase, this functional maturation appears delayed until the new cells have reached the olfactory bulb. In a groundbreaking study, Alan Carleton, Piere-Marie Lledo, and colleagues from Paris applied the same experimental approach chosen by van Praag for the hippocampus and followed migrating enhanced green fluorescent protein (EGFP)-marked neuroblasts from the SVZ through the rostral migratory stream (RMS) to the olfactory bulb (Carleton et al., 2003). Here, too, the expression of GABA receptors preceded the appearance of glutamate receptors. Five distinct stages of neuronal development could be distinguished, beginning with the migratory neuroblasts of the RMS that show immature properties but can already express first glutamate receptors.

For full functional integration, the new neurons have to extend dendrites and axons and form dendritic and axonal synapses in the appropriate target regions. Using retrograde labeling, Stanfield and Trice (1988) were the first to show that the new granule cells in the adult dentate gyrus extend axons along the mossy fiber tract. This study was truly pioneering because it predated the general interest in this question by several years. Axonal projections of new granule cells to CA3 were later confirmed (Hastings and Gould, 1999; Markakis and Gage, 1999). Retrograde labeling consists of injecting a dye, usually fluorogold, into the target region, to which the neurons in question project. Neurons will take up the dye through their axons. Tracers such as fluorogold are retrogradely transported along the axon to the cell soma, where they accumulate. Consequently, all regions that project to the injection site will be visualized with fluorogold. To prove that new hippocampal granule cells project along the mossy fiber tract, animals received BrdU injection to label the new neurons. Several weeks later, fluorogold was injected into CA3. The dye was taken up into the mossy fiber terminals and retrogradely transported to the granule cell layer, where those cells that had incorporated fluorogold became fluorescent. Immunohistochemistry for BrdU clarified whether these cells were newly generated, and in fact a small percentage of them were. The labeling study by Elizabeth Gould's group provided the additional piece of information that the extension of the new axon is very fast and can occur within days after labeling with BrdU (Hastings and Gould, 1999). The labeled cells in these cases will likely be DCX- and calretinin-positive, early postmitotic progenitor cells that had just undergone their last division, but this remains to be confirmed experimentally. After leaving the cell cycle, terminal differentiation is initiated; it seems that axon elongation is an early part of this. This phase of increased plasticity is also characterized by the transient expression of growth cone–associated protein TUC4 (see Chapter 7).

In targeted regenerative neurogenesis in the murine neocortex after a directed ablation of corticothalamic neurons, retrograde labeling similarly confirmed that the new (BrdU-positive) neurons had established normal projections to their physiologic target in the thalamus (Magavi et al., 2000).

In transplantation studies, the implanted cells can be marked with a reporter gene that codes for GFP or β-galactosidase. The reporter protein is anterogradely transported or diffuses into the axon. Contacts between implanted cells and target cells can then be examined. For motoneuron development, for example, the entire regulatory cascade necessary for directed differentiation from embryonic stem cells in vitro can be recapitulated in vitro. After implantation, a reporter gene showed evidence that the neurons formed adequate synapses on the target muscles (Wichterle et al., 2002).

The group of Jonas Frisén in Stockholm used an unusual approach to demonstrate the synaptic integration of newly generated granule cells in the dentate gyrus (Carlen et al., 2002). They infected neurons in the entorhinal cortex, which is the main input structure into the dentate gyrus, with pseudorabies virus. The particular property of rabies viruses is that they are propagated transsynaptically. The virus carried EGFP and after infection in the entorhinal cortex, EGFP expression was found in new neurons of the dentate gyrus and also in pyramidal neurons of CA3 to which the granule cells project, suggesting that the new granule cells became part of the synaptic network. It is not clear how predictive the structural integration of a new neuron is for actual function, but it is an obvious requirement.

Sabrina Wang and Martin Wojtowicz from the University of Toronto were the first to compare the properties of immature neurons in the dentate gyrus with those of older granule cells (Wang et al., 2000). The younger cells were identified by morphology because of their sparser dendritic tree and post hoc by immunohistochemistry against TUC4. The intriguing result was that new neurons showed a higher degree of synaptic plasticity. Long-term potentiation was induced at a lower threshold and the cells were entirely insensitive to $GABA_A$ inhibition (Wang et al., 2000). This finding is in contrast to the finding of early GABAergic innervation of the newly generated cells. However, if one assumes that the new neurons show less inhibition than the more mature cells, LTP induction under superfusion with artificial cerebrospinal fluid should reflect LTP by the new cells, whereas treatment with a blocker of GABAergic synapses should elicit a response from young and old cells. Indeed, LTP induction through stimulation of the medial perforant path showed the facilitated LTP induction supposedly attributable to the immature cells under physiological conditions, and an increase in LTP under GABA blockade that required more stimuli and higher frequency (Snyder et al., 2001).

On the basis of post-hoc immunohistochemistry against PSA-NCAM, Christoph Schmidt-Hieber and coworkers (2004) found that such enhanced synaptic plasticity was due to isolated Ca^{2+} spikes in young neurons that promote fast action potentials. Consequently, there is increasing evidence that immature neurons are highly plastic and particularly prepared to establish and maintain synaptic contacts in an activity-dependent way, as one might predict from the developmental pattern. Low-dose irradiation of the brain prior to the electrophysiological examination in vitro reduced adult hippocampal neurogenesis and abolished the LTP that can be induced by stimulating the medial perforant path (Snyder et al., 2001). Intriguingly, voluntary wheel-running has a parallel effect on LTP induction and adult hippocampal neurogenesis (van Praag et al., 1999), possibly because of an elevation of local brain-derived neurotrophic factor (BDNF) and glutamate receptor expressions (Farmer et al., 2004). Of course, these findings do not imply that there is a generally strict and quantitative relationship between LTP in the dentate gyrus and new neurons; both can be independently influenced by experimental manipulations such as lithium treatment (Son et al., 2003).

Neurogenesis in the adult olfactory system and hippocampus do not primarily feed into a neuronal turnover. Both brain regions grow with increasing age. Net growth could still be accounted for by a turnover and just a lower cell death rate than the production rate of new neurons, but it seems that it is a surplus of new cells that die, not the older granule cells. This net increase has consequences for functional hypotheses at a network and systems level. During adult hippocampal neurogenesis, cell death occurs primarily at the level of early postmitotic cells, presumably at the same stage that shows increased synaptic plasticity. Once the cells have become integrated into the local network and survived a Hebbian selection process, the new neurons are likely to persist for long periods of time in both the hippocampus and olfactory bulb (Winner et al., 2002; Kempermann et al., 2003; Leuner et al., 2004). This early determination and long-term persistence are also reflected in the distribution of new neurons in the adult dentate gyrus. The new cells find their position within the granule cell layer early and the location within the granule cell layer barely changes over time (Kempermann et al., 2003). This temporal and spatial stability of new neurons might be an important prerequisite for function, although from a theoretical perspective, adult neurogenesis could be transient and still be functional.

Compared to our knowledge about functional integration of new neurons into the dentate gyrus, information about the olfactory system is more limited. Both neuronal populations generated in the olfactory bulb project to local targets, which prohibits the use of retrograde tracing techniques. For retrograde labeling the dye has to be injected at some distance from the area in which the nuclei of interest are found. Otherwise, local dye effusion at the injection site overwhelms the fluorescent signal from individual labeled cells that have actively transported the tracer. Also, general knowledge about the electrophysiology of the olfactory bulb is more limited than that of the hippocampus. The first signs of neuronal differentiation are found very early and still within the RMS (Carleton et al., 2003), but spontaneous synaptic activity is detectable only late and spiking activity even later, only after the new neurons are close to their final position in the bulb. Intuitively it makes sense that full functional maturation should be delayed until the cells have entered into the local network structure in which they ultimately have to integrate. When the olfactory nerve was stimulated, synaptic responses were detectable in the new interneurons, indicating that the new cells become functionally integrated (Belluzzi et al., 2003).

The retrovirus-based studies in both hippocampus and olfactory bulb have greatly expanded our knowledge about the functional integration of new neurons. These studies have raised two immediate questions. First, does an entire cohort of new cells become integrated in parallel? The retrovirus-based experiments identified only individual cells. What can be said about functional integration across the entire population of newly generated cells? Second, does functional integration also imply that the new cells would respond to physiological stimuli known to activate the respective neuronal populations into which the new cells are born? Both questions have been addressed with experimental paradigms that make use of the fact that synaptic activation induces fast up-regulation of immediate early genes such as *c-fos*, *zif268*, or *Homer1A*. The transcribed proteins from these genes can be detected immunohistochemically. This allows assessment of the responsiveness of all cells visible in a tissue section. Also, the analysis can be made quantitative by determining the numbers of activated cells.

Systemic injections of kainic acid lead to a generalized synaptic activation of hippocampal granule cells that in turn causes a detectable up-regulation of immediate early proteins in about 80% of the cells (Jessberger and Kempermann, 2003). The activation is likely to be synaptic because an activation of granule cells through the inhibition of local inhibitory circuits by systemic injections of pentylenetetrazole has an identical result. When this type of general activation was applied at different time points after labeling the newborn cells with BrdU, it was found that over a period of weeks the new cells matured into full activity-dependent responsiveness. At 2 weeks after BrdU labeling, kainic acid injections did not lead to any measurable immediate early gene regulation in BrdU-labeled cells. After about 4 weeks roughly half of the new cells responded, and after 7 weeks the rate of 80%, found also in the older granule cells, was detected (Jessberger and Kempermann, 2003).

Immediate early gene regulation can also be used to visualize neuronal activation after specific stimuli. Training in the hippocampus-dependent learning task of the Morris water maze induced c-fos expression in single granule cells, including newly generated cells (Jessberger and Kempermann, 2003).

In the olfactory bulb, Jonas Frisén's group showed that olfactory stimuli evoked an up-regulation of *c-fos* gene expression in newborn neurons, similarly supporting the functional synaptic integration (Carlen et al., 2002).

Between network and systems levels we find studies in which investigators manipulated adult neurogenesis and studied the functional consequences. The general problem with this approach is the same as that with all lesion studies. Eliminating function by destroying parts of the machinery might highlight that a part is important for function, but it does not necessarily elucidate what the function is. By analogy, taking out the accelerator pedal from a car makes driving impossible but does not allow the conclusion that it is the accelerator pedal that propels the car.

This general caveat notwithstanding, correlational evidence for a relationship between adult neurogenesis and function will increasingly come from knockout and transgenic studies. In such cases the cause–effect relationships can become complicated and indirect. Knockout mice with reduced of DNA methylation, for example, had increased genomic instability in neural precursor cells, decreased adult neurogenesis, and reduced LTP in the dentate gyrus (Zhao et al., 2003). Serotonin 1A receptor mutants lacked both the increase in adult neurogenesis and behavioral consequences elicited by selective serotonin reuptake inhibitors (Santarelli et al., 2003).

FUNCTIONAL RELEVANCE OF ADULT-GENERATED NEURONS IN THE HIPPOCAMPUS

Blocking Adult Neurogenesis to Study the Role of New Neurons in Hippocampal Function

A straightforward way to study the functional contribution of adult neurogenesis to hippocampal function is to block adult neurogenesis altogether. So far, the researchers who have chosen this approach have aimed at eliminating the precursor cells as the cellular source for new neurons. This has been achieved by either toxicity or irradiation. Joseph Altman was pioneer in this regard as well. He irradiated the dentate gyrus of rats early postnatally (thus not addressing adult neurogenesis) and found lasting damage to the dentate gyrus and reduced performance in the T-maze (Bayer and Altman, 1975; Gazzara and Altman, 1981) (see also Chapter 9).

One of the most interesting but also most controversially discussed articles in the field of adult neurogenesis is a study by Tracey Shors and Elizabeth Gould that was published in 2001 (Shors et al., 2001). In this study, dividing cells were eliminated by a treatment with methylazoxymethanol acetate (MAM), an antiproliferative drug that acts by methylating the DNA. Because the DNA is exposed, cells that undergo division are sensitive to the effects of cytostatic drugs such as MAM. Cytostatics prevent successful completion of the cell cycle, which causes the death of the dividing cell. They are used in cancer therapy because tumor cells are highly proliferative, but so are precursor cells. Consequently, chemotherapy has side effects such as anemia due to effects on bone marrow stem cells.

In the experiment, MAM blocked precursor cell divisions in the dentate gyrus and led to a down-regulation of adult hippocampal neurogenesis. In the treated animals performance on a hippocampus-dependent learning task (trace conditioning) was disturbed, whereas that on a hippocampus-independent version of the same task was spared (Shors et al., 2001) (Fig. 10.3). The conclusion was that new neurons were needed to mediate the hippocampal contribution to the task. Eye-blink conditioning is a classical conditioning task in which the unconditioned stimulus and the conditioned stimulus can be separated by different time spans. If the two stimuli overlap (and coterminate) the version of the test is called "delay." The delay version of the test is independent of the hippocampus. The information of the unconditioned stimulus remains present for this brief time and can be associated with the conditioned stimulus. In the trace version of the same test the interval between unconditioned and conditioned stimulus is 500 ms and therefore the hippocampus is required to associate unconditioned and conditioned stimulus across the interval. Although the trace version of this task has a hippocampal component, eye-blink conditioning might not adequately represent the complexity of hippocampal function, including higher cognitive processes. It is often used as a test assessing cerebellar function (McCormick et al., 1982; Freeman and Nicholson, 2000). There is a long-standing debate about the information that conditioning tasks provide about hippocampal function and the answer largely depends on the definition of function. Other points of concern are the range of side effects of MAM, which might be impossible to control sufficiently. In fact, the effects of MAM on presumably neurogenesis-dependent hippocampal learning were not detectable or ambiguous on other hippocampal tests, including the Morris water maze (Shors et al., 2002).

A possible functional interpretation of these results is that adult neurogenesis might be particularly important for learning, when trace intervals separate the stimuli that need to be associated. Complex tasks such as spatial navigation, however, consist of many trace situations and it is not clear why adult neurogenesis is necessary for the association of isolated stimuli but not of patterns of stimuli.

Several irradiation experiments have suggested that hippocampal tasks are more sensitive to irradiation and presumably to the irradiation-induced decrease in adult neurogenesis than nonhippocampal learning (Raber et al., 2004; Rola et al., 2004).

Both exposure to an enriched environment (Kempermann et al., 1997) and the experience of specific learning stimuli have stimulated the recruitment of new neurons (Gould et al., 1999a; Leuner et al., 2004). One hypothesis that could be derived from the effects of cytostatics on adult hippocampal neurogenesis and their correlation with functional measures is that immature neurons themselves might play a functional role (see below). Gould and colleagues (1999b) speculated the following:

A rapidly changing population of adult-generated neurons would be particularly suitable as a substrate for such a transient role of the hippocampal formation in memory storage. Neurons produced in adulthood might play a role in information processing related to memory storage

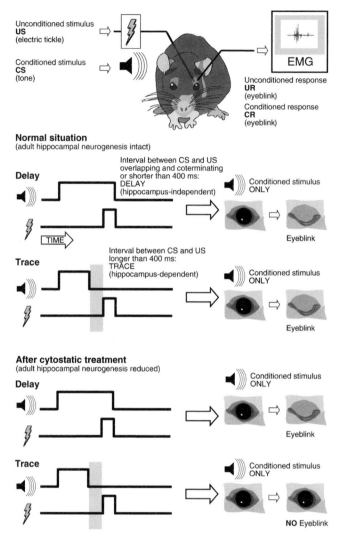

Figure 10–3. Hippocampal neurogenesis in formation of trace memories. Shors et al. (2001) reported that treating rats with cytostatic agent MAM resulted in a defect in acquisition of a hippocampus-dependent version of a learning task (delay eyeblink conditioning), whereas the hippocampus-independent version of the same task (trace eyeblink conditioning) was spared. The finding has been interpreted as evidence for a role of new neurons in learning the hippocampus-dependent task.

during a discrete time after their generation. These cells might then degenerate or undergo changes in connectivity, gene expression, or both, coincident with the end of hippocampal storage of that particular memory.

In contrast to this idea of new neurons as a means of memory storage, the theory favored below proposes that new neurons are recruited during a particularly sensitive phase of their late development and in response to challenges of complexity and novelty in order to cumulatively adapt the network to cope with similar challenges in the future.

Adult Neurogenesis in Animal Models of Depression

One of the most stimulating new ideas in research on adult hippocampal neurogenesis is the hypothesis that failure of adult hippocampal neurogenesis might help to explain the pathogenesis (of at least the hippocampal symptoms) of major depression. We will discuss this theory in greater detail in Chapter 12. Independent of whether this theory will ultimately hold true, it has already provoked a fresh look at the possible function of adult-born neurons. In the present context, the most important aspect of this idea is that its perspective is wider than learning. Depression is a mood disorder that includes cognitive symptoms of hippocampal origin. But the central issue is the link between cognitive contents and emotional contexts that the hippocampus is thought to provide.

Luca Santarelli, René Hen, and colleagues at Columbia University used an irradiation protocol that allowed focusing of the rays on the part of the mouse brain containing the hippocampus (Santarelli et al., 2003) (Fig. 10–4). X-rays are potent inhibitors of proliferation because they interfere with DNA synthesis. The group showed that when the animals underwent a test for anxiety, the effectiveness of antidepressant drugs to improve their performance was dependent on the integrity of the SGZ and thus presumably of adult neurogenesis. Antidepressants have a stimulating effect on adult hippocampal neurogenesis (Malberg et al., 2000), and this effect was absent in the irradiated animals. The study was a major breakthrough in that it extended the question of the functional relevance of adult neurogenesis to include hippocampal function beyond the strict hippocampal learning paradigms. Input from other limbic structures that mediate the emotional contexts of information to be processed in the hippocampus converge at the dentate gyrus and supposedly modulate information processing. At the same time, human emotional memory is associated with enhanced episodic memory, another hippocampal function (Richardson et al., 2004). In addition to ablating dividing cells, however, irradiation affects the stem cell niche in the SGZ and thus alters the integrity of the limbic input as well. Thus, because irradiation damages both the stem cells *and* microenvironment, including the local neuronal network, it is difficult to evaluate how much of the behavioral result was due to the blockade of neural precursor cell activity alone.

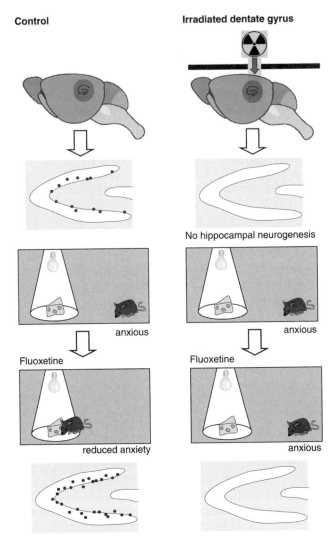

Figure 10–4. Ablation of adult neurogenesis impairs action of antidepressants. Santarelli et al. (2003) irradiated the hippocampal region of mice and thereby wiped out adult neurogenesis. In these mice, the antidepressant fluoxetine, a selective serotonin uptake inhibitor (SSRI), did not reduce anxiety in a task in which the rodents had to cross a brightly lit area to reach food, whereas it did induce it in the nonirradiated animals. In nonirradiated animals, fluoxetine induces an increase in adult hippocampal neurogenesis (compare with Malberg et al., 2000).

Despite all the factual insight derived from these studies, experiments in which damage to the SGZ is used to disrupt adult neurogenesis reveal how difficult it is to directly link an experimental manipulation at the earliest developmental stages of adult neurogenesis to an outcome at the systems level. But the discussion of complex functional pathology, as in the case of major depression, requires an interpretation on both the network *and* the systems levels and beyond. Consequently, the study of adult neurogenesis in animal models of depression has not yet helped much to clarify the situation. Learned helplessness (which is one paradigm for studying depression in rodents), for example, was not associated with a down-regulation of adult neurogenesis (Vollmayr et al., 2003).

Concepts of Hippocampal function

A widely accepted idea is that the hippocampus consolidates memory, meaning that it processes information for long-term storage. Not all types of memory formation require a hippocampal contribution, however. Procedural learning, i.e., the acquisition of motor skills, or priming, i.e., types of instinctive learning, are independent of the hippocampus. One type of learning that requires processing in the hippocampus is the learning of declarative contents. For humans *declarative* can be quite literally explained as information that can be declared or put in words. A more general definition of declarative memory is knowledge of facts and events: knowledge about facts is called "semantic memory," and knowledge about events is called "episodic memory."

To achieve memory consolidation, the hippocampus provides means to link information to contexts and to place it into internal coordinate systems. The hippocampus might also help to identify consistencies across many experiences and thereby prepare the grounds for future association (Eichenbaum, 2003; Wirth et al., 2003). It seems that all these maps, however, are not stored in the hippocampus itself (Eichenbaum et al., 1999). Rather, the processed information is stored primarily elsewhere in the cortex and, together with their coordinates, becomes independent of the hippocampus. The process of consolidation can take days to weeks, and during this time the information to be stored remains sensitive to modification. The hippocampus is also involved in the retrieval of stored information. Again, during recall the stored information can become vulnerable to alterations, further suggesting that the hippocampus plays an active role in this process.

The temporospatial information associated with the stored contents is the basis of episodic memory (Fortin et al., 2002). In addition, the hippocampus allows us to deal with onetime experiences (Nakazawa et al., 2003): in a constantly changing world, most events occur only once. For episodic memory, one-trial learning is indispensable. One-trial learning in turn requires at least transient storage of information in the hippocampus. This transient memory may be located in CA3 (Nakazawa et al., 2003).

Spatial Learning

Spatial navigation is an example of learning that not only is dependent on hippocampal integrity but also exemplifies the necessity of placing information into a set of temporal and spatial coordinates. A path through a new environment is a sequence of temporospatial information. In patients with Alzheimer disease, the hippocampus is affected early and disorientation and lack of spatial memory are typical early symptoms.

Spatial navigation can be tested in rodents and has become the key surrogate measure to assess declarative memory in animals (Morris et al., 1982). This does not imply that the hippocampus is "just for place" (Eichenbaum, 1996).

One of the most widely used tests of spatial memory as a measure of hippocampal function is the Morris water maze (Morris, 1984). Rodents are placed into a circular pool of water and learn to navigate to a small escape platform hidden just below the surface of the water. The time (latency) to find the platform and the distance the animals swim to it can be plotted as a learning curve to describe acquisition of the task. The steeper the slope of the learning curve, the faster the animals have learned the task. Over few days of training, most normal rodents find the platform quickly and with a short swimming distance. If position of the platform is changed in a reversal, most rodents adapt to the new position quickly. The first trial of the reversal can be used as the so-called probe-trial. Here the perseverance of the animals to find the platform at the position where it used to be is taken as a measure of how well the animal learned the task and retained the information or can recall it. Although there are conceptual problems with this interpretation, the probe-trial measures different aspects of learning than the parameters that describe the acquisition period of the task. An animal's ability to navigate the hidden version of the water maze is dependent on the integrity of the hippocampus. If the hidden platform is made visible, the test becomes independent of the hippocampus.

The Morris water maze is one of the most widely used tests of hippocampal function. The idea of a link between spatial learning abilities and hippocampal neurogenesis in humans has been made popular by an imaging study in London taxi drivers was used. It found that taxi-driving in London that poses a considerable challenge to spatial navigation was associated with increased hippocampal volume and that a positive correlation existed between volume and the time spent as a taxi driver (Maguire et al., 2000). Obviously, no conclusions about the nature of these hippocampal changes and thus a potential contribution of adult neurogenesis were possible from this study. Nevertheless, the finding highlighted that activity-dependent changes in gray matter are possible and measurable even in humans, and speculations about the underlying mechanisms were inevitable.

In mice, there was a small but significant correlation between parameters describing the acquisition phase of the water maze and the genetically determined baseline level of adult hippocampal neurogenesis (Kempermann and

Gage, 2002). Similarly, in old rats, water-maze performance predicted levels of adult neurogenesis (Drapeau et al., 2003). On the other hand, elimination of precursor cell activity in the dentate gyrus through cytostatic treatment did not affect water-maze learning (Shors et al., 2002). One confounding problem is that learning the water maze is not an ethologically relevant behavior and places animals under a considerable amount of stress. In the future, better-suited tests of hippocampal functions have to be identified that allow us to relate adult hippocampal neurogenesis more closely to hippocampal function. These tests will have to go beyond the assessment of spatial navigation and appreciate the complexity of hippocampal function and the role of the dentate gyrus within it.

Network Theories of the Dentate gyrus and Hippocampus

The hippocampus has a network architecture that is relatively well understood. It consists of an essentially trisynaptic backbone (Fig. 10–5). The first relay station within this core circuit is the dentate gyrus, the second, CA3; the third, CA1. Excitation follows this path coming from the entorhinal cortex, in which input from many other brain regions, including the sensory areas, converges. From CA1 the flow of information goes via the subiculum back to the entorhinal cortex and from the entorhinal cortex to cortical association areas. Several shortcuts and side paths complicate the general

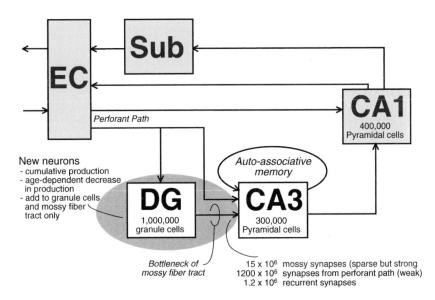

Figure 10–5. The main circuitry of the hippocampus. The input into hippocampal formation from the entorhinal cortex (EC) and dentate gyrus (DG) is a bottleneck within the network of the hippocampus. The numbers are based on a review by Treves and Rolls (1994). Sub, subiculum.

pattern, but for the purpose of most present considerations these complica-
tions seem to be negligible.

Within the trisynaptic path, adult neurogenesis occurs only in the dentate gyrus and thus has a direct influence on only the number of granule
cells in the dentate gyrus and the mossy fiber connection built by the axons
of the granule cells and linking the dentate gyrus with CA3.

The hippocampus is a bottleneck structure into which numerous inputs
converge and from which a wide range of outputs emerge. The entrance
structure for the hippocampus, formed by the entorhinal cortex and the
dentate gyrus, requires a massive reduction in input channels as well as a
reduction in information content. The dentate gyrus thus seems to be involved in compressing data. Firing patterns in the dentate gyrus are sparse,
which is in apparent contrast to the massive flow of information through
this structure. The sparseness of activity is also consistent with the idea that
the dentate gyrus stabilizes neuronal activity flooding into the hippocampus. The underlying assumption is that for complex cognitive functions to
be performed by the hippocampus, a reduction in noise and fluctuations
on very short time scales is necessary.

Judging from the network architecture, CA3, the second station, appears
to serve as a temporary autoassociative memory. The general idea is that the
function of the dentate gyrus is to encode information to make it usable by
CA3. Data compression might be one aspect of this processing, the avoidance
of catastrophic interference a second. *Catastrophic interference* is the problem
that would ensue if a constant flow of information made it impossible to keep
together those pieces of information that belong to each other, leading to a
catastrophic accumulation of useless contents. The dentate gyrus might reduce the overlap, that is, the number of commonly active neurons, between
different input patterns by generating a sparse representation of that information. Since sparse patterns share fewer active neurons at a given time, they
result in less interference, or cross-talk. The avoidance of catastrophic interference would improve reliability of pattern storage and retrieval in CA3. In
contrast to CA3, the dentate gyrus does not have the architectural properties
of a memory network. There is an ongoing debate as to what degree information is actually stored within the hippocampus and not cortical regions.
Clearly, the overall storage capacity of the hippocampus is low compared to
that of the cortex, and within the hippocampus only CA3 has the network
characteristics of a memory device. As mentioned above, this property is
thought to be relevant for the one-trial learning associated with episodic
memory (Nakazawa et al., 2003). Consequently, adult neurogenesis in the
dentate gyrus would add neurons only to a structure that feeds into memory,
but does not seem to be directly involved in building or modifying a structure that can store information.

Independent of the nature of CA3, classical memory formation that is the
transfer or integration of memory contents into the cortex seems to occur
mainly in CA1. This conclusion is based mainly on electrophysiological data

showing that memory correlates best with LTP as the electrophysiological equivalent of learning, in CA1. Episodic memory is also dependent on glutamate action in CA1 (Day et al., 2003). The finding that adult neurogenesis occurs two synaptic relay stations before this step supports the idea that neurogenesis functionally contributes to a processing step independent of the actual storage into the cortex. Adult hippocampal neurogenesis appears to correlate better with parameters describing the acquisition of a hippocampal learning task but not with measures of retention or recall of the stored information (Kempermann and Gage, 2002). The contribution of new neurons to the variance in learning is relatively low, ranging between 10% and 20% in the above study. Thus, there is no strict linear relationship between hippocampal learning and nonspecific inducibility of adult neurogenesis, as it can be achieved, for example, by physical activity (Rhodes et al., 2003). Many factors, not just new neurons, contribute to hippocampal function.

Are New Neurons Needed to Learn or Forget?

It has been hypothesized that new neurons might be necessary to be able to forget, in the sense that they would allow the hippocampus to be cleared of old memory traces (Feng et al., 2001). This idea has received much attention but is so far based only on few experimental data. Mice in which the presenilin-1 gene was knocked out had no overt phenotype in adult hippocampal neurogenesis under normal conditions. When the animals were placed in an enriched environment, however, the up-regulation of adult neurogenesis seen in wild-type mice was reduced by about one third. There were no differences in performance on a hippocampal learning task, including the water maze task. However, in contextual and cued fear conditioning, a task for which the hippocampus is required (Kim et al., 1992), the mutant mice performed better in that they showed more freezing responses to the contextual stimulus. From these results the conclusion was drawn that a "deficit in neurogenesis" was associated with "an enhancement in memory" (McGuire and Davis, 2001) and that neurogenesis might clear those memories from the hippocampus that have been consolidated and transferred to the cortex, thus preparing the hippocampus for new learning experiences (Feng et al., 2001). The idea is generally intriguing: new neurons would free other neurons from processing duties and allow clearing of the system for the next wave of information. Because the lack of presenilin-1 might have many other consequences for hippocampal function, no unambiguous link between the mutation that sparked the hyposthesis and the theory itself can be made. Independent of the specifics of this experiment, however, is difficult to reconcile the theory that new neurons help to clear storage with the generally very low rate of hippocampal neurogenesis throughout most parts of life and especially in old age, or with the fact that it is CA3 and not the dentate gyrus that shows the characteristics of an autoassociative memory network.

The long period of time it takes for a new neuron to mature also argues against the idea that a new neuron might benefit the learning situation that triggered its generation. An alternate possibility, however, is that new neurons are not produced on demand but that the hippocampus and olfactory bulb provide a constant flow of immature cells that could be used in an acute situation. The new cells might exert a specific function in an immature state, just after maturation or even at a lineage-determined progenitor cell stage. During the consolidation process of memory formation, the immature new neurons might form temporary memory that is passed on to long-term storage and might activity-dependently add to the processing network (Deisseroth et al., 2004). After consolidation, the function of the new cells would become obsolete and they would be replaced by the next generation of neurons. The lowered threshold for LTP induction in new granule cells (Wang et al., 2000; Schmidt-Hieber et al., 2004) to some degree argues in favor of such an interpretation. Here, the early neuronal responsiveness might be a relevant property in and of itself and be distinct from what could be perceived as mature neuronal function. This idea would, be primarily consistent with the concept of neuronal turnover in the neurogenic regions and the consequence that the specific function of new neurons would thus be transient. However, the idea that the "time-limited existence [of new neurons] might be related to transient processes thought to be involved in memory" (Gross, 2000) is made problematic by the finding that new neurons, including those generated in response to an acute learning stimulus, survive for long periods of time (Winner et al., 2002; Kempermann et al., 2003; Leuner et al., 2004), and no good evidence of neuronal turnover has been found in the adult dentate gyrus (Bayer et al., 1982; Bayer, 1985; Crespo et al., 1986).

A turnover limited to the population of intermediate cells, however, seems relatively unlikely given the age-dependent decline in adult neurogenesis. This decrease in neurogenesis leads to extremely low numbers of new neurons in aged subjects that nevertheless learn new tasks considerably well (Merrill et al., 2003).

Therefore, the potential contributions of adult neurogenesis to cognition might be found in long-term adaptations of the hippocampal circuitry (or analogously in the olfactory bulb) rather than in acute benefits. The increased synaptic plasticity of immature cells might be necessary to recruit the cells into the network. In that sense the network modification would be immediate but not restricted to that initial period. The specific and distinct early functions of new neurons might be a preparatory step necessary for persistent integration and mature function. Consequently, the two ideas are not necessarily mutually exclusive.

New Gatekeepers at the Gateway to Memory

Strictly speaking, the most narrow connection in the hippocampus with the fewest fibers is the perforant path, linking the entorhinal cortex to the dentate gyrus (Fig. 10–6). Consequently, the input to the dentate gyrus is already sparse. But its output through the mossy fiber tract, which is formed by the axons of both old and new granule cells, is narrow as well. In between lies the information processing provided by the granule cells. The mossy fibers thus convey processed information, still sparse but concentrated in content. While there is principally no explanation for the lack of new neurons to strengthen the perforant path, there is no doubt that the addition of even a small number of neurons to the mossy fiber connection can make a large, relative difference. Among the billions of cortical neurons, the 100,000 new neurons that might ultimately be added to the mouse dentate gyrus throughout life would go unnoticed, but in the mossy fiber tract they account for a net increase by 30% to 40%.

This strategic insertion of new neurons at a narrow, key spot is the basis of the theory "new gatekeepers at the gateway to memory" (Kempermann, 2002; Kempermann and Wiskott, 2004). The assumption is that it is beneficial for the mossy fiber connection to be as sparse as possible while at the same time as strong as necessary. Adult hippocampal neurogenesis would thereby provide a means of optimizing the mossy fiber system to allow efficient processing at a level of information complexity and novelty frequently encountered by the individual. The benefits of an adaptation of the mossy fiber system are cumulative and an investment for the future. This is consistent with the known slow macroscopic changes of the mossy fiber tract over life and their strong dependence on genetic factors. The "new gatekeeper theory" also explains why adult neurogenesis can decrease with increasing age. Normally, younger animals encounter relatively more novel experiences, Whereas older animals have seen it all and thus require less potential for adaptation. If older individuals, however, are challenged by a novel experience, a relatively much stronger induction of adult neurogenesis is possible in the aged brain than in the young brain (Kempermann et al., 1998). Consistent with this theory is the finding that the absolute level of adult neurogenesis at the oldest age alone did not predict performance in the recall phase of the Morris water maze (Bizon and Gallagher, 2003). The new gatekeeper theory links adult hippocampal neurogenesis to the capability of coping with novelty and complexity. Rats bred for strong reaction toward novelty have low levels of adult neurogenesis, presumably because their novelty-seeking behavior compensates for their inability to efficiently and quietly cope with novelty (Lemaire et al., 1999).

FUNCTIONAL RELEVANCE OF ADULT-GENERATED NEURONS IN THE OLFACTORY BULB

Although knowledge about information processing in the olfactory bulb might be even more limited than in the hippocampus, the ethological relevance of olfaction is immense, particularly in rodents. The general network structure of the olfactory bulb and its integration into the olfactory system

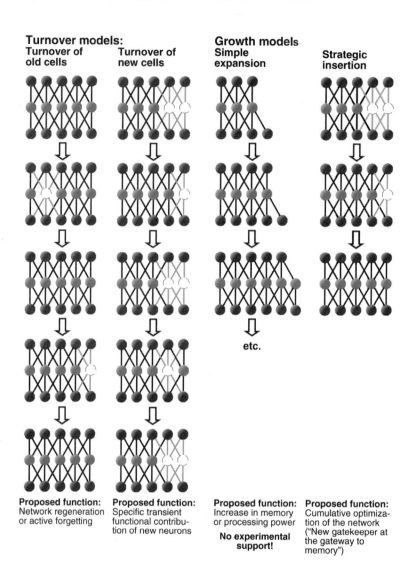

Turnover models:

Turnover of old cells

Turnover of new cells

Growth models

Simple expansion

Strategic insertion

Proposed function:
Network regeneration or active forgetting

Proposed function:
Specific transient functional contribution of new neurons

Proposed function:
Increase in memory or processing power

No experimental support!

Proposed function:
Cumulative optimization of the network ("New gatekeeper at the gateway to memory")

Figure 10–6. Theoretical concepts about the function of new neurons in the hippocampus. Turnover models are opposed to growth models. There is no experimental evidence for plain and general growth of the hippocampus Adult neurogenesis affects only the granule cell layer. In turnover models, two forms can be distinguished. In the first, old cells are replaced because they have been lost. There is little evidence for this idea of a regenerative turnover. Many current theoretical concepts argue in favor instead of a turnover of newly generated cells, which in these concepts would have a particular and transient function. A version of a turnover model is imaginable in which both old and new cells are replaced because the network function requires the turnover of certain neurons. Clearance of the hippocampus for new information or active forgetting might be such functions. The strongest argument against this idea is the very low level of adult hippocampal neurogenesis in old animals, which still have good hippocampal function. We therefore favor a strategic growth model, the model of new gatekeepers at the gateway to memory. This theory states that adult hippocampal neurogenesis strategically inserts new neurons to

has been identified (Hopfield, 1991). Adult neurogenesis generates two types of interneurons in the adult olfactory bulb, most of them in the granule cell layer, and a few percent in the periglomerular regions.

Olfaction plays a major role in regulating neurogenesis in the adult olfactory bulb (Petreanu and Alvarez-Buylla, 2002), but physiologic activators of adult hippocampal neurogenesis, such as voluntary physical activity and exposure to a complex environment, do not affect neurogenesis in the olfactory bulb (Brown et al., 2003). Stimulation of the olfactory nerve resulted in action potentials in newly integrated interneurons in the adult olfactory bulb (Belluzzi et al., 2003).

On the basis of the network structure, the general pattern of regulation and the types of neurons that generate the contribution of new neurons to olfactory bulb function might thus be fundamentally different from their counterparts in the dentate gyrus.

As a first hypothesis, adult neurogenesis allows an activity-dependent adaptation of GABAergic inhibition in the olfactory bulb (Carleton et al., 2002). The olfactory receptor neurons project to the mitral/tufted cells (M/T cells). The synaptic contact between the two cells occurs in the glomeruli of the olfactory bulb. Each glomerulum represents one odor in the sense that all receptors of one type project to the same glomerulum. Periglomerular cells provide inhibitory contacts between different glomeruli. Granule cell interneurons provide inhibitory contacts between different M/T cells.

A first computational model has been developed to explain how new neurons contribute to function of the olfactory bulb (Cecchi et al., 2001). It is based on a simplified network with receptor neurons that project to the M/T cells and with inhibitory granule cell neurons that make pairwise connections with the M/T cells. Consistent with the general ideas applicable to the hippocampus, the underlying assumption was that neural production procedes at a constant and unregulated rate, whereas cell survival is selective and activity-dependent. Within the network model only interneurons were replaced, because adult olfactory neurogenesis affects only interneurons. Survival of the new interneurons was linked to their activity, making more active neurons more likely to survive. Learning in this model was unsupervised—that is, no external instance adjusted key parameters in the course of the training. Even this comparatively simple model revealed

---

adjust the hippocampal network for coping with levels of complexity and novelty frequently encountered by an individual (Kempermann, 2002; Kempermann and Wiskott, 2004). Apparently, the mossy fiber connection should be as sparse as possible but as strong as necessary to work optimally. The effects of adult neurogenesis are thus cumulative and represent long-term adaptation processes. The additional neurons allow the system in the long run to reduce catastrophic interference due to novel stimuli.

that neurogenesis allowed the network to maximize the discrimination of odors (Cecchi et al., 2001).

FUNCTIONAL RELEVANCE OF CELL GENESIS IN NON-NEUROGENIC REGIONS

Few studies on neurogenesis outside the neurogenic regions have included data on the integration of the new cells into the local network (Magavi et al., 2000). Nakatomi and colleagues (2002), who showed growth factor–induced regeneration of CA1 after ischemia, were able to support functionality of the new neurons by electrophysiological measures (field potentials) and behavioral analyses. Outside the well-described hippocampal network, such an attempt would likely have been futile. Consequently, most studies on regenerative neurogenesis do not contain experimental data on the possible functions of the new cells. The technical hurdles are extreme and especially in the cortex, the circuitry into which the new cells would integrate, is exceedingly more complex than in the dentate gyrus and the olfactory bulb. One might argue that no new neuron is new unless it is shown that it functions as one. The fact, however, that it took 35 years to go from initially describing adult hippocampal neurogenesis to proving of neuronal functionality on an electrophysiological level shows that this principally justified requirement must not be overemphasized. However, studies with claims of neurogenesis in non-neurogenic regions or after pathology should clearly state their limitations with regard to functional conclusions.

Adult neurogenesis in general needs to be seen in the larger context of cellular plasticity in the adult brain. The amount of cellular plasticity in general, including cell birth and death, that occurs under physiologic conditions and thus not only in response to pathology is much higher was assumed until recently. Precursor cell biology provides a strong conceptual link between these types of plasticity and adult neurogenesis. Despite the large body of data, though, the functional relevance of constant gliogenesis in the adult brain remains elusive. This gliogenesis is activity-dependently regulated and even microglial proliferation in the cortex is influenced by physical activity (Ehninger and Kempermann, 2003). To date, it remains unclear how brain function relies on this widespread and regulated cellular plasticity. Astrocytes, for example, can receive neuronal input and can modulate synaptic transmission. Oligodendrocytes have a complex physiology and provide more than passive electric isolation. Microglia is increasingly considered to be not only the immune cells of the brain that respond to damage, but also to function as physiologic sensors for needs of plasticity. In this largely uncharted map of cellular plasticity, adult neurogenesis might be only a special case that shares some features but lacks others. Consequently, assessment of the functional relevance of cellular plasticity is a tremendous task that touches on fundamental thoughts about the ways in which brain structure and function are linked.

REFERENCES

Ambrogini P, Lattanzi D, Ciuffoli S, Agostini D, Bertini L, Stocchi V, Santi S, Cuppini R (2004) Morpho-functional characterization of neuronal cells at different stages of maturation in granule cell layer of adult rat dentate gyrus. Brain Res 1017:21–31.

Bayer SA (1985) Neuron production in the hippocampus and olfactory bulb of the adult rat brain: addition or replacement? Ann NY Acad Sci 457:163–172.

Bayer SA, Altman J (1975) The effects of X-irradiation on the postnatally forming granule cell populations in the olfactory bulb, hippocampus, and cerebellum of the rat. Exp Neurol 48:167–174.

Bayer SA, Yackel JW, Puri PS (1982) Neurons in the rat dentate gyrus granular layer substantially increase during juvenile and adult life. Science 216:890–892.

Belluzzi O, Benedusi M, Ackman J, LoTurco JJ (2003) Electrophysiological differentiation of new neurons in the olfactory bulb. J Neurosci 23:10411–10418.

Benninger F, Beck H, Wernig M, Tucker KL, Brustle O, Scheffler B (2003) Functional integration of embryonic stem cell–derived neurons in hippocampal slice cultures. J Neurosci 23:7075–7083.

Bizon JL, Gallagher M (2003) Production of new cells in the rat dentate gyrus over the lifespan: relation to cognitive decline. Eur J Neurosci 18:215–219.

Brown J, Cooper-Kuhn CM, Kempermann G, Van Praag H, Winkler J, Gage FH, Kuhn HG (2003) Enriched environment and physical activity stimulate hippocampal but not olfactory bulb neurogenesis. Eur J Neurosci 17:2042–2046.

Carlen M, Cassidy RM, Brismar H, Smith GA, Enquist LW, Frisen J (2002) Functional integration of adult-born neurons. Curr Biol 12:606–608.

Carleton A, Petreanu LT, Lansford R, Alvarez-Buylla A, Lledo PM (2003) Becoming a new neuron in the adult olfactory bulb. Nat Neurosci 6:507–518.

Carleton A, Rochefort C, Morante-Oria J, Desmaisons D, Vincent JD, Gheusi G, Lledo PM (2002) Making scents of olfactory neurogenesis. J Physiol Paris 96:115–122.

Cecchi GA, Petreanu LT, Alvarez-Buylla A, Magnasco MO (2001) Unsupervised learning and adaptation in a model of adult neurogenesis. J Comput Neurosci 11:175–182.

Crespo D, Stanfield BB, Cowan WM (1986) Evidence that late-generated granule cells do not simply replace earlier formed neurons in the rat dentate gyrus. Exp Brain Res 62:541–548.

Day M, Langston R, Morris RG (2003) Glutamate-receptor-mediated encoding and retrieval of paired-associate learning. Nature 424:205–209.

Deisseroth K, Singla S, Toda H, Monje M, Palmer TD, Malenka RC (2004) Excitation–neurogenesis coupling in adult neural stem/progenitor cells. Neuron 42:535–552.

Drapeau E, Mayo W, Aurousseau C, Le Moal M, Piazza PV, Abrous DN (2003) Spatial memory performances of aged rats in the water maze predict levels of hippocampal neurogenesis. Proc Natl Acad Sci USA 100:14385–14390.

Ehninger D, Kempermann G (2003) Regional effects of wheel running and environmental enrichment on cell genesis and microglia proliferation in the adult murine neocortex. Cereb Cortex 13:845–851.

Eichenbaum H (1996) Is the rodent hippocampus just for "place"? Trends Neurosci 6:187–195.

Eichenbaum H (2003) How does the hippocampus contribute to memory? Trends Cogn Sci 7:427–429.

Eichenbaum H, Dudchenko P, Wood E, Shapiro M, Tanila H (1999) The hippocampus, memory, and place cells: is it spatial memory or a memory space? Neuron 23:209–226.

Farmer J, Zhao X, van Praag H, Wodtke K, Gage FH, Christie BR (2004) Effects of voluntary exercise on synaptic plasticity and gene expression in the dentate gyrus of adult male Sprague-Dawley rats in vivo. Neuroscience 124:71–79.

Feng R, Rampon C, Tang YP, Shrom D, Jin J, Kyin M, Sopher B, Martin GM, Kim SH, Langdon RB, Sisodia SS, Tsien JZ (2001) Deficient neurogenesis in forebrain-specific presenilin-1 knockout mice is associated with reduced clearance of hippocampal memory traces. Neuron 32:911–926.

Filippov V, Kronenberg G, Pivneva T, Reuter K, Steiner B, Wang LP, Yamaguchi M, Kettenmann H, Kempermann G (2003) Subpopulation of nestin-expressing progenitor cells in the adult murine hippocampus shows electrophysiological and morphological characteristics of astrocytes. Mol Cell Neurosci 23:373–382.

Fortin NJ, Agster KL, Eichenbaum HB (2002) Critical role of the hippocampus in memory for sequences of events. Nat Neurosci 5:458–462.

Freeman JH Jr, Nicholson DA (2000) Developmental changes in eye-blink conditioning and neuronal activity in the cerebellar interpositus nucleus. J Neurosci 20:813–819.

Fukuda S, Kato F, Tozuka Y, Yamaguchi M, Miyamoto Y, Hisatsune T (2003) Two distinct subpopulations of nestin-positive cells in adult mouse dentate gyrus. J Neurosci 23:9357–9366.

Gazzara RA, Altman J (1981) Early postnatal X-irradiation of the hippocampus and discrimination learning in adult rats. J Comp Physiol Psychol 95:484–495.

Gould E, Beylin A, Tanapat P, Reeves A, Shors TJ (1999a) Learning enhances adult neurogenesis in the hippocampal formation. Nat Neurosci 2:260–265.

Gould E, Tanapat P, Hastings NB, Shors TJ (1999b) Neurogenesis in adulthood: a possible role in learning. Trends Cogn Sci 3:186–192.

Gross CG (2000) Neurogenesis in the adult brain: death of a dogma. Nat Rev Neurosci 1:67–73.

Hastings NB, Gould E (1999) Rapid extension of axons into the CA3 region by adult-generated granule cells. J Comp Neurol 413:146–154.

Hopfield JJ (1991) Olfactory computation and object perception. Proc Natl Acad Sci USA 88:6462–6466.

Jessberger S, Kempermann G (2003) Adult-born hippocampal neurons mature into activity-dependent responsiveness. Eur J Neurosci 18:2707–2712.

Kempermann G (2002) Why new neurons? Possible functions for adult hippocampal neurogenesis. J Neurosci 22:635–638.

Kempermann G, Gage FH (2002) Genetic determinants of adult hippocampal neurogenesis correlate with acquisition, but not probe trial performance in the water maze task. Eur J Neurosci 16:129–136.

Kempermann G, Gast D, Kronenberg G, Yamaguchi M, Gage FH (2003) Early determination and long-term persistence of adult-generated new neurons in the hippocampus of mice. Development 130:391–399.

Kempermann G, Kuhn HG, Gage FH (1997) More hippocampal neurons in adult mice living in an enriched environment. Nature 386:493–495.

Kempermann G, Kuhn HG, Gage FH (1998) Experience-induced neurogenesis in the senescent dentate gyrus. J Neurosci 18:3206–3212.

Kempermann G, Wiskott L (2004) What is the functional role of new neurons in the adult dentate gyrus? In: Stem Cells in the Nervous System: Function and Clinical Implications (Gage F, Björklund A, Prochiatz A, Christen Y, eds), pp 57–65. Berlin and Heidelberg: Springer.

Kempermann G, Wiskott L, Gage FH (2004) Functional significance of adult neurogenesis. Curr Opin Neurobiol 14:186–191.

Kim JJ, Fanselow MS, DeCola JP, Landeira-Fernandez J (1992) Selective impairment of long-term but not short-term conditional fear by the N-methyl-D-aspartate antagonist APV. Behav Neurosci 106:591–596.

Lemaire V, Aurousseau C, Le Moal M, Abrous DN (1999) Behavioural trait of reactivity to novelty is related to hippocampal neurogenesis. Eur J Neurosci 11:4006–4014.

Leuner B, Mendolia-Loffredo S, Kozorovitskiy Y, Samburg D, Gould E, Shors TJ (2004) Learning enhances the survival of new neurons beyond the time when the hippocampus is required for memory. J Neurosci 24:7477–7481.

Magavi S, Leavitt B, Macklis J (2000) Induction of neurogenesis in the neocortex of adult mice. Nature 405:951–955.

Maguire EA, Gadian DG, Johnsrude IS, Good CD, Ashburner J, Frackowiak RS, Frith CD (2000) Navigation-related structural change in the hippocampi of taxi drivers. Proc Natl Acad Sci USA 97:4398–4403.

Malberg JE, Eisch AJ, Nestler EJ, Duman RS (2000) Chronic antidepressant treatment increases neurogenesis in adult rat hippocampus. J Neurosci 20:9104–9110.

Markakis E, Gage FH (1999) Adult-generated neurons in the dentate gyrus send axonal projections to the field CA3 and are surrounded by synaptic vesicles. J Comp Neurol 406:449–460.

McCormick DA, Clark GA, Lavond DG, Thompson RF (1982) Initial localization of the memory trace for a basic form of learning. Proc Natl Acad Sci USA 79:2731–2735.

McGuire SE, Davis RL (2001) Presenilin-1 and memories of the forebrain. Neuron 32:763–765.

Merrill DA, Karim R, Darraq M, Chiba AA, Tuszynski MH (2003) Hippocampal cell genesis does not correlate with spatial learning ability in aged rats. J Comp Neurol 459:201–207.

Morris R (1984) Developments of a water-maze procedure for studying spatial learning in the rat. J Neurosci Methods 11:47–60.

Morris RG, Garrud P, Rawlins JN, O'Keefe J (1982) Place navigation impaired in rats with hippocampal lesions. Nature 297:681–683.

Nakatomi H, Kuriu T, Okabe S, Yamamoto S, Hatano O, Kawahara N, Tamura A, Kirino T, Nakafuku M (2002) Regeneration of hippocampal pyramidal neurons after ischemic brain injury by recruitment of endogenous neural progenitors. Cell 110:429–441.

Nakazawa K, Sun LD, Quirk MC, Rondi-Reig L, Wilson MA, Tonegawa S (2003) Hippocampal CA3 NMDA receptors are crucial for memory acquisition of one-time experience. Neuron 38:305–315.

Petreanu L, Alvarez-Buylla A (2002) Maturation and death of adult-born olfactory bulb granule neurons: role of olfaction. J Neurosci 22:6106–6113.

Raber J, Fan Y, Matsumori Y, Liu Z, Weinstein PR, Fike JR, Liu J (2004) Irradiation attenuates neurogenesis and exacerbates ischemia-induced deficits. Ann Neurol 55:381–389.

Rakic P (1985) Limits of neurogenesis in primates. Science 227:1054–1056.

Rhodes JS, Van Praag H, Jeffrey S, Girard I, Mitchell GS, Garland T Jr, Gage FH (2003) Exercise increases hippocampal neurogenesis to high levels but does not improve spatial learning in mice bred for increased voluntary wheel running. Behav Neurosci 117:1006–1016.

Richardson MP, Strange BA, Dolan RJ (2004) Encoding of emotional memories depends on amygdala and hippocampus and their interactions. Nat Neurosci 7:278–285.

Rola R, Otsuka S, Obenaus A, Nelson GA, Limoli CL, VandenBerg SR, Fike JR (2004) Indicators of hippocampal neurogenesis are altered by 56Fe-particle irradiation in a dose-dependent manner. Radiat Res 162:442–446.

Santarelli L, Saxe M, Gross C, Surget A, Battaglia F, Dulawa S, Weisstaub N, Lee J, Duman R, Arancio O, Belzung C, Hen R (2003) Requirement of hippocampal neurogenesis for the behavioral effects of antidepressants. Science 301:805–809.

Schmidt-Hieber C, Jonas P, Bischofberger J (2004) Enhanced synaptic plasticity in newly generated granule cells of the adult hippocampus. Nature 429:184–187.

Shors TJ, Miesegaes G, Beylin A, Zhao M, Rydel T, Gould E (2001) Neurogenesis in the adult is involved in the formation of trace memories. Nature 410:372–376.

Shors TJ, Townsend DA, Zhao M, Kozorovitskiy Y, Gould E (2002) Neurogenesis may relate to some but not all types of hippocampal-dependent learning. Hippocampus 12:578–584.

Snyder JS, Kee N, Wojtowicz JM (2001) Effects of adult neurogenesis on synaptic plasticity in the rat dentate gyrus. J Neurophysiol 85:2423–2431.

Son H, Yu IT, Hwang SJ, Kim JS, Lee SH, Lee YS, Kaang BK (2003) Lithium enhances long-term potentiation independently of hippocampal neurogenesis in the rat dentate gyrus. J Neurochem 85:872–881.

Song HJ, Stevens CF, Gage FH (2002) Neural stem cells from adult hippocampus develop essential properties of functional CNS neurons. Nat Neurosci 5:438–445.

Stanfield BB, Trice JE (1988) Evidence that granule cells generated in the dentate gyrus of adult rats extend axonal projections. Exp Brain Res 72:399–406.

Steinhauser C, Kressin K, Kuprijanova E, Weber M, Seifert G (1994) Properties of voltage-activated Na+ and K+ currents in mouse hippocampal glial cells in situ and after acute isolation from tissue slices. Pflugers Arch 428:610–620.

Treves A, Rolls ET (1994) Computational analysis of the role of the hippocampus in memory. Hippocampus 4:374–391.

van Praag H, Christie BR, Sejnowski TJ, Gage FH (1999) Running enhances neurogenesis, learning and long-term potentiation in mice. Proc Natl Acad Sci USA 96:13427–13431.

van Praag H, Schinder AF, Christie BR, Toni N, Palmer TD, Gage FH (2002) Functional neurogenesis in the adult hippocampus. Nature 415:1030–1034.

Vollmayr B, Simonis C, Weber S, Gass P, Henn F (2003) Reduced cell proliferation in the dentate gyrus is not correlated with the development of learned helplessness. Biol Psychiatry 54:1035–1040.

Wang S, Scott BW, Wojtowicz JM (2000) Heterogenous properties of dentate granule neurons in the adult rat. J Neurobiol 42:248–257.

Wichterle H, Lieberam I, Porter JA, Jessell TM (2002) Directed differentiation of embryonic stem cells into motor neurons. Cell 110:385–397.

Winner B, Cooper-Kuhn CM, Aigner R, Winkler J, Kuhn HG (2002) Long-term survival and cell death of newly generated neurons in the adult rat olfactory bulb. Eur J Neurosci 16:1681–1689.

Wirth S, Yanike M, Frank LM, Smith AC, Brown EN, Suzuki WA (2003) Single neurons in the monkey hippocampus and learning of new associations. Science 300:1578–1581.

Zhao X, Ueba T, Christie BR, Barkho B, McConnell MJ, Nakashima K, Lein ES, Eadie BD, Willhoite AR, Muotri AR, Summers RG, Chun J, Lee KF, Gage FH (2003) Mice lacking methyl-CpG binding protein 1 have deficits in adult neurogenesis and hippocampal function. Proc Natl Acad Sci USA 100:6777–6782.

11

Adult Neurogenesis
in Different Animal Species

Lifelong generation of new neurons, something comparable to adult neurogenesis in mammals, is not rare across the animal kingdom. As a general rule, organisms with more primitive nervous systems tend to have a higher level of persisting neurogenesis than those with more complex brains. Overall, during evolution a loss of the ability to undergo abundant adult neurogenesis seems to have been the price paid for higher processing power. With increasing brain complexity the dilemma between plasticity and stability might have forced a decision in favor of more stability.

Both neurogenic regions are part of the limbic system. The fact that both neurogenic regions are phylogenetically old influences concepts: only a few highly specialized yet fundamental and evolutionarily conserved functions might require adult neurogenesis. Just as with increasing brain complexity during the course of evolution the capability of adult neurogenesis seems to have decreased, a similar pattern might also be visible within each species: some older brain parts may have retained lifelong neurogenesis, whereas phylogenetically younger regions have not.

One fundamental difficulty in using a comparative approach to study adult neurogenesis is the not-so-trivial task of determining what is "adult" in different organisms (Rakic, 2002a). One can apply a concept of life periods such as childhood, youth, adulthood, and senescence to all organisms, independent of the actual life span. But although longevity can be assessed in flies, the study of aging is hampered by the fact that it also depends on absolute time scales and not only on those relative to the organism's life expectancy. Even in the oldest fly, the cells are infants compared to longer-living organisms. Adulthood is often equated with sexual maturation, although most biologists would not like to concede that definition to their own children. In mouse research, *adult* often means not more than after weaning—that is, at postnatal day 21, when the pups can be removed from their mothers without ensuing problems. To some degree, this early attribution of adulthood is justified in the context of adult neurogenesis because by that time the germinative matrices have undergone the profound changes that lead to the structure that persists for the rest of the organism's life. Operational definitions of adulthood are useful and often necessary but are limited if extrapolations are made from one species to another. To apply quantitative information from a 4-week-old mouse to an adult human is difficult, if not impossible. A thorough comparative consideration can put such disparities into perspective.

Arguably, in rodents one should speak of adult neurogenesis only after the age of about 3 months, when the rate of newly generated cells has leveled out and has reached the low level that will persist into its oldest age. Alternatively, one could argue that adult hippocampal neurogenesis deserves this name only after all remnants of early postnatal development of the dentate gyrus have ceased. No exact studies exist on this question, but the time point might lie at around 6 to 8 weeks in a mouse.

In species in which adult neurogenesis has been less extensively studied than in rodents, these questions become even more difficult. To avoid the word *adult* in these problematic contexts, Myriam Cayre and colleagues (2002) have proposed using the term *secondary neurogenesis*, which indeed brings some semantic advantage but does not solve the problem of determining whether a continuity between primary and secondary neurogenesis exists.

NONMAMMALS

Because of the lack of specific antibodies for many nonmammalian species (except birds) as well as many other technical challenges, the level of confidence with which adult neurogenesis can be confirmed in these species is sometimes lower than that for the best rodent examples. In many cases, the detection of BrdU-labeled cells has been equated with neurogenesis on the basis of more or less strong circumstantial evidence.

Insects and Crustaceans

Of all insects, the most interesting species in which to study adult neurogenesis is the dew fly, *Drosophila melanogaster*, because *Drosophila* is one of the genetically best characterized organisms. The potential of studying the molecular basis of adult neurogenesis in *Drosophila* is vast. However, there is no evidence of continued neurogenesis in the adult fly brain. Adult neurogenesis has been found in the mushroom bodies, the main processing unit of sensory information in the insect brain in many insect species (Cayre et al., 1996), but (as reviewed in Cayre et al., 2002) neither in *Drosophila* (Ito and Hotta, 1992), bees (Fahrbach et al., 1995), monarch butterflies (Nordlander and Edwards, 1968), nor the migratory locust (Cayre et al., 1996). Especially the latter species, with their fascinating navigational abilities, seem to be good candidates for activity-dependently regulated adult neurogenesis as we know it from rodents and birds. Insect species that show adult neurogenesis in the mushroom bodies include milkweed bugs and crickets (Cayre et al., 1996, 2000). The variability of adult neurogenesis between different insect species and within a structure that serves very similar if not identical purposes in all of these species remains surprising. Environmental enrichment had a stimulating effect on neurogenesis in mushroom bodies of adult crickets (Scotto-Lomassese et al., 2000), whereas unilateral sensory deprivation down-regulated adult neurogenesis ipsilaterally to the damage (Scotto-Lomassese et al., 2002) (Fig. 11–1). Precursor cells form clusters in the calices of the mushroom bodies and generate interneurons in the cortex of the mushroom bodies, the Kenyon cells. Because the effect could be evoked unilaterally, the hypothesis that this regulation is primarily hormonal could be ruled out. Supression of adult neurogenesis in mushroom bodies, on the other hand, affected olfactory learning and memory in the crickets, further supporting a functional role of the new interneurons (Scotto-Lomassese et al., 2003). Ex vivo, precursor cells from adult crickets were inducible by insulin but not fibroblast growth factor-2 (FGF-2). This finding suggests differences from vertebrate precursor cells (Malaterre et al., 2003).

The mushroom body–equivalent in crabs is the hemiellipsoid body that shows adult neurogenesis (Schmidt, 1997). In decapod crustaceans, adult neurogenesis has been described for the olfactory system (Schmidt and Demuth, 1998), where it shows signs of dependency on the sensory input (Hansen and Schmidt, 2001). In crayfish there is also evidence of activity-dependent neurogenesis in the olfactory system (Sandeman and Sandeman, 2000). Lifelong neurogenesis has also been described for the lobster (Harzsch et al., 1999; Schmidt, 2001) and here circadian control of neurogenesis was found (Goergen et al., 2002). Incidentally, the first known scientific work in history

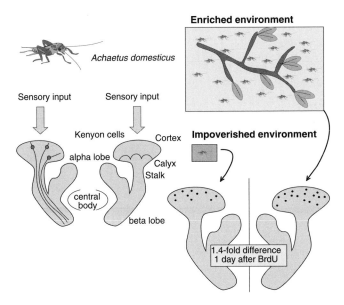

Figure 11–1. Activity-dependent regulation of adult neurogenesis in crickets. Environmental enrichment increased the generation of interneurons in the mushroom bodies of crickets (Scotto-Lomassese et al., 2000). Mushroom bodies are the main integration sites of sensory information in insects. Enrichment consisted of a larger, well-lit cage with more animals and leaves and other objects, whereas impoverished crickets were held in isolation and darkness.

that describes regeneration of lost body parts is an account by René-Antoine Ferchault de Réaumur, who in 1712 reported "Sur les diverses reproductions qui se font dans les écrivesses, les omars, les crabes, etc. et entr'autres sur celles de leurs jambs et de leurs écailles" ("On the diverse reproductions, which are found in crayfish, lobsters, crabs, etc., and among others in their legs and their shells") to the French Royal Academy.

Fish

Zebrafish (*Danio rerio*) is a vertebrate species that can be used for large-scale genetic screens in mutagenesis experiments similar to those done in *Drosophila*. Quite surprisingly, reports on adult neurogenesis in fish covered numerous species before finally showing that adult neurogenesis occurs in the olfactory bulbs of the adult zebrafish (Byrd and Brunjes, 2001). Other regions of sustained proliferative activity (Oehlmann et al., 2004) have not yet been studied in detail. There is considerable theoretical potential of this discovery for studying the genetic bases of adult neurogenesis, although it will be technically challenging to make use of this observation in a fast and simple assay that could be applied to a high-throughput mutant screen.

Neurogenesis in adult fish was described for the goldfish retina as early as 1977 (Johns and Easter, 1977). Another early study reported increasing neuron numbers in the guppy (Birse et al., 1980). The extensive work by Gunther Zupanc and coworkers focused on the gymnotiform fish (teleost), a species that continues to grow throughout life. This continued general growth might put the term *adult* in a different context from a mammalian perspective, but the persistent neurogenesis in the teleost has a number of features that place it in surprisingly close relation to mammalian neurogenesis. The proliferative zones containing the putative precursor cells (on which no ex vivo data exist yet) surround the brain ventricles (Zupanc and Zupanc, 1992) and neurogenesis decreases with age (Kranz and Richter, 1975). Directed migration of new neurons occurs in the zebrafish cerebellum (Zupanc and Horschke, 1995) and cell death can be found in the neurogenic zones. This suggests a similar mechanism of function-dependent selection of newborn cells to that in adult mammalian neurogenesis (Soutschek and Zupanc, 1995, 1996; Zupanc, 1999). Another example of possibly activity-regulated neurogenesis in the adult fish brain is the generation of new neurons in the goldfish tectum, which seems to depend on input from the optic nerves (Raymond and Easter, 1983; Raymond et al., 1983). In addition, there is adult neurogenesis in the goldfish retina, which produces new cone photo receptors (Wu et al., 2001).

Amphibians and Reptiles

Lizards show an amazing degree of brain plasticity and after injury can regrow entire parts of the brain. This was noted by Aristotle, as early as three centuries BC (see Odelberg, 2004).

Adult neurogenesis has been reported for most parts of the lizard fore-brain in a total of three different lizard species (Lopez-Garcia et al., 1988; Perez-Canellas and Garcia-Verdugo, 1996; Font et al., 1997). Cell prolifera-tion occurs in the walls of the ventricles and apparently generates only neurons. The ventricular zone of the adult lizard is subdivided into four sulci (Schulz, 1969) that contain glial fibrillary acidic protein (GFAP)-positive radial glial cells, which can undergo divisions (Font et al., 1995). Analogous to the findings in the adult rodent subventricular zone (SVZ) it is assumed that these radial glial cells serve as the precursor cells for adult cortical neurogenesis in lizards (Garcia-Verdugo et al., 2002; Weissman et al., 2003; Romero-Aleman et al., 2004). Between the germinative sulci the ventricu-lar walls show a simple epithelium without the characteristics of a neuro-genic region. A population of migratory cells has also been identified in lizards, and as in rodents these cells migrate toward the olfactory bulb, where they turn into new interneurons (Perez-Canellas and Garcia-Verdugo, 1996). Other cells from the ventricular zone migrate to the medial cerebral cortex, whose granule cell layer can be considered a homolog to the mam-malian dentate gyrus (Lopez-Garcia et al., 1990).

Because turtles can get very old, they might seem to be particularly prom-ising targets of studies on lifelong brain plasticity. Indeed, neurogenesis has been found in the olfactory system of red-eared slider turtles in a pattern similar to that in lizards (Perez-Canellas et al., 1997).

Birds

Steven A. Goldman and Fernando Nottebohm's first (1983) description of newly generated neurons in the telencephalon of canaries was a true break-through and brought research on adult neurogenesis the long-awaited ac-ceptance of a wider scientific audience. From an anthropocentric point of view, this attention might at first seem surprising because the phylogenetic relation between humans and birds is much less close than that between humans and rodents. Adult neurogenesis had long been reported in ro-dents at first with no lesser evidence but without being able to lose the stigma of curiosity. However, in songbirds adult neurogenesis was found in the higher vocal center (HVC), the brain region responsible for song learning, and the production of new neurons correlated with the seasons in which the birds learn their songs. The researchers had been searching for mechanisms underlying the parallel seasonal changes found in the songs and the volume of the HVC. Because adult neurogenesis added a considerable amount of new neurons to the well-defined neuronal circuit of the HVC, Nottebohm and colleagues were able to verify the birth of new neurons with a variety of methods ranging from microscopical tech-niques, retrograde tracing, and electrophysiological recordings (Kirn et al., 1991; Alvarez-Buylla and Kirn, 1997). The newly generated neurons in the HVC can survive for long periods (Kirn et al., 1991). Their recruitment apparently occurs in an activity-dependent manner: the neurons produced in the spring, when no songs are learned, have a lower chance of survival than those generated in the fall, when song learning peaks (Nottebohm et al., 1994).

Many songbird species, such as zebrafinches need to learn their songs once during a critical period in their youth; some species such as canaries continue to learn songs every year. When a seasonal fluctuation of neurogenesis in the HVC of canaries was found, adult neurogenesis was placed into a context of learning and memory. Unlike adult neurogenesis in rodents, as it had been reported to that date, neurogenesis in adult canaries showed a suggestive relation to a complex brain function. Even more intriguing, song learning is a trait that moves songbirds much closer to humans than rodents, with which humans share larger parts of the genome. Song learning shows many intriguing similarities to speech acquisition in humans, so songbirds are an ideal organism in which to study this particular type of learning (Brainard and Doupe, 2002). Song learning in birds is as close to the human use of language as can be found anywhere in the animal kingdom. Only dolphins, whales, and bats show something similar. No dog, for example, has to learn how to bark. However, the learned vocalizations are not language in that they lack the ability to convey symbolic contents. But in songbirds, as in humans, vocal learning depends on critical periods during which the birds have to hear the songs from adults. The birds also have to hear themselves to adequately learn their songs. Making young birds deaf causes a reduction in the production of new neurons in the HVC (Wang et al., 1999).

The HVC projects to two different brain regions, the motor nucleus in the archistriatum (RA) and the basal ganglia–like area X (Vates and Nottebohm, 1995) (Fig. 11–2). Both types of projection neurons are intermingled with interneurons in the HVC. Only the type of RA-projecting neurons are born in adulthood (Fig. 11–2). Constance Scharff and colleagues from Fernando Nottebohm's group applied a technique developed by Jeffrey Macklis (Macklis, 1993; Madison and Macklis, 1993) to show that selective elimination of the RA projections but not of the area-X projections induced adult neurogenesis (Scharff et al., 2000). This method, called "chromophore-targeted neuronal degeneration," is described in Figure 8–3. It allows the specific elimination of projection neurons and leads to the disappearance of the neuron without a reaction of the surrounding tissue. If area-X projections were killed in young birds, however, neurogenesis was induced, but only RA-projecting neurons were produced. Zebrafinches, which in contrast to canaries learn their songs only in their youth, lose their songs after ablation of the RA-projecting neurons. With recovery of the HVC due to adult neurogenesis, the lost songs returned (Scharff et al., 2000). This indicates that the HVC neurons are not involved in storing song information but are required to use that information. In canaries, the number of new neurons in the HVC-RA projection is so high that the entire system might turnover in 1 year (Nottebohm and Alvarez-Buylla, 1993). In the targeted ablation studies, there was a curious variability in the degree to which the

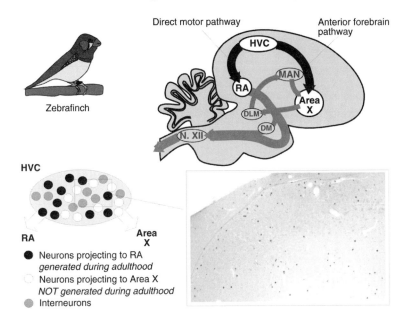

Figure 11–2. Adult neurogenesis in songbirds. In male zebrafinches and other songbirds, adult neurogenesis is found in the higher vocal center (HVC), a brain region centrally involved in song learning. The HVC contains three types of neurons. One projects to the robust nucleus of the archistriatum (RA) and constitutes the output pathway to the motor systems involved in singing. The second population projects to the anterior forebrain, area X. As a third neuronal population the HVC contains interneurons. Only the neurons that project to RA are replaced in adult neurogenesis. The photomicrograph at the bottom shows BrdU-positive cells in the HVC. BrdU-positive cells and cell genesis, however, can be found throughout the entire adult bird brain; the HVC is not highlighted by a particular density of newly generated cells. DLM, dorsolateral thalamic nucleus; DM, dorsomedial nucleus of the intercollicular complex; MAN, magnucellular nucleus of the anterior neostraitum. The schematic drawing is based on Vates et al. (1995). Photomicrograph by Alexander Garthe and Constance Scharff, Berlin.

birds lost their songs and recovered. This finding might indicate that specific projections must be hit to obtain the full effect and that even with induced adult neurogenesis recovery might not be optimal.

Despite these suggestive findings, it is still not known what the exact functional relevance of new neurons is for song learning. In starlings, for example, which, like canaries are open-ended learners, an age-dependent decline in HVC neurogenesis has been noted (Absil et al., 2003), suggesting that the quantity of required new neurons might not be constant. Adult HVC neurogenesis is also constitutively found in zebrafinches, although this species does not have to learn new songs in adulthood, so that in contrast to canaries a functional interpretation is less obvious in this species. Zebra-finches nevertheless show a seasonal fluctuation in incorporating new neu-rons into the HVC (Scharff and Nottebohm, 1991). However, zebrafinches do rely on a persistent auditory feedback of their own songs in order to maintain their song repertoire. This might indicate that new neurons in the adult HVC serve other functions than the mere storage of new songs. This is supported by the finding that in wild canaries, in contrast to the domes-ticated birds of the other experiments, song learning has seasonal patterns, whereas the neuron numbers and HVC volume do not (Leitner et al., 2001). Consequently, in wild canaries, as in zebrafinches, a link between new neurons and learning is neither linear nor mandatory. As an alternative hypothesis, neurogenesis in the HVC might be driven by singing itself and thus represent a form of activity-dependent cellular plasticity (Ball et al., 2002). This hypothesis might help to explain the seasonal changes by making neurogenesis a phenomenon secondary to seasonally fluctuating behavior. However, it does not address the question of the function the new neurons serve. Although adult neurogenesis is much more abundant in birds than in rodents, and at first glance the functional relevance of new neurons seems much more compelling in songbirds than in mammals, adult neurogenesis in the HVC still raises as many functional questions as neurogenesis in the adult hippocampus or olfactory system of mammals. Vocal learning might provide a psychologically plausible explanation for why humans are par-ticularly interested in neurogenesis in adult songbirds. However, so far there is no evidence that adult neurogenesis occurs in brain areas involved in speech generation in humans.

Adult neurogenesis in birds is not limited to the HVC but includes the different parts of the striatum, parolfactory lobe, and hippocampus. As in the HVC, activity-dependent regulation of neurogenesis has been described for the avian hippocampus. In chickadees a navigational challenge appears to be the neurogenic stimulus: adult hippocampal neurogenesis is correlated with seasons in which food-caching chickadees memorize their food stor-age sites for the upcoming winter (Barnea and Nottebohm, 1994, 1996). It has thus been concluded that spatial learning induces adult hippocampal neurogenesis in food-caching birds (Patel et al., 1997). However, as in the case of song learning, not all food-storing bird species, for example, wood-peckers, show this close correlation (Volman et al., 1997). Again, this can-not serve as a general argument against the functional relevance of adult neurogenesis, but these species differences suggest that the adaptive bene-fit provided by new neurons can alternatively be obtained by other means as well.

Neurogenesis in the parolfactory lobe of birds corresponds to some de-gree to the mammalian olfactory system, and as in mammals a large num-ber of new neurons are generated here (Alvarez-Buylla et al., 1994).

Precursor cell proliferation occurs in the avian ventricular zone, but the dividing cells are not evenly distributed. They cluster in proliferative hot spots in the ventricular wall. Similar to the lizard brain, these different domains differ in their cytoarchitecture. The germinative zones show a pseudostratified epithelium. Ependymal cells are interspersed with the radial glia–like B cells that presumably give rise to the migrating neuroblasts (A cells), which are detached from the ventricular lumen. The most proliferation occurs in B cells, which divide with a mitotic spindle perpendicular to the ventricular surface (Alvarez-Buylla et al., 1998). Their nuclei show interkinetic movements with the mitosis occurring close to the ventricular wall. Cell division thus occurs in a highly orchestrated way and differs considerably from that of rodents, despite the existing similarities in cytoarchitecture of the germinative matrix. From the lateral ventricle the new neurons disperse widely throughout the brain and migrate through the brain parenchyma.

The brain centers responsible for song learning are sexually dimorphic in song birds. It is usually the males that sing the complex songs. Female canaries can be masculinized in many aspects of their song behavior by the application of testosterone. The gonadal steroids estradiol and testosterone modulate adult neurogenesis in the HVC. Testosterone does not have an effect on precursor cell proliferation, but increases survival of newly generated cells, presumably through brain–derived neurotrophic factor (BDNF) (Dittrich et al., 1999; Rasika et al., 1999; Li et al., 2000). In addition, testosterone induces angiogenesis in the HVC, possibly by increasing vascular endothelial growth factor (VEGF). Testosterone also increased BDNF secretion from HVC endothelial cells, a result suggesting that through this interaction, testosterone coordinates angiogenesis and neurogenesis in the HVC (Louissaint et al., 2002).

MAMMALS AND MARSUPIALS

Mammals (Other Than Rodents and Primates) and Marsupials

When Altman and Das (1967) first described adult neurogenesis in rodents, the first species after rats and mice they turned to was the guinea pigs. The reason for this choice lies in the fact that in contrast to other rodents, guinea pigs do not have prolonged postnatal brain development and are born with comparatively mature brains. Consequently, the detection of newly generated cells in the adult guinea pig hippocampus supported the idea of truly adult neurogenesis instead of only delayed postnatal brain development.

Adult hippocampal neurogenesis in rabbits was first reported in 1982 (Gueneau et al., 1982). This study was amazingly complete, given the technical limitations of the time, and described a developmental sequence with a putative precursor cell, an intermediate neuroblast, and the new mature neuron. It was thus the first time-course study on adult neurogenesis. Neuronal development reached what was considered the neuroblast stage at about 4 days after the initial division, which is remarkably close to the newer estimates in mice. A more recent article has described migrating immature neurons in the vicinity of the ventricles of rabbits (Luzzati et al., 2003). The surprising aspect of this study is that migration did not seem to occur in the same pattern of chain migration as in rats and mice. This result is particularly interesting in that no signs of chain migration can be detected in the adult human brain either (Sanai et al., 2004).

Initially there was a small controversy over the question of whether marsupials showed adult hippocampal neurogenesis as well (Reynolds et al., 1985; Harman, 1997), but in a classical tritiated thymidine study, Alison Harmann and coworkers (2003) showed that in marsupials, too, hippocampal granule cells are produced in adulthood. In contrast to mice, putting the animals in an enriched environment reduced the survival of the new cells, leaving the proliferation unchanged, an effect possibly attributable to stress (Harman et al., 2003).

Nonhuman Primates

The first signs of DNA synthesis in SVZ cells of adult rhesus monkeys were reported by Michael Kaplen in 1983. However the level of labeling with tritiated thymidine was very low and the evidence remained controversial (Kaplan, 1983).

Other early autoradiographic studies based on tritiated thymidine injections failed to detect adult hippocampal neurogenesis in rhesus monkeys beyond the age of 3 years, which equals postpuberty (Eckenhoff and Rakic, 1988). But in 1997, Elizabeth Gould, Eberhard Fuchs, and colleagues found adult neurogenesis in the dentate gyrus of the adult tree shrew, a species of New World monkeys. Similar to what the group had found earlier in rats, a stress-induced and NMDA receptor–dependent down-regulation of cell proliferation was described, making this study the first to report not only adult neurogenesis in primates (although tree shrews are considered half-primates, phylogenetically located between insectivores and primates) but also its regulation in a species other than rodents thus linking the study to the large body of previous evidence (Gould et al., 1997). In 1999, hippocampal neurogenesis in Old World monkeys (macaques), an undisputed primate species, was independently described by Elizabeth Gould and coworkers and by David Kornack and Pasko Rakic, who used bromodeoxyuridine (BrdU) immunohistochemistry and colocalization of BrdU and neuronal markers (Gould et al., 1999a; Kornack and Rakic, 1999). Neurogenesis was found even in 23-year-old animals (Gould et al., 1999a), but overall levels were reported to be very low (Kornack and Rakic, 1999). Adult hippocampal neurogenesis was also found in young rhesus monkeys (Coe et al., 2003). Prenatal stress had long-lasting effects on hippocampal neurogenesis in these monkeys.

Olfactory bulb neurogenesis was detected in macaque and rhesus monkeys in patterns similar to that known from rodents (Kornack and Rakic, 2001b; Pencea et al., 2001) (Fig. 11–3, Color Plate 13). In addition, olfactory

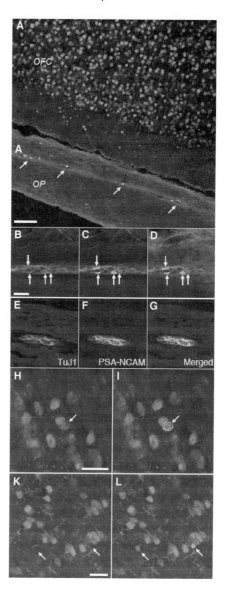

Figure 11–3 (Color Plate 13). Neurogenesis in the olfactory bulb of adult monkeys. Kornack and Rakic (2001b) reported newly generated neurons in the olfactory bulb of macaque monkeys.
A: Below the orbitofrontal cortex (OFC) the rostral migratory stream (arrows) is visible in the olfactory peduncle (OP). BrdU-labeled cells (green) ar found in the GFAP-positive (blue) pathway.
B–D: b-III-tubulin-expressing cells are in the stream (B, red), a few of which are BrdU-labeled (C, green); D again shows the GFAP-positive environment (blue) E and F: β-III-tubulin-labeling coincides with expression of PSA-NCAM. H and I: A newly generated neuron in the olfactory bulb of a macaque monkey is shown, 97 days after the last injection of BrdU (NeuN, red; BrdU, green; GFAP, blue) K and L: An example of a newly generated, non-neuronal cell in the same region. Scale bars, 100 μm for A; 25 μm for B–G; 20 μm for H–L. Reprinted with kind permission of the authors and the Copyright 2001 National Academy of Sciences, U.S.A.

bulb neurogenesis was found in squirrel monkeys, a New World species (Bedard et al., 2002).

Global ischemia induced the proliferation of Musahi- and nestin-positive cells in the dentate gyrus and the SVZ of macaque monkeys (Tonchev et al., 2003a, 2003b). This finding suggested a responsiveness of the precursor cells similar to the situation found in rodents.

The controversy over reports on neocortical neurogenesis in macaques was covered in Chapter 8. The initial report about a robust and steady stream of new cortical neurons originating from the SVZ (Gould et al., 1999b), was not confirmed by other groups (Kornack and Rakic, 2001a; Koketsu et al., 2003); mostly methodical concerns have been raised (Rakic, 2002b). A number of additional studies have implied that neurogenesis could occur outside the canonical neurogenic regions of primates—for example, in the amygdala and adjacent temporal cortex (Bernier et al., 2002) or olfactory tubercle (Bedard et al., 2002). Neither study could conclusively dispel the concerns regarding the validity of marker co-localization. These reports therefore invite further investigations; they should neither be plainly dismissed nor blindly taken as evidence.

In summary, it is generally accepted at present that adult neurogenesis is found in the neurogenic regions of the adult monkey brain, but claims of adult neurogenesis in other brain regions still raise the same questions as those discussed for rodents.

HUMANS

From a justifiable if not somewhat superficial perspective, the value of research on adult neurogenesis (and with it the value of this book) rises and falls with the findings covered below. How much of what has been described in the previous chapters is relevant to the human situation? This question is important because research on adult neurogenesis is to a large degree justified to funding agencies and the tax-paying public by the belief that adult neurogenesis occurs, or can occur, in humans and that its exploration will lead to progress in medicine.

Adult neurogenesis can be found in humans. The proof of principle, in terms of the standards set by research in rodents, has been led by Peter Eriksson in a 1998 landmark study (Eriksson et al., 1998). Eriksson, a neurologist in Gothenburg, Sweden, identified a group of patients suffering from throat carcinomas who, as part of their treatment regimen, had received a single BrdU infusion to allow staging of the tumor after its surgical removal. Eriksson reasoned that the BrdU would have labeled not only the dividing tumor cells but also the proliferating precursor cells in the brain. He obtained informed consent from the patients to perform a brain autopsy after their death. The five patients died at the ages of 57, 58, 67, 68, and 72 years, between 2 weeks and 2 years after the BrdU injection. The same method that had been established for the analysis of adult hippocampal neurogenesis in rodents was applied to the examination of these patients' brains. Because no complete series through the entire dentate gyrus could be obtained, no absolute counts of BrdU-labeled neurons could be generated. The numbers of BrdU-marked neurons per cubic millimeter ranged between about 2 and 40 cells. Given that the patients in this studies were of older age, that the human dentate gyrus contains 50 times as many granule cells as in a mouse (15 million vs. 300,000), and that, as in rodents, human adult hippocampal neurogenesis is likely to decline with increasing age, this detected rate of adult hippocampal neurogenesis in the five patients appeared substantial.

Unfortunately, the olfactory bulbs of the same patients could not be investigated. Because the Eriksson study has remained unique in that it used patients who had received BrdU and were willing to donate their brain for examination after their death, it is not known whether adult neurogenesis can also be found in the adult human olfactory bulb. However, two studies that searched for markers associated with neurogenesis in the adult human olfactory bulb found dividing cells that expressed nestin, doublecortin, NeuroD, vimentin, calretinin, or β-III-tubulin (Liu and Martin, 2003; Bedard and Parent, 2004).

A number of ex vivo studies have shown that the adult human brain contains precursor cells. Most of these experiments were done on brain tissue that had be surgically removed. The indication for the operation was usually pharmacologically intractable epilepsy, for which a unilateral temporal lobectomy (removal of the part of the temporal lobe that contains the hippocampus) was performed. A unilateral resection of the hippocampus can be compensated for functionally; only a bilateral removal would lead to complete anterograde amnesia. Other samples were taken from resections that had become necessary to decompress a swelling brain after hemorrhage and stroke. In any case, most of the presently available evidence about precursor cells in the adult human brain has been obtained from brains that were not healthy. However, the concern that precursor cells in the adult human brain are only a consequence of brain pathology seems unlikely to be true, given the evidence from animal studies including primates. Nevertheless, the caveat has to be taken seriously until precursor cells can be directly derived from normal adult human brain. To date, the oldest documented human individual from whom precursor cells were isolated in the absence of brain pathology, but postmortem, was only 11 months old (Palmer et al., 2001).

A series of detailed experiments about neural precursor cells in the adult human brain came from Steven Goldman's group at Cornell University in New York. Their first study in 1994 indicated that dividing cells from the human ventricular wall could give rise to neurons in vitro (Kirschenbaum et al., 1994). In a similar study from 1998, the same group used explant cultures from the adult human SVZ to show that over a period of weeks new neurons would grow out of the explant and that this outgrowth could be boosted by the application of BDNF and FGF-2. This study also contained histological analyses of the human SVZ, where putative precursor cells were identified by their expression of Musashi and Hu antigens (Pincus et al., 1998).

The first experiments that included assays to determine stemness in cells isolated from human brain samples came from Dennis A. Steindler and colleagues, who in 1999 showed that both the SVZ and hippocampus contained precursor cells that formed primary and secondary neurospheres after cultivation at clonal density (Kukekov et al., 1999). The spheres also expressed transcription factor Pax6, which in rodents is found in astrocyte-like precursor cells both in vivo and in vitro. In this study, the individuals were 24 to 57 years old.

At the same time, S.F. Pagano and colleagues in Milan isolated precursor cells from the adult human olfactory bulb (Pagano et al., 2000). Finally, in a series of elegant experiments, N.S. Roy and colleagues from Steven Goldman's laboratory gave further evidence of precursor cells in the human hippocampus (Roy et al., 2000b) and SVZ (Roy et al., 2000a). In these studies, precursor cells were isolated from the surgical specimens by transfecting the cultured cells with plasmid DNA encoding the green fluorescent protein (GFP) under precursor cell–relevant promoters such as Tα1–tubulin or nestin. Precursor cells from the human (as well as rodent) SVZ showed some regional differences in growth and differentiation parameters in vitro (Bernier et al., 2000; Ostenfeld et al., 2002).

Arturo Alvarez-Buylla and colleagues investigated the adult human SVZ in the most extensive study thus far (Sanai et al., 2004). They examined a total of 110 surgical and postmortem samples that allowed good spatial resolution of different regions of the SVZ. The precursor cells isolated from the adult human SVZ had astrocytic properties. Through transfection of isolated cells with GFP under the GFAP promoter and sorting for GFP-positive cells, a population of multipotent cells was identified. In vivo, a band of astrocytes could be detected below the ependyma, representing a structure that is not present in the adult rodent SVZ. A certain percentage of these astrocytes were proliferatively active. The GFAP-expressing precursor cells ex vivo might correspond to these dividing astrocytes in vivo, but formal proof for this will be difficult to obtain.

Intriguingly, only a very few migrating neuroblasts were found in vivo, and those that were identified did not show the characteristic pattern of chain migration. With this finding the study did not categorically disprove the existence of SVZ-derived neurogenesis in the adult human olfactory bulb but questioned its potential quantity. In absolute terms, the human rostral migratory stream is about two orders of magnitude longer than that in a mouse, whereas the human olfactory bulb is, relative to the rest of the brain and the body, much smaller than in a mouse. In addition to these traits, the fact that humans do not rely heavily on olfaction (they are a microsmatic species and might thus have relatively less adult olfactory neurogenesis) and that an age-dependent decline in olfactory neurogenesis is to be expected might account for a considerable dilution effect in the potential migratory route to the human olfactory bulb. Only comparatively very few cells might actually migrate in humans and still maintain a low level of adult olfactory neurogenesis. Neural precursor cells have been isolated from the human olfactory bulb, but these might also be resident precursor cells. Consequently, Sanai and colleagues (2004) concluded that their "findings raise the unexpected possibility that migration from the SVZ to the olfactory bulb does not take place in humans or, if it does, precursors migrate as individual cells."

There is conflicting evidence about neural precursor cells in the human cortex. Whereas two ex vivo studies detected precursor cells in cortical regions (Arsenijevic et al., 2001; Palmer et al., 2001), others did not (Kirschenbaum et al., 1994; Sanai et al., 2004).

Many of these studies reported that neural precursor cells from the adult human brain differed from their rodent counterparts in vitro. For example, human precursor cells showed a preference for laminin as coating of the surface on which the cells were plated out for differentiation. Also, expansion of human precursor cells can be promoted by the presence of leukemia inhibiting factor (LIF), which has no effect in rodents. Human neural precursor cells can differentiate in the presence of growth factors, whereas in mice growth factors have to be withdrawn to induce proliferation. The growth factor effects themselves showed differences as well. For example, platelet-derived growth factor (PDGF) increases oligodendrocytic differentiation in rodents but has no such effect on human precursor cells (Arsenijevic et al., 2001).

The human corpus callosum contains parenchymal precursor cells that generate neurons in cell culture (Roy et al., 1999). Neuronal nature was determined not only immunocytochemically but also electrophysiologically and the production of neurons was even found shortly after the isolation of precursor cells from the intraoperative specimens. This immediacy is important because it minimizes the chance that the neurogenic potential is induced only by culture conditions. The neurogenic potential was further confirmed after xenografting the cells into the developing rat brain, where they incorporated into the neurogenic regions and formed neurons.

Precursor cells from the adult human brain cannot be propagated indefinitely in vitro, prohibiting the use of the term *stem cell* for them. After a maximum of about 30 doublings the cells appear to turn into senescence. To date it is not clear whether this result reflects a technical problem or a fundamental biological principle. It is conceivable that all studies were successful in expanding not true stem cells but selective populations of progenitor cells with a limited capability for expansion. On the other hand, expandability of fetal human progenitor cells could be greatly enhanced by maintaining cell–cell contacts in the cultures. Clive Svendsen, Maeve Caldwell, and colleagues from Cambridge "chopped" the neurospheres in quarters instead of triturating them to single-cell suspensions. This treatment increased not only the number of possible cell doublings (Svendsen et al., 1998) but also the number of neurons per sphere (Caldwell et al., 2001). The proposed explanation was that cell–cell contacts were maintained through this method. Interestingly, this method did not work in rodents, adding further support to the idea that some fundamental differences exist between rodent and human precursor cell biology.

Neuronal outgrowth from dividing cells in biopsies taken from the olfactory epithelium of adult humans confirmed the existence of neurogenesis

(Murrell et al., 1996) to the same degree as had been done by the pioneering 1994 study by Kirschenbaum, Goldman, and colleagues for the human
SVZ. Surprisingly, further detailed studies on precursor cell properties (most
notably clonal expansion) in cells isolated from the adult human olfactory
epithelium are still lacking, and so is an in vivo study. Despite these short-
comings, however, the fact that human neuronal development in the olfactory epithelium is accessible by comparatively simple biopsy in the adult
has raised a number of interesting speculations (see Chapter 5).

REFERENCES

Absil P, Pinxten R, Balthazart J, Eens M (2003) Effect of age and testosterone on
    autumnal neurogenesis in male European starlings (*Sturnus vulgaris*). Behav
    Brain Res 143:15–30.
Altman J, Das GD (1967) Postnatal neurogenesis in the guinea-pig. Nature 214:1098–
    1101.
Alvarez-Buylla A, Garcia-Verdugo JM, Mateo AS, Merchant-Larios H (1998) Pri-
    mary neural precursors and intermitotic nuclear migration in the ventricu-
    lar zone of adult canaries. J Neurosci 18:1020–1037.
Alvarez-Buylla A, Kirn JR (1997) Birth, migration, incorporation, and death of vocal
    control neurons in adult songbirds. J Neurobiol 33:585–601.
Alvarez-Buylla A, Ling CY, Yu WS (1994) Contribution of neurons born during
    embryonic, juvenile, and adult life to the brain of adult canaries: regional
    specificity and delayed birth of neurons in the song-control nuclei. J Comp
    Neurol 347:233–248.
Arsenijevic Y, Villemure JG, Brunet JF, Bloch JJ, Deglon N, Kostic C, Zurn A,
    Aebischer P (2001) Isolation of multipotent neural precursors residing in
    the cortex of the adult human brain. Exp Neurol 170:48–62.
Ball GF, Riters LV, Balthazart J (2002) Neuroendocrinology of song behavior and
    avian brain plasticity: multiple sites of action of sex steroid hormones. Front
    Neuroendocrinol 23:137–178.
Barnea A, Nottebohm F (1994) Seasonal recruitment of hippocampal neurons in adult
    free-ranging black-capped chickadees. Proc Natl Acad Sci USA 91:11217–11221.
Barnea A, Nottebohm F (1996) Recruitment and replacement of hippocampal neu-
    rons in young and adult chickadees: an addition to the theory of hippocam-
    pal learning. Proc Natl Acad Sci USA 93:714–718.
Bedard A, Levesque M, Bernier PJ, Parent A (2002) The rostral migratory stream in
    adult squirrel monkeys: contribution of new neurons to the olfactory tubercle
    and involvement of the antiapoptotic protein Bcl-2. Eur J Neurosci 16:1917–
    1924.
Bedard A, Parent A (2004) Evidence of newly generated neurons in the human ol-
    factory bulb. Brain Res Dev Brain Res 151:159–168.
Bernier PJ, Bedard A, Vinet J, Levesque M, Parent A (2002) Newly generated neu-
    rons in the amygdala and adjoining cortex of adult primates. Proc Natl Acad
    Sci USA 99:11464–11469.
Bernier PJ, Vinet J, Cossette M, Parent A (2000) Characterization of the subventricular
    zone of the adult human brain: evidence for the involvement of Bcl-2. Neurosci
    Res 37:67–78.
Birse SC, Leonard RB, Coggeshall RE (1980) Neuronal increase in various areas of
    the nervous system of the guppy, *Lebistes*. J Comp Neurol 194:291–301.
Brainard MS, Doupe AJ (2002) What songbirds teach us about learning. Nature
    417:351–358.

Byrd CA, Brunjes PC (2001) Neurogenesis in the olfactory bulb of adult zebrafish. Neuroscience 105:793–801.

Caldwell MA, He X, Wilkie N, Pollack S, Marshall G, Wafford KA, Svendsen CN (2001) Growth factors regulate the survival and fate of cells derived from human neurospheres. Nat Biotechnol 19:475–479.

Cayre M, Malaterre J, Charpin P, Strambi C, Strambi A (2000) Fate of neuroblast progeny during postembryonic development of mushroom bodies in the house cricket, *Acheta domesticus*. J Insect Physiol 46:313–319.

Cayre M, Malaterre J, Scotto-Lomassese S, Strambi C, Strambi A (2002) The common properties of neurogenesis in the adult brain: from invertebrates to vertebrates. Comp Biochem Physiol B Biochem Mol Biol 132:1–15.

Cayre M, Strambi C, Charpin P, Augier R, Meyer MR, Edwards JS, Strambi A (1996) Neurogenesis in adult insect mushroom bodies. J Comp Neurol 371:300–310.

Coe CL, Kramer M, Czeh B, Gould E, Reeves AJ, Kirschbaum C, Fuchs E (2003) Prenatal stress diminishes neurogenesis in the dentate gyrus of juvenile rhesus monkeys. Biol Psychiatry 54:1025–1034.

Dittrich F, Feng Y, Metzdorf R, Gahr M (1999) Estrogen-inducible, sex-specific expression of brain-derived neurotrophic factor mRNA in a forebrain song control nucleus of the juvenile zebra finch. Proc Natl Acad Sci USA 96:8241–8246.

Eckenhoff MF, Rakic P (1988) Nature and fate of proliferative cells in the hippocampal dentate gyrus during the life span of the rhesus monkey. J Neurosci 8:2729–2747.

Eriksson PS, Perfilieva E, Björk-Eriksson T, Alborn AM, Nordborg C, Peterson DA, Gage FH (1998) Neurogenesis in the adult human hippocampus. Nat Med 4:1313–1317.

Fahrbach SE, Strande JL, Robinson GE (1995) Neurogenesis is absent in the brains of adult honey bees and does not explain behavioral neuroplasticity. Neurosci Lett 197:145–148.

Font E, Desfilis E, Perez-Canellas M, Alcantara S, Garcia-Verdugo JM (1997) 3-Acetylpyridine-induced degeneration and regeneration in the adult lizard brain: a qualitative and quantitative analysis. Brain Res 754:245–259.

Font E, Garcia-Verdugo JM, Desfilis E, Perez-Canellas M (1995) Neuron–glia interrelations during 3–acetylpyridine-induced degeneration and regeneration in the adult lizard brain. In: Neuron–Glia Interrelations During Phylogeny (Vernadakis A, Roots B, eds), pp 275–302. Totowa: Humana.

Garcia-Verdugo JM, Ferron S, Flames N, Collado L, Desfilis E, Font E (2002) The proliferative ventricular zone in adult vertebrates: a comparative study using reptiles, birds, and mammals. Brain Res Bull 57:765–775.

Goergen EM, Bagay LA, Rehm K, Benton JL, Beltz BS (2002) Circadian control of neurogenesis. J Neurobiol 53:90–95.

Goldman SA, Nottebohm F (1983) Neuronal production, migration and differentiation in a vocal control nucleus of the adult female canary brain. Proc Acad Sci USA 80:2390–2394.

Gould E, McEwen BS, Tanapat P, Galea LAM, Fuchs E (1997) Neurogenesis in the dentate gyrus of the adult tree shrew is regulated by psychosocial stress and NMDA receptor activation. J Neurosci 17:2492–2498.

Gould E, Reeves AJ, Fallah M, Tanapat P, Gross CG, Fuchs E (1999a) Hippocampal neurogenesis in adult old world primates. Proc Natl Acad Sci USA 96:5263–5267.

Gould E, Reeves AJ, Graziano MS, Gross CG (1999b) Neurogenesis in the neocortex of adult primates. Science 286:548–552.

Gueneau G, Privat A, Drouet J, Court L (1982) Subgranular zone of the dentate gyrus of young rabbits as a secondary matrix. A high-resolution autoradiographic study. Dev Neurosci 5:345–358.

Hansen A, Schmidt M (2001) Neurogenesis in the central olfactory pathway of the adult shore crab *Carcinus maenas* is controlled by sensory afferents. J Comp Neurol 441:223–233.

Harman A, Meyer P, Ahmat A (2003) Neurogenesis in the hippocampus of an adult marsupial. Brain Behav Evol 62:1–12.

Harman AM (1997) Development and cell generation in the hippocampus of a marsupial, the quokka wallaby (*Setonix brachyurus*). Brain Res Dev Brain Res 104:41–54.

Harzsch S, Miller J, Benton J, Beltz B (1999) From embryo to adult: persistent neurogenesis and apoptotic cell death shape the lobster deutocerebrum. J Neurosci 19:3472–3485.

Ito K, Hotta Y (1992) Proliferation pattern of postembryonic neuroblasts in the brain of *Drosophila melanogaster*. Dev Biol 149:134–148.

Johns PR, Easter SS Jr. (1977) Growth of the adult goldfish eye. II. Increase in retinal cell number. J Comp Neurol 176:331–341.

Kaplan MS (1983) Proliferation of subependymal cells in the adult primate CNS: differential uptake of DNA labelled precursors. J Hirnforsch 24:23–33.

Kirn JR, Alvarez-Buylla A, Nottebohm F (1991) Production and survival of projection neurons in a forebrain vocal center of adult male canaries. J Neurosci 11:1756–1762.

Kirschenbaum B, Nedergaard M, Preuss A, Barami K, Fraser RA, Goldman SA (1994) In vitro neuronal production and differentiation by precursor cells derived from the adult human forebrain. Cereb Cortex 6:576–589.

Koketsu D, Mikami A, Miyamoto Y, Hisatsune T (2003) Nonrenewal of neurons in the cerebral neocortex of adult macaque monkeys. J Neurosci 23:937–942.

Kornack DR, Rakic P (1999) Continuation of neurogenesis in the hippocampus of the macaque monkey. Proc Natl Acad Sci USA 96:5768–5773.

Kornack DR, Rakic P (2001a) Cell proliferation without neurogenesis in adult primate neocortex. Science 294:2127–2130.

Kornack DR, Rakic P (2001b) The generation, migration, and differentiation of olfactory neurons in the adult primate brain. Proc Natl Acad Sci USA 98:4752–4757.

Kranz VD, Richter W (1975) [Neurogenesis and regeneration in the brain of teleosts in relation to age. (Autoradiographic studies)]. Z Alternsforsch 30:371–382.

Kukekov VG, Laywell ED, Suslov O, Davies K, Scheffler B, Thomas LB, O'Brien TF, Kusakabe M, Steindler DA (1999) Multipotent stem/progenitor cells with similar properties arise from two neurogenic regions of adult human brain. Exp Neurol 156:333–344.

Leitner S, Voigt C, Garcia-Segura LM, Van't Hof T, Gahr M (2001) Seasonal activation and inactivation of song motor memories in wild canaries is not reflected in neuroanatomical changes of forebrain song areas. Horm Behav 40:160–168.

Li XC, Jarvis ED, Alvarez-Borda B, Lim DA, Nottebohm F (2000) A relationship between behavior, neurotrophin expression, and new neuron survival. Proc Natl Acad Sci USA 97:8584–8589.

Liu Z, Martin LJ (2003) Olfactory bulb core is a rich source of neural progenitor and stem cells in adult rodent and human. J Comp Neurol 459:368–391.

Lopez-Garcia C, Molowny A, Garcia-Verdugo JM, Ferrer I (1988) Delayed postnatal neurogenesis in the cerebral cortex of lizards. Brain Res 471:167–174.

Lopez-Garcia C, Molowny A, Garcia-Verdugo JM, Perez-Sanchez F, Martinez-Guijarro FJ (1990) Postnatal neurogenesis in the brain of the lizard *Podarcis hispanica*. In: The Forebrain in Non-mammals: New Aspects of Structure and Development. (Schwerdtfeger WK, Germroth P, eds), pp 103–117. Berlin: Springer.

Louissaint A Jr, Rao S, Leventhal C, Goldman SA (2002) Coordinated interaction of neurogenesis and angiogenesis in the adult songbird brain. Neuron 34:945–960.

Luzzati F, Peretto P, Aimar P, Ponti G, Fasolo A, Bonfanti L (2003) Glia-independent chains of neuroblasts through the subcortical parenchyma of the adult rabbit brain. Proc Natl Acad Sci USA 100:13036–13041.

Macklis JD (1993) Transplanted neocortical neurons migrate selectively into regions of neuronal degeneration produced by chromophore-targeted laser photolysis. J Neurosci 13:3848–3863.

Madison RD, Macklis JD (1993) Noninvasively induced degeneration of neocortical pyramidal neurons *in vivo*: selective targeting by laser activation of retrogradely transported photolytic chromophore. Exp Neurol 121:153–159.

Malaterre J, Strambi C, Aouane A, Strambi A, Rougon G, Cayre M (2003) Effect of hormones and growth factors on the proliferation of adult cricket neural progenitor cells in vitro. J Neurobiol 56:387–397.

Murrell W, Bushell GR, Livesey J, McGrath J, MacDonald KP, Bates PR, Mackay-Sim A (1996) Neurogenesis in adult human. Neuroreport 7:1189–1194.

Nordlander RH, Edwards JS (1968) Morphology of the larval and adult brains of the monarch butterfly, *Danaus plexippus plexippus*, L. J Morphol 126:67–94.

Nottebohm F, Alvarez-Buylla A (1993) Neurogenesis and neuronal replacement in adult birds. In: Neuronal Cell Death and Repair (Cuello AC, ed), pp 227–236. Amsterdam: Elsevier.

Nottebohm F, O'Loughlin B, Gould K, Yohay K, Alvarez-Buylla A (1994) The life span of new neurons in a song control nucleus of the adult canary brain depends on time of year when these cells are born. Proc Natl Acad Sci USA 91:7849–7853.

Odelberg SJ (2004) Unraveling the molecular basis for regenerative cellular plasticity. PLoS Biol 2:E232.

Oehlmann VD, Berger S, Sterner C, Korsching SI (2004) Zebrafish beta-tubulin-1 expression is limited to the nervous system throughout development, and in the adult brain is restricted to a subset of proliferative regions. Gene Expr Patterns 4:191–198.

Ostenfeld T, Joly E, Tai YT, Peters A, Caldwell M, Jauniaux E, Svendsen CN (2002) Regional specification of rodent and human neurospheres. Brain Res Dev Brain Res 134:43–55.

Pagano SF, Impagnatiello F, Girelli M, Cova L, Grioni E, Onofri M, Cavallaro M, Etteri S, Vitello F, Giombini S, Solero CL, Parati EA (2000) Isolation and characterization of neural stem cells from the adult human olfactory bulb. Stem Cells 18:295–300.

Palmer TD, Schwartz PH, Taupin P, Kaspar B, Stein SA, Gage FH (2001) Cell culture. Progenitor cells from human brain after death. Nature 411:42–43.

Patel SN, Clayton NS, Krebs JR (1997) Spatial learning induces neurogenesis in the avian brain. Behav Brain Res 89:115–128.

Pencea V, Bingaman KD, Freedman LJ, Luskin MB (2001) Neurogenesis in the subventricular zone and rostral migratory stream of the neonatal and adult primate forebrain. Exp Neurol 172:1–16.

Perez-Canellas MM, Font E, Garcia-Verdugo JM (1997) Postnatal neurogenesis in the telencephalon of turtles: evidence for nonradial migration of new neurons from distant proliferative ventricular zones to the olfactory bulbs. Brain Res Dev Brain Res 101:125–137.

Perez-Canellas MM, Garcia-Verdugo JM (1996) Adult neurogenesis in the telencephalon of a lizard: a [3H]thymidine autoradiographic and bromodeoxyuridine immunocytochemical study. Brain Res Dev Brain Res 93:49–61.

Pincus DW, Keyoung HM, Harrison-Restelli C, Goodman RR, Fraser RA, Edgar M, Sakakibara S, Okano H, Nedergaard M, Goldman SA (1998) Fibroblast growth factor-2/brain-derived neurotrophic factor-associated maturation of new neurons generated from adult human subependymal cells. Ann Neurol 43:576–585.

Rakic P (2002a) Adult neurogenesis in mammals: an identity crisis. J Neurosci 22:614–618.

Rakic P (2002b) Neurogenesis in adult primate neocortex: an evaluation of the evidence. Nat Rev Neurosci 3:65–71.

Rasika S, Alvarez-Buylla A, Nottebohm F (1999) BDNF mediates the effects of testosterone on the survival of new neurons in an adult brain. Neuron 22:53–62.

Raymond PA, Easter SS Jr. (1983) Postembryonic growth of the optic tectum in goldfish. I. Location of germinal cells and numbers of neurons produced. J Neurosci 3:1077–1091.

Raymond PA, Easter SS Jr, Burnham JA, Powers MK (1983) Postembryonic growth of the optic tectum in goldfish. II. Modulation of cell proliferation by retinal fiber input. J Neurosci 3:1092–1099.

Reynolds ML, Cavanagh ME, Dziegielewska KM, Hinds LA, Saunders NR, Tyndale-Biscoe CH (1985) Postnatal development of the telencephalon of the tammar wallaby (*Macropus eugenii*). An accessible model of neocortical differentiation. Anat Embryol (Berl) 173:81–94.

Romero-Aleman MM, Monzon-Mayor M, Yanes C, Lang D (2004) Radial glial cells, proliferating periventricular cells, and microglia might contribute to successful structural repair in the cerebral cortex of the lizard *Gallotia galloti*. Exp Neurol 188:74–85.

Roy NS, Benraiss A, Wang S, Fraser RA, Goodman R, Couldwell WT, Nedergaard M, Kawaguchi A, Okano H, Goldman SA (2000a) Promoter-targeted selection and isolation of neural progenitor cells from the adult human ventricular zone. J Neurosci Res 59:321–331.

Roy NS, Wang S, Harrison-Restelli C, Benraiss A, Fraser RA, Gravel M, Braun PE, Goldman SA (1999) Identification, isolation, and promoter-defined separation of mitotic oligodendrocyte progenitor cells from the adult human subcortical white matter. J Neurosci 19:9986–9995.

Roy NS, Wang S, Jiang L, Kang J, Benraiss A, Harrison-Restelli C, Fraser RA, Couldwell WT, Kawaguchi A, Okano H, Nedergaard M, Goldman SA (2000b) In vitro neurogenesis by progenitor cells isolated from the adult human hippocampus. Nat Med 6:271–277.

Sanai N, Tramontin AD, Quinones-Hinojosa A, Barbaro NM, Gupta N, Kunwar S, Lawton MT, McDermott MW, Parsa AT, Manuel-Garcia Verdugo J, Berger MS, AlvarezBuylla A (2004) Unique astrocyte ribbon in adult human brain contains neural stem cells but lacks chain migration. Nature 427:740–744.

Sandeman R, Sandeman D (2000) "Impoverished" and "enriched" living conditions influence the proliferation and survival of neurons in crayfish brain. J Neurobiol 45:215–226.

Scharff C, Kirn JR, Grossman M, Macklis JD, Nottebohm F (2000) Targeted neuronal death affects neuronal replacement and vocal behavior in adult songbirds. Neuron 25:481–492.

Scharff C, Nottebohm F (1991) A comparative study of the behavioral deficits following lesions of various parts of the zebra finch song system: implications for vocal learning. J Neurosci 11:2896–2913.

Schmidt M (1997) Continuous neurogenesis in the olfactory brain of adult shore crabs, *Carcinus maenas*. Brain Res 762:131–143.

Schmidt M (2001) Neuronal differentiation and long-term survival of newly generated cells in the olfactory midbrain of the adult spiny lobster, *Panulirus argus*. J Neurobiol 48:181–203.

Schmidt M, Demuth S (1998) Neurogenesis in the central olfactory pathway of adult decapod crustaceans. Ann NY Acad Sci 855:277–280.

Schulz E (1969) [Postnatal biomorphosis of the ependyma in the telencephalon of *Lacerta agilis agilis* (L.)]. Z Mikrosk Anat Forsch 81:111–152.

Scotto-Lomassese S, Strambi C, Aouane A, Strambi A, Cayre M (2002) Sensory inputs stimulate progenitor cell proliferation in an adult insect brain. Curr Biol 12:1001–1005.

Scotto-Lomassese S, Strambi C, Strambi A, Aouane A, Augier R, Rougon G, Cayre M (2003) Suppression of adult neurogenesis impairs olfactory learning and memory in an adult insect. J Neurosci 23:9289–9296.

Scotto-Lomassese S, Strambi C, Strambi A, Charpin P, Augier R, Aouane A, Cayre M (2000) Influence of environmental stimulation on neurogenesis in the adult insect brain. J Neurobiol 45:162–171.

Soutschek J, Zupanc GK (1995) Apoptosis as a regulator of cell proliferation in the central posterior/prepacemaker nucleus of adult gymnotiform fish, *Apteronotus leptorhynchus*. Neurosci Lett 202:133–136.

Soutschek J, Zupanc GK (1996) Apoptosis in the cerebellum of adult teleost fish, *Apteronotus leptorhynchus*. Brain Res Dev Brain Res 97:279–286.

Svendsen CN, ter Borg MG, Armstrong RJ, Rosser AE, Chandran S, Ostenfeld T, Caldwell MA (1998) A new method for the rapid and long-term growth of human neural precursor cells. J Neurosci Methods 85:141–152.

Tonchev AB, Yamashima T, Zhao L, Okano H (2003a) Differential proliferative response in the postischemic hippocampus, temporal cortex, and olfactory bulb of young adult macaque monkeys. Glia 42:209–224.

Tonchev AB, Yamashima T, Zhao L, Okano HJ, Okano H (2003b) Proliferation of neural and neuronal progenitors after global brain ischemia in young adult macaque monkeys. Mol Cell Neurosci 23:292–301.

Vates GE, Nottebohm F (1995) Feedback circuitry within a song-learning pathway. Proc Natl Acad Sci USA 92:5139–5143.

Volman SF, Grubb TC Jr, Schuett KC (1997) Relative hippocampal volume in relation to food-storing behavior in four species of woodpeckers. Brain Behav Evol 49:110–120.

Wang N, Aviram R, Kirn JR (1999) Deafening alters neuron turnover within the telencephalic motor pathway for song control in adult zebra finches. J Neurosci 19:10554–10561.

Weissman T, Noctor SC, Clinton BK, Honig LS, Kriegstein AR (2003) Neurogenic radial glial cells in reptile, rodent and human: from mitosis to migration. Cereb Cortex 13:550–559.

Wu DM, Schneiderman T, Burgett J, Gokhale P, Barthel L, Raymond PA (2001) Cones regenerate from retinal stem cells sequestered in the inner nuclear layer of adult goldfish retina. Invest Ophthalmol Vis Sci 42:2115–2124.

Zupanc GK (1999) Neurogenesis, cell death and regeneration in the adult gymnotiform brain. J Exp Biol 202 (Pt 10):1435–1446.

Zupanc GK, Horschke I (1995) Proliferation zones in the brain of adult gymnotiform fish: a quantitative mapping study. J Comp Neurol 353:213–233.

Zupanc GK, Zupanc MM (1992) Birth and migration of neurons in the central posterior/prepacemaker nucleus during adulthood in weakly electric knifefish (*Eigenmannia* sp.). Proc Natl Acad Sci USA 89:9539–9543.

12

Medicine

Research on adult neurogenesis and neural stem cells is often justified to funding agencies, policy makers, and taxpayers by its potential benefit to medicine. The general tenor of these justifications is the aim of replacing lost neurons in cases of neuronal loss. In this chapter we will review what is known about the contributions that adult neurogenesis can make toward this goal. But we will also see that in many circumstances this important goal is somewhat at odds with the realities of adult neurogenesis.

In the previous chapter we have seen that our present knowledge about adult neurogenesis in humans is still limited and that there is even some evidence that human adult neurogenesis might differ considerably if not principally from adult neurogenesis in rodents. The architecture of the subventricular zone (SVZ) and rostral migratory stream (RMS) in humans, for example, is substantially different from its rodent counterpart (Rakic, 2004; Sanai et al., 2004). Still, neural precursor cells can be isolated from the human SVZ and subgranular zone (SGZ), and adult hippocampal neurogenesis has been shown to occur in humans (see Chapter 11). These findings justify subdued enthusiasm and much further research, but the presently available data ask more questions about the applicability of rodent data to the human situation than they answer. With respect to regulation and function, two key aspects of adult neurogenesis, we know next to nothing about the situation in humans. This lack of knowledge does not disqualify the hopes for human therapy based on results obtained in rodents or even primate species, but it cautions us to consider the animal data as what they are—models. It remains to be established how good these models are. The fact that neural stem cells and adult neurogenesis generally exist in the adult human brain justifies the use of the models. On the other hand, the data obtained in rodents have to be carefully evaluated for their relevance to the human situation if they are to be used toward clinical applications.

This caveat is important because after what has been perceived as the dissolution of the "no-new-neurons dogma" (see Chapter 1 on the problems with this term), the common perception seems to have swung to the other extreme. The few signs of adult human neurogenesis, together with the much more suggestive therapeutic findings in rodents, have led to the misconception that in neuroregeneration everything should be generally possible. Quite surprisingly, neural stem cells have sometimes been greeted as the last missing link in an otherwise obviously coherent picture of what would constitute successful neuroregeneration. As with the discovery of precursor cells and adult neurogenesis, everything should fall into place and neuroregeneration become suddenly possible. However, the adult brain still regenerates poorly. It does so *despite* the presence of neural stem cells and not, as was previously thought, because of their absence.

Premature clinical trials based on idealistic concepts and slim experimental evidence have already brought adult neurogenesis to the patient. Especially the idea of transdifferentiation has elicited clinical trials in which, for example, bone marrow cells were infused into stroke patients.

There is no conclusive experimental evidence showing that bone marrow–derived cells would incorporate into an ischemic area and lead to structural restoration. Not surprisingly, the therapeutic success of such human experiments is limited if not absent. For obvious good reasons, double-blind studies are lacking and in prospective trials on individual patients the magnitude of the placebo effect is difficult to estimate. In most cases, no attempts have been made to elucidate the underlying biology and thus learn anything from these trials other than a confirmation of one's own vision and prejudice. In a case of sensational failure this haste into the clinic threatens to bring the entire field into discredit. An ill-designed trial in gene therapy that resulted in the death of the victim has paralyzed progress in many other, thoroughly planned attempts to bring gene therapy to the clinic. Cell therapy has seen some worrying examples of problematic strategies, too. There has been a clinical trial for neuronal replacement in stroke patients with cells derived from a human teratocarcinoma cell line. Luckily, in this attempt no patients developed tumors, but a thorough risk assessment and understanding of the biology of these cells appears difficult to achieve (Kleppner et al., 1995; Kondziolka et al., 2000).

Besides the imminent dangers in premature clinical applications, a second threat to cell-based therapy in neurology and psychiatry arises from those for whom development is still not fast enough. There are voices that categorically question the value of stem cell research in general because of the present lack of convincing clinical success and because of the general difficulties in transfering promising results from rodents to the human situation. Both those who leap into clinic and the pessimistic critics, however, miss the point that the relevance of adult neurogenesis and neural stem cell biology go far beyond cell replacement strategies.

In this book we have considered adult neurogenesis to be neuronal development in the adult brain. We have emphasized the point that the rise of stem cell biology has led to a fundamental paradigm shift: the profound insight that brain development never ends. Precursor cells with their accessible genetic potential persist in the adult brain and make lifelong contributions to brain plasticity. We are only at the beginning of grasping the consequences of this paradigm shift. Neural stem cell biology adds an important next step to the concept of brain plasticity, just as the idea of plasticity had revolutionized neurobiology in the previous few decades. Admittedly,

immediate clinical consequences of this revolution have been rather limited thus far. But patience and thorough, basic work will pay off.

One reason for the lack of existing therapies based on the plasticity concept is that knowledge of neural precursor cells, the obvious cellular targets
for therapeutic measures and from which regeneration based on plasticity could originate, has been missing. Consideration of plasticity as a form
of persistent cellular brain development, however, might change this situation. Entire cells become part of the equation, and plasticity goes beyond
neurites or synapses. This does not reduce the value of, for example, the
exploration of synaptic plasticity, but synaptic and other subcellular aspects
of plasticity alone have not yet proven to be successful targets for neurological therapies. For the general effects demanded in therapy they might
be too far downstream of the necessary structural events that would allow
true reconstitution.

Seen within this concept of precursor cell–based plasticity, the generation
of new neurons is just one, albeit important, aspect. Many important insights
can be expected from glial biology. Consequently, the medical consequences
of adult neurogenesis and neural stem cell biology will not necessarily lie in
neuronal cell replacement but in a profound change in understanding how
the brain maintains its structural identity. The neurogenic regions are privileged regions in this sense and therefore cellular plasticity of neurons will
play a larger role in these areas than in the non-neurogenic regions. Neurogenesis is possible in nonneurogenic regions under exceptional conditions
and this potential might become exploitable in the future. In addition, however, precursor cell–based plasticity will be otherwise involved in the brain's
response to disease, and this function might harbor even greater potential
for therapy.

A classic concept states that precursor cells could contribute to neuro-
regenerative therapies in the following two ways (Bjorklund and Lindvall,
2000):

- Replace lost cells
- Provide a pro-regenerative microenvironment for other cells.

This concept includes therapeutic strategies based on neurotransplantation. In the context of transplantation, neural stem cell biology is seen
primarily as a tool for generating transplantable cells. Most strategies rely
on predifferentiating donor cells in vitro before implantation. Nevertheless,
the cellular environment in the host brain will influence graft survival and
function. Insights from research on adult neurogenesis in vivo can help to
understand the neurogenic requirements in the host brain to promote graft
function.

It is often stated that stimulation of an endogenous potential for regeneration is the great alternative to transplanting neurons to the brain. In reality, evidence for this claim is scant, partially because our knowledge about
the potential of cell replacement therapies in the adult brain is generally

rather limited. Targeted neurogenesis is a fascinating strategy (Chapter 8) and one day its therapeutic potential might indeed be tapped (Arlotta et al., 2003). Precursor cells in vivo have the necessary potential for targeted neurogenesis, although the regenerative potential of endogenous precursor cells in different models of disease has varied greatly across conditions and species.

Thus, the obstacles to inducing regenerative neurogenesis remain high; at present the available experimental evidence from animal models provides impressive proofs of principle but no direct access to clinical solutions. However, this perspective reduces adult neurogenesis to just an endogenous variant of cell replacement. This is not the most radical orientation possible, based on our increasing knowledge about adult neurogenesis. Considering the facts that (1) brain development never ends, and (2) precursor cells are carriers of cellular brain plasticity, the following two related aspects can be added to the classical perspective. Neural precursor cells might also be of clinical relevance because

- a failure of normal precursor cell activity might underlie or contribute to brain pathology, and
- prevention and therapy strategies might therefore target precursor cells to reconstitute normal brain plasticity.

These two aspects are two sides of the same coin, but both together are considerably different from a direct cell-replacement strategy. As exemplified in the work of Jeffrey Macklis at Harvard University, cell replacement strategies can merge with the developmental approach and blur the conceptional boundaries.

Pathologies in general tend to have a strong, acute effect on cell proliferation in both the SGZ and the SVZ. As exemplified in the deafferentation of the olfactory bulb, the initial increase in cell proliferation is followed by a lasting decrease (Corotto et al., 1994; Jankovski et al., 1998; Mandairon et al., 2003). Thus, acute effects have to be distinguished from chronic consequences of pathology. The principle seems to be the following: acute damages causes a (transient) effect on cell proliferation; chronic damage results in a lasting decrease in adult neurogenesis.

FAILING PRECURSOR CELL FUNCTION AND ADULT NEUROGENESIS

Brain Tumors

Because precursor cells are proliferating cells with developmental potential, control of both proliferation and development might fail and lead to tumors (Noble and Dietrich, 2004).

The first tumors for which a connection between precursor cell activity and tumorigenesis was proposed were subependymomas, relatively rare tumors of the ventricular wall. At the time when this idea was first phrased (Globus and Kuhlenbeck, 1944), precursor cells in the adult brain had not yet been discovered, but a hypothetical link to persistently dividing cells in the walls of the ventricles could be made. Thus, a neurooncological report became one of the first comments on continued cell division in the adult brain.

A connection between brain precursor cells and tumorigenesis seems so immediately plausible that the initial lack of studies tracking this hint is surprising. The most relevant class of brain tumors are gliomas, that is tumors with signs of glial differentiation. Gliomas show a large variability of neuropathological appearance, and its most malignant variant, glioblastoma multiforme (GBM), is the most frequent brain tumor. As the name "multiforme" alludes to, GBM are characterized by a mix of differently differentiated cell types, vascularization, necrosis, and lymphocytic reaction. Most GBM are dominated by astrocyte-like differentiation, but forms with intermingled oligodendrocytic and mesenchymal differentiation exist. Even signs of neuronal differentiation have been found in tumor cells (Labrakakis et al., 1997). The notion that these neuronal features originate from resident neurons that become enclosed by growing tumor has been largely abandoned. This range of differentiation patterns within one tumor is best explained if one assumes that the origin is from a cell with a wide potential for differentiation. Gene defects known to result in tumorigenic transformation concern genes that also often play prominent roles in stem cell biology and can be used to transform neural precursor cells experimentally (Holland et al., 2000; Uhrbom et al., 2002; Seoane et al., 2004). From human glioma samples, a CD133-positive population of cells could be isolated that behaved as stem cells in vitro and caused tumor formation in a xenograft model (Singh et al., 2004). Currently this is the strongest argument in favor of the stem cell hypothesis of tumorigenesis.

In this context, tumors in which neuronal differentiation goes beyond the expression of some marker proteins, such as in neurocytomas or gangliocytomas, are particularly interesting. Both are very rare entities. Because differentiated neurons cannot divide, the idea of a neuronal origin of neurocytomas and gangliocytomas seemed improbable. The unproven hypothesis that they develop from a type of precursor cell is more plausible but requires further molecular analysis.

Nestin is expressed in neuroectodermal tumors and provided an early hint at potential precursor cells in brain tumors (Tohyama et al., 1992; Kashima et al., 1993). However, the specificity of this finding remains low. From neuroblastoma samples and glioblastoma cell lines a side population has been isolated by fluorescence-activated cell sorting (FACS) (Hirschmann-Jax et al., 2004). This population is characterized by a high efflux of dye, a property that coincides with stem cell qualities in bone marrow.

More available data concern the possible role of oligodendrocyte precursor cells in the genesis of gliomas (Noble, 1997). Human gliomas, for example, express many genes that are active in the oligodendrocyte lineage (Kashima et al., 1993). Transforming O2A progenitor cells with oncogenes *c-myc* and *Ras* resulted in gliomas after implantation in the mouse brain (Barnett et al., 1998). Similarly, activation of Akt and Ras in neural precursor cells led to the development of glioblastoma-like tumors in mice (Holland et al., 2000).

Classical stem cell tumors, in particular teratomas and teratocarcinomas, can affect the brain as well. Another category of dysontogenetic tumors is primitive neuroectodermal tumors (PNET) and medulloblastomas, malignant childhood tumors mostly of the hindbrain with a uniform undifferentiated growth pattern and a still unknown origin. There might be no such cell as a medulloblast, but the transformed cell might still be a neuroepithelial precursor cell. A precursor cell line with the properties of this proposed cellular identity has been described (Valtz et al., 1991). In many transplantation studies involving neural precursor cells, tumor formation has been found; this was largely considered only a technical problem and a potentially confounding side effect. These "accidents," however, harbor great potential for brain tumor biology and deserve to be analyzed neuropathologically. Novel tumor models could be developed from precursor cells that mirror the properties of human gliomas and other brain tumors better than the existing lines.

Side Effects of Tumor Irradiation and Chemotherapy

Irradiation and chemotherapy are known to be associated with cognitive dysfunction (Kramer et al., 1992; Crossen et al., 1994; Abayomi, 1996). Children who received high-dose irradiation prior to bone marrow transplantation for acute myeloic leukemia often have learning difficulties later. In one study, children who underwent chemotherapy for similar diagnoses took up an academic profession less often than their healthy peers (Kingma et al., 2000).

Both chemotherapy and irradiation target proliferating cells, and common side effects consequently affect highly proliferating tissues, most notably bone marrow. Neural precursor cell dysfunction underlying cognitive impairment after irradiation might be an as yet underestimated side effect of cancer treatment (Monje et al., 2002). Precursor cells in the adult SVZ and SGZ have been found to be particularly sensitive to irradiation (Shinohara et al., 1997; Parent et al., 1999; Peissner et al., 1999) and are most likely eliminated by apoptotic cell death (Limoli et al., 2004). In one study, precursor cell proliferation in the dentate gyrus decreased by up to 95% at all doses above 1 Gy and led to a long-lasting reduction in neurogenesis but, interestingly, not gliogenesis (Mizumatsu et al., 2003). Irradiation was associated with a strong inflammatory response in the hippocampus. Treatment of the irradiated animals concomitantly with anti-inflammatory agents rescued adult hippocampal neurogenesis, a finding suggesting that part of the precursor cell damage is secondary and due to the inflammatory reaction (Monje et al., 2003).

Blockade of adult hippocampal neurogenesis by irradiation correlated with reduced performance on a hippocampus-dependent learning task, whereas hippocampus-independent learning was spared (Madsen et al., 2003). Irradiated animals also showed more anxious behavior, and this effect could not be resolved with antidepressive therapy (Santarelli et al., 2003). Although that study was primarily designed to show that hippocampal neurogenesis is necessary for the function of antidepressants, it also showed how irradiation alters behavior connected with adult hippocampal neurogenesis.

Cytostatic treatment shows similar effects on adult neurogenesis. Procarbazin and cytosine arabinoside (Ara-C) have been used to experimentally reduce precursor cell activity in the adult brain (Doetsch et al., 1999; Seri et al., 2001). Similarly, the clinically less relevant methylazoxymethanol (MAM), a drug with many side effects, acutely diminished cell proliferation in the dentate gyrus. This decrease was associated with impaired performance on some but not other hippocampal learning tasks. Again, hippocampus-independent cognitive abilities were spared (Shors et al., 2001, 2002).

The dentate gyrus can recover from acute and short-term treatment with cytostatics quite well. Most likely, the rarely dividing stem cells are not hit by the antiproliferative drug and can repopulate the germinative matrix of the SGZ (Seri et al., 2001; Ciaroni et al., 2002). If the damage occurs early, compensation from this source can be complete (Ciaroni et al., 2002). The apparent difference between the long-term effects of irradiation, which did not allow recovery even after 4 months (Tada et al., 2000), and chemotherapy is most likely not a principal difference but a matter of dosage.

Infection

Infection with human herpesvirus 6 is detectable in 70% of all brain samples that come to autopsy (Sanders et al., 1996). In most cases the infection is benign and does not lead to a clinical phenotype. However, herpesvirus 6 infection can also lead to leukencephalopathy with severe demyelination. In vitro, herpesvirus 6 infected human glial precursor cells and caused cell cycle arrest and premature oligodendrocytic differentiation (Dietrich et al., 2004). On the one hand this finding raises the possibility that failing precursor cell function could be part of the pathogenesis of manifest herpesvirus 6 infection. On the other hand, the vulnerability of precursor cells to a common pathogen might prevent attempts to recruit these cells for regeneration. Classical herpes encephalitis can affect the temporal lobes and thus might exert some of its signs of hippocampal dysfunction through damage to adult neurogenesis, but this possibility has not yet been studied specifically. Neonatal infection with the lymphocytic choriomeningitis virus caused a reduction in granule cell numbers, a decrease in proliferating cells and Mash1–positive cells in the SGZ, and a lasting reduction in adult neurogenesis (Sharma et al., 2002).

After bacterial meningeal infection, which tends to be much more acute than the often latent infection with herpesvirus 6, cell proliferation was increased in the dentate gyrus of mice and rabbits. At later time points the number of cells expressing immature neuronal markers remained elevated (Gerber et al., 2003).

Seizures and Epilepsy

The temporal lobe is frequently the site of origin for epileptic seizures, typically psychomotoric seizures, with their wide spectrum of symptoms, adequately reflecting the range of functions of the temporal lobe. Temporal lobe epilepsy is associated with sclerosis of the hippocampus in about 90% of operated cases and a characteristic dispersion of granule cells in the dentate gyrus in about 40% of cases (Houser, 1990; Thom et al., 2002). In 10% of cases the granule cell dispersion shows a bilaminar pattern similar to that doublecortex syndrome, a developmental disorder caused by mutations in the doublecortin gene (hence the name). Whether doublecortin expression in the migrating, newly generated granule cells is responsible for this coincidence has to be further examined. The organization of the granule cell layer itself can thus be profoundly disturbed in temporal lobe epilepsy (Houser, 1990; Lurton et al., 1997, 1998; El Bahh et al., 1999). It is not clear, however, whether a preexisting hippocampal abnormality is responsible for the development of the seizures (Blumcke et al., 2002). Magnetic resonance imaging (MRI) studies in families with febrile convulsions suggest this link (Fernandez et al., 1998). It has also been postulated that Cajal-Retzius neurons persist in the epileptic dentate gyrus, which might be indicative of disturbed development (Blumcke et al., 1999, 2001; Thom et al., 2002). More severe cases of epilepsy tend to have fewer Cajal-Retzius cells in the molecular layer of the adult dentate gyrus than in milder cases but still more than controls (Thom et al., 2002).

In an experimental setting, seizures robustly increase adult neurogenesis in both neurogenic regions (Bengzon et al., 1997; Parent et al., 1997, 1999, 2002a). The induction of cell proliferation is massive and has been shown in several models of epilepsy. The first group of models contains chemoconvulsant-dependent seizures—that is, seizures that are pharmacologically induced. Injections of kainic acid and pilocarpine elicit seizures via excitation of glutamate receptors (Bengzon et al., 1997; Parent et al., 1997; Gray and Sundstrom, 1998; Covolan et al., 2000), whereas pentylene tetrazole acts by inhibiting GABAergic inhibition (Jiang et al., 2003). Seizures can also be induced directly by external electrodes in animal models of electroconvulsive therapy (Madsen et al., 2000) and by kindling, i.e., by subthreshold stimulation from an intraparenchymal electrode (Parent et al., 1998; Scott et al., 1998; Nakagawa et al., 2000; Auvergne et al., 2002; Ferland et al., 2002). Kindling in which an inserted needle provides a sort of epileptic focus might be closest to the situation in patients with temporal lobe epilepsy. In general, the models will only reflect single aspects of the disease. Most importantly, with respect to the open question of whether the seizures or the neurogenic dysregulation comes first, these models necessarily take a biased stand.

All seizure models lead to a similar response in adult hippocampal neurogenesis. Cell proliferation increases 8- to 10-fold within a few days after the seizures. Labeling proliferative cells prior to the induction of seizures revealed that it is not a quiescent population that responds to the stimulus but one that is highly dividing (Parent et al., 1999). In seizures elicited by kindling in the amygdala the total number of PSA-NCAM-expressing cells in the dentate gyrus increased (Saegusa et al., 2004). This increase correlated with an increase in PSA-NCAM-positive mossy fibers in CA3. In contrast to this finding, others have reported that seizures primarily induced proliferation of radial glia–like astrocytes in the dentate gyrus (Huttmann et al., 2003).

The involvement of the late precursor cells in response to ictogenic stimuli might be indicative of a certain stage of maturation that the new cells need to acquire before they can be stimulated by excitation. Because these cells express doublecortin and because doublecortin is associated with cell migration, a potential dysregulation of migration in response to seizure activity may occur at this stage. In a model of electroconvulsive seizures it was also found that endothelial proliferation was increased along the division of SGZ precursor cells (Hellsten et al., 2004). Given the close connection of precursor cells and blood vessels in the stem cell niche, this finding suggests of a concerted effect. The induction of endothelial proliferation was not restricted to the SGZ, but the clusters of proliferating cells in the SGZ contained more dividing endothelia.

The long-term effects of seizures on adult hippocampal neurogenesis depends on the severity of the seizures. Both partial and full status eplilepticus caused a similar increase in cell proliferation, but in full status epilepticus survival of the newly generated neurons was reduced (Mohapel et al., 2004). This result might be due to increased damage to the permissive microenvironment in the SGZ under this condition.

Prolonged seizures also affected neurogenesis in the SVZ and olfactory bulb. Most of the newly generated cells took the normal path of migration to the olfactory bulb; a certain percentage, however, prematurely left the RMS and were found in other forebrain regions (Parent et al., 2002a). Neuronal development also appeared to be accelerated under normal conditions, further supporting the idea of a developmental dysregulation. In both the hippocampus and olfactory system it thus seems that seizures speed up development and disconnect migration from the appropriate maturation. Cells might receive inappropriate developmental cues, leading to ectopically

placed cells and incorrect connections. The molecular mechanisms underlying these disturbances are unknown. Chronic seizures resulted in a lasting decrease in adult neurogenesis months after induction of the seizures
(Hattiangady et al., 2004).

Seizure activity can induce cell death, which in turn might be involved
in triggering the neurogenic response. In chronic temporal-lobe epilepsy,
a substantial loss of hippocampal neurons is found (Thom et al., 2002).
However, mechanisms independent of cell death must also exist, because
in C57Bl/6 mice kainic acid does not induce cell death but strongly increases neurogenesis. Also, in amygdala kindling, tissue damage is mini-
mized, compared to that in other models, without losing a strong induction
of neurogenesis (Ferland et al., 2002). The proliferative response, is dose-
dependent and single seizures are still able to induce division of the precursor cells (Ferland et al., 2002) and a long-lasting response after status
epilepticus.

It remains unclear to what degree the neurogenic response to seizures
is an attempt at regeneration or part of the pathology itself. Ectopic new
neurons can be found in the hilus of rats and mice with seizure-induced
neurogenesis. Trains of migrating cells have been described to lead from
the SGZ into the hilus (Parent et al., 1999), suggesting that these ectopic cells
originate from the dividing precursor cells of the SGZ. Such ectopic hilar
granule cells fire with CA3 pyramidal neurons and not with granule cells,
further supporting their incorrect integration (Scharfman et al., 2000). In
specimens from human patients with chronic temporal lobe epilepsy, ectopic granule-like cells in hilus and CA3 were found in about 18% of cases
(Thom et al., 2002). In their 1997 report on seizure-induced neurogenesis
(Parent et al., 1997), Jack Parent and Daniel Lowenstein speculated that the
seizure-induced new neurons might be responsible for the aberrant axonal
sprouting found in temporal lobe epilepsy (Houser et al., 1990; Lurton et al.,
1997) and its animal models (Tauck and Nadler, 1985; Mello et al., 1993).
They reported that axons of newly generated granule cells contributed to
mossy fiber sprouting in both CA3 and the inner molecular layer. However,
they also found that inhibiting neurogenesis through irradiation did not
prevent axonal sprouting, suggesting that sprouting might originate from
both new and old cells (Parent et al., 1999).

Often the ectopic new granule cells retain a basal dendrite that is normally absent in mature granule cells (Ribak et al., 2000). Developing granule cells in the adult go through a period during which they possess basal
dendrites (Ribak et al., 2004). In the ectopic granule cells the number of
excitatory synapses on these dendrites was increased, further supporting
the idea that these cells are involved in the generation or propagation of
seizures (Ribak et al., 2000).

On a side note, valproic acid, one classical antiepileptic drug, has direct effects on precursor cells. Jenny Hsieh and colleagues from Fred H. Gage's group
at the Salk Institute found that valproic acid promoted the differentiation

of neurons and suppressed a glial cell fate through the induction of NeuroD (Hsieh et al., 2004).

Alzheimer Disease

The possible functional relevance of adult neurogenesis discussed in Chapter 10 can be reconsidered in the context of possible causes underlying hippocampal dysfunction. If the gatekeeper theory holds (Kempermann, 2002), it might explain how disturbed adult hippocampal neurogenesis could lead to a maladaptation of hippocampal circuitry to cognitive challenges. It is unlikely that this theory will explain dementias completely. However, if considered in the larger contexts of normal and disturbed brain plasticity, it might be that adult neurogenesis plays a particularly prominent role in a more general contribution of precursor cells to brain plasticity.

Dementia is an acquired, irreversible decrease in cognitive abilities. Besides the cognitive impairment after antiproliferative treatment discussed above and reversible (pseudo-) dementia in the context of depression, dealt with below, Alzheimer disease (AD) has received the most attention in the context of a potential contribution of precursor cell dysfunction to pathogenesis and the course of cognitive decline. Alzheimer disease is a common cause of dementia in the elderly. The initial symptoms of AD often concern the hippocampus. Patients have memory problems and become disorientated. Structural alterations in the brains of AD patients include neuronal and glial pathology. Degenerating neurons show neurofibrillary tangles; glial dysfunction is associated with the extracellular accumulation of β-amyloid, leading to the formation of the characteristic plaques.

It has been noted that cell cycle–dependent markers are expressed in the hippocampus of AD patients (Nagy et al., 1997a, 1997b, 2000). This observation led to the hypothesis that in the course of AD, as in other cases of neuronal damage such as ischemia (Katchanov et al., 2001; Kuan et al., 2004), postmitotic neurons might be induced to enter into cell cycle that cannot be completed and results in their death (Nagy, 2000; Herrup and Yang, 2001; Yang et al., 2001, 2003). In contrast to this hypothesis, doublecortin immunohistochemistry showed that adult hippocampal neurogenesis might be increased in AD patients (Jin et al., 2004b). However, quantification is problematic in postmortem samples (see Chapter 7). The neurodegenerative disorder might have reduced the volume of the granule cell layer, consistent with the atrophy found in AD. A reduced volume with the same or even decreased number of cells might lead to an increased cell number because the cells are closer to each other and thus more likely to be visible in one section plane. Western blot analysis confirmed the presence of markers associated with adult neurogenesis such as doublecortin, PSA-NCAM, and NeuroD. The immature cells had a condensed morphology, though, and it was speculated that they might undergo apoptotic cell death before maturing into granule cells.

In mouse models, the reaction of precursor cells to AD-like pathology was ambiguous. In a transgenic mouse model overexpressing a mutated form of the amyloid precursor protein APP, the enzymatic breakdown of APP leads to the presence of β-amyloid, which accumulates and leads to an AD-like plaque load (Sturchler-Pierrat et al., 1997). Such APP overexpression interferes with neurogenesis in both the SGZ and SVZ (Haughey et al., 2002a, 2002b). In other studies, however, increased hippocampal neurogenesis (Jin et al., 2004a) and increased proliferation in the SVZ (Caille et al., 2004) were found. In vitro, APP was able to stimulate the proliferation of neural precursor cells in one study (Ohsawa et al., 1999), but not in another (Haughey et al., 2002b). In old transgenic mice, an up to six-fold increase in cortical cell genesis was found, but none of the new cells exhibited a neuronal phenotype (Bondolfi et al., 2002) and most of the new cells were microglia. β-Amyloid, the product of APP splicing that accumulates in AD, is not generally inhibitory or toxic to precursor cells. To the contrary, a dose-dependent increase in the number of neuronal progeny was found in an in vitro assay (Lopez-Toledano and Shelanski, 2004) and in one transgenic mouse model an increase in adult hippocampal neurogenesis was reported in vivo as well (Jin et al., 2004a). These divergent findings might indicate that adult neurogenesis is differentially affected by different pathological factors associated with the disease.

Presenilins are a family of membrane proteins whose mutation can underlie familiar cases of early-onset AD. Presenilin-1 is expressed in nestin-positive and nestin-negative precursor cells of the SGZ (Wen et al., 2002). In a conditional mutant for presenilin-1, normal adult hippocampal neurogenesis was unaffected but the increase in response to exposure to environmental enrichment was reduced by one-third (Feng et al., 2001), which might reflect reduced plasticity.

Overall, it seems likely that precursor cell plasticity in AD models is impaired and that any regenerative attempts are abortive, potentially leading to the impression of proliferative cells and shrunken immature neurons in human tissue samples from AD patients. In this scenario disturbed adult neurogenesis might contribute to the hippocampal cognitive deficits found in AD patients.

Parkinson Disease

Dopaminergic denervation of the striatum and hippocampus leads to a decrease in local precursor cell proliferation. In the SVZ, C cells have been identified as the targets. In a report on adult precursor cells in Parkinson disease (PD), Gunter Höglinger and colleagues speculated that patients with PD who lack dopaminergic innervation might consequently face a loss of precursor cells in the SVZ and SGZ (Hoglinger et al., 2004). Data from human postmortem samples even suggested that patients with PD have indeed reduced levels of cells expressing precursor cell markers (Hoglinger et al.,

2004). This technically challenging part of the study will have to be replicated with more samples, stereological methods, and with more markers, but the initial finding is suggestive and should encourage further studies. In patients with PD, often a loss or alteration of smell is found (Berendse et al., 2001) and hippocampal atrophy is associated with signs of dementia (Laakso et al., 1996; Riekkinen et al., 1998; Camicioli et al., 2003). One neuropathological feature of PD is the accumulation of α-synuclein in so-called Lewy bodies. Overexpression of α-synuclein impaired survival of newly generated cells in the RMS and olfactory bulb without affecting cell proliferation (Winner et al., 2004).

Major Depression and Schizophrenia

The hypothesis that a failure of adult hippocampal neurogenesis might underlie the pathogenesis of major depression is based on three different lines of reasoning: one empirical, one experimental, and one theoretical. First, patients with chronic depression have hippocampal symptoms and sometimes show hippocampal atrophy. Second, all known antidepressants stimulate adult neurogenesis and some antidepressants might not be effective in the absence of adult neurogenesis. Third, on the basis of functional interpretation of adult neurogenesis as outlined in Chapter 10, a theory can be developed that explains how a lack of adult neurogenesis might contribute to the clinical picture of major depression.

Both MRI studies and postmortem data confirm that patients with chronic depression can have atrophied hippocampi (Sheline et al., 1996; Rajkowska et al., 1999; Rajkowska, 2000; Sheline, 2000). At first glance this site of pathology coincides well with the location of adult neurogenesis, but adult hippocampal neurogenesis affects only the dentate gyrus, and the low rates in the production of new neurons in adult humans are unlikely to generate enough neurons that their absence would become discernible by MRI. Because patients with major depression have a disturbed regulation of cortisol levels, chronically elevated and dysregulated serum cortisol might be responsible for both signs of atrophy in the entire hippocampus and the diminished level of adult hippocampal neurogenesis. In animal models of depression, however, this straightforward connection has not yet been unambiguously confirmed (Malberg and Duman, 2003; Vollmayr et al., 2003). As discussed in Chapter 9, the role of stress and stress hormone corticosterone in the regulation of adult neurogenesis is complex. Also, models such as learned helplessness, in which rodents are exposed to nonpredictable stress that ultimately makes them resigned with many symptoms and biochemical parameters of depression, do not mirror the very long time scales of the human disease. Barry Jacobs from Princeton University, who first developed the neurogenesis hypothesis of depression, proposed that the "waxing and waning of adult hippocampal neurogenesis" could underlie the fluctuating nature of the disease (Jacobs et al., 2000). However, one ar-

gument against this idea is that adult hippocampal neurogenesis is cumulative and neuronal development takes several weeks. Consequently, this
take on a role of adult neurogenesis in depression would be linked to the
idea that cognitive function relevant to depression could be assigned to the
precursor cells or immature neurons and not just to the fully matured new
cells (Jacobs, 2002; Leuner et al., 2004; Shors, 2004; see Chapter 10).

Patients with major depression have a number of hippocampal symptoms. For example, they can show pseudodementia, that is, a reversible
impairment of learning and memory, and a reduced ability to assign emotional values to content that has to be learned. For depressed patients the
entire world is gray and even simple cognitive tasks involving learning
and memory become arduous. These and other symptoms do not make
major depression a hippocampal disorder, though. To causally link major
depression and adult hippocampal neurogenesis, not only a central role
of the hippocampus in major depression would have to be shown but also
an indispensable contribution of new neurons to this relevant function
(Kempermann and Kronenberg, 2003).

On the other hand, antidepressants of various types positively affect adult
hippocampal neurogenesis. The finding that selective serotonin reuptake
inhibitors (SSRI) such as fluoxetine increase neurogenesis is in line with the
positive correlation of serotonergic input to the dentate gyrus with the level
of adult neurogenesis (Malberg et al., 2000; Radley and Jacobs, 2002; Malberg
and Duman, 2003; Santarelli et al., 2003). The negative effects of inescapable stress on cell proliferation in the adult hippocampus were reversed by
fluoxetine (Malberg and Duman, 2003). Specifically, serotonin receptor 1A
appears to mediate the effect: specific antagonists decreased cell proliferation in the adult dentate gyrus (Radley and Jacobs, 2002). In serotonin receptor 1A knockouts, the effect on adult neurogenesis and the behavioral
effects of fluoxetine were abolished (Santarelli et al., 2003). When adult hippocampal neurogenesis was blocked by irradiation, the fluoxetine effects
on behavior were similarly prevented, a finding suggesting that adult neurogenesis is necessary for the action of fluoxetine. Substances of other classes
also increase adult neurogenesis, among them atypic antidepressant drugs
such as tianeptine, which paradoxically blocks serotonergic action (Fuchs
et al., 2002). Tianeptine robustly diminished the behavioral consequences
of chronic psychosocial stress and reduced the parallel loss of cell proliferation in the dentate gyrus. The effect on cell proliferation, however, was found
only in stressed animals, not in normal animals (Czeh et al., 2001). In a different study, tianeptine was found to reduce apoptotic cell death in the dentate
gyrus of normal and stressed tree shrews (Lucassen et al., 2004). Because essentially all dying cells in the normal dentate gyrus are newly generated neurons that are not recruited for long-term survival and functional integration,
it is conceivable that tianeptine has some effects on cell survival.

Other antidepressant measures with effects on adult hippocampal neurogenesis are classical tricyclic antidepressants such as desipramine and

imipramine (Malberg et al., 2000; Santarelli et al., 2003), electroconvulsive therapy (Madsen et al., 2000), and general measures such as physical activity (van Praag et al., 1999). The psychopharmacological interventions showed the typical latency of 2 to 4 weeks to reach their full effectiveness, a period of time coinciding with the latency known from antidepressant therapy in patients. (Malberg et al., 2000). Only transcranial magnetic stimulation, which had good effects on reversing the consequences of chronic psychosocial stress and the associated disturbances in the hypothalamic-pituitary-adrenocortical system, did not disinhibit adult neurogenesis and had further negative effects on cell survival (Czeh et al., 2002).

Because major depression is not primarily a hippocampal disorder but affects cognitive function in many brain regions, most notably but not exclusively structures involved in mood processing, a narrow pathogenetic interpretation of these date might not be justified. To accomododate the complexity of the disorder, it might be necessary to broaden the neurogenesis hypothesis of depression to a neuroplasticity hypothesis. Adult hippocampal neurogenesis might be the most visible aspect of a more general precursor cell–based plasticity that also includes glial cells in many brain regions, neurogenic or not (Kempermann and Kronenberg, 2003). Many growth factors, most notably brain-derived neurotrophic factor (BDNF), hormones, and neurotransmitters have an effect on adult neurogenesis, but their possible role in depression goes beyond this local effect (D'Sa and Duman, 2002). Serotonergic innervation, for example, is active throughout the brain, not just in the SGZ. In depressed patients, cellular plasticity, including adult hippocampal neurogenesis (but not limited to it), might thus be chronically and severely disturbed. Coping with the many situations of complexity and novelty in everyday life might constantly work at its limits, probably for a long time without clinical symptoms. In the brains of these patients, form can no longer follow function. A depressive episode might be a functional decompensation from this precious and increasingly fragile balance, to which a brain lacking mechanisms of plasticity cannot easily return.

Of all hypotheses linking adult neurogenesis to disease, the theory for major depression is so far the most elaborate. Despite its highly stimulating effect on the scientific community and many interesting results on adult neurogenesis, however, it still remains largely unproven.

Similar thoughts have also been raised in the context of schizophrenia. Here, too, a hippocampal pathology can be found, but the structural damage to the hippocampus is less clear. In one of the few established rodent models of schizophrenia, based on a transient toxic lesion of the developing hippocampus, no alteration in adult hippocampal neurogenesis was found (Lipska, 2004). Also, the classic antipsychotic agent, haloperidol, a dopamine antagonist, did not affect adult hippocampal neurogenesis (Malberg et al., 2000; Halim et al., 2004). Atypical antipsychotics, in contrast, affected cell proliferation. Olanzapine and risperidon increased cell divisions in the SVZ (Wakade et al., 2002) and in the prefrontal cortex (Wang et al., 2004).

The theory that a chronic hypofunction of NMDA receptors might underlie schizophrenia is similar to the neuroplasticity hypothesis of depression,
which consequently one day might be more aptly phrased a "neuroplasticity
hypothesis of affective disorders."

Alcohol

In contrast to the drugs of abuse discussed in Chapter 9, in the case of alcohol it cannot be assumed that any seen effect on precursor cell function is
specific. Alcohol does not serve a physiological regulatory function. However, susceptibility to alcohol-related toxicity differs among various cell
populations and brain regions, thus explaining the sequence of symptoms
after acute alcohol intake. There may be a link to adult neurogenesis because
chronic alcohol abuse causes learning and memory problems and decreased
olfaction in late stages of the disease. Chronic alcoholism in mice, for example, results in atrophy of the dentate gyrus (Walker et al., 1980). MRI
studies in humans have shown fluctuations in hippocampal volume under
alcohol abuse (White et al., 2000). A highly speculative hypothesis is that
these consequences of alcohol abuse might be caused by alcohol-related
negative effects on adult neurogenesis.

Acute alcohol consumption (binge drinking) of 1 or 4 days acutely reduced cell proliferation in the SGZ; the 4-day treatment also reduced cell
survival (Nixon and Crews, 2002). Physical exercise was able to counteract
these effects to some degree (Crews et al., 2004). Chronic alcohol intake for
6 weeks at moderate doses decreased the number of newly generated neurons in the adult dentate gyrus of rats but not in the olfactory bulb. This
decrease was due to a reduction in cell survival, whereas cell proliferation
was not impaired. Intake of Ebselen, an antioxidative agent, together with
alcohol prevented the damage (Herrera et al., 2003), which indicates that
the damage might be due to oxidative stress. Abstinence from alcohol after
4 days of binge alcohol intake caused a strong rebound in cell proliferation
(Nixon and Crews, 2004).

Alcohol thus seems to have an acute down-regulating effect on SGZ precursor cells that can be compensated for unless the damage is prolonged,
which leads to a sustained net reduction in adult neurogenesis. It is not
yet known whether the toxic effects are direct or indirect by affecting the
neurogenic niche.

ENDOGENOUS PRECURSOR CELLS IN BRAIN REPAIR

Targeted Neurogenesis

Visions of making medical use of the endogenous potential for neurogenesis
tend to leave the boundaries of the neurogenic zones. In the previous section of this chapter we have seen that adult neurogenesis can be linked with

several disorders that affect the neurogenic zones, primarily the hippocampus. In this context it is straightforward to envision therapeutic strategies by trying to reverse diminished neurogenesis as a potential basis of major depression, or diminish disturbed neurogenesis in temporal lobe epilepsy. Nevertheless, therapeutic visions based on endogenous neural precursor cells and adult neurogenesis have been most prominently put forth for situations in which a pathogenic involvement of precursor cells and neurogenesis is much less obvious. In the absence of a clear link to normal precursor cell function, the proposed therapies thus become more utopian than in the case of tumor, epilepsy, dementia, or depression.

In such therapies precursor cells are here primarily considered a resource for endogenous cell replacement. However, both endogenously recruited and exogenously expanded and implanted cells face the environment of a diseased brain that in general is more or less adverse to neuronal regeneration and neurogenesis. In non-neurogenic regions the key issue is the lack of neurogenic permissiveness, not the absence (or promoted presence) of neural precursor cells. Regenerative neurogenesis in non-neurogenic regions has to overcome this inhibition. In some cases it seems that the pathology itself induces a pattern change. In models of Striatal ischemia, for example, a low number of new neurons has been found (Arvidsson et al., 2002; Parent et al., 2002b).

It also seems that inhibitory and promoting stimuli are competing, with the promoting factors being easily overwhelmed by the inhibitory influences. The experiments by Sanjay S. Magavi, Jeffrey D. Macklis, and colleagues from Harvard University have demonstrated that targeted lesions of individual neuronal populations (as described in detail in Chapter 8), leading to the apoptotic death of single cells without reaction from the local environment, can induce neuronal replacement, probably from resident cortical precursor cells (Magavi et al., 2000; Chen et al., 2004). In some sense these studies embody the quintessential goal of all attempts to achieve regenerative neurogenesis. The finding that death of the cell was sufficient to trigger neurogenesis is ambivalent. On the encouraging side it shows that conducive clues can be expressed by the adult brain; on the discouraging side it indicates that unless the lesion is so discrete that it does not trigger an adverse tissue response, the competing antineurogenic signals are stronger. That the apoptotic elimination of single neurons can indeed induce changes that locally transform the non-neurogenic adult cortex into a neurogenic zone is supported by the finding that, under the condition of targeted apoptosis, exogenous precursor cells implanted into the cortex also differentiate into neurons (Sheen and Macklis, 1995; Snyder et al., 1997; Shin et al., 2000).

Stroke

Given the clinical relevance of stroke, it is no surprise that a large number of experiments are aimed at identifying an endogenous neurogenic response to ischemic brain damage. Stroke generally leads to necrotic tissue loss that cannot be replaced. Transplantation with the goal of reconstructing the entire lost structure is an unlikely option because of the typical size of the lesion and the complexity of the destroyed brain structure. Cell therapy, however, might aid in retaining tissue that would otherwise succumb to secondary loss and might provide trophic or other support to the spared structures. In theory, this benefit could also be obtained from endogenous resources.

Consequently, a promising long-term therapeutic strategy might be to promote endogenous attempts for regeneration to improve outcome after stroke. Does the adult brain show a precursor cell–based response to ischemia that could be exploited to develop novel strategies to overcome persistent structural damage of brain tissue after stroke?

Clinically, two major forms of ischemic damage can be distinguished: stroke and hemorrhage. Stroke is the complete or partial interruption of cerebral blood flow; hemorrhage is due to bleeding into the parenchyma, for example, from a ruptured aneurysm or a subarachnoidal artery. If the entire carotid artery is occluded or blood flow is abruptly stopped after cardiac arrest, the result is global ischemia; if single cerebral arteries are occluded by a thrombus, focal ischemia is found. One fundamental difference between the forms of ischemic brain damage lies in the amount and distribution of spared tissue. Also, the kind and severity of cell damage and its distribution can greatly vary among different types of ischemia. This variation has important consequences for the interpretation of studies dealing with the effects of ischemic brain damage on adult neurogenesis.

On a phenomenological level, both global (Liu et al., 1998; Takagi et al., 1999; Iwai et al., 2001; Kee et al., 2001; Yagita et al., 2001) and focal (Arvidsson et al., 2001; Jin et al., 2001; Komitova et al., 2002; Takasawa et al., 2002) ischemia models robustly induce cell proliferation in the SGZ. In contrast, an acute decrease with consecutive recovery of cell proliferation in the SGZ and SVZ has been found after subarachnoid hemorrhage (Mino et al., 2003). In none of these cases was it resolved whether the newly generated cells actively participated in structural reconstitution. The increase in hippocampal neurogenesis also occurs in the absence of direct (at least visible) hippocampal damage (Arvidsson et al., 2001), suggesting a relatively nonspecific mechanism. There was also no sign of cell migration out of the SGZ toward ischemic regions.

In partial contrast to these results Hirofumi Nakatomi and Masato Nakafuko from Tokyo University showed that precursor cells migrating from the SVZ into the hippocampus can reconstitute ischemic damage in CA1 if this process is supported by massive growth factor infusions (Nakatomi et al., 2002). Unfortunately, the study lacked an absolute quantification of both the initial damage and the consecutive regeneration. The correlational link to an improvement in functional outcome has also been criticized. Methodological questions in this context have been discussed in previous chapters. Irrespective of these issues, however, the study led to a profound change in perspective: endogenous regenerative attempts can be exogenously supported and can lead to substantial reconstitution. It will be important to further characterize how the incoming immature cells can take the place of the deceased predecessors.

From the perspective of human disease, the hippocampus is not of primary interest in the context of stroke. Most studies have thus focused on a neurogenic response to ischemia in the SVZ because it is close to the striatum. In humans, stroke most frequently affects the internal capsule and striatal tissue.

Focal cerebral ischemia after middle cerebral artery occlusion (MCAO) caused an increase in cell proliferation in the SVZ (Jin et al., 2001; Zhang et al., 2001), possibly of late progenitor cells (C cells), because immature neuronal markers were detected in the dividing cells (Jin et al., 2001). The study on regenerative striatal neurogenesis was discussed in Chapter 9 (Arvidsson et al., 2002) (Fig. 9–6).

Whereas Nakatomi and colleagues reported a large structural reconstitution of CA1, in the Arvidsson study, only 0.2% of the lost striatal neurons were replaced, making it unlikely that these cells alone would be able to carry substantial functional recovery.

Focal ischemia also had an effect on cortical cell proliferation and on the migration of cells from the SVZ and RMS into the cortex (Jin et al., 2001; Zhang et al., 2001). The degree to which these cells acquire a functional phenotype remains to be discovered. But these studies indicate that ischemia can induce a complex response from SVZ precursor cells that is not restricted to the normal path toward olfactory bulb neurogenesis. The response includes unusual pathways of migration, which might indeed provide a basis for regeneration outside the neurogenic regions. Independent of neurogenesis, this plastic response might harbor important potential for regeneration or be involved in existing but underestimated regeneration.

Neurodegenerative Disorders

We discussed above the hypothesis that adult neurogenesis might be stimulated in AD, potentially by the amyloid precursor protein itself. In contrast to AD, the brain damage in PD is not as generalized. Although many brain areas are afflicted during the course of the disease, the primarily degenerating neurons are dopaminergic neurons in the substantia nigra of the midbrain. This relatively circumscribed cell loss has made PD the prime case for attempts of transplanting neurons. The question of whether physiologically adult neurogenesis can be found in the adult substantia nigra, has been controversially discussed. Most studies did not find evidence of new neurons in the adult substantia nigra, but the initial positive report by Zhao et al. (2003) was unusual in its range of methods. The exact reasons for the discrepancy in findings are not known, but currently it appears that the claim of neurogenesis in the adult substantia nigra cannot be generally maintained (Lie et al., 2002; Frielingsdorf et al., 2004).

The classical animal models of PD are lesions of the medial forebrain bundle, the axonal projection of substantia nigra neurons to the striatum, by injections of 6-hydroxydopamine, and the degeneration of substantia nigra neurons by the toxin MPTP. Neither of these models has been unambiguously shown to induce regenerative neurogenesis, neither in the substantia nigra nor the striatum. In the debated report of neurogenesis in the substantia nigra, MPTP induced a strong increase in the generation of new dopaminergic neurons (Zhao et al., 2003).

The 6-hydroxdopamine lesion induced cell proliferation in the substantia nigra, but only glial cells developed (Lie et al., 2002). Precursor cells could, however, be isolated from the substantia nigra and were able to generate neurons in vitro and after implantation into a neurogenic region (Lie et al., 2002). Thus not all pathological stimuli seem to be sufficient to elicit degrees of neurogenic permissiveness.

The 6-hydroxydopamine model of PD causes a dopaminergic deafferentation of the striatum. This pathological stimulus induced directed migration of SVZ precursor cells into the striatum and neuronal differentiation could be boosted by the infusion of transforming growth factor-α (Fallon et al., 2000). Apomorphine-induced rotations, the typical behavioral readout in this type of study, was improved in the infused rats. It seems that unlike the ischemic striatum, where a low level of regenerative neurogenesis was constitutively found (Arvidsson et al., 2002), adult striatal neurogenesis of SVZ origin in response to dopaminergic deafferentation could only be induced by the infusion of an appropriate growth factor in addition to the intrinsic effect of the pathogenic stimulus. Neuronal damage itself seems to be a necessary trigger for regenerative neurogenesis and neuroregeneration, although additional support by exogenously applied factors is necessary to actually elicit a measurable response. Striatal neurogenesis in the absence of pathology was also induced by a combination of adenovirally applied BDNF and the local overexpression of bone morphogenic protein (BMP) antagonist noggin (Chmielnicki et al., 2004), further supporting the idea that at least in the striatum, reactive neurogenesis is possible and might have certain therapeutic potential. In the neurogenic regions reduced neurogenesis was found in models of PD and no signs of induced regeneration (Hoglinger et al., 2004).

Huntington disease is an autosomal-dominant disorder leading to the primary degeneration of medium spiny neurons in the striatum. Injection of quinolinic acid into the striatum of rodents mimics some aspects of the pathological features of the disease, but not its complex pathogenesis, which includes protein aggregates. In a quinolinic-acid model of Huntington disease, the lesion induced cell proliferation in the neighboring SVZ and migration of doublecortin-positive cells toward the lesion (Tattersfield et al., 2004). The study thus reflected a traumatic lesion to the striatum and its consequences on precursor cell activity in the SVZ, not the situation in Huntington disease. In the brain of deceased Huntington patients, increased levels of subventricular cell proliferation were detected and the presence of β-III-tubulin in such cells was taken as sign of increased neurogenesis (Curtis et al., 2003). Although this conclusion is problematic (see Chapter 7), the finding fits in the context of other examples of signs of increased cellular plasticity in cases of human neurodegenerative disorders. All of these findings require more studies.

Demyelinating Disorders

Multiple sclerosis is characterized by autoimmunity against myelin, leading to foci of demyelination and consecutive axonal damage as well as to direct neuronal damage. Despite this damage to neurons, oligodendrocytes that could remyelinate demyelinated axons are in the focus of attempts to treat multiple sclerosis with cell therapy.

In cell culture, precursor cells isolated from adult brain are multipotent and produce neurons, glia, and oligodendrocytes. In vivo, only a few new oligodendrocytes are generated in the neurogenic zones. New oligodendrocytes in the adult brain appear to originate from specified oligodendrocyte precursor cells. These precursor cells were first identified by Mark Noble and Martin Raff in 1983 and named O2A progenitor cells (Raff et al., 1983), because they could generate oligodendrocytes (O) and type-II astrocytes (2A) in vitro. Some if not all O2A precursor cells express NG2. In Chapter 8 we reviewed the difficulties in determining the exact nature and identity of NG2 cells. Concepts developed primarily from observations of cells isolated from the fetal spinal cord suggest a direct lineage relationship between NG2 cells or O2A cells and neuroepithelial precursor cells. Ex vivo, NG2 cells apparently can be multipotent (Belachew et al., 2003), but it is not clear whether this is also true in vivo. At least a subpopulation of NG2 cells can express antigens from astroglial and neuronal lineages. Independent of the limits of NG2 as a specific marker, oligodendrocyte precursor cells can be isolated from the adult rodent (Ffrench-Constant and Raff, 1986; Wolswijk and Noble, 1989; Gensert and Goldman, 1996) and human brain (Armstrong et al., 1992; Gogate et al., 1994; Scolding et al., 1995; Roy et al., 1999). In the normal adult brain, only relatively few new oligodendrocytes are generated (McCarthy and Leblond, 1988; Ehninger and Kempermann, 2003), but after demyelinating injury they can give rise to new oligodendrocytes (Redwine and Armstrong, 1998; Levine and Reynolds, 1999). Oligodendrocyte precursor cells have also been found near plaques in multiple sclerosis (Scolding et al., 1998; Maeda et al., 2001). But in advanced stages of the disease, which are probably associated with increasing axonal damage, they become ineffective in remyelinating the axons (Wolswijk, 1998). Demyelinating lesions in the corpus callosum attract precursor cells from the SVZ, but it is not clear to what degree they can contribute to remyelination (Nait-Oumesmar et al.,

1999). With increasing age of the animals in the experiment, this response decreases but can be reconstituted by growth factor injections (Decker et al., 2002). Demyelination due to chemical injury induced an SVZ response leading to astrogenesis, possibly indicating lineage-specific regulation (Nait-Oumesmar et al., 1999).

Because demyelination does not seem to attract oligodendrocyte precursor cells from far-away brain regions and only precursors at the plaque site participate in remyelination, damage to the precursor cells efficiently prevents further endogenous repair (Gensert and Goldman, 1997). Consequently, to achieve increased remyelination from intrinsic oligodendrocyte progenitor or multipotent precursor cells, the rescuing cells have to be attracted to the lesion, protected from damage, and induced to remyelinate over prolonged periods of time, barring no progression of the underlying disease.

Demyelination due to inflammation as seen in the classical model of multiple sclerosis, experimental autoimmune encephalitis (EAE), directly induced changes in precursor cells. Under the influence of interferon-γ or tumor necrosis factor-α, the precursor cells expressed markers such as CD80 and CD86, which are normally found on pluripotent cells. Cross-linking of CD80 on isolated EAE-induced precursor cells caused apoptotic cell death, a result suggesting that inflammation in EAE might directly damage neural precursor cells (Imitola et al., 2004). This finding is in accordance with the others that inflammation is detrimental to precursor cells.

Trauma

Trauma is mechanical injury to the brain. Besides the direct damage by cuts or shear force, trauma includes indirect secondary damage from axonopathies, ischemia, hypoxia, and toxicity from free radicals and excitatory amino acids. Traumatic injury thus comprises several types of cellular damage, each of which might harm precursor cells. The overall net effect is determined by the relative contribution of the individual damaging stimuli. Consequently, plasticity in response to trauma is variable and thus far no unique reaction of precursor cells to trauma has been identified. The response to trauma in neurogenic vs. the non-neurogenic regions differs, and in contrast to ischemia, in which a few new neurons become detectable in the striatum, no cases of trauma-induced neurogenesis outside the neurogenic regions have been described thus far. Some migration of cells expressing neuronal marker Hu into the damaged regions has been reported (Lu et al., 2003).

It has been noted early that the adult SVZ responds to ipsilateral cortical injury with increased cell proliferation (Altman, 1962; Reznikov, 1975). This increase includes both a microglial response (Tzeng and Wu, 1999) and an increase in PSA-NCAM-expressing cells (Szele and Chesselet, 1996). The response has not yet been specified with respect to the precursor cell types in the SVZ. In a fluid percussion model of traumatic brain injury, induction of cell proliferation in both the SVZ and hippocampus was found (Dash et al., 2001; Chirumamilla et al., 2002); in the hippocampus this led to a net increase in neurogenesis (Dash et al., 2001). Induction of proliferation by this contusion-type trauma was not limited to the neurogenic regions but included the damaged cortex surrounding the injury site as well. Most of the dividing cells expressed nestin or glial fibrillary acidic protein (GFAP) (Kernie et al., 2001). Whereas in the hippocampus cortical injury robustly induced the generation of neurons by a factors of 4 or 5, cell genesis in the cortex produced mostly astrocytes. These results suggest that this type of proliferation builds the glial scar found late after injury (Kernie et al., 2001). Interestingly, the induction of hippocampal neurogenesis also occurred contralateral to the injury (Kernie et al., 2001; Lu et al., 2003) and even pre-dated the ipsilateral response (Kernie et al., 2001). When neural precursor cells were implanted into the lesioned adult brain, the cells differentiated along the neuronal and astroglial lineage on the ipsilateral side. Surprisingly, only neuronal but no astroglia differentiation was found on the contralat-eral side (Riess et al., 2002).

The long-term fate of trauma-induced newborn cells in the SVZ is not yet clear. Percussion trauma induces cell division in the SVZ, which leads to increased astrogenesis (Holmin et al., 1997). However, it is not known whether brain injury nonspecifically induces neurogenesis in the olfactory bulb as it does in the hippocampus. Damage to the olfactory bulb itself induces cell proliferation in the SVZ, which can only lead to abortive neurogenesis because the target of cell migration is missing (Kirschenbaum et al., 1999; Li et al., 2002b). Immature migratory cells build up in the RMS. Limited migration from the SVZ to the corpus callosum and into the stria-tum has also been reported (Lu et al., 2003).

One of the central concepts in neurodegeneration is excitatory toxicity. An overload of glutamate (or under experimental conditions its agonists) triggers cell death and specific receptor-dependent tissue responses. In-creased glutamate concentrations in the parenchyma can be found in many pathological circumstances. The injection of NMDA receptor agonist ibutenic acid can be used to model strong excitatory toxicity. In a first step, it leads to the degeneration of neuronal populations sensitive to glutamate. In the den-tate gyrus, ibutenic acid injections induced both cell death and cell prolifera-tion (Gould and Tanapat, 1997). In the RMS, ibutenic acid down-regulated proliferation and the number of calretinin-expressing cells. This finding might indicate that the calretinin stage is particularly sensitive to excitatory damage. Two weeks after the injury cell proliferation rebounded, suggest-ing an attempt of compensation (Li et al., 2002b).

The trauma-induced neurogenic response in the dentate gyrus is reduced in FGF-2-deficient mice and can be stimulated by gene transfer with FGF-2 (Yoshimura et al., 2003). Similarly, a nitric oxide donor induced the endoge-nous neurogenic response (Lu et al., 2003). The migration of precursor cells to the site of injury is mediated by stem cell factor (SCF) and dependent on

SCF-receptor c-kit on the precursor cells (Sun et al., 2004). Both findings support the idea that neurogenesis after trauma (and possibly other aspects of precursor cell–based plasticity) can be supported exogenously, thereby opening a window for therapeutic interventions.

Spinal Cord Injury

Spinal cord injury is a special case of brain trauma, in that its most prominent symptoms are due to white matter damage. Consequently, regeneration has to originate from neurons whose cell bodies are at long distances from the injury site. For regeneration to occur, the local microenvironment must become primarily permissive axonal regrowth. Neuronal cell replacement at the damage site is a lesser issue. To enable regeneration it is necessary to prevent scar formation, support and promote axonal elongation and path finding, and remyelinate the regenerating axons. In therapeutic strategies developed toward this goal, precursor cells play diverse roles but few have focused on the contribution of endogenous precursor cells (Horner and Gage, 2000). Whereas in the normal spinal cord a number of oligodendrocytes are produced, no further strong induction of oligodendrocytes has been found after damage. Transplantation studies confirmed that the normal and injured adult spinal cord is not permissive for neuronal differentiation and only partially permissive for oligodendrocytic differentiation (Horner et al., 2000; Shihabuddin et al., 2000; Cao et al., 2002). Astrocytes isolated from the adult spinal cord were not able to induce neurogenesis, whereas astrocytes from the neurogenic regions were (Song et al., 2002).

Although the adult rodent spinal cord contains multipotent precursor cells that can generate neurons after implantation into neurogenic regions (Shihabuddin et al., 1997, 2000), no adult neurogenesis is found in the spinal cord; it also appears to remain absent after injury. Precursor cells are found near the central canal and within the gray and white matter, particularly the substantia gelatinosa (Horner et al., 2000). Both areas responded to traumatic injury with increased proliferation and generated primarily astrocytes (Yamamoto et al., 2001; Takahashi et al., 2003).

TRANSPLANTATION

Replacing Lost Neuronal or Glial Populations

Precursor cells have been successfully transplanted into a number of animal models of neurological disease, including traumatic brain injury (Riess et al., 2002), spinal cord injury (McDonald et al., 1999; Ogawa et al., 2002), and PD (Bjorklund et al., 2002). In these studies, integration of the graft into the host tissue was shown, functionality of the grafted cells could be visualized, and improvements in functional tests could be correlated with the engraftment.

Together these findings proved that precursor cell–based cell therapy is generally possible in the brain. In humans there is much experience with the transplantation of fetal mesencaphalic tissue into patients with PD. Some of these patients showed extraordinary improvements and have not required any PD medication for many years (Lindvall et al., 1987; Wenning et al., 1997). Double-blind studies of cell therapy in PD, have indicated, however, that not all patients benefit from transplantation and that side effects such as dyskinesias can occur—that is, a hypermotility typically seen after long treatment with dopamine (Freed et al., 2001; Hagell et al., 2002). Clinical trials are also under way for Huntington disease, which shares with PD the trait that a relatively circumscribed population of neurons is primarily affected, in this case medium spiny interneurons in the striatum (Bachoud-Levi et al., 2000).

The use of stem cells as a source for transplantable cells is highly desirable and thus at the focus of research in many laboratories worldwide. Stem cells would alleviate the logistic and ethical problems associated with the use of fetal cells that have to be obtained from aborted human fetuses.

Precursor Cell Therapy for Diffuse Cell Losses

Implantation of wild-type embryonic stem cells into genetic models of disease, for example, an inherited demyelinating disorder, demonstrated that particularly if introduced during development, grafted stem cells can widely distribute and lead to almost complete structural reconstitution (Brustle et al., 1999). Because multiple sclerosis has a strong inflammatory component and is not a developmental disorder, cell-based treatment strategies face considerable technical difficulties in this instance. Neurospheres injected into mice with chronic EAE, however, caused remyelination and even functional recovery (Pluchino et al., 2003).

Despite such reports of successful transplantation strategies, diffuse pathologies seem to call for the induced recruitment of endogenous precursor cells. Endogenous precursor cells are distributed throughout the brain and could realize their migratory potential to reach the sites of pathology. As outlined above, this hope might not be entirely justified, because both the amount of migration and appropriate differentiation are low and would have to be boosted tremendously to achieve functional restitution.

One theoretical solution to the problem of directed migration is the diffuse application of exogenous precursor cells. The simplest strategy is to distribute precursor cells through the blood stream, although in this case the cells have to cross the blood–brain barrier. Only a few reporter gene–labeled bone marrow or blood cells have been detected in the intact brain after intravenous infusion (Priller et al., 2001a). In stroke, however, or at other sites of pathology, the blood–brain barrier is open, allowing the transition of blood cells into the brain parenchyma. In such cases most of the cells found after infusion of marked bone marrow cells are microglia, which originate from blood monocytes. The low number of neuronal cells taken as signs of transdifferentiation of bone marrow cells (see Chapter 3) are now largely explained by cell fusion.

Infusion of bone marrow cells into rodent models of ischemia were nevertheless associated with some therapeutic benefit (Li et al., 2001, 2002a; Kurozumi et al., 2004). Infusion of bone marrow cells into patients with myocardic infaction resulted in a small clinical improvement (Assmus et al., 2002; Wollert et al., 2004), but data remained ambiguous. One study found that the beneficial effect occurred independent of whether the peripherally administered precursor cells entered the brain (Borlongan et al., 2004). The analogous application of stem cells for stroke therapy has been widely discussed (Savitz et al., 2002; Agoston, 2004) and several clinical studies are currently under way. Whether the rodent data were indeed sound enough to allow clinical application is questionable. A beneficial effect is unlikely to be due to neurogenesis or even gliogenesis from the infused cells because no evidence exists of functionally relevant neurogenesis after systemic precursor cell applications. This would not necessarily argue against systemic cell therapy in general, because in addition to replacing lost cells, the goal might be to stimulate a microenvironment that provided trophic support for damaged but still rescuable neurons. More research is needed, however, to understand trophic actions of bone marrow–derived precursor cells and to estimate the riskbenefit ratio of systemic cell therapies.

Problems in Using Stem Cells for Human Therapy

The use of stem cells expanded in cell culture for therapy is hindered by a number of problems. Embryonic stem cells are easily expandable. Their isolation from human embryos, however, is ethically controversial. They also have to be predifferentiated and the implant has to be absolutely free of pluripotent stem cells to avoid the development of teratomas (Langa et al., 2000; Reubinoff et al., 2000; Asano et al., 2003). In some contexts, there are useful concepts for achieving differentiation from embryonic stem cells into specific, desired neuronal phenotypes (Castelo-Branco et al., 2003; Perrier and Studer, 2003), but for many other cell types no protocols exist yet. In the case of dopaminergic differentiation, the desired phenotype for the treatment of PD, several strategies have been developed to yield dopaminergic neurons, but no application in human therapy has been achieved. Some lineages of cell development might require such complex series of concerted manipulations that the entire process would turn out to be unfeasible if not impossible.

Adult neural stem cells, by contrast, are by definition predifferentiated and less tumorigenic, but do not seem to readily differentiate into many of the different phenotypes of interest. Because the periglomerular interneurons generated in adult olfactory bulb neurogenesis use dopamine as their transmitter, a dopaminergic phenotype (albeit in an inkineuron) seems to lie within the spectrum of adult SVZ precursor cells. So far, this differentiation has not been replicated in vitro. In addition, neural precursor cells are difficult to obtain from the adult human brain and cannot be expanded readily to sufficiently large numbers. Their main advantage is that they are isogenic and thus avoid immunological problems. On the other hand, if isolated from a patient, precursor cells will carry the genetic profile associated with the disease they are supposed to cure. The impact of this problem, which would also apply to somatic nuclear transfer, will vary with the diseases and their different genetic causes.

Great hopes had been placed on the therapeutic use of easily accessible stem cells from bone marrow, cord blood, or skin in the treatment of neurological disorders. The reported findings of a transdifferentiation of such cells into neurons, however, were later explained by cell fusion, resulting in polyploid cells of combined host and graft phenotype (see Chapter 3). This fusion showed a striking tropism, and only very few cell populations were identified as being able to fuse with hematopoetic cells. In the brain, it was Purkinje cells that fused with the transplanted cells from bone marrow (Priller et al., 2001b; Alvarez-Dolado et al., 2003). Whereas analogous cell fusion in the liver, where bone marrow cells can fuse with hepatocytes, might have therapeutic potential of its own (Willenbring et al., 2004; Willenbring and Grompe, 2004), this is not necessarily possible for cerebellar Purkinje neurons.

The most fundamental problem in stem cell therapy remains the identity of stem cells. To develop standardized and reliable forms of therapy in which risk and benefit can be precisely determined, stem cells have to become definable beyond their degree of self-renewal plus multipotency and even beyond a marker profile. Stem cells are the most difficult cells in our body because they represent the open genome. Hope and danger are very closely related in using stem cells for therapy. "Know thy stem cell" is one of the strategies for avoiding risks and using its potential.

Research on adult neurogenesis and on neural precursor cells in neurogenic and non-neurogenic zones can help to overcome some of the obstacles seen in the more applied tissue-engineering aspects of neural stem cell biology. These goals include the definition of precursor cell identities, identification of parameters defining neurogenic permissiveness, and description of neuronal development and maturation to functionality under the conditions of the healthy and diseased human brain. All of these endeavors are necessary for transplantation-based approaches for neurological therapy as well, although some details and preferences will vary.

Somatic Nuclear Transfer (Therapeutic Cloning)

The application of somatic nuclear transfer (McGrath and Solter, 1983) aims at obtaining cells with the pluripotency of embryonic stem cells from an adult individual. For cell therapy, these cells would avoid immunological problems such as graft rejection and allow development of a patient's personal stem cell lines. These could at least theoretically be developed into many different types of cells and enable realization of even the most advanced ideas of cell replacement.

In somatic nuclear transfer, the nucleus of a body cell of the patient is removed from the cell and inserted into a similarly enucleated egg cell from a female donor. The resulting cell is diploid, but contains only nuclear genetic information from the patient. The mitochondrial DNA, however, always originates from the egg, but this minute "contamination" can probably be ignored for most purposes. One then initiates division of the hybrid cell. If successful, the resulting embryoid body is allowed to develop to the blastocyst stage, when embryonic stem cells containing the patient's genetic makeup can be isolated from the inner cell mass. These cells would at least in theory have all the advantages (and disadvantages) of pluripotent cells, but would be derived from an adult individual, thus in some sense allowing a turning back of the biological clock.

Somatic nuclear transfer is in principal possible in rodents and even humans (Rideout et al., 2002; Hwang et al., 2004). The efficiency is still extremely low and very limited information is available about the health and normality of the obtained stem cell lines. The technique is considered ethically problematic by many people because it involves a step of totipotency and thus the potential generation of an entire human being if the hybrid cell were implanted into a uterus. This proximity to reproductive cloning, in addition to general ethical concerns regarding the moral status of the human embryo, has brought somatic nuclear transfer into discussion. We cannot address this controversy and the scientific issues around somatic nuclear transfer here. However, the general option exists and will influence medicine and stem cell biology in the future. The perspective of somatic nuclear transfer and the use of pluripotent autogenic cells in cell therapy are part of the context in which neural precursor cell biology, especially its medical applications, has to be seen.

DISEASE MODELING IN STEM CELLS

One can argue that even if transplantation therapy based on stem cells one day became feasible, its technical and logistic complexities would prevent it from turning into a treatment option for large numbers of patients worldwide. Depending on the means of achieving this goal, enhancing or maintaining precursor cell–based plasticity as a tool of therapy might be better positioned to become broadly used. However, enhancement of endogenous cellular plasticity might not be able to offer concrete and powerful solutions in many disorders. Some researchers thus believe that the strongest impact of stem cell biology on medicine might ultimately come from the possibility of developing strong and specific models of human disease (Jakel et al., 2004). These models could be used to discover novel drugs, they would in relative terms reduce the number of animal studies, and they would remove the uncertainties associated with transferring insights from animal studies to the human situation.

Transgenic and knockout mouse models, as well as a number of spontaneous mutations and selective breeding in rats, have generated a number of very useful animal models of disease (Norgren, 2004). Despite much insight from these models, their ultimate reach is limited. They are most powerful for single-gene defects, but these account for only a minority of human disorders. Rodents have a life span of only a 40th of a human's, with the consequence that especially chronic disorders or slowly progressing storage disorders must be studied, if they can be modeled at all, in a much accelerated fashion. Even in the oldest mouse the cells are chronologically not older than in a human infant. Life span–related differences are laid down in the genome. Many disorders common in humans naturally do not occur in rodents, Alzheimer disease and Parkinson disease being prominent neurological examples. Also, as long as the exact pathogenesis of many disorders is unknown to a certain degree the development of models remains guesswork. Models thus usually only mirror aspects of the disease, and targeted mutations affect only genes whose relevance to the disease is already assumed. Alternatively, a mutation generated for other purposes shows symptoms and signs of a human disorder, which might open a new path of research, but again might only mirror one aspect of the disease. None of the animal models of Parkinson disease, for example, show the classical clinical trias of human Parkinson disease: rigor, tremor, and akinesia. The models reflect the consequences of destructed dopaminergic neurons in the substantia nigra, not the underlying molecular and cellular defects.

Some of these problems could be circumvented if human cells from patients with the disease could be propagated, developed into appropriate phenotypes, and tested for their behavior in vitro or by xenografting them into a rodent host. The range of diseases that could be studied by this means would be considerably larger, although the approach would of course still favor those diseases in which the genetic component is relatively strong.

Besides the clear familiar cases with single-gene mutations Parkinson disease in general has a genetic component, that makes dopaminergic neurons vulnerable to degeneration and even isolated dopaminergic neurons might show this sensitivity and would allow studying its mechanisms. Dopaminergic neurons from human patients, however, are not accessible. Tissue engineering from stem cells would make it possible to develop and expand human cells that adequately reflect a genotype and a line and stage of differentiation relevant to a disease. Genes of interest could be introduced by viral vectors or homologous recombination that is the site-specific, nonrandom insertion of a gene (Belteki et al., 2003; Zwaka and Thomson, 2003).

In general, all types of stem cells—embryonic, fetal or adult—could be used for this approach. If combined with the technology of somatic nuclear transfer and thus some sort of diagnostic cloning, it would be possible to even personalize disease models. Interindividual differences could be studied in vitro and drugs could be designed to suit exactly the needs of a patient.

These tools, should they become available, would enables us to study aspects of human neuronal development in vitro. In a book on adult neurogenesis, this perspective is only briefly mentioned because of its potential relevance to neurological disease and because it is becoming an important aspect of precursor cell–related neurobiology.

REFERENCES

Abayomi OK (1996) Pathogenesis of irradiation-induced cognitive dysfunction. Acta Oncol 35:659–663.

Agoston H (2004) Stem cells show promise as stroke therapy. Lancet Neurol 3:575.

Altman J (1962) Autoradiographic study of degenerative and regenerative proliferation of neuroglia cells with tritiated thymidine. Exp Neurol 5:302–318.

Alvarez-Dolado M, Pardal R, Garcia-Verdugo JM, Fike JR, Lee HO, Pfeffer K, Lois C, Morrison SJ, Alvarez-Buylla A (2003) Fusion of bone-marrow-derived cells with Purkinje neurons, cardiomyocytes and hepatocytes. Nature 425:968–973.

Arlotta P, Magavi SS, Macklis JD (2003) Induction of adult neurogenesis: molecular manipulation of neural precursors in situ. Ann NY Acad Sci 991:229–236.

Armstrong RC, Dorn HH, Kufta CV, Friedman E, Dubois-Dalcq ME (1992) Preoligodendrocytes from adult human CNS. J Neurosci 12:1538–1547.

Arvidsson A, Collin T, Kirik D, Kokaia Z, Lindvall O (2002) Neuronal replacement from endogenous precursors in the adult brain after stroke. Nat Med 8:963–970.

Arvidsson A, Kokaia Z, Lindvall O (2001) N-methyl-D-aspartate receptor-mediated increase of neurogenesis in adult rat dentate gyrus following stroke. Eur J Neurosci 14:10–18.

Asano T, Ageyama N, Takeuchi K, Momoeda M, Kitano Y, Sasaki K, Ueda Y, Suzuki Y, Kondo Y, Torii R, Hasegawa M, Ookawara S, Harii K, Terao K, Ozawa K, Hanazono Y (2003) Engraftment and tumor formation after allogeneic in utero transplantation of primate embryonic stem cells. Transplantation 76:1061–1067.

Assmus B, Schachinger V, Teupe C, Britten M, Lehmann R, Dobert N, Grunwald F, Aicher A, Urbich C, Martin H, Hoelzer D, Dimmeler S, Zeiher AM (2002) Transplantation of progenitor cells and regeneration enhancement in acute myocardial infarction (TOPCARE-AMI). Circulation 106:3009–3017.

Auvergne R, Lere C, El Bahh B, Arthaud S, Lespinet V, Rougier A, Le Gal La Salle G (2002) Delayed kindling epileptogenesis and increased neurogenesis in adult rats housed in an enriched environment. Brain Res 954:277–285.

Bachoud-Levi AC, Remy P, Nguyen JP, Brugieres P, Lefaucheur JP, Bourdet C, Baudic S, Gaura V, Maison P, Haddad B, Boisse MF, Grandmougin T, Jeny R, Bartolomeo P, Dalla Barba G, Degos JD, Lisovoski F, Ergis AM, Pailhous E, Cesaro P, Hantraye P, Peschanski M (2000) Motor and cognitive improvements in patients with Huntington's disease after neural transplantation. Lancet 356:1975–1979.

Barnett SC, Robertson L, Graham D, Allan D, Rampling R (1998) Oligodendrocyte-type-2 astrocyte (O-2A) progenitor cells transformed with c-myc and H-ras form high-grade glioma after stereotactic injection into the rat brain. Carcinogenesis 19:1529–1537.

Belachew S, Chittajallu R, Aguirre AA, Yuan X, Kirby M, Anderson S, Gallo V (2003) Postnatal NG2 proteoglycan-expressing progenitor cells are intrinsically multipotent and generate functional neurons. J Cell Biol 161:169–186.

Belteki G, Gertsenstein M, Ow DW, Nagy A (2003) Site-specific cassette exchange and germline transmission with mouse ES cells expressing phiC31 integrase. Nat Biotechnol 21:321–324.

Bengzon J, Kokaia Z, Elmér E, Nanobashvili A, Kokaia M, Lindvall O (1997) Apoptosis and proliferation of dentate gyrus neurons after single and intermittent limbic seizures. Proc Natl Acad Sci USA 94:10432–10437.

Berendse HW, Booij J, Francot CM, Bergmans PL, Hijman R, Stoof JC, Wolters EC (2001) Subclinical dopaminergic dysfunction in asymptomatic Parkinson's disease patients' relatives with a decreased sense of smell. Ann Neurol 50:34–41.

Bjorklund A, Lindvall O (2000) Cell replacement therapies for central nervous system disorders. Nat Neurosci 3:537–544.

Bjorklund LM, Sanchez-Pernaute R, Chung S, Andersson T, Chen IY, McNaught KS, Brownell AL, Jenkins BG, Wahlestedt C, Kim KS, Isacson O (2002) Embryonic stem cells develop into functional dopaminergic neurons after transplantation in a Parkinson rat model. Proc Natl Acad Sci USA 8:8.

Blumcke I, Beck H, Suter B, Hoffmann D, Fodisch HJ, Wolf HK, Schramm J, Elger CE, Wiestler OD (1999) An increase of hippocampal calretinin-immunoreactive neurons correlates with early febrile seizures in temporal lobe epilepsy. Acta Neuropathol (Berl) 97:31–39.

Blumcke I, Schewe JC, Normann S, Brustle O, Schramm J, Elger CE, Wiestler OD (2001) Increase of nestin-immunoreactive neural precursor cells in the dentate gyrus of pediatric patients with early-onset temporal lobe epilepsy. Hippocampus 11:311–321.

Blumcke I, Thom M, Wiestler OD (2002) Ammon's horn sclerosis: a maldevelopmental disorder associated with temporal lobe epilepsy. Brain Pathol 12:199–211.

Bondolfi L, Calhoun M, Ermini F, Kuhn HG, Wiederhold KH, Walker L, Staufenbiel M, Jucker M (2002) Amyloid-associated neuron loss and gliogenesis in the neocortex of amyloid precursor protein transgenic mice. J Neurosci 22:515–522.

Borlongan CV, Hadman M, Sanberg CD, Sanberg PR (2004) Central nervous system entry of peripherally injected umbilical cord blood cells is not required for neuroprotection in stroke. Stroke 35:2385–2389.

Brustle O, Jones KN, Learish RD, Karram K, Choudhary K, Wiestler OD, Duncan ID, McKay RD (1999) Embryonic stem cell–derived glial precursors: a source of myelinating transplants. Science 285:754–756.

Caille I, Allinquant B, Dupont E, Bouillot C, Langer A, Muller U, Prochiantz A (2004) Soluble form of amyloid precursor protein regulates proliferation of progenitors in the adult subventricular zone. Development 131:2173–2181.

Camicioli R, Moore MM, Kinney A, Corbridge E, Glassberg K, Kaye JA (2003) Parkinson's disease is associated with hippocampal atrophy. Mov Disord 18:784–790.

Cao QL, Howard RM, Dennison JB, Whittemore SR (2002) Differentiation of engrafted neuronal-restricted precursor cells is inhibited in the traumatically injured spinal cord. Exp Neurol 177:349–359.

Castelo-Branco G, Wagner J, Rodriguez FJ, Kele J, Sousa K, Rawal N, Pasolli HA, Fuchs E, Kitajewski J, Arenas E (2003) Differential regulation of midbrain dopaminergic neuron development by Wnt-1, Wnt-3a, and Wnt-5a. Proc Natl Acad Sci USA 100:12747–12752.

Chen J, Magavi SS, Macklis JD (2004) Neurogenesis of corticospinal motor neurons extending spinal projections in adult mice. Proc Natl Acad Sci USA 101:16357–16362.

Chirumamilla S, Sun D, Bullock MR, Colello RJ (2002) Traumatic brain injury induced cell proliferation in the adult mammalian central nervous system. J Neurotrauma 19:693–703.

Chmielnicki E, Benraiss A, Economides AN, Goldman SA (2004) Adenovirally expressed noggin and brain-derived neurotrophic factor cooperate to induce new medium spiny neurons from resident progenitor cells in the adult striatal ventricular zone. J Neurosci 24:2133–2142.

Ciaroni S, Cecchini T, Ferri P, Ambrogini P, Cuppini R, Riccio M, Lombardelli G, Papa S, Del Grande P (2002) Impairment of neural precursor proliferation increases survival of cell progeny in the adult rat dentate gyrus. Mech Ageing Dev 123:1341–1352.

Corotto FS, Henegar JR, Maruniak JA (1994) Odor deprivation leads to reduced neurogenesis and reduced neuronal survival in the olfactory bulb of the adult mouse. Neuroscience 61:739–744.

Covolan L, Ribeiro LT, Longo BM, Mello LE (2000) Cell damage and neurogenesis in the dentate granule cell layer of adult rats after pilocarpine- or kainate-induced status epilepticus. Hippocampus 10:169–180.

Crews FT, Nixon K, Wilkie ME (2004) Exercise reverses ethanol inhibition of neural stem cell proliferation. Alcohol 33:63–71.

Crossen JR, Garwood D, Glatstein E, Neuwelt EA (1994) Neurobehavioral sequelae of cranial irradiation in adults: a review of radiation-induced encephalopathy. J Clin Oncol 12:627–642.

Curtis MA, Penney EB, Pearson AG, van Roon-Mom WM, Butterworth NJ, Dragunow M, Connor B, Faull RL (2003) Increased cell proliferation and neurogenesis in the adult human Huntington's disease brain. Proc Natl Acad Sci USA 100:9023–9027.

Czeh B, Michaelis T, Watanabe T, Frahm J, de Biurrun G, van Kampen M, Bartolomucci A, Fuchs E (2001) Stress-induced changes in cerebral metabolites, hippocampal volume, and cell proliferation are prevented by antidepressant treatment with tianeptine. Proc Natl Acad Sci USA 98:12796–12801.

Czeh B, Welt T, Fischer AK, Erhardt A, Schmitt W, Muller MB, Toschi N, Fuchs E, Keck ME (2002) Chronic psychosocial stress and concomitant repetitive transcranial magnetic stimulation: effects on stress hormone levels and adult hippocampal neurogenesis. Biol Psychiatry 52:1057–1065.

Dash PK, Mach SA, Moore AN (2001) Enhanced neurogenesis in the rodent hippocampus following traumatic brain injury. J Neurosci Res 63:313–319.

Decker L, Picard-Riera N, Lachapelle F, Baron-Van Evercooren A (2002) Growth factor treatment promotes mobilization of young but not aged adult subventricular zone precursors in response to demyelination. J Neurosci Res 69:763–771.

Dietrich J, Blumberg BM, Roshal M, Baker JV, Hurley SD, Mayer-Proschel M, Mock DJ (2004) Infection with an endemic human herpesvirus disrupts critical glial precursor cell properties. J Neurosci 24:4875–4883.

Doetsch F, Garcia-Verdugo JM, Alvarez-Buylla A (1999) Regeneration of a germinal layer in the adult mammalian brain. Proc Natl Acad Sci USA 96:11619–11624.

D'Sa C, Duman RS (2002) Antidepressants and neuroplasticity. Bipolar Disord 4:183–194.

Ehninger D, Kempermann G (2003) Regional effects of wheel running and environmental enrichment on cell genesis and microglia proliferation in the adult murine neocortex. Cereb Cortex 13:845–851.

El Bahh B, Lespinet V, Lurton D, Coussemacq M, Le Gal La Salle G, Rougier A (1999) Correlations between granule cell dispersion, mossy fiber sprouting, and hippocampal cell loss in temporal lobe epilepsy. Epilepsia 40:1393–1401.

Fallon J, Reid S, Kinyamu R, Opole I, Opole R, Baratta J, Korc M, Endo TL, Duong A, Nguyen G, Karkehabadhi M, Twardzik D, Patel S, Loughlin S (2000) In vivo induction of massive proliferation, directed migration, and differentiation of neural cells in the adult mammalian brain. Proc Natl Acad Sci USA 97:14686–14691.

Feng R, Rampon C, Tang YP, Shrom D, Jin J, Kyin M, Sopher B, Martin GM, Kim SH, Langdon RB, Sisodia SS, Tsien JZ (2001) Deficient neurogenesis in forebrain-specific presenilin-1 knockout mice is associated with reduced clearance of hippocampal memory traces. Neuron 32:911–926.

Ferland RJ, Gross RA, Applegate CD (2002) Increased mitotic activity in the dentate gyrus of the hippocampus of adult C57BL/6J mice exposed to the flurothyl kindling model of epileptogenesis. Neuroscience 115:669–683.

Fernandez G, Effenberger O, Vinz B, Steinlein O, Elger CE, Dohring W, Heinze HJ (1998) Hippocampal malformation as a cause of familial febrile convulsions and subsequent hippocampal sclerosis. Neurology 50:909–917.

Ffrench-Constant C, Raff MC (1986) Proliferating bipotential glial progenitor cells in adult rat optic nerve. Nature 319:499–502.

Freed CR, Greene PE, Breeze RE, Tsai WY, DuMouchel W, Kao R, Dillon S, Winfield H, Culver S, Trojanowski JQ, Eidelberg D, Fahn S (2001) Transplantation of embryonic dopamine neurons for severe Parkinson's disease. N Engl J Med 344:710–719.

Frielingsdorf H, Schwarz K, Brundin P, Mohapel P (2004) No evidence for new dopaminergic neurons in the adult mammalian substantia nigra. Proc Natl Acad Sci USA 101:10177–10182.

Fuchs E, Czeh B, Michaelis T, de Biurrun G, Watanabe T, Frahm J (2002) Synaptic plasticity and tianeptine: structural regulation. Eur Psychiatry 17 (Suppl 3):311–317.

Gensert JM, Goldman JE (1996) In vivo characterization of endogenous proliferating cells in adult rat subcortical white matter. Glia 17:39–51.

Gensert JM, Goldman JE (1997) Endogenous progenitors remyelinate demyelinated axons in the adult CNS. Neuron 19:197–203.

Gerber J, Bottcher T, Bering J, Bunkowski S, Bruck W, Kuhnt U, Nau R (2003) Increased neurogenesis after experimental *Streptococcus pneumoniae* meningitis. J Neurosci Res 73:441–446.

Globus JH, Kuhlenbeck H (1944) The subependymal cell plate (matrix) and its relationship to brain tumors of the ependymal type. J Neuropathol Exp Neurol 3:1–35.

Gogate N, Verma L, Zhou JM, Milward E, Rusten R, O'Connor M, Kufta C, Kim J, Hudson L, Dubois-Dalcq M (1994) Plasticity in the adult human oligodendrocyte lineage. J Neurosci 14:4571–4587.

Gould E, Tanapat P (1997) Lesion-induced proliferation of neuronal progenitor cells in the dentate gyrus of the adult rat. Neuroscience 80:427–436.

Gray WP, Sundstrom LE (1998) Kainic acid increases the proliferation of granule cell progenitors in the dentate gyrus of the adult rat. Brain Res 790:52–59.

Hagell P, Piccini P, Bjorklund A, Brundin P, Rehncrona S, Widner H, Crabb L, Pavese N, Oertel WH, Quinn N, Brooks DJ, Lindvall O (2002) Dyskinesias following neural transplantation in Parkinson's disease. Nat Neurosci 5:627–628.

Halim ND, Weickert CS, McClintock BW, Weinberger DR, Lipska BK (2004) Effects of chronic haloperidol and clozapine treatment on neurogenesis in the adult rat hippocampus. Neuropsychopharmacology 29:1063–1069.

Hattiangady B, Rao MS, Shetty AK (2004) Chronic temporal lobe epilepsy is associated with severely declined dentate neurogenesis in the adult hippocampus. Neurobiol Dis 17:473–490.

Haughey NJ, Liu D, Nath A, Borchard AC, Mattson MP (2002a) Disruption of neurogenesis in the subventricular zone of adult mice, and in human cortical neuronal precursor cells in culture, by amyloid beta-peptide: implications for the pathogenesis of Alzheimer's disease. Neuromol Med 1:125–135.

Haughey NJ, Nath A, Chan SL, Borchard AC, Rao MS, Mattson MP (2002b) Disruption of neurogenesis by amyloid beta-peptide, and perturbed neural progenitor cell homeostasis, in models of Alzheimer's disease. J Neurochem 83:1509–1524.

Hellsten J, Wennstrom M, Bengzon J, Mohapel P, Tingstrom A (2004) Electroconvulsive seizures induce endothelial cell proliferation in adult rat hippocampus. Biol Psychiatry 55:420–427.

Herrera DG, Yague AG, Johnsen-Soriano S, Bosch-Morell F, Collado-Morente L, Muriach M, Romero FJ, Garcia-Verdugo JM (2003) Selective impairment of hippocampal neurogenesis by chronic alcoholism: protective effects of an antioxidant. Proc Natl Acad Sci USA 100:7919–7924.

Herrup K, Yang Y (2001) Pictures in molecular medicine: contemplating Alzheimer's disease as cancer: a loss of cell-cycle control. Trends Mol Med 7:527.

Hirschmann-Jax C, Foster AE, Wulf GG, Nuchtern JG, Jax TW, Gobel U, Goodell MA, Brenner MK (2004) A distinct "side population" of cells with high drug efflux capacity in human tumor cells. Proc Natl Acad Sci USA 101:14228–14233.

Hoglinger GU, Rizk P, Muriel MP, Duyckaerts C, Oertel WH, Caille I, Hirsch EC (2004) Dopamine depletion impairs precursor cell proliferation in Parkinson disease. Nat Neurosci 7:726–735.

Holland EC, Celestino J, Dai C, Schaefer L, Sawaya RE, Fuller GN (2000) Combined activation of Ras and Akt in neural progenitors induces glioblastoma formation in mice. Nat Genet 25:55–57.

Holmin S, Almqvist P, Lendahl U, Mathiesen T (1997) Adult nestin-expressing subependymal cells differentiate to astrocytes in response to brain injury. Eur J Neurosci 9:65–75.

Horner PJ, Gage FH (2000) Regenerating the damaged central nervous system. Nature 407:963–970.

Horner PJ, Power AE, Kempermann G, Kuhn HG, Palmer TD, Winkler J, Thal LJ, Gage FH (2000) Proliferation and differentiation of progenitor cells throughout the intact adult rat spinal cord. J Neurosci 20:2218–2228.

Houser CR (1990) Granule cell dispersion in the dentate gyrus of humans with temporal lobe epilepsy. Brain Res 535:195–204.

Houser CR, Miyashiro JE, Swartz BE, Walsh GO, Rich JR, Delgado-Escueta AV (1990) Altered patterns of dynorphin immunoreactivity suggest mossy fiber reorganization in human hippocampal epilepsy. J Neurosci 10:267–282.

Hsieh J, Nakashima K, Kuwabara T, Mejia E, Gage FH (2004) Histone deacetylase inhibition-mediated neuronal differentiation of multipotent adult neural progenitor cells. Proc Natl Acad Sci USA 101:16659–16664.

Huttmann K, Sadgrove M, Wallraff A, Hinterkeuser S, Kirchhoff F, Steinhauser C, Gray WP (2003) Seizures preferentially stimulate proliferation of radial glia–like astrocytes in the adult dentate gyrus: functional and immunocytochemical analysis. Eur J Neurosci 18:2769–2778.

Hwang WS, Ryu YJ, Park JH, Park ES, Lee EG, Koo JM, Jeon HY, Lee BC, Kang SK, Kim SJ, Ahn C, Hwang JH, Park KY, Cibelli JB, Moon SY (2004) Evidence of a pluripotent human embryonic stem cell line derived from a cloned blastocyst. Science 303:1669–1674.

Imitola J, Comabella M, Chandraker AK, Dangond F, Sayegh MH, Snyder EY, Khoury SJ (2004) Neural stem/progenitor cells express costimulatory molecules that are differentially regulated by inflammatory and apoptotic stimuli. Am J Pathol 164:1615–1625.

Iwai M, Hayashi T, Zhang WR, Sato K, Manabe Y, Abe K (2001) Induction of highly polysialylated neural cell adhesion molecule (PSA-NCAM) in postischemic gerbil hippocampus mainly dissociated with neural stem cell proliferation. Brain Res 902:288–293.

Jacobs BL (2002) Adult brain neurogenesis and depression. Brain Behav Immun 16:602–609.

Jacobs BL, Praag H, Gage FH (2000) Adult brain neurogenesis and psychiatry: a novel theory of depression. Mol Psychiatry 5:262–269.

Jakel RJ, Schneider BL, Svendsen CN (2004) Using human neural stem cells to model neurological disease. Nat Rev Genet 5:136–144.

Jankovski A, Garcia C, Soriano E, Sotelo C (1998) Proliferation, migration and differentiation of neuronal progenitor cells in the adult mouse subventricular zone surgically separated from its olfactory bulb. Eur J Neurosci 10:3853–3868.

Jiang W, Wan Q, Zhang ZJ, Wang WD, Huang YG, Rao ZR, Zhang X (2003) Dentate granule cell neurogenesis after seizures induced by pentylenetrazol in rats. Brain Res 977:141–148.

Jin K, Galvan V, Xie L, Mao XO, Gorostiza OF, Bredesen DE, Greenberg DA (2004a) Enhanced neurogenesis in Alzheimer's disease transgenic (PDGF-APPSw,Ind) mice. Proc Natl Acad Sci USA 101:13363–13367.

Jin K, Minami M, Lan JQ, Mao XO, Batteur S, Simon RP, Greenberg DA (2001) Neurogenesis in dentate subgranular zone and rostral subventricular zone after focal cerebral ischemia in the rat. Proc Natl Acad Sci USA 98:4710–4715.

Jin K, Peel AL, Mao XO, Xie L, Cottrell BA, Henshall DC, Greenberg DA (2004b) Increased hippocampal neurogenesis in Alzheimer's disease. Proc Natl Acad Sci USA 101:343–347.

Kashima T, Tiu SN, Merrill JE, Vinters HV, Dawson G, Campagnoni AT (1993) Expression of oligodendrocyte-associated genes in cell lines derived from human gliomas and neuroblastomas. Cancer Res 53:170–175.

Katchanov J, Harms C, Gertz K, Hauck L, Waeber C, Hirt L, Priller J, von Harsdorf R, Bruck W, Hortnagl H, Dirnagl U, Bhide PG, Endres M (2001) Mild cerebral ischemia induces loss of cyclin-dependent kinase inhibitors and activation of cell cycle machinery before delayed neuronal cell death. J Neurosci 21:5045–5053.

Kee NJ, Preston E, Wojtowicz JM (2001) Enhanced neurogenesis after transient global ischemia in the dentate gyrus of the rat. Exp Brain Res 136:313–320.

Kempermann G (2002) Why new neurons? Possible functions for adult hippocampal neurogenesis. J Neurosci 22:635–638.

Kempermann G, Kronenberg G (2003) Depressed new neurons?—Adult hippocampal neurogenesis and a cellular plasticity hypothesis of major depression. Biol Psychiatry 54:499–503.

Kernie SG, Erwin TM, Parada LF (2001) Brain remodeling due to neuronal and astrocytic proliferation after controlled cortical injury in mice. J Neurosci Res 66:317–326.

Kingma A, Rammeloo LA, van Der Does-van den Berg A, Rekers-Mombarg L, Postma A (2000) Academic career after treatment for acute lymphoblastic leukaemia. Arch Dis Child 82:353–357.

Kirschenbaum B, Doetsch F, Lois C, Alvarez-Buylla A (1999) Adult subventricular zone neuronal precursors continue to proliferate and migrate in the absence of the olfactory bulb. J Neurosci 19:2171–2180.

Kleppner SR, Robinson KA, Trojanowski JQ, Lee VM (1995) Transplanted human neurons derived from a teratocarcinoma cell line (NTera-2) mature, integrate, and survive for over 1 year in the nude mouse brain. J Comp Neurol 357:618–632.

Komitova M, Perfilieva E, Mattsson B, Eriksson PS, Johansson BB (2002) Effects of cortical ischemia and postischemic environmental enrichment on hippocampal cell genesis and differentiation in the adult rat. J Cereb Blood Flow Metab 22:852–860.

Kondziolka D, Wechsler L, Goldstein S, Meltzer C, Thulborn KR, Gebel J, Jannetta P, DeCesare S, Elder EM, McGrogan M, Reitman MA, Bynum L (2000) Transplantation of cultured human neuronal cells for patients with stroke. Neurology 55:565–569.

Kramer JH, Crittenden MR, Halberg FE, Wara WM, Cowan MJ (1992) A prospective study of cognitive functioning following low-dose cranial radiation for bone marrow transplantation. Pediatrics 90:447–450.

Kuan CY, Schloemer AJ, Lu A, Burns KA, Weng WL, Williams MT, Strauss KI, Vorhees CV, Flavell RA, Davis RJ, Sharp FR, Rakic P (2004) Hypoxia-ischemia induces DNA synthesis without cell proliferation in dying neurons in adult rodent brain. J Neurosci 24:10763–10772.

Kurozumi K, Nakamura K, Tamiya T, Kawano Y, Kobune M, Hirai S, Uchida H, Sasaki K, Ito Y, Kato K, Honmou O, Houkin K, Date I, Hamada H (2004) BDNF gene-modified mesenchymal stem cells promote functional recovery and reduce infarct size in the rat middle cerebral artery occlusion model. Mol Ther 9:189–197.

Laakso MP, Partanen K, Riekkinen P, Lehtovirta M, Helkala EL, Hallikainen M, Hanninen T, Vainio P, Soininen H (1996) Hippocampal volumes in Alzheimer's disease, Parkinson's disease with and without dementia, and in vascular dementia: an MRI study. Neurology 46:678–681.

Labrakakis C, Patt S, Weydt P, Cervos-Navarro J, Meyer R, Kettenmann H (1997) Action potential–generating cells in human glioblastomas. J Neuropathol Exp Neurol 56:243–254.

Langa F, Kress C, Colucci-Guyon E, Khun H, Vandormael-Pournin S, Huerre M, Babinet C (2000) Teratocarcinomas induced by embryonic stem (ES) cells lacking vimentin: an approach to study the role of vimentin in tumorigenesis. J Cell Sci 113(Pt 19):3463–3472.

Leuner B, Mendolia-Loffredo S, Kozorovitskiy Y, Samburg D, Gould E, Shors TJ (2004) Learning enhances the survival of new neurons beyond the time when the hippocampus is required for memory. J Neurosci 24:7477–7481.

Levine JM, Reynolds R (1999) Activation and proliferation of endogenous oligodendrocyte precursor cells during ethidium bromide–induced demyelination. Exp Neurol 160:333–347.

Li Y, Chen J, Chen XG, Wang L, Gautam SC, Xu YX, Katakowski M, Zhang LJ, Lu M, Janakiraman N, Chopp M (2002a) Human marrow stromal cell therapy for stroke in rat: neurotrophins and functional recovery. Neurology 59:514–523.

Li Y, Chen J, Wang L, Lu M, Chopp M (2001) Treatment of stroke in rat with intracarotid administration of marrow stromal cells. Neurology 56:1666–1672.

Li Z, Kato T, Kawagishi K, Fukushima N, Yokouchi K, Moriizumi T (2002b) Cell dynamics of calretinin-immunoreactive neurons in the rostral migratory stream after ibotenate-induced lesions in the forebrain. Neurosci Res 42:123–132.

Lie DC, Dziewczapolski G, Willhoite AR, Kaspar BK, Shults CW, Gage FH (2002) The adult substantia nigra contains progenitor cells with neurogenic potential. J Neurosci 22:6639–6649.

Limoli CL, Giedzinski E, Rola R, Otsuka S, Palmer TD, Fike JR (2004) Radiation response of neural precursor cells: linking cellular sensitivity to cell cycle checkpoints, apoptosis and oxidative stress. Radiat Res 161:17–27.

Lindvall O, Backlund EO, Farde L, Sedvall G, Freedman R, Hoffer B, Nobin A, Seiger A, Olson L (1987) Transplantation in Parkinson's disease: two cases of adrenal medullary grafts to the putamen. Ann Neurol 22:457–468.

Lipska BK (2004) Using animal models to test a neurodevelopmental hypothesis of schizophrenia. J Psychiatry Neurosci 29:282–286.

Liu J, Solway K, Messing RO, Sharp FR (1998) Increased neurogenesis in the dentate gyrus after transient ischemia in gerbils. J Neurosci 18:7768–7778.

Lopez-Toledano MA, Shelanski ML (2004) Neurogenic effect of beta-amyloid peptide in the development of neural stem cells. J Neurosci 24:5439–5444.

Lu D, Mahmood A, Zhang R, Copp M (2003) Upregulation of neurogenesis and reduction in functional deficits following administration of DEtA/NONOate, a nitric oxide donor, after traumatic brain injury in rats. J Neurosurg 99:351–361.

Lucassen PJ, Fuchs E, Czeh B (2004) Antidepressant treatment with tianeptine reduces apoptosis in the hippocampal dentate gyrus and temporal cortex. Biol Psychiatry 55:789–796.

Lurton D, El Bahh B, Sundstrom L, Rougier A (1998) Granule cell dispersion is correlated with early epileptic events in human temporal lobe epilepsy. J Neurol Sci 154:133–136.

Lurton D, Sundstrom L, Brana C, Bloch B, Rougier A (1997) Possible mechanisms inducing granule cell dispersion in humans with temporal lobe epilepsy. Epilepsy Res 26:351–361.

Madsen TM, Kristjansen PE, Bolwig TG, Wortwein G (2003) Arrested neuronal proliferation and impaired hippocampal function following fractionated brain irradiation in the adult rat. Neuroscience 119:635–642.

Madsen TM, Treschow A, Bengzon J, Bolwig TG, Lindvall O, Tingstrom A (2000) Increased neurogenesis in a model of electroconvulsive therapy. Biol Psychiatry 47:1043–1049.

Maeda Y, Solanky M, Menonna J, Chapin J, Li W, Dowling P (2001) Platelet-derived growth factor-alpha receptor-positive oligodendroglia are frequent in multiple sclerosis lesions. Ann Neurol 49:776–785.

Magavi S, Leavitt B, Macklis J (2000) Induction of neurogenesis in the neocortex of adult mice. Nature 405:951–955.

Malberg JE, Duman RS (2003) Cell proliferation in adult hippocampus is decreased by inescapable stress: reversal by fluoxetine treatment. Neuropsychopharmacology 28:1562–1571.

Malberg JE, Eisch AJ, Nestler EJ, Duman RS (2000) Chronic antidepressant treatment increases neurogenesis in adult rat hippocampus. J Neurosci 20:9104–9110.

Mandairon N, Jourdan F, Didier A (2003) Deprivation of sensory inputs to the olfactory bulb up-regulates cell death and proliferation in the subventricular zone of adult mice. Neuroscience 119:507–516.

McCarthy GF, Leblond CP (1988) Radioautographic evidence for slow astrocyte turnover and modest oligodendrocyte production in the corpus callosum of adult mice infused with 3H-thymidine. J Comp Neurol 271:589–603.

McDonald JW, Liu XZ, Qu Y, Liu S, Mickey SK, Turetsky D, Gottlieb DI, Choi DW (1999) Transplanted embryonic stem cells survive, differentiate and promote recovery in injured rat spinal cord. Nat Med 5:1410–1412.

McGrath J, Solter D (1983) Nuclear transplantation in the mouse embryo by microsurgery and cell fusion. Science 220:1300–1302.

Mello LE, Cavalheiro EA, Tan AM, Kupfer WR, Pretorius JK, Babb TL, Finch DM (1993) Circuit mechanisms of seizures in the pilocarpine model of chronic epilepsy: cell loss and mossy fiber sprouting. Epilepsia 34:985–995.

Mino M, Kamii H, Fujimura M, Kondo T, Takasawa S, Okamoto H, Yoshimoto T (2003) Temporal changes of neurogenesis in the mouse hippocampus after experimental subarachnoid hemorrhage. Neurol Res 25:839–845.

Mizumatsu S, Monje ML, Morhardt DR, Rola R, Palmer TD, Fike JR (2003) Extreme sensitivity of adult neurogenesis to low doses of X-irradiation. Cancer Res 63:4021–4027.

Mohapel P, Ekdahl CT, Lindvall O (2004) Status epilepticus severity influences the long-term outcome of neurogenesis in the adult dentate gyrus. Neurobiol Dis 15:196–205.

Monje ML, Mizumatsu S, Fike JR, Palmer TD (2002) Irradiation induces neural precursor-cell dysfunction. Nat Med 8:955–962.

Monje ML, Toda H, Palmer TD (2003) Inflammatory blockade restores adult hippocampal neurogenesis. Science 302:1760–1765.

Nagy Z (2000) Cell cycle regulatory failure in neurones: causes and consequences. Neurobiol Aging 21:761–769.

Nagy Z, Esiri MM, Cato AM, Smith AD (1997a) Cell cycle markers in the hippocampus in Alzheimer's disease. Acta Neuropathol (Berl) 94:6–15.

Nagy Z, Esiri MM, Smith AD (1997b) Expression of cell division markers in the hippocampus in Alzheimer's disease and other neurodegenerative conditions. Acta Neuropathol (Berl) 93:294–300.

Nait-Oumesmar B, Decker L, Lachapelle F, Avellana-Adalid V, Bachelin C, Van Evercooren AB (1999) Progenitor cells of the adult mouse subventricular zone proliferate, migrate and differentiate into oligodendrocytes after demyelination. Eur J Neurosci 11:4357–4366.

Nakagawa E, Aimi Y, Yasuhara O, Tooyama I, Shimada M, McGeer PL, Kimura H (2000) Enhancement of progenitor cell division in the dentate gyrus triggered by initial limbic seizures in rat models of epilepsy. Epilepsia 41:10–18.

Nakatomi H, Kuriu T, Okabe S, Yamamoto S, Hatano O, Kawahara N, Tamura A, Kirino T, Nakafuku M (2002) Regeneration of hippocampal pyramidal neurons after ischemic brain injury by recruitment of endogenous neural progenitors. Cell 110:429–441.

Nixon K, Crews FT (2002) Binge ethanol exposure decreases neurogenesis in adult rat hippocampus. J Neurochem 83:1087–1093.

Nixon K, Crews FT (2004) Temporally specific burst in cell proliferation increases hippocampal neurogenesis in protracted abstinence from alcohol. J Neurosci 24:9714–9722.

Noble M (1997) The oligodendrocyte-type-2 astrocyte lineage: in vitro and in vivo studies on development, tissue repair and neoplasia. In: Isolation, Characterization and Utilization of CNS Stem Cells (Gage FH, Christen Y, eds), pp 101–128. Berlin, Heidelberg: Springer.

Noble M, Dietrich J (2004) The complex identity of brain tumors: emerging concerns regarding origin, diversity and plasticity. Trends Neurosci 27:148–154.

Norgren RB Jr. (2004) Creation of non-human primate neurogenetic disease models by gene targeting and nuclear transfer. Reprod Biol Endocrinol 2:40.

Ogawa Y, Sawamoto K, Miyata T, Miyao S, Watanabe M, Nakamura M, Bregman BS, Koike M, Uchiyama Y, Toyama Y, Okano H (2002) Transplantation of in vitro–expanded fetal neural progenitor cells results in neurogenesis and functional recovery after spinal cord contusion injury in adult rats. J Neurosci Res 69:925–933.

Ohsawa I, Takamura C, Morimoto T, Ishiguro M, Kohsaka S (1999) Amino-terminal region of secreted form of amyloid precursor protein stimulates proliferation of neural stem cells. Eur J Neurosci 11:1907–1913.

Parent JM, Janumpalli S, McNamara JO, Lowenstein DH (1998) Increased dentate granule cell neurogenesis following amygdala kindling in the adult rat. Neurosci Lett 247:9–12.

Parent JM, Tada E, Fike JR, Lowenstein DH (1999) Inhibition of dentate granule cell neurogenesis with brain irradiation does not prevent seizure-induced mossy fiber synaptic reorganization in the rat. J Neurosci 19:4508–4519.

Parent JM, Valentin VV, Lowenstein DH (2002a) Prolonged seizures increase proliferating neuroblasts in the adult rat subventricular zone–olfactory bulb pathway. J Neurosci 22:3174–3188.

Parent JM, Vexler ZS, Gong C, Derugin N, Ferriero DM (2002b) Rat forebrain neurogenesis and striatal neuron replacement after focal stroke. Ann Neurol 52:802–813.

Parent JM, Yu TW, Leibowitz RT, Geschwind DH, Sloviter RS, Lowenstein DH (1997) Dentate granule cell neurogenesis is increased by seizures and contributes to aberrant network reorganization in the adult rat hippocampus. J Neurosci 17:3727–3738.

Peissner W, Kocher M, Treuer H, Gillardon F (1999) Ionizing radiation-induced apoptosis of proliferating stem cells in the dentate gyrus of the adult rat hippocampus. Brain Res Mol Brain Res 71:61–68.

Perrier AL, Studer L (2003) Making and repairing the mammalian brain—in vitro production of dopaminergic neurons. Semin Cell Dev Biol 14:181–189.

Pluchino S, Quattrini A, Brambilla E, Gritti A, Salani G, Dina G, Galli R, Del Carro U, Amadio S, Bergami A, Furlan R, Comi G, Vescovi AL, Martino G (2003) Injection of adult neurospheres induces recovery in a chronic model of multiple sclerosis. Nature 422:688–694.

Priller J, Flugel A, Wehner T, Boentert M, Haas CA, Prinz M, Fernandez-Klett F, Prass K, Bechmann I, de Boer BA, Frotscher M, Kreutzberg GW, Persons DA, Dirnagl U (2001a) Targeting gene-modified hematopoietic cells to the central nervous system: use of green fluorescent protein uncovers microglial engraftment. Nat Med 7:1356–1361.

Priller J, Persons DA, Klett FF, Kempermann G, Kreutzberg GW, Dirnagl U (2001b) Neogenesis of cerebellar Purkinje neurons from gene-marked bone marrow cells in vivo. J Cell Biol 155:733–738.

Radley JJ, Jacobs BL (2002) 5–HT1A receptor antagonist administration decreases cell proliferation in the dentate gyrus. Brain Res 955:264–267.

Raff MC, Miller RH, Noble M (1983) A glial progenitor cell that develops in vitro into an astrocyte or an oligodendrocyte depending on culture medium. Nature 303:390–396.

Rajkowska G (2000) Postmortem studies in mood disorders indicate altered numbers of neurons and glial cells. Biol Psychiatry 48:766–777.

Rajkowska G, Miguel-Hidalgo JJ, Wei J, Dilley G, Pittman SD, Meltzer HY, Overholser JC, Roth BL, Stockmeier CA (1999) Morphometric evidence for neuronal and glial prefrontal cell pathology in major depression. Biol Psychiatry 45:1085–1098.

Rakic P (2004) Neuroscience: immigration denied. Nature 427:685–686.

Redwine JM, Armstrong RC (1998) In vivo proliferation of oligodendrocyte progenitors expressing PDGFalphaR during early remyelination. J Neurobiol 37:413–428.

Reubinoff BE, Pera MF, Fong CY, Trounson A, Bongso A (2000) Embryonic stem cell lines from human blastocysts: somatic differentiation in vitro. Nat Biotechnol 18:399–404.

Reznikov K (1975) [Incorporation of 3H-thymidine into glial cells of the parietal region and cells of the subependymal zone of two-week and adult mice under normal conditions and following brain injury]. Ontogenez 6:169–176.

Ribak CE, Korn MJ, Shan Z, Obenaus A (2004) Dendritic growth cones and recurrent basal dendrites are typical features of newly generated dentate granule cells in the adult hippocampus. Brain Res 1000:195–199.

Ribak CE, Tran PH, Spigelman I, Okazaki MM, Nadler JV (2000) Status epilepticus-induced hilar basal dendrites on rodent granule cells contribute to recurrent excitatory circuitry. J Comp Neurol 428:240–253.

Rideout WM 3rd, Hochedlinger K, Kyba M, Daley GQ, Jaenisch R (2002) Correction of a genetic defect by nuclear transplantation and combined cell and gene therapy. Cell 109:17–27.

Riekkinen P, Jr., Kejonen K, Laakso MP, Soininen H, Partanen K, Riekkinen M (1998) Hippocampal atrophy is related to impaired memory, but not frontal functions in non-demented Parkinson's disease patients. Neuroreport 9:1507–1511.

Riess P, Zhang C, Saatman KE, Laurer HL, Longhi LG, Raghupathi R, Lenzlinger PM, Lifshitz J, Boockvar J, Neugebauer E, Snyder EY, McIntosh TK (2002) Transplanted neural stem cells survive, differentiate, and improve neurological motor function after experimental traumatic brain injury. Neurosurgery 51:1043–1052; discussion 1052–1044.

Roy NS, Wang S, Harrison-Restelli C, Benraiss A, Fraser RA, Gravel M, Braun PE, Goldman SA (1999) Identification, isolation, and promoter-defined separation of mitotic oligodendrocyte progenitor cells from the adult human subcortical white matter. J Neurosci 19:9986–9995.

Saegusa T, Mine S, Iwasa H, Murai H, Seki T, Yamaura A, Yuasa S (2004) Involvement of highly polysialylated neural cell adhesion molecule (PSA-NCAM)-positive granule cells in the amygdaloid-kindling-induced sprouting of a hippocampal mossy fiber trajectory. Neurosci Res 48:185–194.

Sanai N, Tramontin AD, Quinones-Hinojosa A, Barbaro NM, Gupta N, Kunwar S, Lawton MT, McDermott MW, Parsa AT, Manuel-Garcia Verdugo J, Berger MS, Alvarez-Buylla A (2004) Unique astrocyte ribbon in adult human brain contains neural stem cells but lacks chain migration. Nature 427:740–744.

Sanders VJ, Felisan S, Waddell A, Tourtellotte WW (1996) Detection of herpesviridae in postmortem multiple sclerosis brain tissue and controls by polymerase chain reaction. J Neurovirol 2:249–258.

Santarelli L, Saxe M, Gross C, Surget A, Battaglia F, Dulawa S, Weisstaub N, Lee J, Duman R, Arancio O, Belzung C, Hen R (2003) Requirement of hippocampal neurogenesis for the behavioral effects of antidepressants. Science 301:805–809.

Savitz SI, Rosenbaum DM, Dinsmore JH, Wechsler LR, Caplan LR (2002) Cell transplantation for stroke. Ann Neurol 52:266–275.

Scharfman HE, Goodman JH, Sollas AL (2000) Granule-like neurons at the hilar/CA3 border after status epilepticus and their synchrony with area CA3 pyramidal cells: functional implications of seizure-induced neurogenesis. J Neurosci 20:6144–6158.

Scolding N, Franklin R, Stevens S, Heldin CH, Compston A, Newcombe J (1998) Oligodendrocyte progenitors are present in the normal adult human CNS and in the lesions of multiple sclerosis. Brain 121(Pt 12):2221–2228.

Scolding NJ, Rayner PJ, Sussman J, Shaw C, Compston DA (1995) A proliferative adult human oligodendrocyte progenitor. Neuroreport 6:441–445.

Scott BW, Wang S, Burnham WM, De Boni U, Wojtowicz JM (1998) Kindling-induced neurogenesis in the dentate gyrus of the rat. Neurosci Lett 248:73–76.

Seoane J, Le HV, Shen L, Anderson SA, Massague J (2004) Integration of Smad and forkhead pathways in the control of neuroepithelial and glioblastoma cell proliferation. Cell 117:211–223.

Seri B, Garcia-Verdugo JM, McEwen BS, Alvarez-Buylla A (2001) Astrocytes give rise to new neurons in the adult mammalian hippocampus. J Neurosci 21:7153–7160.

Sharma A, Valadi N, Miller AH, Pearce BD (2002) Neonatal viral infection decreases neuronal progenitors and impairs adult neurogenesis in the hippocampus. Neurobiol Dis 11:246–256.

Sheen VL, Macklis JD (1995) Targeted neocortical cell death in adult mice guides migration and differentiation of transplanted embryonic neurons. J Neurosci 15:8378–8392.

Sheline YI (2000) 3D MRI studies of neuroanatomic changes in unipolar major depression: the role of stress and medical comorbidity. Biol Psychiatry 48:791–800.

Sheline YI, Wang PW, Gado MH, Csernansky JG, Vannier MW (1996) Hippocampal atrophy in recurrent major depression. Proc Natl Acad Sci USA 93:3908–3913.

Shihabuddin LS, Horner PJ, Ray J, Gage FH (2000) Adult spinal cord stem cells generate neurons after transplantation in the adult dentate gyrus. J Neurosci 20:8727–8735.

Shihabuddin LS, Ray J, Gage FH (1997) FGF-2 is sufficient to isolate progenitors found in the adult mammalian spinal cord. Exp Neurol 148:577–586.

Shin JJ, Fricker-Gates RA, Perez FA, Leavitt BR, Zurakowski D, Macklis JD (2000) Transplanted neuroblasts differentiate appropriately into projection neurons with correct neurotransmitter and receptor phenotype in neocortex undergoing targeted projection neuron degeneration. J Neurosci 20:7404–7416.

Shinohara C, Gobbel GT, Lamborn KR, Tada E, Fike JR (1997) Apoptosis in the subependyma of young adult rats after single and fractionated doses of X-rays. Cancer Res 57:2694–2702.

Shors TJ (2004) Memory traces of trace memories: neurogenesis, synaptogenesis and awareness. Trends Neurosci 27:250–256.

Shors TJ, Miesegaes G, Beylin A, Zhao M, Rydel T, Gould E (2001) Neurogenesis in the adult is involved in the formation of trace memories. Nature 410:372–376.

Shors TJ, Townsend DA, Zhao M, Kozorovitskiy Y, Gould E (2002) Neurogenesis may relate to some but not all types of hippocampal-dependent learning. Hippocampus 12:578–584.

Singh SK, Hawkins C, Clarke ID, Squire JA, Bayani J, Hide T, Henkelman RM, Cusimano MD, Dirks PB (2004) Identification of human brain tumour initiating cells. Nature 432:396–401.

Snyder EY, Yoon C, Flax JD, Macklis JD (1997) Multipotent neural precursors can differentiate toward replacement of neurons undergoing targeted apoptotic degeneration in adult mouse neocortex. Proc Natl Acad Sci USA 94:11663–11668.

Song H, Stevens CF, Gage FH (2002) Astroglia induce neurogenesis from adult neural stem cells. Nature 417:39–44.

Sturchler-Pierrat C, Abramowski D, Duke M, Wiederhold KH, Mistl C, Rothacher S, Ledermann B, Burki K, Frey P, Paganetti PA, Waridel C, Calhoun ME, Jucker M, Probst A, Staufenbiel M, Sommer B (1997) Two amyloid precursor protein transgenic mouse models with Alzheimer disease–like pathology. Proc Natl Acad Sci USA 94:13287–13292.

Sun L, Lee J, Fine HA (2004) Neuronally expressed stem cell factor induces neural stem cell migration to areas of brain injury. J Clin Invest 113:1364–1374.

Szele FG, Chesselet M-F (1996) Cortical lesions induce an increase in cell number and PSA-NCAM expression in the subventricular zone of adult rats. Comp Neurol 368:439–454.

Tada E, Parent JM, Lowenstein DH, Fike JR (2000) X-irradiation causes a prolonged reduction in cell proliferation in the dentate gyrus of adult rats. Neuroscience 99:33–41.

Takagi Y, Nozaki K, Takahashi J, Yodoi J, Ishikawa M, Hashimoto N (1999) Proliferation of neuronal precursor cells in the dentate gyrus is accelerated after transient forebrain ischemia in mice. Brain Res 831:283–287.

Takahashi M, Arai Y, Kurosawa H, Sueyoshi N, Shirai S (2003) Ependymal cell reactions in spinal cord segments after compression injury in adult rat. J Neuropathol Exp Neurol 62:185–194.

Takasawa K, Kitagawa K, Yagita Y, Sasaki T, Tanaka S, Matsushita K, Ohstuki T, Miyata T, Okano H, Hori M, Matsumoto M (2002) Increased proliferation of neural progenitor cells but reduced survival of newborn cells in the contralateral hippocampus after focal cerebral ischemia in rats. J Cereb Blood Flow Metab 22:299–307.

Tattersfield AS, Croon RJ, Liu YW, Kells AP, Faull RL, Connor B (2004) Neurogenesis in the striatum of the quinolinic acid lesion model of Huntington's disease. Neuroscience 127:319–332.

Tauck DL, Nadler JV (1985) Evidence of functional mossy fiber sprouting in hippocampal formation of kainic acid–treated rats. J Neurosci 5:1016–1022.

Thom M, Sisodiya SM, Beckett A, Martinian L, Lin WR, Harkness W, Mitchell TN, Craig J, Duncan J, Scaravilli F (2002) Cytoarchitectural abnormalities in hippocampal sclerosis. J Neuropathol Exp Neurol 61:510–519.

Tohyama T, Lee VM, Rorke LB, Marvin M, McKay RD, Trojanowski JQ (1992) Nestin expression in embryonic human neuroepithelium and in human neuroepithelial tumor cells. Lab Invest 66:303–313.

Tzeng SF, Wu JP (1999) Responses of microglia and neural progenitors to mechanical brain injury. Neuroreport 10:2287–2292.

Uhrbom L, Dai C, Celestino JC, Rosenblum MK, Fuller GN, Holland EC (2002) Ink4a-Arf loss cooperates with KRas activation in astrocytes and neural progenitors to generate glioblastomas of various morphologies depending on activated Akt. Cancer Res 62:5551–5558.

Valtz NL, Hayes TE, Norregaard T, Liu SM, McKay RD (1991) An embryonic origin for medulloblastoma. New Biol 3:364–371.

van Praag H, Kempermann G, Gage FH (1999) Running increases cell proliferation and neurogenesis in the adult mouse dentate gyrus. Nat Neurosci 2:266–270.

Vollmayr B, Simonis C, Weber S, Gass P, Henn F (2003) Reduced cell proliferation in the dentate gyrus is not correlated with the development of learned helplessness. Biol Psychiatry 54:1035–1040.

Wakade CG, Mahadik SP, Waller JL, Chiu FC (2002) Atypical neuroleptics stimulate neurogenesis in adult rat brain. J Neurosci Res 69:72–79.

Walker DW, Barnes DE, Zornetzer SF, Hunter BE, Kubanis P (1980) Neuronal loss in hippocampus induced by prolonged ethanol consumption in rats. Science 209:711–713.

Wang HD, Dunnavant FD, Jarman T, Deutch AY (2004) Effects of antipsychotic drugs on neurogenesis in the forebrain of the adult rat. Neuropsychopharmacology 29:1230–1238.

Wen PH, Friedrich VL, Jr., Shioi J, Robakis NK, Elder GA (2002) Presenilin-1 is expressed in neural progenitor cells in the hippocampus of adult mice. Neurosci Lett 318:53–56.

Wenning GK, Odin P, Morrish P, Rehncrona S, Widner H, Brundin P, Rothwell JC, Brown R, Gustavii B, Hagell P, Jahanshahi M, Sawle G, Bjorklund A, Brooks DJ, Marsden CD, Quinn NP, Lindvall O (1997) Short- and long-term survival and function of unilateral intrastriatal dopaminergic grafts in Parkinson's disease. Ann Neurol 42:95–107.

White AM, Matthews DB, Best PJ (2000) Ethanol, memory, and hippocampal function: a review of recent findings. Hippocampus 10:88–93.

Willenbring H, Bailey AS, Foster M, Akkari Y, Dorrell C, Olson S, Finegold M, Fleming WH, Grompe M (2004) Myelomonocytic cells are sufficient for therapeutic cell fusion in liver. Nat Med 10:744–748.

Willenbring H, Grompe M (2004) Delineating the hepatocyte's hematopoietic fusion partner. Cell Cycle 3:1489–1496.

Winner B, Lie DC, Rockenstein E, Aigner R, Aigner L, Masliah E, Kuhn HG, Winkler J (2004) Human wild-type alpha-synuclein impairs neurogenesis. J Neuropathol Exp Neurol 63:1155–1166.

Wollert KC, Meyer GP, Lotz J, Ringes-Lichtenberg S, Lippolt P, Breidenbach C, Fichtner S, Korte T, Hornig B, Messinger D, Arseniev L, Hertenstein B, Ganser A, Drexler H (2004) Intracoronary autologous bone-marrow cell transfer after myocardial infarction: the BOOST randomised controlled clinical trial. Lancet 364:141–148.

Wolswijk G (1998) Chronic stage multiple sclerosis lesions contain a relatively quiescent population of oligodendrocyte precursor cells. J Neurosci 18:601–609.

Wolswijk G, Noble M (1989) Identification of an adult-specific glial progenitor cell. Development 105:387–400.

Yagita Y, Kitagawa K, Ohtsuki T, Takasawa K, Miyata T, Okano H, Hori M, Matsumoto M (2001) Neurogenesis by progenitor cells in the ischemic adult rat hippocampus. Stroke 32:1890–1896.

Yamamoto S, Yamamoto N, Kitamura T, Nakamura K, Nakafuku M (2001) Proliferation of parenchymal neural progenitors in response to injury in the adult rat spinal cord. Exp Neurol 172:115–127.

Yang Y, Geldmacher DS, Herrup K (2001) DNA replication precedes neuronal cell death in Alzheimer's disease. J Neurosci 21:2661–2668.

Yang Y, Mufson EJ, Herrup K (2003) Neuronal cell death is preceded by cell cycle events at all stages of Alzheimer's disease. J Neurosci 23:2557–2563.

Yoshimura S, Teramoto T, Whalen MJ, Irizarry MC, Takagi Y, Qiu J, Harada J, Waeber C, Breakefield XO, Moskowitz MA (2003) FGF-2 regulates neurogenesis and degeneration in the dentate gyrus after traumatic brain injury in mice. J Clin Invest 112:1202–1210.

Zhang RL, Zhang ZG, Zhang L, Chopp M (2001) Proliferation and differentiation of progenitor cells in the cortex and the subventricular zone in the adult rat after focal cerebral ischemia. Neuroscience 105:33–41.

Zhao M, Momma S, Delfani K, Carlen M, Cassidy RM, Johansson CB, Brismar H, Shupliakov O, Frisen J, Janson AM (2003) Evidence for neurogenesis in the adult mammalian substantia nigra. Proc Natl Acad Sci USA 100:7925–7930.

Zwaka TP, Thomson JA (2003) Homologous recombination in human embryonic stem cells. Nat Biotechnol 21:319–321.

Index